Reader's Digest

Guide to
DRUGS
and Supplements

D1517141

Reader's Digest

The Reader's Digest Association, Inc.
Pleasantville, New York / Montreal

Copyright © 2004 The Reader's Digest Association, Inc.
Copyright © 2004 The Reader's Digest Association (Canada) Ltd.
Copyright © 2004 Reader's Digest Association Far East Ltd.
Philippine Copyright © 2004 Reader's Digest Association Far East Ltd.

Library of Congress Cataloging-in-Publication Data

Reader's digest guide to drugs and supplements / Reader's Digest.
    p. cm.
Includes bibliographical references and index.
 ISBN 0-7621-0504-6 (Softcover)
1. Drugs–Popular works. 2. Dietary supplements–Popular works. I.
Reader's Digest Association.
 RM301.15.R43 2004
 615'.1–dc22

                                        2003023747

US 4403/T

Address any comments about *Reader's Digest Guide to Drugs and Supplements* to:
The Reader's Digest Association, Inc.
Managing Editor, Home & Health Books
Reader's Digest Road
Pleasantville, NY 10570-7000

To order copies of *Reader's Digest Guide to Drugs and Supplements*,
call 1-800-846-2100.

Visit our website at www.rd.com

Printed in the United States

1 3 5 7 9 10 8 6 4 2

The editors, writers, medical consultants, and publisher have conscientiously and carefully tried to ensure that recommended measures and drug dosages in this book are accurate and conform to the standards that prevailed at the time of publication. The reader is advised, however, to consult with his or her doctors, pharmacists, and other health-care professionals and to refer to any product information sheets that accompany the medications, whether they are prescription or over-the-counter. This advice should be taken with particular seriousness if the drug is a new one or one that is infrequently used. Because of the uniqueness of each patient, the need to take into account many clinical factors, and the continually evolving nature of drug information, use this book only as a general guide— along with the advice of your doctor, pharmacist, and other health-care professionals—to help make informed medical decisions.

Reader's Digest Project Staff

Senior Editor	Marianne Wait
Senior Design Director	Elizabeth Tunnicliffe
Production Technology Manager	Douglas A. Croll
Manufacturing Manager	John L. Cassidy

Reader's Digest Health Publishing

Editor-in-Chief and Publishing Director	Neil Wertheimer
Managing Editor	Suzanne G. Beason
Art Director	Michele Laseau
Marketing Director	Dawn Nelson
Vice President and General Manager	Keira Krausz

The Reader's Digest Association, Inc.

President, North America	
Global Editor-in-Chief	Eric W. Schrier

Reader's Digest Guide to Drugs and Supplements produced by

NOVA Graphic Services, Inc.
2370 York Road, Suite A9A
Jamison, PA 18929
(215) 542-3900
http://www.novagrafics.com

President
David Davenport

Editorial Director
Robin C. Bonner

Composition Manager
Steve Magnin

Associate Project Editor
Linnea Hermanson

CONTENTS

▼

A-TO-Z PRESCRIPTION DRUG PROFILES

Find the information you need about a particular prescription drug and its proper use, including why it's prescribed, how it works, dosage guidelines, precautions, side effects, what to do in the case of an overdose, and food and drug interactions.

A-TO-Z OVER-THE-COUNTER DRUG PROFILES

Choose the correct over-the-counter medication for you or your family and learn how to use these drugs safely and effectively. Find out how each drug works, dosage guidelines, precautions, side effects, what to do in the case of an overdose, and food and drug interactions.

CONTENTS

▼

A-TO-Z SUPPLEMENT PROFILES ... 323

New research has documented the healing powers of many dietary supplements, and this chapter will help you decide which vitamins, minerals, and herbs could be best for you. Learn how to use them safely and effectively, how supplements interact with medications, and important precautions you need to know.

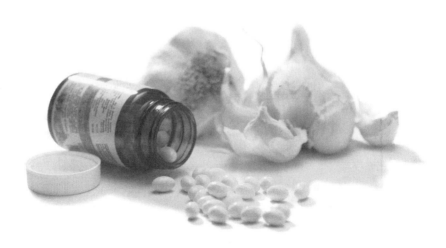

INTRODUCTION

▼

A WORLD OF MEDICINE

Each fall, college campuses are filled with freshman students who have visions of future doctorhood dancing in their hearts and minds. Colleges, being the gentle towers of learning that they are, immediately try to disillusion and/or weed out the majority of these students, in the knowledge that only a few will ever have what it takes to actually become doctors.

The method for weeding students out? Organic Chemistry. It is a brutally tough course that is often mandated in the first year of pre-med studies. On the first day of class, the professor makes clear that out of the hundreds of students filling the room, by the end of the semester, many will be gone, and only a few will get the "B" or "A" that indicates they are on the right career path. Those who do battle with the course are intellectually savaged and ravaged. As promised, only a few emerge at the end with a good grade and the positive attitude needed to continue on the road toward doctorhood.

Why use organic chemistry as the first rigorous screen for future doctors? Simple. Modern healthcare, boiled down, focuses on two healing approaches. The more extreme and specialized method is called "invasive"—actually entering the body and fixing things via surgical techniques. Obviously, you can't screen freshmen by asking them to do surgery. The other, more common healing approach is using medicine to battle disease, manage symptoms, and correct physiological imbalances.

With this perspective, it makes sense to screen out would-be doctors using the science of chemistry. After all, so much of modern healing is exactly that: the science of medicine and its interaction with your body.

THE REALM OF MEDICATIONS

The chemistry of medicine is undoubtedly complex. But even more challenging is the art and science of proper diagnosis and prescription. There are thousands of pills available to a doctor, and millions of pill combinations. If each of us responded the same way to the same medicine, it would be challenging enough, but we are all quite individual, with different reactions and responses to medicine. A doctor needs to factor the individual into every medicinal choice. It should make you glad that Organic Chemistry is so hard.

Not to say that nondoctors can't have a good grasp on the medicine. No one expects anyone except a doctor or pharmacist to understand the chemical reactions an aspirin triggers in the body, but we all know that it does a good job killing pain. Most of us also know that aspirin is an acid and thus shouldn't be taken in excess if you don't want holes in your stomach. And some of us even know that it thins the blood slightly, meaning it can have a nice side benefit of being heart healthy when carefully administered in small dosages. And that is certainly a lot of relevant knowledge.

Life is good if all we ever use is the occasional aspirin. But most of us will progress through many medicines in our lives. From simple painkillers to an herbal cold remedy to an antibiotic to the more powerful controllers of chronic disease, we mark our days by the pills we take. And knowing what they are doing is crucial, both to our bodies and our minds. Hence this book.

Reduced to the simplest of forms, there are just three categories of medicines. The gentlest (which is not to say that they are all gentle) are natural supplements: herbs, vitamins, minerals, amino acids, and so forth. Because their primary ingredients are drawn directly from plants or natural ingredients, supplements are regulated as foods, not medicine. The agreement between the government and manufacturers is pretty simple: Don't make medical claims for your product, and we'll let you sell them without a lot of scrutiny. Thus, you won't find any type of health claim on a bottle of vitamins or echinacea. This is a double-edged sword. Lacking close regulation, the supplements you buy are of variable quality. Plus, their lack of "drug" status incorrectly suggests all are mild and safe. In truth, some supplements are quite strong, with potentially serious side effects, especially when taken with drugs or other supplements.

The second category of medicine is popularly termed "OTC." That means "over the counter" and refers to medicines that are available for sale to any adult at any time. You know—it is the medicine on the shelves at the drug store for pain, colds, flu, stomachaches, and so on. These are regulated by the government, meaning a few things:

• All have clinical research to prove that they work.
• All are produced with a high level of accuracy and consistency.
• All have specific usages for which they are made.
• All carry full disclosure of side effects, usages, expiration dates, and so on.

The third category is prescription drugs. These are only available if a doctor says in writing you are to have this medicine. The same four criteria for OTC drugs hold for prescription drugs. However, prescription drugs are far stronger, more specialized, and often have greater side effects. Their usage must be closely monitored. One should never be haphazard with a prescription medication.

Although the regulation and sale of medicines in these three categories are distinct, all three are really just part of a single spectrum, starting with the gentlest and ending with the strongest course of healing. For mild conditions or preventive care, we start with safe, natural remedies. We step up to over-the-counter drugs for more serious health concerns. And when strong and direct healing is necessary, we add prescription drugs to the equation.

HOW TO USE THIS BOOK

This book presents the essential facts on roughly 1,300 of the most common supplements, OTC medicines, and prescription drugs in use today. We'll tell you what they do, how they do it, the best way to take them, how to store them, side effects to watch for—most everything that is important to know about the pills you take. Knowing this for the pills you and your family take is an important responsibility. In this world of fast, move-'em-through health care, we consumers have more responsibility than ever to understand the health care we are receiving. Merely trusting the doctor, or trusting the pill, is no longer a good option. We may not wish it were so, but it is.

We've built the book in three sections:

A General Medication Overview. The introductory portion of the book contains essential information to help you use medicines wisely. It has practical advice on understanding your medications, including valuable tips on drug safety, traveling with medications, proper storage, as well as dozens of other relevant topics. It also features a comprehensive listing of common disorders and the drugs prescribed for them.

A-to-Z Individual Drug and Supplement Profiles. The core of this book is three A-to-Z resources. First are more than 180 of the most common prescription drugs; next are more than 85 of the most popular OTC medicines; then come more than 85 natural supplements that are used for healing. Each entry is thoroughly researched, up-to-date, and reviewed by health experts to make sure they are as useful and accurate as possible.

A Drug Interactions Chart, Directories, Glossary, and Index. The back pages of the book contain a discussion of drug interactions, a state-by-state directory of certified poison control centers, a directory of health information organizations, a comprehensive glossary of drug terms, and an index to help you quickly and easily find the appropriate drug profile.

A note about drug names: Just as cola is to Pepsi, aspirin is to Anacin. Every drug and supplement has a generic name (aspirin). Most every drug and supplement is sold by for-profit companies using fancy brand names they came up with (Anacin). Through this book, we organize the drugs by their generic names, even though the brand names are often more recognizable. However, we give all the brand names of the drug in each entry, and if you only know a drug by its brand name, a quick look in the index will tell you where to find it.

THE HEALTH-CARE TEAM

Remember, you are part of a health-care team. While it is the doctor's responsibility to recommend the right medicine for you, it is your responsibility to understand the medicine, to monitor its effects, and to ultimately make sure you are doing what's right for your body. We hope this book provides you with the knowledge and assurances you need to take your medicine safely, effectively, and with confidence.

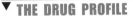

▼ THE DRUG PROFILE

Each of the prescription or over-the-counter medications covered in this book is given a drug profile, which contains the essential facts about it in an easy-to-follow, standardized, one- or two-page format. The profile will give you the various names and formulations for a drug, information on its proper use or uses, guidelines for taking the drug, side effects and precautions associated with the drug, any potentially dangerous interactions with food or other medicines, and additional facts that you need to know to manage your medications.

The individual components of each drug profile are discussed in the following sections, with a brief description of the topics covered under each heading. General tips and suggestions for using your medicines safely and effectively are given here as well. You can use this overview to get acquainted with how the profiles are organized and to obtain important general advice about your medications. Refer to it again to answer any questions you may have about general drug safety after consulting a specific drug profile or whenever you begin a new course of medication.

◆ *Generic and Brand Names*

The drug profile identifies each drug by its generic name—a unique and standardized scientific designation that is recognized worldwide—in large, bold type at the top of the page. In addition, many drugs are commonly known by one or more brand names—the name that the drug manufacturer selects to market its product. For example, ibuprofen is the generic designation for a commonly used pain reliever; Motrin, Nuprin, Medipren, and Advil are four of the brand names for ibuprofen. The drug profile includes brand names that are commonly available in the United States. Unlike generic designations, brand names (also referred to as trade names) may vary from country to country.

Generic drug names are listed alphabetically in the main section of the book. If you know the generic name of a drug, you can use this A-to-Z resource to quickly locate the relevant information. Note that some profiles include combinations of two or more generic drugs formulated as a single preparation.

GENERIC VERSUS BRAND NAME: WHICH IS BETTER?

Generic drugs have become increasingly popular since the 1980s, when the generic drug approval process was expanded and safety guidelines were issued by the Food and Drug Administration (FDA). About 250 new generic drugs are approved by the FDA each year. Generics are less expensive than brand name drugs—but are they as effective?

Ongoing supervision by the FDA helps ensure that generics sold in this country *are* as safe and effective as their brand name counterparts. The FDA requires that all generic drugs be bioequivalent to their brand name counterparts—that is, they must deliver the same amount of active ingredient to the body in a similar time frame. Furthermore, they must have similar chemical stability, so that they maintain their potency under normal circumstances for an equivalent period of time.

In addition, all drugs, including generics, must meet specifications set by the U.S. Pharmacopeial Convention, a private scientific organization that sets standards for drugs and drug products in the United States. Although there are stories in the media from time to time about the sale of substandard generic drugs, such occurrences are rare. The FDA maintains strict standards and inspection practices as well as extensive testing and monitoring of all drug manufacturing processes. About 80% of generic drugs sold in this country are manufactured by brand name firms in state-of-the-art plants.

You and your doctor can discuss whether generic or brand name drugs are right for you. Once you have started on a new drug therapy, it's best to stick with what you've been using—whether it's generic or name brand—unless your doctor says it's okay to change. There are subtle variations between some generic and brand name drugs that may make one type preferable for your situation. Switching from one form to the other could slightly alter the dose that your doctor has determined to be most suitable for your needs.

Also, terms such as "hydrochloride" or "sodium" are sometimes included in a generic drug's name. In many instances the modified formulation (sometimes called a "salt") is not important, because the drug will break down into a single active ingredient in the body.

The pain reliever naproxen, for example, is sold by prescription simply as naproxen, whereas the version of the drug that has been approved for nonprescription use is formulated as naproxen sodium; both versions act identically once the common active ingredient (naproxen) is released in the body, and hence both have a single, over-the-counter drug profile.

In other cases, though, a chemical modification is significant. For example, magnesium citrate, magnesium oxide, and magnesium sulfate will all act differently enough in the body to qualify as separate drugs, so each one has its own drug profile. The same holds true for acetaminophen with codeine phosphate, acetaminophen and oxycodone, and acetaminophen and propoxyphene.

If you know a drug by its brand name, you can find its profile quickly by consulting the index at the back of the book, which lists both generic and brand names for drugs and the appropriate page number for their profiles. Of course, because of space constraints, not every medicine sold around the world is included in this book. We have selected the generic and brand name drugs most commonly used in the United States today.

◆ *Available Forms*

The drug profile lists the available forms of a drug, such as tablet, capsule, liquid, or inhalant. Each form has certain prop-

TIPS FOR TAKING YOUR MEDICATIONS

TABLETS AND CAPSULES

Tablets come in many forms besides the standard round pill. Capsules and caplets (oblong-shaped tablets) are preferred by some people because they are easier to swallow than most round tablets. Chewable tablets are good for those who have trouble swallowing any type of pill; they should be chewed thoroughly to avoid stomach upset and should not be given to children younger than 2 years (who can't chew them properly).

Some people prefer crushing tablets and mixing them with juice, water, or soft foods such as applesauce to make them easier to swallow. This may be okay for some drugs, but certain medications are not designed for this. Enteric-coated tablets, for example, have a protective layer that allows the pill to dissolve in the intestine rather than in the stomach. Crushing the tablet could cause stomach irritation.

Pills that have a sustained-release, timed-release, or extended-release formulation are also designed to disintegrate slowly within the body and should be swallowed whole. Capsules, too, are not supposed to be broken up or cut into pieces. Check with your doctor or pharmacist before crushing any pills or tablets.

Additional Tips

• To make a pill easier to swallow, drink some water before taking it and a glass of water after. It's also a good idea to stand up while swallowing.

• If a pill gets stuck in your throat, try eating a soft food such as a banana. Swallowing the food may help carry the pill down.

EYE AND EAR MEDICATIONS

Always wash your hands before and after administering eye (ophthalmic) or ear (otic) medications. In addition, be careful not to touch the tip of the dropper or applicator to any surface, including the ear canal or eye lids, to avoid contamination. Additional tips for applying these medications follow.

Using an Eyedropper

• Tilt your head back.

• Pull your lower eyelid downward using a finger or by pinching and pulling with your thumb and index finger, creating a pocket between the eye and lower lid.

• Drop the medication into this eyelid pocket. Blink to disperse.

Applying Eye Ointments

• Pull your lower eyelid downward using a finger or by pinching and pulling with your thumb and index finger to create a pocket.

• Squeeze the tube and apply a thin strip (about a third of an inch) of ointment into this eyelid pocket. Blink to disperse.

Administering Ear Drops

• Lie down or tilt your head so that the affected ear faces up.

• For adults, pull your earlobe up and back to straighten the ear canal. For young children, pull the earlobe down and back.

• Drop the medication into your ear canal, but don't insert the tip of the dropper any deeper than the outer ear.

• Keep your ear facing up for a few minutes so the medication can reach the bottom of the ear canal.

RECTAL SUPPOSITORIES

A rectal suppository is a relatively large, bullet-shaped drug preparation that is designed to be inserted into the rectum. Once inside, it melts with body heat and the drug is released. Suppositories may be useful for very ill patients, young children, or others who cannot take oral medications. Lubricant suppositories may also be helpful for the treatment of constipation.

Inserting a Rectal Suppository

• The suppository should not be too soft or it will be difficult to insert. If necessary, before removing the foil wrapper, run the suppository under cold water or chill it in the refrigerator for about a half hour, until it is firm.

• Wearing a latex glove, unwrap the suppository and moisten it with water. Lie on your side and gently push the suppository, rounded end first, well up into the rectum with your finger.

• For children, gently insert the suppository no more than 3 inches into the rectum.

• Lie still and try to retain the suppository for at least 20 minutes so that the drug is absorbed.

VAGINAL MEDICATIONS

Use the special applicator that comes with your medicine and follow the directions carefully. To administer the medicine, lie on your back with your knees pulled up. Insert the applicator into the vagina as far as you can without forcing it and then press the plunger to release the medicine. After you withdraw the applicator, wash it with soap and warm water.

INHALERS AND SPACERS

Many people who have asthma or related respiratory disorders need to use a metered-dose inhaler (also known as a nebulizer). This pressurized container propels aerosolized medication into the mouth and down the throat, where it can be delivered to the airways. The inhaler must be used properly to ensure that enough of the medication is delivered to the airways, where it will exert its therapeutic effect, rather than to the sides of the mouth and throat.

Using an Inhaler Correctly

• Shake the inhaler well before use.

• Tilt your head back slightly and hold the mouthpiece a half an inch from your mouth. The bottom of the nebulizer bottle should be pointing up.

• Exhale normally. At the end of the exhalation, inhale slowly over 5 seconds while firmly pressing the bottle against the mouthpiece, which releases the drug. Slow inhalation is the key to getting an effective dose. Hold your breath for 5 to 10 seconds.

• If your doctor wants you to receive more than one dose of the drug, wait a few minutes and then repeat the steps above.

A spacer—a plastic chamber or holding bag that attaches to the inhaler and acts as a reservoir to hold the mist—may make the job easier by allowing you to inhale at a comfortable rate. Follow the doctor's instructions for how much of the drug to take and how often, and have the doctor check your technique from time to time to be sure it is correct.

NASAL MEDICATIONS

Blow your nose gently before administering nasal medications. After use, rinse the tip of the applicator with hot water and dry it with a clean tissue. To avoid spreading infection, don't share medications with others.

Administering Nose Drops

• Tilt your head back and place the recommended number of drops in each nostril. Keep your head back for several minutes to allow the medicine to spread through the nasal passages.

Administering Nasal Sprays

• Keep your head upright and squeeze bottle firmly to spray medicine into each nostril while sniffing in briskly. Hold your breath for a few seconds, then breathe out through the mouth.

LIQUID MEDICATIONS

Measure the liquid carefully. Don't use ordinary kitchen spoons to measure out a dose; instead, use the measuring device that comes with the drug, or ask your pharmacist for one.

INJECTIONS

Some drugs (for example, insulin for diabetes or an anaphylaxis medication for life-threatening allergic reactions) are best administered by injection. Injections are given intravenously (into a vein), intramuscularly (into a muscle), or subcutaneously (under the skin). If you need to give yourself or someone else home injections, go over the correct procedure with your doctor or other health educator. Don't be reluctant to ask questions, and return for periodic reviews.

erties that may make it preferable for your condition or that can make taking your medications easier, safer, or more effective. If you have a skin infection, for example, you may need an antibiotic skin cream; an eye or ear infection, on the other hand, may call for ophthalmic or otic drops or ointment.

A distinction is sometimes made between local and systemic drugs. Local drugs tend to exert their effects over a limited area of the body. They include topical preparations–which are applied to the skin, eyes, ears, hair, or mucous membranes (lips, nasal passages, vagina, and rectum, for example)–and certain types of injections into the skin, muscles, or joints.

In contrast, systemic drugs are absorbed by the bloodstream and circulated through many of the body's organ systems. This category includes oral preparations that are taken by mouth (such as tablets, capsules, or liquids) as well as injections into a vein. Locally acting formulations tend to cause fewer and less-serious side effects (for example, a limited skin rash) than systemic drugs, although local drugs can cause widespread reactions as well.

The type of formulation can also affect how rapidly a drug is absorbed, how much of the drug is absorbed, or how quickly it can take effect. An injection of a medication directly into a vein takes effect almost immediately and can be critical during emergency situations. At the other end of the spectrum are the controlled-release, timed-release, sustained-release, or prolonged-action preparations, including specially formulated capsules or transdermal skin patches. These are made specifically to provide slow, uniform absorption of a drug over a period of 8 hours or longer. Enteric-

 ## DRUG NAMES **THAT LOOK OR SOUND ALIKE**

Marketers continue to think up new brand names for drugs. Every year, however, a certain number of these are rejected by regulators because the proposed brand name looks or sounds too similar to existing names—which may lead to errors when a drug prescription is filled. Even so, mix-ups continue to occur, in part because prescriptions are all too often scribbled in semi-legible script or quickly phoned in to a pharmacy. Review the common name-related errors below (brand names are in upper case), which are based on reports to the Food and Drug Administration (FDA). This is only a small sample, so be on guard the next time you have a prescription filled!

Accutane (for acne) ....Accupril (for hypertension)

acetazolamide (for glaucoma, ...acetohexamide (for diabetes)
    seizures, heart failure)

Altace (for hypertension).........................Artane (for Parkinson's disease)

Ambien (for insomnia)..............................Amen (for menstrual disorders)

Asacol (for bowel disease)........................Os-Cal (calcium supplement)

Ativan (for anxiety)...................................Atarax (for allergies, anxiety)

Cardene (for angina)................................codeine (for pain relief)

Cardura (for hypertension, ...Coumadin (for blood clots)
    prostate enlargement)

Cardene SR (for angina) ....Cardizem SR (for heart disease)

Celebrex (for pain relief) ....Celexa (for depression)

codeine (for pain relief)............................Lodine (for pain relief)

cycloserine (for tuberculosis) ....cyclosporine (for organ transplants)

Darvon (for pain relief).............................Diovan (for hypertension)

Levoxine (for thyroid disease) ....Lanoxin (for heart disease)

Lorabid (for infections) ....Lortab (for pain relief)

Luvox (for obsessive-...............................Lasix (for heart disease)
    compulsive disorder)

Naprosyn (for pain relief)..........................Naprelan (for pain relief)

Ocuflox (for eye infections) ....Ocufen (for eye disorders)

penicillamine (for arthritis) ....penicillin (for infections)

pindolol (for hypertension) ....Plendil (for hypertension)

Plendil (for hypertension).........................Prinivil (for heart disease)

Prilosec (for ulcer, heartburn) ....Prozac (for depression)

Prozac (for depression).............................Proscar (for prostate enlargement)

Verelan (for heart disease) ....Virilon (for hormone disorders)

Zantac (for digestive disorders)...............Xanax (for anxiety)

coated oral preparations are designed to keep the drug from being dissolved by stomach acids, lessening the likelihood of gastrointestinal side effects.

Other drug formulations include sublingual preparations (which are placed under the tongue and then rapidly absorbed), nasal and inhalant preparations (breathed in through the nose or mouth), rectal suppositories, and vaginal creams or suppositories. Many additional drug preparations are

SELECTING **OVER-THE-COUNTER DRUGS**

Over-the-counter (OTC) drugs should not be taken lightly. All drugs have side effects and need to be taken as directed—whether that direction comes from your doctor, a pharmacist, or the back of the package. To help avoid mishaps, follow the steps listed below when choosing an OTC preparation.

1. Read the label. All OTC drugs sold in the United States must meet strict labeling requirements. Follow all directions carefully.

2. Check for ingredients. Many products with similar-sounding brand names actually contain different active ingredients. Nondrowsy formulas, for example, may contain different drugs than regular formulas. Be sure to check inactive ingredients too. Some products contain dyes or fillers that can cause allergic reactions. People who are allergic to aspirin, for example, will also be allergic to the dye Yellow No. 5.

3. Be aware of combination products. Many OTC products contain multiple active ingredients, some of which may not be appropriate for you. Patients with liver disease, for example, should be wary of products that contain acetaminophen, a common ingredient in many OTC preparations.

4. Protect against tampering. Learn about the product's tamper-evident features from the label, and check the package for signs of tampering, such as broken seals, puncture holes, or open or damaged wrapping. Never take medicine that is discolored, has an unusual odor, or seems suspicious in some other way. Return suspicious medicine to the store manager or pharmacist.

5. Save money by buying generics. These products are as safe and effective as their brand name counterparts and are much less costly.

6. Be cautious when shopping overseas. Many foreign countries do not have the strict guidelines required in the United States for ensuring drug quality.

7. Check the expiration date. You do not want to buy a product that will soon expire, although you can safely use some OTC drugs past their expiration date. If stored under good conditions, most OTC drugs retain 70 to 80% of their potency for 1 or 2 years after the expiration date, even if the package has been opened. (Prescription drugs should never be used past their expiration date.)

8. Buy the right strength. Many OTC medications are available in multiple strengths or concentrations. Check with your doctor for advice on the potency that's right for you.

9. Watch for product reformulations. Brand name OTC drugs occasionally are reformulated with different ingredients but retain their popular name. If you regularly take a particular OTC drug, periodically check the ingredients to be sure you are getting the same medication.

10. Don't confuse products. In addition to making different products that have similar-sounding brand names, some drug manufacturers also wrap their products in similar packaging. Double-check the label when you buy a product and again when you take it to make sure you are getting the right medication.

---

available. Your doctor can advise which form of medication is best for you.

◆*Available OTC?*
Most new drugs are available only by prescription initially and later may become available over-the-counter (OTC). Each prescription drug profile indicates whether or not a drug is also available OTC–that is, obtainable without a prescription in a drugstore, supermarket, or other store. Common categories of OTC drugs include some laxatives; diet pills; vitamins; cold

medicine; aspirin or other pain, headache, or fever medicine; cough medicine; allergy relief medicine; antacids; and sleeping pills.

A prescription drug is granted OTC status by the FDA after a panel of experts determines that it can be used safely and effectively without a doctor's supervision, although all drugs carry at least a few risks.

Many medications continue as prescription drugs even after an OTC version becomes available. Typically, the OTC form has a different brand name,

a lower dosage, and more limited uses. OTC drugs must be taken with the same caution as prescriptions. Always read the labels for proper dosing and possible food or drug interactions.

◆*Available as Generic?*
The drug profile tells you whether or not a drug is available in a generic form. A generic drug is a copycat version of a brand name drug–it should not be confused with the generic name for a drug (see page 8). All medications have a scientific, or generic, name,

but only certain drugs are available in generic versions.

Typically, a pharmaceutical company will conduct exhaustive research and testing to launch a pioneer drug, or the first version of a new drug. In return, the company usually has patents and an exclusive license to sell that new drug for a set period of time, normally about 20 years from the time testing begins. The drug is usually marketed under a brand name. Once that license expires, other drug companies are free to make generic versions of that drug—provided the copy is as safe and effective as the original.

The FDA estimates that about three-fourths of generic drugs are made by the same manufacturers who make the brand name drug. Generic drugs are usually sold under their generic, or scientific, name, often at half the price of the brand name version. Often there are many generic versions of a popular parent drug, and generics are available for both prescription and OTC drugs.

◆ Drug Class

Each drug is classified according to its drug class—a group of drugs that have similar chemical structures or similar actions on the body. For example, a drug that reduces blood pressure falls into the antihypertensive class; one that kills infectious bacteria belongs in the antibiotic class. A drug that reduces fever falls into the antipyretic class; one that relieves pain belongs in the analgesic class. Some drugs have multiple functions and may therefore belong to more than one drug class. In general, however, drugs with similar chemical structures have somewhat similar effects on the body.

If you're having a problem with one medication, an alternative from the same drug group may be an appropriate option to discuss with your doctor.

▼ USAGE INFORMATION

◆ Why It's Prescribed or Taken

The specific conditions, disorders, diseases, or symptoms for which a drug is prescribed are known as its indications. All drugs—prescription and OTC—must be approved specifically for one or more indications before they are brought to market; additional indications may later be approved by the FDA after appropriate studies have been conducted.

For OTC drugs, all indications listed on the drug's label must be approved by the FDA. Hence, you will sometimes see OTC indications referred to as "FDA-approved uses" or simply "approved uses."

The situation is slightly different for prescription drugs. Once a drug has been approved for at least one indication, doctors are free to prescribe it for any purpose they deem appropriate—a common practice known as "off-label use." For example, various antibiotics that are not specifically approved for Lyme disease are often used to treat it and other infectious diseases. Indeed, about half of all prescriptions are written for off-label purposes.

Approved indications for specific drugs are included in each drug profile under the heading "Why It's Prescribed." In addition, beginning on page 24 you will find a listing of "Common Disorders and the Drugs Prescribed for Them." Here you can look up a disease or ailment and find a list of drugs that have been specifically

approved by the FDA for that condition. Off-label uses are not noted in either location, because their use is unofficial. If you're taking a particular drug but don't see its indication listed, you may be following an off-label prescription. You should discuss any concerns you may have about this with your doctor or pharmacist.

◆ How It Works

This section of the drug profile briefly describes how a medicine acts on or within your body to achieve its desired therapeutic effect. Some drug actions are well understood. For many drugs, however, the precise mechanism of action is unknown.

▼ DOSAGE GUIDELINES

The first safety rule for any medicine—be it prescription or OTC—is to take the correct dose at the right intervals. You should be very careful to precisely follow the dosage instructions of your doctor or pharmacist and to read the label on the package. Never take more or less than the recommended dose without talking to your doctor first.

◆ Range and Frequency

The drug profile lists the usual dosage ranges for each drug. Use these figures as general guidelines, but don't be alarmed if your doctor recommends a dosage that is slightly above or below the range given. The correct dosage will vary from person to person and will depend on many factors, including your age, weight, state of health, kidney and liver function, and use of other medications.

All these factors can affect how much of the drug your body absorbs, how it is distributed in your body, how long it stays there, and the amount needed for a response. Your doctor will determine the right dosage for you. If you have any questions or concerns or suspect a dosing error, do not hesitate to contact your doctor or other health-care professional.

Note that drug dosages are often given in metric units of weight, such as grams (g); milligrams (mg, or one-thousandth of a gram); or micrograms (μg, or one-millionth of a gram). Dosages for some medications, including vitamins, may be given in milliequivalents (mEq), a standard chemical unit of measure. Sometimes drug dosages are prescribed per pound of body weight; this method is especially useful in determining the optimal dosage for children.

◆ Onset of Effect

Many drugs exert their effects within minutes. Common analgesics such as aspirin or acetaminophen, for example, begin to relieve pain within an hour. Often, though, you must take multiple doses of a drug before levels have built up enough in your body to be effective. Usually this will occur within a day or two; for certain drugs, such as some antidepressants, however, it may take several weeks for the drug to exert a noticeable effect.

◆ Duration of Effect

How long a drug exerts its effects depends on the individual medication. Some can stay in your system for days or even much longer; others will last only a few hours. The body metabolizes different drugs at different rates. In general, the faster a medication is metabolized, the more frequently you will need to take another dose.

The drug profile indicates how long, on average, a medication may

 ## AVOIDING **PRESCRIPTION ERRORS**

Prescription errors can—and do—occur. There are a number of easy steps you can take to help avoid these errors. First, make sure you understand the prescription fully, including what drug has been prescribed as well as its generic and, if applicable, brand name. Ask your doctor to write legibly and carefully check prescription refills and renewals. Many doctors use Latin abbreviations and other notations when writing out a drug prescription; below is a list of some commonly used terms. It may also be a good idea to have the doctor include the intended use of the drug (for example, by indicating that it is for diabetes or hypertension) on the prescription.

READING A PRESCRIPTION

TERM	ABBREVIATION	MEANING
ante cibum	ac	before meals
bis in die	bid	twice a day
gutta	gtt	drop
hora somni	hs	at bedtime
milligrams	mg	
milliliters	ml	
oculus dexter	od	right eye
oculus sinister	os	left eye
per os	po	by mouth
post cibum	pc	after meals
pro re nata	prn	as needed
quaque 3 hora	q3h	every 3 hours
quaque die	qd	every day
quattuor in die	qid	4 times a day
ter in die	tid	3 times a day

The Brown Bag Review

Another measure to help avoid prescription errors, especially if you're taking several drugs on a regular basis, is to have an annual "brown bag review." Once a year, bring in all the medications you are taking, both prescription and over-the-counter, so that your doctor can evaluate them and, if needed, modify your regimen. In addition, keep thorough records, and clearly indicate any medications you are taking to any new doctors who may be prescribing additional drugs. Finally, check refills and renewals carefully. A refill or renewal of a generic drug may be a different color, shape, or size because the drug comes from a different manufacturer; it can also mean an error has been made. If you have any doubts, don't hesitate to ask your doctor or pharmacist.

remain in your system. Various factors, including your general health, kidney or liver function, and food or drug interactions, can significantly increase or decrease a drug's duration of action.

◆ Dietary Advice

The drug profile tells you if a medication should be taken with or without food. Food can affect how much of the drug will be absorbed into your body, and how quickly.

Many drugs should be taken with a meal, especially with foods that contain some protein and fat. Food delays the emptying of stomach contents, allowing more time for a pill or capsule to be dissolved before entering the intestines, where many drugs are absorbed. In addition, some drugs can irritate the stomach lining if taken on an empty stomach. Taking them with food or even a glass of milk can help minimize the likelihood of stomach upset or other gastrointestinal disturbances. Avoid taking drugs with coffee, tea, or other hot beverages, however, because heat can inactivate or alter some medications.

Other drugs should be taken on an empty stomach—which means at least 1 hour before or 2 hours after a meal. In general, such drugs are poorly absorbed if they're taken with food. They should, however, be taken with a glass of water.

Specific foods and drinks, including alcohol, can also interact with individual drugs. These effects are discussed under "Precautions" (see page 18) and "Food Interactions" (see page 22).

◆ *Storage*

Requirements for storing medicines should be clearly indicated on the label. In general, it is recommended that most medications be kept in a cool, dry place. This usually precludes the bathroom medicine cabinet, because bathrooms tend to be humid. Drugs also should not be kept near a hot kitchen stove. A bedroom or kitchen closet, which tends to be cooler and drier, may be preferable.

Some liquid medicines, such as insulin or antibiotics for children's use, may need to be refrigerated. Unless your doctor or pharmacist tells you otherwise, though, it is not necessary

TRAVELING **WITH YOUR MEDICATIONS**

• Make sure you bring enough medications to last your entire trip, plus an extra supply to cover unexpected travel delays. Don't pack medications in suitcases that you plan to check; the luggage might be delayed or lost. If you carry syringes or certain drugs like narcotic pain relievers, it's wise to carry a note from your doctor that clearly explains your health history and medication requirements; in some countries, these might be confiscated at customs.

• Keep drugs in their original, labeled containers. Pill bottles should be stuffed with cotton to prevent damage during transit; liquid medications should be stored in self-sealing plastic bags.

• Carry extra copies of any prescriptions in case you need to obtain additional medicine during your trip. Prescriptions should be typed, with the generic drug name included, because drugs may be known by different brand names outside of the United States.

• Be up to date on your immunizations. You may need additional shots or medications for travel to certain exotic locales. Consult your doctor or a doctor who specializes in travel medicine at least 6 weeks prior to your trip about the need for any new vaccinations or drugs. You may also want to check beforehand about where to obtain emergency medical help while traveling.

• Be aware that a change in climate may bring on unwelcome drug side effects. In hot climates, for example, diuretics may cause some dizziness at first, but such side effects usually pass quickly. Other drugs, such as antihistamines, cold preparations, and tranquilizers, can decrease your ability to perspire.

• If you are crossing several time zones and are on a fixed dosage schedule (for example, for insulin injections), you may have to make dosing adjustments. Discuss these and any other concerns with your doctor before you depart.

to refrigerate most medications.

It's always a good idea to store drugs in their original containers. Discard the cotton at the top of pill bottles; once it is touched, it can quickly become contaminated with the bacteria on your skin. If you need to use a pill organizer, check with your doctor or pharmacist to make sure that the amount of light or moisture it lets through will not adversely affect any of your medicines.

If young children are around the house, be sure to store medicines in containers with childproof caps and well out of a child's reach. In addition,

don't store medications near any dangerous substances that might be taken by mistake.

◆ *Missed Dose*

Everyone misses a dose of medication now and then. The drug profile tells you what to do when this occurs. For some drugs, the missed dose should be taken right away. For others, you can modify your schedule or wait until the next scheduled dose. In general, it's better not to simply double up on missed doses because you run the risk of raising the drug concentration in your body to dangerously high levels.

TRAVELER'S **MEDICAL KIT**

Wherever you plan to travel, it's a good idea to pack certain essential items. What goes into a medical travel kit will obviously depend on where you're going, how long you're staying, and the general health condition and ages of those traveling. There are certain basic items, however, that it's prudent for almost all travelers to have. The list below outlines some items that might be included in a basic medical kit. Review these and decide which might be appropriate for you to bring along. It's best to be prepared so that an unexpected injury or ailment doesn't spoil a much-anticipated trip.

HEALTH CONCERN	WHAT TO PACK
Allergies and allergic reactions	An antihistamine, such as diphenhydramine hydrochloride.
Children's and infants' special needs	Syrup of ipecac and activated charcoal (antidotes for some cases of accidental poisoning, fluid replacement formula, ear drops and antibiotic creams (in case of bacterial infection). Keep any medications in childproof containers and out of reach.
Constipation	A laxative.
Colds, cough, or sinus congestion	Throat lozenges, gargle solution, cough syrup. For air travel, a decongestant taken a half-hour before takeoff and landing can help ease sinus and ear discomfort.
Cuts and scrapes/ skin infections	Topical antibiotic ointment, such as iodine antiseptic or bacitracin.
Diarrhea, indigestion	Bismuth subsalicylate, loperamide, antacids, or antigas preparations.
Eye care	A spare pair of eyeglasses or contact lenses, along with cleaning supplies, and a copy of your lens prescription.
Fever, headache, minor aches and pains	Aspirin, acetaminophen, naproxen, or ibuprofen.
First-aid supplies	Bandages, gauze, tape, scissors, tweezers, pocket knife, safety pins, alcohol wipes, thermometer—stored in a waterproof case. Don't forget to bring along any health insurance or medical alert cards.
Insects	Insect repellent containing DEET or permethrin.
Itches, bites, skin rashes	A topical corticosteroid cream, such as hydrocortisone 1%; an antihistamine.
Motion sickness	An over-the-counter antihistamine, such as dimenhydrinate or meclizine, or a prescription scopolamine skin patch.
Nasal congestion caused by colds or allergies	A decongestant, such as pseudoephedrine, or an antihistamine.
Sprains and strains	An elastic bandage along with an antiinflammatory pain reliever, such as aspirin or ibuprofen.
Sun protection	Sunscreen and lip balm with an SPF of 15 or higher.
Water impurities	Water purification tablets.

Products that help remind you to take your medicines on a proper schedule are available. These items, sometimes called compliance aids, include containers with sections for daily doses, check-off calendars, electronic devices that beep when it's time for a dose, and computerized pill dispensers. If you need help selecting one of these aids, check with your doctor or pharmacist.

◆ *Stopping the Drug*

Never stop taking a prescribed drug, even if you're feeling better, without consulting your doctor. For example, even a minor infection that appears to have cleared up with a few days worth of antibiotics usually requires a full course of therapy (often 2 weeks). If you stop taking the antibiotic too soon, resistant bacteria can multiply and cause an even more serious infection. Abrupt changes in dosage of some drugs can also be dangerous. For example, a narcotic pain reliever may have to be reduced gradually to avoid withdrawal symptoms. If a hypertensive medicine is stopped suddenly, blood pressure may soar.

For all drugs, it's important that you follow through with the recommended course of therapy. Some drugs may take months to produce their full benefit. Others may need to be continued on a long-term basis. If you experience bothersome side effects or don't think that a drug is having the intended effect, talk to your doctor or pharmacist; don't change your medication schedule on your own.

◆ *Prolonged Use*

If you require a drug for a chronic condition, you may need to take it for extended periods or even a lifetime. Regular checkups or periodic testing may be required to make sure the drug is not causing any hidden or slowly developing adverse effects.

▼ SIDE EFFECTS

Along with their desired effect, drugs typically exert other effects on the body, many of which are undesirable. Such side effects can occur with virtually all prescription and over-the-counter drugs, even when they're taken properly. Keep in mind, though, that only a small percentage of patients who are taking a drug actually experience significant side effects, even the relatively common ones.

The drug profile lists the side effects as serious, common, and less common. Serious side effects are those that may be life-threatening or otherwise have a significant impact on your well-being. You should seek immediate medical assistance if you experience a serious side effect from a drug. Of course, even a mild one is significant if it has a negative impact on your quality of life.

It's a good idea to call your doctor if you are concerned about any side effect, even a seemingly minor one. Write down any problems you have with your medicine so you'll remember them when you talk with your doctor or pharmacist, and don't be afraid to ask questions.

▼ PRECAUTIONS

◆ *Over 60*

Drugs should be used with special caution by people over age 60. Physiological changes brought on by aging—including reduced kidney and liver function, an increase in the ratio of fat to muscle, and a decrease in the amount of water in the tissues of the body—act to concentrate drugs and prevent them from being eliminated at a normal rate. For this reason, older adults may require lower dosages than the amounts usually recommended.

According to the FDA, 17% of all hospitalizations among older adults are caused by the side effects of prescription medications—six times more than for the general population. Drug side effects, as well as drug and food interactions and overdoses, are more common in older patients in part because they are much more likely than younger people to be taking medications in the first place.

The problem is compounded when multiple medicines are involved, particularly when drugs are prescribed by different doctors, who are not always aware of other medications (especially OTC drugs) the patient is taking. In addition, studies have shown that a sizeable percentage of elderly patients are prescribed drugs that should not be used by those in their age group.

It's important to tell your doctors about all the medications you are taking—whether prescription or OTC—and to learn as much as possible about these drugs. As a general rule, don't attribute any changes in mood or any new or unusual reactions or physical changes simply to old age; they may actually be drug side effects or even dangerous interactions.

◆ *Driving and Hazardous Work*

Because some medications may cause drowsiness or confusion, they should not be used when driving, working with dangerous tools or machinery, or in other situations in which a lapse in concentration could cause serious injury. If a drug makes you drowsy, talk to your doctor about scheduling doses near your bedtime or ask about other drugs that might be substituted. Always check to see if a drug may affect alertness and concentration before driving or engaging in a potentially hazardous activity.

◆ *Alcohol*

Certain medications, including many OTC drugs, can be dangerous if taken with alcohol. It's important for you to know whether you should avoid alcohol whenever you begin taking a new drug.

Common signs of alcohol-drug interactions include excessive sleepiness, difficulty breathing, and stomach irritation. When in doubt, it is always a good idea to give up alcoholic beverages entirely while you are taking a medication. According to the FDA, "Of the 100 medicines most commonly prescribed, more than half contain at least one substance that reacts badly with alcohol."

◆ *Pregnancy*

Some drugs are known to be harmful during pregnancy and should unequivocally be avoided during that time. A few have been shown to be safe, but for most drugs, not enough studies have been conducted for researchers to know for sure if the drug is truly dangerous to the fetus.

In general, it's a good idea to minimize the use of prescription and OTC drugs during pregnancy (although certain medications, such as vitamin supplements, may be recommended by your doctor). This precaution should extend to the use of alcohol (present in some drug preparations), which most experts recommend avoiding. Your specific medical needs—as assessed by your doctor—will determine whether a drug is absolutely necessary. Keep in

---

BASIC MEDICINE SAFETY TIPS

1. Follow instructions carefully. It's essential that you take the correct dose at the proper time intervals and avoid potential food and drug interactions.

2. Keep a log of your medicines and let your doctor know your drug and medical history. It's a good idea to review your medications, including both prescription and OTC drugs, with your primary care doctor annually.

3. Try to have prescriptions filled at one pharmacy. The pharmacist will get to know you and your medicines and will be more likely to detect any possible prescription errors.

4. Store medicines properly, away from sunlight, heat, and humidity. The bathroom medicine cabinet is not a good location because of the humidity. A locked closet—away from the reach and sight of children—is ideal.

5. Discard outdated medicines. Prescription drugs should not be used past their expiration date. Some drugs lose their potency with time; other outdated medicines, such as the tetracycline antibiotics, may have dangerous side effects. Ask your pharmacist to label your prescription container with an expiration date and regularly discard old medicines down the toilet.

6. Don't share prescription drugs or borrow them from others. What's good for one person may be harmful to another.

7. Don't take medicines in the dark. You could take the wrong pill by accident. Read the label carefully each time you take a drug to be sure you are getting the right medicine.

8. Keep emergency phone numbers handy. You should have the numbers of your doctor, emergency medical services, and the nearest poison control center readily available in case a medical emergency arises.

9. Don't be afraid to ask questions. Understand your medicines as thoroughly as possible. Know why you are taking them, how and when they should be taken, and things to look out for. People who ask questions are more satisfied with their medical care.

10. Alert your doctor to any side effects or changes in your condition. He or she may be able to adjust your dosage or give you a substitute medication.

---

mind that the benefits of many drugs, when indicated, far outweigh the slight possible risk to mother or fetus.

◆ *Breast Feeding*

Check with your doctor before taking any prescription or OTC medicine if you are nursing. Most drugs (including vitamins and herbal supplements) pass into breast milk to some extent, although some do so more readily than others. Most medications have little or no apparent effect on the nursing infant, but some—such as anticancer drugs—are dangerous.

The drug profile indicates whether a specific drug should be avoided by nursing mothers. In general, as with pregnancy, it's a good idea to minimize the use of medications during this time. Most experts recommend avoiding or strictly limiting alcohol intake as well. For mild pain relief, ibuprofen may be preferable to aspirin or other analgesics, although most analgesics can be used relatively safely while breast feeding; check with your doctor about the best choice for you.

Of course, your medical condition may require that you take certain medications while breast feeding. Ask your doctor to help you to weigh the risks and benefits of drug therapy. In some cases, a drug regimen can be suspended during the nursing period, breast feeding can be stopped if a drug is needed for only a short time, the dosing regimen can be modified, or a substitute drug can be used.

◆ Infants and Children

Children are more sensitive than adults to many drugs. If a drug is indicated for use by children, be very attentive to adverse reactions. If you have any concerns, talk to your doctor, pediatrician, or pharmacist.

OTC drugs, like all medications, should be given with caution to children. To begin, thoroughly study the label of any OTC medicine you're considering for a child to make sure the drug is indeed child-safe. If the label does not have a pediatric dose listed, don't administer it to any child under age 12 years. OTC drugs should not be given to any child younger than age 2 years without a doctor's or pharmacist's approval. Avoid combining children's OTC remedies. Many preparations contain more than one active ingredient, and giving your child two or more different remedies can more easily lead to side effects or overdose.

Important note: Aspirin and other salicylates should not be given to children under age 16 years unless your doctor instructs otherwise. When used to treat chicken pox or the flu, these drugs have been associated with Reye's syndrome, a rare but potentially fatal liver disorder. Use acetaminophen or ibuprofen instead.

Remember that many OTC medications contain alcohol, which can be dangerous for small children.

◆ Special Concerns

The drug profile notes any additional special concerns that you should be aware of. One such possibility is an allergic drug reaction, which occurs when the immune system mounts a response against a particular medication. Allergic reactions can occur with almost any drug, although they are most common with penicillin and related antibiotics. Other common allergens include sulfa drugs, barbiturates, anticonvulsants, certain insulin preparations, and local anesthetics.

Allergic reactions can also occur with OTC medications. For example, some people are allergic to NSAIDs (nonsteroidal antiinflammatory drugs), to certain insulin preparations, and even to some antibacterial skin creams.

Common signs of an allergic drug reaction include a skin rash, hives, and itching. Very severe reactions, known medically as anaphylaxis, can result in swelling of the face, tongue, lips, arms, or legs; swelling can also extend to the airways, making breathing difficult—a life-threatening emergency that requires immediate medical attention.

Call the doctor if you develop any signs of an allergic reaction to a drug. Most drug allergies respond readily to treatment. Antihistamines or topi-

---

 DRUGS AND CHILDREN: **SPECIAL SAFETY MEASURES**

• Keep all prescription and over-the-counter medications out of the reach of children. Some medicines, such as iron supplements, are very toxic to youngsters.

• Use child-resistant caps, and never leave containers open.

• Never give medicine to children unless it is recommended for them on the label or by a doctor.

• Check with the doctor or pharmacist before giving a child more than one medicine at a time.

• Examine dose cups carefully. Cups may be marked with various standard abbreviations. Follow label directions.

• When using a dosing syringe that has a cap, discard the cap before using the syringe.

• Never guess when converting measuring units—from teaspoons or tablespoons to ounces, for example. Consult a reliable source, such as a pharmacist.

• Don't try to remember the dose used during previous illnesses; read the label each time.

• Never use medicine for purposes not mentioned on the label unless so directed by a doctor.

• Check with the doctor before giving a child aspirin products. Never give aspirin to a child or teenager who has or is recovering from chicken pox or has flu symptoms (nausea, vomiting, or fever). Aspirin may be associated in such patients with an increased risk of Reye's syndrome, a rare but serious illness.

FDA Consumer

cal corticosteroids may be advised for skin rashes, hives, or itching. Bronchodilators can make breathing easier. Epinephrine relieves severe reactions. In some cases, a doctor may improve your tolerance to a particular drug, such as penicillin, by giving you a series of slightly increasing doses of that drug—a treatment process that is known medically as desensitization.

Take note of the drug that caused the reaction and let doctors, dentists, and other health-care professionals know about it in the future. You should be careful to avoid taking that drug again, because the allergic reaction may be more serious with subsequent doses.

A medical alert tag, worn as a bracelet or necklace or carried as a card, may also be helpful. The tag states the medical problem and often includes a telephone number that can be dialed for a detailed medical history; you can discuss this option with your doctor.

◆ *Overdose: Symptoms and What to Do*

Virtually any drug can be toxic if taken in high enough doses, but the seriousness will depend on the individual and the particular drug taken. Every profile includes a discussion of the symptoms that are typical of an overdose and what to do if one occurs.

Accidental poisonings are of particular concern for infants and children. Prescription and OTC diet pills, stimulants, and decongestants and prescription antidepressants are common causes of childhood poisoning. Supplements that contain iron are a leading cause of death in young children, who cannot metabolize this mineral well. With certain drugs, even a single tablet can be life-threatening to a small child.

Be sure to store all medications in child-resistant containers and keep them out of the reach—and sight—of children. Remember that a child-resistant container is designed so that it takes longer than 5 minutes for 80% of 5-year-olds to open the bottle. Child-resistant does not mean completely childproof!

The elderly are also at increased risk for overdose. They are more sensitive to some drugs or may forget when they took their last dose.

An intentional overdose, commonly associated with suicide attempts, is a concern in depressed patients of any age, who may have access to large quantities of potentially lethal antidepressant medications.

Most drug poisonings work fairly quickly, although some overdose effects can take weeks to appear. Signs and symptoms of an overdose vary widely and may include listlessness, rolling eyes, confusion, breathing difficulties, unusual sleepiness, or stomach upset. If a child is involved, look for open drug containers around the house or stains around the mouth, and check for a strange breath odor.

If you suspect an overdose, don't panic. Call your poison control center immediately. Depending on the drug, an antidote such as ipecac syrup may be recommended. It's a good idea to keep a bottle of ipecac on hand (safely stored); it induces vomiting and helps rid the body of the drug. Some experts also recommend activated charcoal (available in drugstores, usually in liquid form) for overdose. It absorbs the poison, preventing it from spreading through the body. (Activated charcoal should not be given with ipecac syrup, because the charcoal will absorb ipecac).

For both antidotes, the patient must be conscious. Unconscious victims need immediate professional attention. Neither antidote should be used until you have talked with a doctor or poison control center, because in some cases, ipecac or charcoal can make a patient worse.

▼ INTERACTIONS

Drugs can interact with other drugs or particular foods or can be affected by certain diseases. The drug profile indicates specific interactions to watch for. Effects can range from extremely mild to life-threatening. People over age 60 are especially prone to these drug interactions and should exercise special caution.

◆ *Drug Interactions*

Drug interactions occur when two or more medications react with one another, causing adverse effects. Some drugs can decrease the effectiveness of others; conversely, some bolster another medication's actions. Drug interactions may be felt almost immediately, or they can take days, weeks, or even months to develop.

It's important to note that the effects of drug interactions vary from person to person. Most patients who receive drugs that could interact do not develop notable adverse effects. On the other hand, a few patients experience life-threatening reactions and require immediate treatment.

Anyone who is on multiple medications should take special care, especially if the drugs are prescribed by different doctors. In some cases, however, a doctor will knowingly prescribe two potentially interacting drugs after deciding that the benefits they provide sufficiently outweigh the drawbacks of a possible interaction between them.

Check with your doctor if you are concerned about possible drug interactions or notice unusual symptoms. Take care with OTC drugs as well; they may interact with prescription drugs or with other OTC preparations. For example, don't automatically take an OTC antacid if another drug causes stomach upset, because antacids can alter the effectiveness of certain drugs. Similarly, some vitamin, mineral, or herbal supplements can interact with drugs (see box at right).

◆ Food Interactions

Certain drugs should be taken on an empty stomach, whereas others should be taken with food. For some, it doesn't make a great deal of difference whether you eat or don't eat when you take them. These general dietary recommendations are covered in the drug profile under "Dietary Advice" (see page 15).

Listed in this section are specific foods or drinks that can interact with a particular drug. For example, dairy products can inactivate certain antibiotics. Peculiar interactions have likewise been noted between certain drugs and specific foods such as grapefruit juice (but not orange juice).

The list of potential food interactions is long and drug-specific. Pay close attention to the food or drink interactions for your medications to ensure that you don't interfere with the proper course of your drug therapy.

◆ Disease Interactions

The final section of each drug profile details specific diseases that can have a significant impact on the effects of a particular medication. Kidney or liver disease, for example, can dramatically

DRUGS & HERBAL SUPPLEMENTS: **SOME CAVEATS**

Drug-Herb Interactions

Although there are entire databases documenting how drugs may interact with other drugs, few studies have been done on how drugs interact with herbal supplements. Furthermore, unlike prescription and OTC drugs, herbal products are not regulated by the FDA. Many consumers therefore are unaware of the potentially serious risks of mixing botanicals with other pharmaceutical products.

The main drugs to worry about are known as narrow therapeutic index (NTI) agents. These drugs require precise dosages in order to be effective without being toxic. The anticoagulant drug warfarin (Coumadin) is one example. Too little is ineffective; too much can cause life-threatening bleeding episodes. Supplements such as feverfew, fish oils, garlic, pau d'arco, devil's claw, dong quai, papaya enzyme, and vitamins E and K can dangerously alter blood levels of anticoagulants.

Other Notable Examples

Ginkgo biloba—when taken with aspirin, acetaminophen, pain relievers containing caffeine, or anticoagulants—may lead to bleeding complications such as hyphema (bleeding into the front chamber of the eye) or hemorrhagic stroke (bleeding into the brain).

Licorice can interfere with blood pressure medications, diuretics, hormone replacement therapy, and corticosteroids and can cause serious complications in women who are taking oral contraceptives.

Ginseng may interact adversely with MAO inhibitors (a class of antidepressant) and digoxin (a heart drug).

St. John's wort may be hazardous to people taking selective serotonin reuptake inhibitors (SSRIs) for depression, and it may interfere with the action of warfarin, digoxin, oral contraceptives, and cyclosporine (an immunosuppressant drug taken for organ transplantation).

Some supplements pose such significant risks that they should be avoided altogether. These include comfrey, coltsfoot, chaparral, ephedra (ephedrine or ma huang), sassafras, and yohimbe.

Avoiding Problems

• Tell your doctor about any supplements you take, and ask him or her or a pharmacist about risks of specific herb-drug interactions. People taking medication for such chronic conditions as diabetes, heart disease, or hypertension should be especially cautious.

• Avoid supplements if you are pregnant, trying to conceive, or are breast feeding. Do not give herbal preparations to children without first checking with their doctor.

• Discontinue herbal supplements 2 to 3 weeks prior to and following surgery. Certain supplements may promote unwanted bleeding and other complications.

• Don't take an herb and a drug for the same condition; it would be risky, for example, to use both St. John's wort and Prozac for depression. Side effects might increase.

• Don't abruptly start or stop taking herbs or drugs; this may produce unpredictable and potentially harmful fluctuations in the blood levels of your medications.

• Stop taking supplements immediately if you experience side effects.

affect drug levels in your system. Many drugs, including OTC medications, are metabolized in the liver and excreted by way of the kidneys. If either of these organs is impaired, an excess of a drug may build up in your body.

Many other disorders, such as diabetes mellitus or heart disease, may also affect your body's response to medication—including the OTC drugs you regularly take for such unrelated conditions as allergies or headaches.

It's important to tell your doctor about all diseases or conditions that you have, even if they are not related to your immediate medical concerns.

COMMON DISORDERS *and* THE DRUGS PRESCRIBED FOR THEM

As a rule, your doctor can choose from a variety of drugs to treat a particular medical condition. He or she will determine which drug or combination of drugs should be right for you based on a number of factors: the duration and severity of your illness, other medications you may be taking, your age and general health, any accompanying medical problems, and drug allergies or past experiences you've had with particular medications.

If you think that a drug is not working well or you cannot tolerate its side effects, consult your doctor about trying another medication. Do not discontinue the drug on your own, and never borrow prescription medicines from others.

The drugs covered in this book are grouped below according to the specific diseases, disorders, symptoms, and conditions for which they are typically used. The list is not exhaustive; it is meant to be a general resource so you can explore which drugs may be useful for specific medical concerns.

Don't be alarmed if a drug you are taking is not listed under your condition. Only indications that have been approved by the Food and Drug Administration (FDA) are included here. It's important to note that once a drug has been FDA-approved for one indication, doctors are free to prescribe it for other purposes—a common and often effective practice known as "off-label use."

ACID INDIGESTION AND UPSET STOMACH
Famotidine
Nizatidine
Omeprazole
Ranitidine

ACNE
Tetracycline hydrochloride
Tretinoin

AIDS (HIV INFECTION)
Indinavir
Interferon beta-1b
Saquinavir
Zidovudine (AZT)

ALCOHOL WITHDRAWAL
Diazepam

ALLERGIES AND ALLERGIC REACTIONS
Beclomethasone inhalant and nasal
Cetirizine
Dexamethasone systemic
Fexofenadine
Fexofenadine/ pseudoephedrine
Loratadine
Loratadine/pseudoephedrine
Methylprednisolone
Mometasone furoate nasal
Prednisone

Promethazine hydrochloride
Triamcinolone inhalant and nasal

ALZHEIMER'S DISEASE
Donepezil
Rivastigmine tartrate
Tacrine

ANEMIA
Dexamethasone systemic
Folic acid
Methylprednisolone
Prednisone

ANGINA PECTORIS
Amlodipine
Atenolol
Diltiazem hydrochloride
Isosorbide mononitrate
Metoprolol
Nifedipine
Nitroglycerin
Propranolol hydrochloride
Verapamil hydrochloride

ANXIETY
Alprazolam
Buspirone hydrochloride
Diazepam
Lorazepam

ARTHRITIS
Celecoxib

Dexamethasone systemic
Diclofenac/misoprostol
Ibuprofen
Methotrexate
Methylprednisolone
Nabumetone
Naproxen
Oxaprozin
Prednisone
Rofecoxib

ASTHMA
Albuterol
Beclomethasone inhalant and nasal
Dexamethasone systemic
Methylprednisolone
Montelukast
Prednisone
Salmeterol xinafoate
Theophylline
Triamcinolone inhalant
Zafirlukast

ATHLETE'S FOOT
Terbinafine hydrochloride

ATTENTION DEFICIT HYPERACTIVITY DISORDER (ADHD)
Amphetamine/ dextroamphetamine
Methylphenidate hydrochloride

BEHAVIOR PROBLEMS IN CHILDREN
Haloperidol

BLEEDING, ABNORMAL UTERINE
Estradiol
Estrogens, conjugated
Estrogens, conjugated/med- roxyprogesterone acetate
Medroxyprogesterone acetate

BLOOD CLOTS AND DISORDERS
Clopidogrel bisulfate
Warfarin

BRONCHITIS
Albuterol
Amoxicillin
Azithromycin
Cefprozil
Cefuroxime
Ciprofloxacin systemic
Clarithromycin
Erythromycin systemic
Ipratropium bromide
Levofloxacin
Penicillin V
Tetracycline hydrochloride
Theophylline
Trimethoprim/ sulfamethoxazole

BURSITIS AND JOINT INFLAMMATION

Dexamethasone systemic
Methylprednisolone

CANCER

Estradiol
Estrogens, conjugated
Interferon beta-1b
Levothyroxine sodium
Medroxyprogesterone
  acetate
Methotrexate
Tamoxifen citrate

CHLAMYDIA

Azithromycin
Erythromycin systemic

CHOLESTEROL, HIGH LEVELS OF

Atorvastatin
Fluvastatin
Gemfibrozil
Lovastatin
Pravastatin
Simvastatin

COLDS AND COUGH

Codeine
Promethazine hydrochloride

CONGESTION, NASAL AND SINUS

Loratadine
Mometasone furoate nasal
Promethazine hydrochloride

CONGESTIVE HEART FAILURE

Digoxin
Enalapril maleate
Lisinopril
Metoprolol
Nitroglycerin

CONJUNCTIVITIS (ITCHY EYES) DUE TO ALLERGIES

Cetirizine
Dexamethasone systemic
Loratadine
Methylprednisolone
Mometasone furoate nasal
Prednisone
Promethazine hydrochloride

CONTRACEPTION

Contraceptives, oral (combination products)
Levonorgestrel implants
Medroxyprogesterone
  acetate

COUGHING

Codeine
Promethazine hydrochloride

CUSHING'S DISEASE/SYNDROME

Dexamethasone systemic

DEMENTIA

Tacrine

DEPRESSION

Amitriptyline hydrochloride
Bupropion hydrochloride
Citalopram hydrobromide
Fluoxetine hydrochloride
Nefazodone hydrochloride
Paroxetine hydrochloride
Sertraline hydrochloride
Trazodone
Venlafaxine

DIABETES

Acarbose
Glimepiride
Glipizide
Glyburide
Insulin glargine (rDNA
  origin)
Insulin lispro (rDNA origin)
Metformin

Repaglinide
Rosiglitazone maleate

DIZZINESS (VERTIGO)

Promethazine hydrochloride

EAR INFECTIONS

Amoxicillin
Amoxicillin/potassium clavu-
  lanate
Cefprozil
Cefuroxime
Cephalexin
Clarithromycin
Erythromycin systemic
Penicillin V
Tetracycline hydrochloride
Trimethoprim/
  sulfamethoxazole

EPILEPSY AND SEIZURES

Carbamazepine
Clonazepam
Gabapentin
Phenytoin
Valproic acid (valproate;
  divalproex sodium)

ERECTILE DYSFUNCTION

Alprostadil injection
Sildenafil citrate

EYE INFECTIONS AND INFLAMMATION

Dexamethasone systemic
Fexofenadine
Fexofenadine/
  pseudoephedrine
Loratadine
Loratadine/
  pseudoephedrine
Methylprednisolone
Mometasone furoate nasal
Neomycin/polymyxin B/
  hydrocortisone
  ophthalmic and otic
Prednisone
Promethazine hydrochloride

FEVER

Ibuprofen
Naproxen

FLU

Oseltamivir phosphate
Rimantadine hydrochloride
Zanamavir

FLUID RETENTION

Furosemide
Hydrochlorothiazide
Hydrochlorothiazide/
  triamterene

FUNGAL INFECTIONS

Betamethasone/clotrimazole
Fluconazole
Terbinafine hydrochloride

GINGIVITIS AND GUM DISEASE

Penicillin V
Tetracycline hydrochloride

GLAUCOMA

Brimonidine tartrate
Latanoprost

GOITER

Levothyroxine sodium

GONORRHEA

Amoxicillin
Cefuroxime
Erythromycin systemic

GOUT

Allopurinol
Dexamethasone systemic
Methylprednisolone
Naproxen
Prednisone

HEADACHES— MIGRAINE, SINUS, TENSION, VASCULAR

Naratriptan hydrochloride

Nifedipine
Propranolol hydrochloride
Sumatriptan succinate
Valproic acid (valproate; divalproex sodium)
Zolmitriptan

HEART ATTACK PREVENTION
Atenolol
Clopidogrel bisulfate
Metoprolol
Propranolol hydrochloride
Warfarin

HEARTBURN
Famotidine
Nizatadine
Omeprazole
Ranitidine

HEART RHYTHM DISORDERS
Digoxin
Diltiazem hydrochloride
Propranolol hydrochloride
Verapamil hydrochloride

HEPATITIS
Interferon beta-1b

HIGH BLOOD PRESSURE
Amlodipine
Atenolol
Benazepril hydrochloride
Bisoprolol fumarate/ hydrochlorothiazide
Clonidine hydrochloride
Diltiazem hydrochloride
Doxazosin mesylate
Enalapril maleate
Felodipine
Fosinopril sodium
Furosemide
Hydrochlorothiazide
Hydrochlorothiazide/ triamterene
Irbesartan

Lisinopril
Lisinopril/ hydrochlorothiazide
Losartan potassium
Metoprolol
Nifedipine
Propranolol hydrochloride
Quinapril hydrochloride
Ramipril
Terazosin
Valsartan
Verapamil hydrochloride

HIVES
Cetirizine
Fexofenadine
Fexofenadine/ pseudoephedrine
Loratadine
Loratadine/ pseudoephedrine
Mometasone furoate nasal
Promethazine hydrochloride

HYPOTHYROIDISM
Levothyroxine sodium

IMPETIGO
Mupirocin

INFLAMMATORY BOWEL DISEASE
Dexamethasone systemic
Methylprednisolone
Prednisone

INSOMNIA
Diazepam
Lorazepam
Temazepam
Zaleplon
Zolpidem tartrate

JOCK ITCH
Terbinafine hydrochloride

KIDNEY STONES
Allopurinol

LEGIONNAIRES' DISEASE
Erythromycin systemic

LEUKEMIA
Dexamethasone systemic
Methotrexate
Methylprednisolone
Prednisone
Tretinoin

LUNG DISEASE
Albuterol
Ipratropium bromide
Theophylline

LUPUS
Dexamethasone systemic
Fluticasone
Methylprednisolone

LYME DISEASE
Cefuroxime
Lyme disease vaccine (recombinant OspA)

MALARIA
Mefloquine hydrochloride

MELANOMA
Interferon beta-1b

MENOPAUSE
Estradiol
Estrogens, conjugated
Estrogens, conjugated/med- roxyprogesterone acetate

MENSTRUAL CRAMPS
Ibuprofen
Naproxen

MENSTRUAL PERIODS, REGULATION OF
Medroxyprogesterone acetate

MOTION SICKNESS
Promethazine hydrochloride

MULTIPLE SCLEROSIS
Dexamethasone systemic
Interferon beta-1b
Methylprednisolone
Prednisone

MUSCLE SPASM
Carisoprodol
Cyclobenzaprine

NAIL FUNGUS
Terbinafine hydrochloride

NARCOLEPSY
Amphetamine/ dextroamphetamine
Methylphenidate hydrochloride

NASAL POLYPS
Beclomethasone inhalant and nasal
Dexamethasone systemic
Methylprednisolone
Prednisone

NAUSEA AND VOMITING
Promethazine hydrochloride

OBESITY
Orlistat
Sibutramine hydrochloride monohydrate

OBSESSIVE-COMPULSIVE DISORDERS
Fluoxetine hydrochloride
Paroxetine hydrochloride

OSTEOPOROSIS
Alendronate sodium
Calcitonin (salmon)
Estrogens, conjugated
Estrogens, conjugated/med- roxyprogesterone acetate
Estradiol
Raloxifene hydrochloride
Risedronate sodium

PAGET'S DISEASE
Alendronate sodium
Calcitonin (salmon)
Risedronate sodium

PAIN RELIEVERS
Acetaminophen with
  codeine phosphate
Clonidine hydrochloride
Codeine
Hydrocodone bitartrate/
  acetaminophen
Ibuprofen
Naproxen
Oxycodone
Oxycodone/
  acetaminophen
Promethazine hydrochloride
Propoxyphene/
  acetaminophen
Rofecoxib
Tramadol hydrochloride

PANIC ATTACKS
Alprazolam
Paroxetine hydrochloride

PARKINSON'S DISEASE
Levodopa

PERTUSSIS (WHOOPING COUGH)
Erythromycin systemic

PNEUMONIA
Amoxicillin
Amoxicillin/potassium
  clavulanate
Azithromycin
Cefuroxime
Cephalexin
Ciprofloxacin systemic
Clarithromycin
Erythromycin systemic
Levofloxacin
Tetracycline hydrochloride
Trimethoprim/
  sulfamethoxazole

PROSTATE ENLARGEMENT, BENIGN
Doxazosin mesylate
Finasteride
Terazosin

PSORIASIS
Fluticasone

PSYCHOTIC DISORDERS
Haloperidol
Olanzapine
Risperidone

RHEUMATIC FEVER
Erythromycin systemic
Penicillin V

ROCKY MOUNTAIN SPOTTED FEVER
Tetracycline hydrochloride

RUNNY NOSE AND POSTNASAL DRIP
Cetirizine
Ipratropium bromide
Loratadine
Mometasone furoate nasal
Promethazine hydrochloride

SCHIZOPHRENIA
Olanzapine

SINUS INFECTION
Amoxicillin
Amoxicillin/potassium
  clavulanate
Clarithromycin
Erythromycin systemic
Levofloxacin
Tetracycline hydrochloride

SKIN IRRITATIONS, INFLAMMATION, RASHES
Betamethasone/
  clotrimazole
Dexamethasone systemic
Fluticasone

Methylprednisolone
Prednisone

SNEEZING
Fexofenadine
Fexofenadine/
  pseudoephedrine
Loratadine
Loratadine/
  pseudoephedrine
Mometasone furoate nasal
Promethazine hydrochloride

STREP THROAT
Azithromycin
Clarithromycin
Erythromycin systemic

SUNBURN
Fluticasone

SYPHILIS
Erythromycin systemic
Tetracycline hydrochloride

THRUSH
Fluconazole

THYROID HORMONE DEFICIENCY
Levothyroxine sodium

TONSILLITIS
Cefprozil
Cefuroxime

TOURETTE'S SYNDROME
Haloperidol

TRAVELER'S DIARRHEA
Trimethoprim/
  sulfamethoxazole

TRIGEMINAL NEURALGIA
Carbamazepine

TYPHOID FEVER
Ciprofloxacin systemic

TYPHUS FEVER
Tetracycline hydrochloride

ULCERS
Clarithromycin
Famotidine
Lansoprazole
Nizatidine
Omeprazole
Ranitidine

URINARY TRACT INFECTIONS
Amoxicillin
Amoxicillin/potassium
  clavulanate
Cefuroxime
Cephalexin
Ciprofloxacin systemic
Levofloxacin
Nitrofurantoin
Tetracycline hydrochloride
Trimethoprim/
  sulfamethoxazole

VAGINAL IRRITATION OR INFECTION
Estradiol
Estrogens, conjugated
Estrogens, conjugated/med-
  roxyprogesterone acetate
Medroxyprogesterone
  acetate

VOMITING
Promethazine hydrochloride

WRINKLES
Tretinoin

YEAST INFECTIONS, VAGINAL
Fluconazole

THE NEW AGE OF NUTRITIONAL MEDICINES

▼ THE CHANGING VIEW OF SUPPLEMENTS

The substances and products that we classify as supplements are by no means entirely new. Vitamins in pill form have been available for more than 50 years. Herbs, also known as botanicals or phytomedicines (*phyto* means "plant" in Latin), have been staples in the sickroom and the kitchen for centuries and were the primary form of medicine in the United States until this century. Yet only a decade ago, most vitamin pills were fairly uniform "one-a-day" formulas, and herbal remedies often had to be concocted at home or purchased in out-of-the-way health food stores.

◆ *Revived Interest*
Today in the United States, "dietary supplements," as they are officially called, encompass a dizzying array of vitamins, minerals, and herbs, as well as other compounds that have been extracted or created from natural sources. (These compounds carry names such as glucosamine, coenzyme Q10, and lycopene.)

Available without a prescription, supplements are sold in virtually every American supermarket and drugstore. Many malls and shopping areas have stores devoted entirely to supplements, and they can also be bought through catalogs and over the Internet. Annual supplement sales now exceed $34 billion and are expected to grow markedly in the future.

Newspapers, TV, and radio regularly highlight evidence of supplements' benefits—whether it is a review of 23 studies of St. John's wort for mild depression, a survey of the effects of ginkgo biloba on patients with dementia, or an article noting that the standard treatment for enlarged prostate in many European countries is not a conventional prescription drug but rather the herb saw palmetto. Another recent article tells of vitamin A being prescribed to stave off throat cancer.

With all this attention and the rising sales of supplements, it isn't surprising that millions of Americans, including many doctors and scientists, have come to realize that substances such as garlic, echinacea, and grape seed extract, along with vitamins and minerals, are as beneficial to health as low-fat foods, exercise, and aspirin.

According to a number of surveys, one-third to one-half of all Americans now regularly use various forms of supplements as preventive medicine or as therapies for a wide range of ailments—from common complaints such as colds and headaches to more serious concerns, including arthritis, depression, heart disease, and even cancer.

The fact that so many people are eager to try supplements, even when it is often hard to find reliable information, shows that major changes in health care have brought herbal and nutritional remedies closer to mainstream medicine. Traditionally, the medical community has been skeptical of these remedies and of alternative medicine. That is changing.

◆ *Increased Research*
Since the 1990s, nutritional research has produced a flood of studies offering compelling evidence that specific foods and nutrients may help prevent, slow, or even reverse serious diseases.

For example, several large-scale studies from Harvard University have provided strong evidence that vitamin E supplementation is linked to lower rates of heart disease in men and women. From these results, experts have concluded that a higher level of vitamin E than is found in the average American diet (or can possibly be obtained from food alone) very likely offers some protection against heart disease.

These and similar studies cited throughout this book have changed the opinions of many scientists and other experts who were skeptics. They now believe that supplementation with reasonable amounts of vitamins and minerals may increase a person's chances of preventing disease and enjoying optimal health.

◆ *Learning from Europe*
Although research into herbal remedies has lagged in the United States, in Europe herbs have been widely studied and scrutinized over the past 25 years, and standards have been established for their effectiveness and safety.

In Germany a special body of scientists and health professionals known as Commission E has been investigating the usefulness and safety of herbal remedies since 1978, gathering information from scientific literature, clinical trials, and medical associations. It has issued reports on some 300 herbs—and has found about two-thirds of them to be safe and effective.

This information about the way herbs are used elsewhere has persuaded more American doctors and scientists to take a less dismissive view of herbal remedies.

◆ *Better Studies Still Needed*

Despite more extensive research, however, a number of benefits attributed to vitamins, minerals, and herbs remain unproven and controversial. Many doctors and researchers insist the studies on alternative remedies are not sufficiently rigorous. Furthermore, extreme claims of therapeutic benefits draw fire from critics—either because they are without merit or because they leave the impression that anything "natural" is harmless, which is not always the case. Many of the studies have been small in scale, and most don't offer a long-term evaluation of benefits and side effects.

On the other hand, as more studies are conducted, some impressive evidence is accumulating. In the research on the herb St. John's wort for mild to moderate depression, for example, 15 studies have compared an extract of the herb to a placebo, or neutral pill, in order to test for a placebo effect (an improvement in symptoms that some people experience because they believe they are receiving treatment, even though the pill is inactive).

In these studies, St. John's wort was found to be more effective than a placebo in treating relatively mild (although not severe) depressive symptoms. Other studies have shown that the herb works as well as standard prescription medications for treating mild depression. Moreover, side effects were infrequent and relatively innocuous—which is part of the appeal of many herbs.

◆ *Emphasis on Prevention*

There is increasing emphasis—backed by growing numbers of medical experts—on lifestyle choices as a critical factor in staying well. This has led more people to pay attention to diet,

exercise, and weight control, which can help prevent or relieve common complaints, including backache and constipation. Many people have also quit smoking and limited their alcohol intake. All these changes can reduce the risk of serious ailments such as heart disease and cancer. (Researchers now think that three-quarters of all cancers result mainly from things people eat, drink, smoke, or encounter in the environment.)

Vitamins, minerals, and herbs can reinforce and enhance the benefit of these self-care measures, which are also essential for enjoying what might be termed optimal health—not simply the absence of illness, but the capacity to lead a full, vital, and productive life.

◆ *New Regulations*

In 1994, the U.S. government passed a new set of regulations called the Dietary Supplement Health and Education Act, which eased restrictions on the selling of vitamin, mineral, and herbal supplements. Reflecting and reinforcing the demands of consumers, the regulations have allowed

supplement manufacturers to make certain claims about a product's health benefits without absolute proof of its therapeutic effects. The freedom to make these claims has been a key factor in the enormous number and variety of supplements that have come on the market.

▼ INTEGRATIVE HEALING

In recent years, Americans—including many consumers and some doctors—have become increasingly aware of the limitations of conventional medicine. Although medical science has found cures for many troubling health problems (including some infectious diseases that caused sickness and premature death on a grand scale), it has been less successful in combating chronic illnesses such as heart disease, cancer, and diabetes. Drugs often offer potent treatments for many ailments, but they also pose the risk of powerful and distressing side effects. In addition, medications can be very expensive, and the cost may be prohibitive for many patients.

HEALTH PROFESSIONALS AND SUPPLEMENTS

Many doctors and nurses (as well as dietitians and other health professionals) who practice conventional medicine may act skeptical about alternative therapies. As it turns out, however, many use vitamin and mineral supplements themselves.

In one survey of 181 cardiologists, nearly half were taking antioxidant vitamins. These included vitamins C and E,

which have been linked to the prevention of heart disease and certain forms of cancer, as well as to control of a host of other ailments. A smaller percentage of the physicians (37%), however, recommended antioxidants routinely to their patients.

Another survey of 665 dietitians in Washington State found that nearly 60% took some nutritional supplement either daily or occasionally.

◆ *Beyond Managed Care*

A good number of patients and doctors have been frustrated by the growth of health maintenance organizations (HMOs) and similar managed-care health plans. Such plans have forced thousands of Americans, often against their will, to change doctors and at the same time have restricted their choice. Doctors, in turn, chafe because their time with patients is limited. In fact, surveys show that more people are now complaining that their doctors don't pay enough attention to them. Furthermore, many managed-care plans don't provide the same level of coverage that traditional insurers once did, so patients frequently have to pay more out of their own pockets for services rendered.

As awareness of these shortcomings has grown, consumers have become more enthusiastic about alternative approaches to treating ailments. Generally these methods—which include therapies such as chiropractic care, acupuncture, and massage, as well as supplements—are considered less invasive and more "holistic" (treating the whole person rather than simply suppressing symptoms) than conventional treatments. As you read this book, you will see that supplements often act to enhance the body's own defenses. An herb you take to help treat an infection, for example, often doesn't directly kill bacteria (as an antibiotic would) but rather strengthens your immune system so your body can kill the bacteria.

Alternative therapies are also typically less expensive than conventional treatments; supplements, in particular, usually cost far less than prescription drugs and may even be cheaper than some over-the-counter medications. Alternative therapies, such as acupuncture and chiropractic care, are now covered by some health-care plans.

Behind many of these alternative choices in healing is a common perspective: The body has amazing powers of self-repair. According to this view, supplements, when used wisely, can bolster the body's immune system to prevent disease. If a health problem does occur, they can enhance and accelerate self-healing.

◆ *Doctors Reassess*

Consumers have shown that they want to try alternative approaches, and physicians are slowly responding to demands from patients. Rather than thinking of supplements and other less-established remedies as "alternatives" that exclude conventional treatments, however, some doctors are attempting to integrate the two, so alternative medicine options can work hand in hand with Western medicine. (Recognizing this development, the federal government in 1992 established an Office of Alternative Medicine, which funds serious research at major medical centers to study complementary and alternative treatments for a variety of ailments.)

In an integrative approach, ideally, you and your doctor work together to reach a decision about which supplement or other therapy to use for treating your particular health problem (see the box opposite). On the other hand, many doctors and other members of the medical establishment are still resistant to complementary healing methods. Thus, there is no single reliable entity to supply advice about these remedies. In the end, it is up to consumers to acquaint themselves with the various types of complementary therapies, including supplements, that are now available.

▼ SUPPLEMENTS—OR DRUGS?

One reflection of the mainstream popularity of herbal and nutritional supplements is that most drugstores in the United States stock them, and these products are often shelved right next to over-the-counter drugs. Both types of products make health-related claims, and both are supplied in forms such as capsules, tablets, or powders—so a consumer may well ask, what's the difference?

◆ *No Simple Answer*

Concerned about the marketing of supplements, legislators have made a concerted effort to distinguish them from pharmaceutical drugs. By law, manufacturers of drugs (both over-the-counter and prescription) can make explicit claims about a product's ability to prevent or treat a recognized medical condition—for example, alleviating headaches or relieving heartburn. Such claims can be made only after a lengthy approval process by the Food and Drug Administration (FDA), which verifies the drug's safety and effectiveness.

According to the Dietary Supplement Health and Education Act, which regulates the marketing of such products, supplements are intended to "supplement the diet" and must contain one or more of the following: vitamins, minerals, herbs (also called botanicals), amino acids, or other nutritional substances. Supplements are not subjected to the rigorous testing and scrutiny that drugs receive; therefore the labels on supplements cannot promise to cure or prevent diseases. The labels *can* list potential benefits that affect bodily functions, such as "promoting healthy cholesterol" or "aiding digestion."

YOU AND YOUR DOCTOR: SOME GUIDELINES

A growing number of doctors and patients are embracing an integrative, or complementary, approach to treating health problems. This entails carefully weighing both conventional and alternative methods in order to create a strategy best suited to a patient's particular needs.

For example, a person with high blood pressure finds that the side effects from a prescription drug are intolerable, so patient and doctor decide on a course of therapy that combines supplements with other lifestyle adjustments to see if it can effectively lower the blood pressure with fewer side effects.

Traditionally, medical schools teach their students very little about nutritional and herbal therapies. Because professional journals and postgraduate courses for physicians are giving these forms of treatment increasing attention, however, many doctors are becoming better acquainted with them.

Be sure to keep the following guidelines in mind when considering various treatment options and working with your doctor:

• **Don't diagnose yourself.** If you have symptoms that suggest an illness, see a doctor—an M.D., a D.O. (doctor of osteopathic medicine), or a trained and licensed doctor of naturopathy.

• **Talk to your doctor.** Be sure to report all of your symptoms; never hide anything from your doctor. Also, be sure to tell your doctor about any supplements that you are now taking, because some of them might not interact well with conventional drugs that you may be asked to try. Even if your doctor isn't receptive to nutritional remedies, you should discuss any supplements you are already taking or thinking of using, particularly if you have a chronic condition such as asthma, diabetes, migraine, heart disease, or high blood pressure.

• **Don't stop treatment.** Some supplements may complement, or even replace, conventional drugs. You should never discontinue or alter the dosage of any prescribed medication without first consulting your doctor.

• **Recognize when conventional methods are best.** It can be foolish—and sometimes even dangerous—to seek alternative options for medical conditions that Western-trained doctors excel in treating or preventing. These include medical and surgical emergencies, physical injuries, acute infections, sexually transmitted diseases, kidney infections, reconstructive surgery, and serious illnesses, such as polio and diphtheria, that can be prevented with immunizations.

Of course, such statements (which are called "structure-function claims") usually imply treatment for a particular health problem. People who are worried about high cholesterol levels and heart disease, for example, are more likely to respond to anything promoting "healthy" cholesterol. Such links are frequently spelled out in manufacturers' brochures and in supplement sales materials, as well as in news reports and various publications.

◆ *Truthfulness of Claims*

Whether the assertions on supplement labels are always true is an issue that regulators have wrestled with but not resolved. The law states that all claims must be "truthful and not misleading,"

and in many cases, there is some scientific basis for such claims. Supplement manufacturers don't have to submit any data in advance of making a claim, however; they merely need to have the evidence on hand. Hence, labels must contain a statement that the claims " . . . have not been evaluated by the Food and Drug Administration."

So, if many supplements do, in fact, act like drugs and are often used as drugs, why aren't they tested and marketed as drugs? It's because vitamins, minerals, herbs, and other supplements can be derived directly from plants and other natural sources—and therefore can't be patented. Thus, there is little financial incentive for drug or supplement makers to spend

millions on the research and approval process required for a nutrient to obtain the status of a drug. Once an herb or herb component receives FDA approval, any company can sell the same product.

Government regulation of supplements will no doubt evolve as their use grows and as more is learned about their effects. At some point, U.S. regulations and practices may move closer to those of a number of European countries, where herbal remedies are examined and formulated with more rigor. For now, it is helpful to remember that the claims made on most supplement labels are not equivalent to—or as stringent as—those on most drug labels.

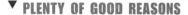

▼

▼ PLENTY OF GOOD REASONS

Many people take a multivitamin supplement as nutritional "insurance" against deficiencies. Research has provided additional reasons for using a variety of supplements, including herbs, and indicates that optimal levels may be higher than conventional wisdom has long dictated.

If you're basically healthy, should you take supplements on a regular basis? If you develop an ailment, can you really expect supplements to help? What follows is a summary of the major benefits most people can expect from using the supplements covered in this book.

▼ ENHANCING YOUR DIET

Conventional wisdom holds that as long as people who are healthy eat well enough to avoid specific nutri-

tional deficiencies, they don't need to supplement their diet. The only thing they have to do is consume foods that meet the RDAs—Recommended Dietary (or Daily) Allowances—and other guidelines for vitamin and mineral intakes developed by the federal government (see the box on page 35).

Even if one accepts the government's standards for vitamin and mineral intake as adequate for good health, however, the evidence is overwhelming that most people don't come close to meeting those nutritional requirements. Surveys show that only 9% of Americans eat 5 daily servings of fresh fruits and vegetables—the amount recommended for obtaining the minimum level of nutrients believed necessary to prevent illness.

Average calcium consumption in the United States and Canada is estimated to be about 60% of the current suggested level of 1,000 mg for adults

ages 19 to 50—and far below the 1,200 mg recommended for men and women ages 51 to 70 and older.

According to a review of national data by experts at the University of California, Berkeley, people often make food choices that are nutritionally poor. They are more likely to select french fries than broccoli as a vegetable and will typically opt for a soft drink over a glass of skim milk as a beverage. Not only can these and other foods contribute too much fat and sugar to the diet, they can also result in less than optimal intakes of vitamins, minerals, and disease-fighting phytochemicals. The diets of many Americans, these experts note, contain just half the recommended amounts of magnesium and folic acid. Vitamins A, C, and B_6, as well as iron and zinc, are other nutrients that surveys show are at low levels in the American diet.

ANTIOXIDANTS: POWERFUL FREE RADICAL FIGHTERS

Although oxygen is essential for life, it can also have adverse effects on your body. In the normal process of using oxygen, chemical changes that create reactive unstable oxygen molecules called free radicals occur in the body; these free radicals can damage cells and structures within cells, including genetic material (DNA).

Free radicals also may form in response to external factors (cigarette smoke and alcohol), pollutants (nitrogen oxide and ozone), and ultraviolet light and other forms of radiation (including X rays). If the genetic material in cells is affected, it can be replicated in new cells, contributing to cancer and other serious health problems. Free radicals may also weaken artery walls, allowing fatty deposits that can lead to heart disease to collect.

Cells have special agents for combating free radicals and repairing molecular damage. These are called antioxidants. A good deal of research suggests that antioxidants may play important roles in preventing or delaying heart disease, cancer, and other ills and may even slow the effects of aging.

Vitamins C and E are perhaps the best-known antioxidants. The mineral selenium is also an antioxidant, as are carotenoids such as beta-carotene and lycopene. Enzymes and certain other compounds (such as glutathione) manufactured by the cells themselves also act as antioxidants. A number of other substances, including certain herbs, may act as antioxidants as well. For example, green tea, grape seed extract, and ginkgo biloba (among others) are all thought to have antioxidant properties.

◆ Filling Nutritional Gaps

Even with the best nutritional planning, it is difficult to maintain a diet that meets the RDAs for all nutrients. For example, vegetarians, who as a group are healthier than meat eaters (and who tend to avoid junk foods low in vitamins and minerals), still may be deficient in some nutrients, such as iron, calcium, and vitamin B$_{12}$. Most people who want to maintain a healthy low-fat diet will have a problem obtaining the recommended amounts of vitamin E from their food alone, because so many of the food sources for vitamin E are high in fat.

Another complication is that a balanced diet may not contain the more specialized substances—fish oils, soy isoflavones, or alpha-lipoic acid—that researchers think may promote health. For generally healthy people who can't eat a well-balanced diet every day, a supplement can fill in these nutritional gaps or boost the nutrients they consume from adequate to optimal.

There are various other reasons why people who maintain good eating habits might benefit from a daily supplement. Some experts now believe that exposure to environmental pollutants—from car emissions to industrial chemicals and wastes—can cause damage in myriad ways inside the body at the cellular level, destroying tissues and depleting the body of nutrients. Many supplements, particularly those that act as antioxidants, can help control the cell and tissue damage that follows toxic exposure (see the box opposite). Some evidence also indicates that certain medications, excess alcohol, smoking, and persistent stress may interfere with the absorption of certain key nutrients. Even an excellent diet would be unable to make up for such a shortfall.

TOO MANY BENEFITS: **TOO GOOD TO BE TRUE?**

When you see a supplement label that lists a variety of functions and benefits for a single herb or substance, you might wonder if this is more marketing hype than facts. You can't rely entirely on label claims, because they aren't scrutinized for accuracy by the government or any other agency. As you will see in reading this book, however, some supplements do have multiple effects that are well documented.

Consider an herb such as green tea. According to many studies, its benefits may include helping control several cancers, including colon and pancreatic cancer; protecting against heart disease; inhibiting the action of bacteria; and acting as an anti-oxidant to bolster the immune system. All of these benefits aren't too surprising given that researchers have identified various active components in green tea.

You should be aware that many common medications were initially developed for one purpose. As more people take the drugs and their effects are studied, new uses come to light. Imagine a drug that can cure headaches, relieve arthritis, help prevent heart disease, ease the pain of athletic injuries, and reduce the risk of colon cancer. It's aspirin, of course—and its precursor came from an herbal source, the bark of the white willow tree.

▼ PREVENTING DISEASE AND SLOWING AGING

For many years, it was thought that a lack of nutrients was linked only to specific deficiency diseases such as scurvy, a condition marked by soft gums and loose teeth that is caused by too little vitamin C. In the past three decades, however, thousands of scientific studies have indicated that specific nutrients appear to play key roles in the prevention of a number of chronic ailments common in contemporary Western societies.

Many studies highlighting the disease-fighting potential of different nutrients are mentioned in this book. What most of these studies reveal is that the level of nutrients associated with disease prevention is often significantly higher than the current RDIs or RDAs. To achieve these higher levels, the participants in these studies often had to depend on using supplements.

◆ The Role of Antioxidants

In slowing or preventing the development of disease, some experts suggest that nutrients, particularly antioxidants, can also delay the wear and tear of aging by reducing the damage done to cells. This idea does not mean vitamin E or coenzyme Q10, for example, are "youth potions." Several studies, including work done at the Nutritional Immunological Laboratory at Tufts University, however, have found that supplementation with single nutrients, such as vitamin E, or with multivitamin and mineral formulas, appears to improve immune response among older people.

For example, the results of a study of 11,178 elderly subjects conducted by researchers at the National Institute on Aging showed that the use of vitamin E was associated with a lowered risk of total mortality and especially of death from heart disease. In fact, vitamin E users were only half as likely to die of heart disease as those taking no supplements. In addition, there is evidence that antioxidant supplements are effective in lowering the risk of cataracts and macular degeneration, two age-related vision conditions.

Other supplements that serve as high-potency antioxidants against aging disorders include the mineral selenium, carotenoids, flavonoids, certain amino acids, and coenzyme Q10. Some experts also believe that the herb ginkgo biloba may improve many age-related symptoms, especially those involving reduced blood flow, such as dizziness, impotence, and short-term memory loss. Substances found in echinacea and other herbs are reported to strengthen the immune system, and phytoestrogens such as soy isoflavones are thought to help delay or forestall some of the effects of menopause, as well as to help prevent cancer and heart disease.

▼ TREATING AILMENTS

Practitioners of complementary medicine often recommend supplements for a wide range of health problems affecting virtually every body system. For most of these conditions, conventional physicians would be more likely to prescribe drugs. Some disorders, however, routinely require supplements. For example, iron may be prescribed for some types of anemia, vitamin A (in the drug isotretinoin, or Accutane) for severe acne, and high doses of the B vitamin niacin for reducing high cholesterol levels.

In this book, certain vitamins and minerals are suggested for the treatment of specific ailments. Still, the use of supplements as remedies, especially for serious conditions, is controversial. Most doctors practicing conventional medicine are skeptical of supplements' efficacy and believe it is sometimes dangerous to rely on them. Based on published data and their own clinical observations, however, nutritionally oriented physicians and practitioners think the use of these supplements is justified—and that to wait years for unequivocal proof to appear would be wasting valuable time. Even so, until there is more consistent evidence available, you should be careful about depending on nutritional supplements alone to treat any serious ailment.

◆ Age-old Remedies

Despite these cautions, it is important to note that for thousands of years, various cultures have employed herbs for soothing, relieving, or even curing many common health problems, a fact not ignored by medical science. The pharmaceutical industry, after all, arose as a consequence of people using herbs as medicine. Some studies suggest that a number of the claims made for herbs have validity, and the pharmacological actions of the herbs covered in this book are often well documented by clinical studies as well as historical practice. In Europe, a number of herbal remedies, including St. John's wort, ginkgo biloba, and saw palmetto, now are accepted and prescribed as medications for treating disorders such as allergies, depression, impotence, and even heart disease. Of course, even herbs and other supplements with proven therapeutic effects should be used judiciously (see the safety guidelines box on page 41).

▼ WHAT SUPPLEMENTS WON'T DO

Despite the many promising benefits that supplements offer, it's important to note their limits—and to question some of the extravagant claims currently being made for them.

◆ Not Food Stand-Ins

As the word itself suggests, supplements are not meant to replace the nutrients available from foods. They can't counteract a high intake of saturated fat (which has been linked to an increased risk of heart disease and cancer), and they can't replace nutrients found in foods you ignore. Also, although scientists have extracted a number of disease-fighting phytochemical compounds from fruits, vegetables, and other foods, there may be many others that are yet undiscovered—ones you can get only from foods. In addition, some of the known compounds may work only in combination with others in various foods rather than as single isolated ingredients in supplement form.

◆ Not Magic Lifestyle Bullets

Supplements won't compensate for habits known to contribute to ill health, such as smoking or a lack of exercise. Optimal health requires a wholesome lifestyle—particularly if, as people get older, they are intent on aging well.

◆ Not Weight Loss Miracles

Weight loss preparations may be popular, but it's questionable whether any of them can help you shed pounds without the right food choices and regular exercise. Products that claim to "burn fat" won't burn enough on their own for significant weight loss.

◆ *Not Performance Boosters*

Claims of improving performance, whether physical or mental, are also very difficult to back up—and any "enhancement" will be a limited one at best in a healthy person. Although a supplement may boost mental functioning in someone experiencing mild to severe memory loss, it may have a negligible effect on the memory or concentration of most adults. Likewise, a supplement that combats fatigue isn't going to turn the average jogger into an endurance athlete. Nor is it clear that "aphrodisiac" supplements favored by many men today are effective for enhancing sexual performance if you aren't suffering from some form of sexual dysfunction.

◆ *Not Cure-Alls*

To date, no supplements have been found to cure any serious diseases—including cancer, heart disease, high blood pressure, diabetes, or AIDS. The right supplement, however, may help improve a chronic condition, such as migraine or osteoarthritis, and it may also help relieve symptoms such as pain or inflammation. Supplements are also good for treating minor wounds and burns.

The important thing to remember is that before using supplements for any ailment, you first need to consult a health professional for treatment.

 RDAs, DVs, RDIs, AIs: **WHAT DO THOSE NUMBERS MEAN?**

Over the years, government-sponsored committees of nutritional experts, including those in the National Academy of Sciences and the Food and Drug Administration, have established various guidelines for the amounts of vitamins and minerals needed by most individuals to achieve and maintain good health. Understanding what these different standards signify can be confusing. All of them, however, represent similar values based on the "gold standard" of vitamin and mineral intake: the RDAs, or Recommended Dietary (or Daily) Allowances.

Early standards
The first RDAs were developed in 1941 and have been revised periodically by the Food and Nutrition Board of the National Research Council. The RDAs are different for men, women, and children; for different age groups; and for pregnant or lactating women. Some years ago, a new standard, the Reference Daily Intake, or RDI, was created for each nutrient. The RDIs are intended to represent nutrient needs of an average healthy person. In most cases they are the highest levels of adult RDAs, although they also take into account other guidelines.

On many labels of vitamin and mineral supplements (as well as on food labels), you will see a set of figures under the heading "% Daily Value," or DV. The Daily Value is simply a percentage of the RDI. It tells you how much of a particular nutrient is supplied by a dose of the supplement (or, in the case of food labels, by a serving of food). The sample label on page 39 shows how the DV typically appears.

The RDIs replace an older value called the U.S. RDA. Although this value is no longer used for foods, some supplement labels continue to state nutrient values as a percentage of the U.S. RDA.

Slightly revised guidelines
The Food and Nutrition Board has introduced a new set of values called Dietary Reference Intakes (DRIs). These include RDAs as well as Adequate Intakes (AIs) for certain nutrients for which there is not enough evidence to establish an RDA. In releasing new recommendations, the board raised some RDA levels to take into account the prevention of disorders other than deficiency diseases. For example, the latest recommendation for folic acid for women age 18 and older has been raised from 180 µg to 400 µg—a level thought to protect against certain birth defects and heart disease.

In each of the vitamin and mineral profiles (under "How Much You Need"), you'll find the RDA or AI for that nutrient. Deficiencies from getting too little and adverse effects from getting too much are indicated when known.

Are they enough?
Remember that the RDAs, RDIs, and DRIs are recommendations, not requirements, for large groups of people. The values are at a level assumed to supply the nutrient needs of most people, plus a generous margin of safety. Many experts, however, think RDAs (especially those for vitamins) are still far too low for maintaining optimal health or for treating certain diseases. Also, the values don't take into account such variables as smoking, alcohol consumption, exposure to pollutants, and medication use, which can interfere with nutrient absorption.

▼ TYPES OF SUPPLEMENTS

Anyone who has strolled down a dietary supplement aisle is aware of—and possibly overwhelmed by—the huge variety of products available. Counting different brands and combinations of supplements, there are now literally thousands of choices. Although you'll hardly encounter this many products in any one location, even the relatively limited selection in your local supermarket can be very confusing.

One reason for so much variety is that marketers are constantly trying to make their own brands stand out, so they devise different dosages, new combinations of ingredients, and creatively worded claims for their products. At the same time, scientists have found new and better ways of extracting nutritional components from plants and synthesizing nutrients in a laboratory—discoveries that have resulted in many new products.

To make informed decisions, it's essential to understand the terms used on supplement labels (see the box on page 39), as well as the properties and characteristics of specific supplements, which you will find in the individual supplement profiles (beginning on page 323). To avoid feeling overwhelmed by all the choices facing you, it's first useful to learn about the basic types of supplements that are available and the key functions they perform in helping keep you healthy.

◆ Vitamins
Vitamins are chemically organic substances (meaning they contain carbon) essential for regulating both the metabolic functions within the cells and the biochemical processes that release energy from food. In addition, evidence is accumulating that certain vitamins also act as antioxidants—substances that protect tissues from cell damage and possibly help prevent a number of degenerative diseases (see pages 32 to 34).

With a few exceptions (notably vitamins D and K), the body cannot manufacture vitamins on its own, so they must be ingested in food or nutritional supplements. There are 13 known vitamins that can be categorized as either fat-soluble (A, D, E, and K) or water-soluble (8 B vitamins and vitamin C). The distinction is important because the body stores fat-soluble vitamins for relatively long periods (months or even years); on the other hand, water-soluble vitamins (except for vitamin B_{12}) remain in the body for a short period of time and must be replenished more frequently.

◆ Minerals
Minerals are present in your body in small amounts. All together, they add up to only 4% of body weight. Yet these inorganic substances, which are found in the earth's crust as well as in many foods, are essential for a wide range of vital processes, from basic bone formation to the normal functioning of the heart and digestive system. A number of minerals have also been linked to the prevention of cancer, osteoporosis, and other chronic illnesses.

Just as with vitamins, people must replenish their mineral supply either through foods or through supplements. The body contains more than 60 different minerals, but only 22 are thought to be essential. Of these, 7—including calcium, chloride, magnesium, phosphorus, potassium, sodium, and sulfur—are usually designated as macrominerals, or major minerals. The other 15 minerals are called trace minerals, or microminerals, because the amount that the body requires each day for good health is extremely tiny (usually it's measured in micrograms, or millionths of a gram).

◆ Herbs
Herbal supplements are prepared from plants—often using the leaves, stems, roots, or bark, as well as the buds and flowers. Known for centuries as medicinal agents, many plant parts can be used in their natural form, or they can be refined into tablets, capsules, powders, liquids, and other supplement formulations.

Many herbs have several active compounds that interact with one another to produce a therapeutic effect. An herbal supplement may contain all of the compounds found in a plant, or just one or two of the isolated compounds that have been successfully extracted. For some herbs, however, the active agents simply haven't been identified, so using the complete herb is necessary to obtain all its benefits.

Of the hundreds of remedies that are surfacing in the current rebirth of herbal medicines, the majority are being used to treat chronic or mild health problems. Increasingly, herbs are also being employed to attain or maintain good health—for example, to enhance the immune system, to help maintain low blood cholesterol levels, and to safeguard against fatigue. Less commonly, some herbs are now recommended as complementary therapy for acute or severe diseases.

◆ *Nutritional Supplements*

These nutrients include a diverse group of supplement products. Some, such as fish oils, are food substances that scientists have concluded possess disease-fighting potential. Flavonoids, soy isoflavones, and carotenoids are phytochemicals—compounds found in fruits and vegetables that work to lower the risk of disease and that may, in addition, alleviate symptoms of some ailments, such as heart disease and menopausal problems.

Other nutritional supplements, such as DHEA, melatonin, and coenzyme Q10, are substances present in the body that can be recreated synthetically in a laboratory. A similar example is acidophilus, a "friendly" bacterium in the body that, taken as a supplement, may aid in the treatment of digestive disorders. Amino acids, which are building blocks for proteins and may play a role in strengthening the immune system and in promoting health in other ways, have been known to scientists for many years. Only fairly recently, however, have they been marketed as individual dietary supplements.

The many choices available today allow you to find supplements that are safe, effective, and convenient. Some of these "special" formulations, however, appear to provide little additional benefit, and they are frequently not worth the extra expense.

Supplements come in a variety of forms that affect both their ease of use and, in some cases, their rate of absorption by the body. (Each supplement profile lists the available forms for that supplement.)

▼ COMMON FORMS

In general, tablets and capsules are the most convenient forms of vitamin, mineral, or nutritional supplements to take, but there are other options as well. You can purchase whole herbs and make up your own formulations. Most of the prepackaged forms described here are readily available in drugstores, supermarkets, and health food stores. Whole herbs can be purchased at herb stores and some health food stores.

Tablets and Capsules Stored away from heat and light, tablets and capsules will generally keep longer than other supplement forms. It's important to be aware that vitamin tablets often contain generally inert additives known as excipients, in addition to the vitamin itself. These compounds bind, preserve, or give bulk to the supplement and help the tablets break down more quickly in your stomach. Increasingly, supplements are also available in capsule-shaped, easy-to-swallow tablets called "caplets."

The fat-soluble vitamins A, D, and E are typically packaged in "softgel" capsules. Other vitamins and minerals are processed into powders or liquids and then encapsulated. Like tablets, capsules are easy to use and store. They also tend to have fewer additives than

 ABOUT **THE LABEL CLAIMS**

Advertising claims imply that vitamins derived from "natural" sources (such as vitamin E from soybeans) are better than "synthetic" vitamins created chemically in a laboratory. They may state that their natural products are more potent or more efficiently absorbed—and manufacturers generally charge more for natural products—but what is "natural"?

Actually, most supplements, no matter what their source, undergo processing with chemicals in laboratories. Some products labeled "natural" are really synthetic vitamins with plant extracts or minute amounts of naturally derived vitamins mixed in. Hence, "vitamin C from rose hips" may be mostly synthetic. Even the most natural products must be refined and processed, so they contain some additives. In any case, there's no difference chemically between natural and synthetic vitamins—nor can your body distinguish between the two.

Some researchers consider natural sources of vitamin E more effective than synthetic versions. The International Units (IUs) used to measure vitamin E's potency take this into account, so a capsule designated to provide 400 IUs will have that potency no matter what its source.

Generally, there's no reason to pay more for supplements advertised as "natural." The cheapest synthetic vitamin or mineral supplement will give you the same benefit. Of course, the cheapest supplement isn't always the best. You should check the excipients, or additives, in a supplement to be sure that you aren't allergic to any—and you may have to pay more for a supplement with fewer of these inert filler ingredients.

tablets, and there is some evidence that they dissolve more readily (although this doesn't mean they are better absorbed by the body—just that they may be absorbed more quickly).

If you are taking herbs, you can avoid the taste of the herb (which some people don't like) if you use tablets or capsules. Herbal tablets and capsules are prepared using either a whole herb or an extract of the herb containing a high concentration of the herb's active components. In either of these forms, the constituents are ground into a powder that can then be pressed into tablets or encapsulated.

Some herbs come in enteric-coated capsules, which pass through the stomach to the small intestine before dissolving. This minimizes potential gastrointestinal discomfort and, for some herbs, enhances their absorption into the bloodstream.

Sublingual Tablets A few supplements, such as vitamin B$_{12}$, are formulated to dissolve under the tongue. This process provides quick absorption into the bloodstream without interference from stomach acids and digestive enzymes.

Powders People who find pills hard to swallow can use powders, which can be mixed into juice or water or stirred into food and taken with meals. (Ground seeds such as psyllium and flaxseed often come in powdered form.) Powders also allow dosages to be adjusted easily. Because they may have fewer binders or additives than tablets or capsules, powders are useful for those individuals who are allergic to certain substances. In addition, powders are often cheaper than tablets or capsules.

Tinctures and Liquid Extracts Tinctures are made by soaking the whole herb or parts of it in water and ethyl alcohol. The alcohol extracts and concentrates the herb's active components. (Nonalcoholic concentrations can be made using glycerin.)

Liquid extracts are more concentrated than tinctures. Again, the herb is soaked in a solvent such as water and alcohol, but then the alcohol is distilled away, usually by a vacuum process that doesn't heat the herb and change its potency.

Chewables Such supplements (usually packaged as flavored wafers) are particularly recommended for those who have trouble getting pills down. In this book, the most common wafer form is DGL, a licorice preparation. DGL is activated by saliva, so the wafers must be chewed, not simply swallowed.

Lozenges A number of supplements are available as lozenges or drops. These are intended to dissolve gradually in the mouth, either for ease of use or, in the case of zinc lozenges, to help in the treatment of colds and the flu.

Oils Oils extracted from herbs can be commercially distilled to form potent concentrations for external use. These so-called essential oils are placed in a neutral "carrier" oil, such as almond oil, before use on the skin. Essential herbal oils should never be ingested. The exception is peppermint oil. A few drops on the tongue are recommended for bad breath, and capsules can be beneficial for an irritable colon.

Gels, Ointments, and Creams Gels and ointments, made from fats or oils of aromatic herbs, can be applied to the skin to soothe rashes, heal bruises

or wounds, and serve other therapeutic purposes. Creams are light mixtures of oil and water that are partially absorbed by the skin, allowing it to breathe while keeping in moisture. Creams can be used for moisturizing dry skin, cleansing, and relieving rashes, insect bites, or sunburn.

Tea Infusions and Decoctions Less concentrated than liquid forms, herbal tea infusions are brewed from the softer parts of the herb—the fresh or dried flowers or the stems or leaves. These can be purchased in bulk or in tea bags. Be sure to use very hot (not boiling) water when preparing a tea infusion to preserve the beneficial oils that can be dissipated by the steam of boiling water. Also, let the tea sit covered for 5 to 10 minutes. Decoctions, which use the tougher parts of an herb (roots, twigs, or bark), are simmered for at least half an hour.

For maximum potency, drink herbal teas soon after brewing them or store them in tightly sealed glass jars in the refrigerator for up to 3 days.

◆ *Special Formulations*
You will usually pay more for a supplement if the label says "timed-release" or "chelated." Does it provide extra benefits? Not often, according to available data. If you do decide to purchase one of these products keep the following information in mind:

Timed-Release Formulas These formulas contain microcapsules that gradually break down to release the vitamin steadily into the bloodstream over roughly 2 to 10 hours, depending on the product. ("Sustained-release" describes the same process.)

There are no reliable studies showing that timed-release formulas are

HOW TO READ **A SUPPLEMENT LABEL**

It wasn't that long ago that labels on dietary supplements provided scant information and made unsubstantiated claims. Rulings by the Food and Drug Administration (FDA), however, have now changed all that.

All supplement labels now are required to carry a "Supplement Facts" box listing ingredients by weight. For those nutrients with an established Reference Daily Intake (RDI), the percentage must be listed and expressed as Percent Daily Value (DV). In the case of plant (or herbal) medicines, the label must identify the part used.

In addition, a number of other requirements must be followed. The information accompanying the label shown here explains some of the key FDA rulings.

It is important to note that the FDA requirements are aimed at providing consumers with more reliable and consistent information about the tens of thousands of products designed to "supplement" the diet, such as vitamins, minerals, herbs, and amino acids.

The new labeling requirements do not, however, mean that supplements must withstand strict government scrutiny, as do prescription and over-the-counter drugs. Supplement manufacturers are expected to ensure that their preparations are safe, but most products need not undergo an elaborate testing and review process. The government can step in only if a supplement appears to pose a health risk or makes drug-like claims for treating disease.

The bottom line: Stick with products made by reputable manufacturers that you trust. Never use products with labels that do not give you enough information for careful use.

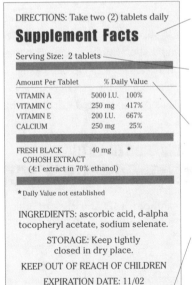

HIGH POTENCY FORMULA FOR WOMEN

Antioxidant dietary supplement

STRENGTHENS CELLS, SUPPORTS BONE HEALTH, PROTECTS AGAINST OXIDATIVE DAMAGE*

*This statement has not been evaluated by the Food and Drug Administration. This product is not intended to diagnose, treat, cure, or prevent any disease.

Antioxidant vitamins C and E

100 tablets

DIRECTIONS: Take two (2) tablets daily

Supplement Facts

Serving Size: 2 tablets

Amount Per Tablet		% Daily Value
VITAMIN A	5000 I.U.	100%
VITAMIN C	250 mg	417%
VITAMIN E	200 I.U.	667%
CALCIUM	250 mg	25%
FRESH BLACK COHOSH EXTRACT (4:1 extract in 70% ethanol)	40 mg	*

* Daily Value not established

INGREDIENTS: ascorbic acid, d-alpha tocopheryl acetate, sodium selenate.

STORAGE: Keep tightly closed in dry place.

KEEP OUT OF REACH OF CHILDREN

EXPIRATION DATE: 11/02

Manufacturer or distributor's name, address, and zip code

A high-potency label can be added to a product, such as this antioxidant formula, if at least two-thirds of the nutrients meet the Daily Value—and those nutrients must be identified. A single-nutrient product must contain 100% or more of the nutrients that meet the Daily Value. Most vitamin and mineral supplements easily meet this standard. For herbs, no Daily Value has been established.

Structure and function claims can describe only a product's effects on the body's structure or function and not its potential health benefits.

A standard FDA disclaimer must accompany the vague and often meaningless structure-function claims that are allowed.

The Supplement Facts box, similar to the Nutrition Facts box on foods, lists key ingredients by weight.

Serving size notes the amount per serving, which may be one, or many, tablets.

The % Daily Value is essentially the same as the "U.S. RDA," which used to appear on labels. It tells you the minimum amount of a specific nutrient you need but not the higher doses often required for therapeutic benefits.

Contact the manufacturer for verification of a product's safety or effectiveness. Many manufacturers now have websites and toll-free telephone numbers. Buy brands only from a company you trust.

more efficiently utilized by the body than conventional capsules or tablets. In fact, the gellike substance that acts to delay the release may actually interfere with the absorption of fat-soluble vitamins, such as vitamin A.

Although timed-release versions of niacin (vitamin B$_3$) may help prevent unpleasant side effects, this formulation is generally not recommended because of the potential risk of liver damage.

Chelated Minerals Chelation is a process in which a mineral is bonded to another substance, or "chelator"— usually an amino acid. This attached substance is supposed to enhance the body's absorption of the mineral. In most cases, there's no proof that chelated minerals are absorbed any better or any quicker than nonchelated minerals. In fact, there is no solid information that any process or added ingredients improve the absorption of vitamins or most minerals.

◆ *Standardized Extracts*

When herbs are recommended in this book, we often suggest that you look for "standardized extracts." Herbalists and manufacturers use this term to describe the consistency of a product. When creating an herbal supplement, manufacturers can extract the active components from the whole herb. These active ingredients—for example, the allicin in garlic or the ginsenosides in ginseng—are then concentrated and made into a supplement (tablets, capsules, tinctures, or liquid extracts). They are standardized in order to supply you with a precise amount of key substances in each dose.

Sometimes, instead of standardized extracts, manufacturers process the whole, or crude, herb. In this case, the whole herb is simply air- or freeze-dried, made into a powder, and then packaged into a supplement—again a capsule, tablet, tincture, liquid extract, or other form.

Whether a standardized extract or the whole herb is better is an ongoing controversy among herbalists. Supporters of whole herb supplements contend that the entire herb may contain still-unidentified active ingredients and that only through ingesting the entire herb can all the benefits be obtained. On the other hand, advocates of standardized extracts argue that the active ingredients in whole herbs can vary greatly depending on where they're grown and how the herbs are harvested and processed. Proponents of standardization say that the only way to be sure you're receiving a consistent amount of active ingredients is by taking only standardized extracts.

Although standardized products are indeed more consistent from batch to batch, this fact doesn't guarantee that they are more effective than whole-herb products. In many cases, however, you would have to use a much greater amount of a whole herb to achieve a similar therapeutic effect. More to the point, reliability and consistency can be of great value, particularly when a product proves to be beneficial for a specific disorder.

◆ *Multisupplements*

Many herbs have traditionally been paired in combination products to enhance their benefits. The most straightforward pairings team herbs with similar effects, such as valerian and chamomile, which both act as sedatives. Other formulas include several herbs that address different symptoms of an ailment, not unlike a combination cold remedy that has one ingredient for congestion and another for sore throat. Still others feature an array of substances touted as antioxidant "cocktails." Supplement manufacturers have also marketed herbs with vitamins and other nutritional supplements such as amino acids.

Some of these combinations can promote health and may also save you money. In addition, you may find that fewer pills are needed. For example, liver detoxifying products called lipotropic combinations often include the nutrients choline, inositol, and

 WHEN YOU BUY **STANDARDIZED EXTRACTS**

The amount of an active or main ingredient in a standardized herbal extract is often expressed as a percentage. Milk thistle "standardized to contain 80% silymarin" means that 80% of the extract contains that ingredient. Accordingly, recommendations in this book for most standardized products are given as percentages. For example, a 150-mg dose of milk thistle standardized to contain 80% silymarin contains 120 mg of silymarin (150 X .80 = 120).

Sometimes, though, a standardized extract product will simply state the actual amount of active ingredient you're getting (e.g., 120 mg silymarin) rather than listing a percentage. This is fine, too.

methionine, as well as the herb milk thistle—all of which, in a blend, assist liver function. These formulas cost less and are more convenient to take than individual supplements.

In some combination products, however, certain ingredients are present in such small quantities that their therapeutic effect is doubtful. They are there simply to promote the product. It pays to check the label to determine the amount of each ingredient.

▼ SUPPLEMENT SAFETY

Although supplement manufacturers are prohibited by the Food and Drug Administration (FDA) from making direct claims about curing or treating diseases, the FDA has otherwise given them great leeway, and the safety or effectiveness of a supplement doesn't have to be demonstrated as it does with drugs.

Responsible manufacturers are careful to print instructions about proper use on their labels, but you may encounter many brands that do not supply them. Therefore, you need to read the supplement profiles in this book carefully and also keep the following guidelines mind.

◆ *The Proper Amounts*
Dietary supplements are generally safe in the appropriate dosages. Remember, though, that more isn't necessarily better—and sometimes it can be worse. For example, the mineral selenium has many recommended uses, from treating cataracts to preventing cancer. Taking doses even slightly higher than recommended can cause hair loss and other toxic reactions. When using supplements, it's a good idea to avoid high doses, particularly very high ones ("megadoses").

Vitamins and Minerals Most vitamins can be taken in significantly higher doses than their RDAs without producing adverse reactions. Some fat-soluble vitamins, however, which are stored in the body rather than excreted, may be toxic at high doses. Overloading on vitamin A or D is particularly dangerous. And although the body naturally excretes extra water-soluble vitamins such as vitamin C, avoid extremely high doses. Toxic reactions can occur. Reducing the dosage usually remedies the situation.

Some minerals, when taken in large doses or over a long period of time, can block the absorption of other minerals. Zinc, for example, can hamper the absorption of copper. Also, large amounts of certain minerals have been linked to disease—several studies show that too much iron in men increases their risk of heart disease. For these reasons, even doctors who believe that the RDAs for many vitamins are too low also think that the levels for minerals are generally adequate for optimal health.

Herbs According to reviews by experts in pharmacology and toxicology, serious side effects or toxic reactions associated with herbal medicines are

---

 SAFETY GUIDELINES

Because supplements, especially herbs, can have potent primary effects and side effects, keep these points in mind when using them:

• **Shop carefully.** Because there is no independent guarantee of purity or potency, it's your responsibility to select brands with a reputation for quality.

• **Take the recommended dosages.** As with conventional drugs, overdosing with a supplement can have serious consequences. With herbs and nutritional supplements, always start with the lowest dose when a dosage range is given.

• **Monitor your reactions.** At the first sign of an adverse reaction, stop using the supplement. Also stop if the herb doesn't seem to be working for you (give it

time, though—some herbs may take a month or more to have a noticeable effect).

• **Take a break.** Doctors using conventional medications typically recommend "drug holidays" for certain non-life-threatening conditions such as a persistent headache, eczema, or mild depression. The same wisdom applies to supplements; it's best to take them for specified periods and then stop temporarily to see if the condition has improved. If the problem returns, you may need to take the supplement long term as a "maintenance" medication.

• **Avoid risks.** If you have symptoms that indicate a serious problem, don't self-treat it with supplements. See a doctor or other trained health professional. Also, ask about interactions with any drugs you are taking.

rare. Still, some once-popular medicinal herbs, such as foxglove and chaparral, are now recognized as toxic. Occasionally, some people exhibit serious allergic reactions to an herb, which may include hives or some other rash or difficulty breathing.

Furthermore, because no uniform quality control for herbal preparations exists, the chemical composition of an herbal remedy can vary greatly from batch to batch, and it may contain potentially toxic contaminants and other ingredients that can influence side effects or effectiveness. Products that contain standardized extracts may be more reliable than those that don't in terms of getting a proper dose of a particular supplement. Still, whenever you buy a supplement you still rely on the manufacturer's integrity.

In addition, using some herbs can be risky for people with certain health conditions or for those on particular medications (see pages 498 to 500). Garlic, for example, may intensify the effects of anticoagulant drugs, and licorice—which aids digestive problems and enhances the immune system—can raise blood pressure.

Other herbs may have no immediate adverse effects but may cause side effects or prove harmful when taken long term. When using supplements, always follow the dosage recommendations closely. In addition, notify your doctor at once if any serious adverse reactions develop.

▼ QUALITY CONTROL

How do you know what a product actually contains? The best way to find out is to call the manufacturer of a particular supplement and ask how the supplement's potency is ensured. You should also check how long the company has been in business. Established supplement manufacturers have a reputation to protect and therefore take measures to ensure that their products contain what is stated on the labels.

You can also ask your doctor or another health professional (such as a dietitian or nutritionist) who uses supplements for recommendations of reliable products.

A FINAL WORD

◆ About the Dosages
The dosage suggestions in each profile are the total daily amount that you'll need to treat a disorder. They are based on findings from hundreds of research studies and the clinical experience of the consulting doctors for this book. You may have to adjust these numbers to factor in amounts found in your daily multivitamin or in individual supplements you're already using for other health reasons.

Although every effort has been made to include widely available dosages, the strengths of individual products vary greatly. Many qualified people—health professionals, pharmacists, health food store staff—can help you find products with equivalent doses.

◆ Special Exceptions
The recommendations in this book do not apply to pregnant or breast-feeding women, who have specific needs and restrictions, or to children under age 16 years, whose growth and development vary widely. Individuals in these groups can still benefit from using supplements, but they should always consult a doctor before deciding what supplements to take.

◆ Talk to Your Doctor
You should talk with your doctor before trying the supplements discussed here, particularly if you have a serious health problem, such as heart disease or diabetes. The book's goal is to inform you about the numerous benefits that can come from taking supplements wisely. This means using them as a complement to—not as a substitute for—responsible medical care.

A-to-Z
Prescription
Drug Profiles

ACARBOSE

Precose

Available in: Tablets
Available OTC? No   **As Generic?** No
Drug Class: Antidiabetic agent

▼ USAGE INFORMATION

WHY IT'S PRESCRIBED
As an adjunct (supplemental) therapy in patients with diabetes who do not require insulin injections but are unable to control their blood glucose levels with diet alone or with other medications.

HOW IT WORKS
Acarbose inhibits the activity of enzymes that are required to break down carbohydrates into simple sugars in the intestine. This effect delays the digestion of carbohydrates and thus reduces the rise in blood sugar that typically occurs after meals.

▼ DOSAGE GUIDELINES

RANGE AND FREQUENCY
Initially, 25 mg 1 to 3 times a day. The dose may be increased (at 4- to 8-week intervals) to a maximum of 100 mg 3 times daily.

ONSET OF EFFECT
Within 1 hour.

DURATION OF ACTION
Up to 2 hours.

DIETARY ADVICE
This medicine should be taken with the first bite of breakfast, lunch, and dinner. Follow your doctor's advice regarding diet, weight loss, and exercise.

STORAGE
Keep in a tightly sealed container away from heat and direct light.

MISSED DOSE
If you have finished a meal without taking the medication, skip the missed dose and resume your regular dosing schedule with the next meal. Do not double the next dose.

STOPPING THE DRUG
Take this medication as prescribed for the full treatment period.

PROLONGED USE
Non-insulin-dependent diabetes is a chronic condition, so use of acarbose will be ongoing. Blood glucose levels should be checked regularly during treatment so that the dosage may be adjusted if necessary.

▼ PRECAUTIONS

Over 60: No special precautions required.

Driving and Hazardous Work: Acarbose should not impair your ability to perform such tasks safely.

Alcohol: Drink only in moderation when taking acarbose.

Pregnancy: Consult your doctor for advice. Insulin is usually the treatment of choice for women with diabetes who are pregnant.

Breast Feeding: Trace amounts of acarbose can be found in breast milk; however, adverse effects in infants have not been documented. Consult your doctor for advice.

Infants and Children: Safety and effectiveness have not been established for patients under 18 years of age. Consult your doctor for more specific advice.

Special Concerns: You should not take acarbose if you've had an allergic reaction to this drug in the past or if you are taking, or took within the past 14 days, a monoamine oxidase (MAO) inhibitor (a class of antidepressant drugs).

OVERDOSE
Symptoms: Increased gas, diarrhea, and stomach pain.

What to Do: These symptoms usually subside on their own within a short period of time. If they do not, consult your doctor for more specific advice. Symptoms of hypoglycemia should not occur when taking acarbose alone but may occur if a patient is also taking sulfonylurea or insulin for diabetes.

▼ INTERACTIONS

DRUG INTERACTIONS
Do not take acarbose if you are taking, or took within the past 14 days, an MAO inhibitor. Consult your doctor for specific advice if you are taking any of the following drugs that may interact with acarbose: digestive enzyme preparations containing amylase or pancreatin, intestinal absorbents (such as charcoal), insulin, or sulfonylureas (oral antidiabetic agents).

FOOD INTERACTIONS
Avoid foods that contain large amounts of sugar (for example, cake, cookies, candy, and acidic fruits). Closely follow the diet your doctor has prescribed.

DISEASE INTERACTIONS
Acarbose should not be taken by patients with a history of any of the following disorders: diabetic ketoacidosis, intestinal disorders (including malabsorption or obstruction), inflammatory bowel disease (for example, Crohn's disease or ulcerative colitis), liver disease, kidney disease, or gastric ulcers.

≡ SIDE EFFECTS ≡

SERIOUS
There are no serious side effects associated with acarbose.

COMMON
Feelings of bloating, gas, abdominal discomfort, diarrhea. These symptoms tend to decrease over time.

LESS COMMON
Increase in liver enzymes, causing yellowish tinge to eyes or skin (jaundice), when maximal dose is exceeded. When used in combination with sulfonylureas, may cause symptoms of low blood sugar, which include sweating, tremor, anxiety, hunger, confusion, seizures, rapid heartbeat, vision changes, dizziness, headache, loss of consciousness. Hypoglycemia must be treated by ingestion of glucose (dextrose). Sucrose (table sugar) and foods or drinks containing sugars or starches are ineffective because acarbose prevents their breakdown and absorption.

ACETAMINOPHEN WITH CODEINE PHOSPHATE

Available in: Capsules, tablets, oral solution, oral suspension
Available OTC? No **As Generic?** Yes
Drug Class: Opioid (narcotic) analgesic/antipyretic

▼ USAGE INFORMATION

WHY IT'S PRESCRIBED
To relieve mild to severe pain when nonprescription pain relievers prove inadequate. A narcotic analgesic, such as codeine, in combination with acetaminophen may provide better pain relief than either medicine used alone. In addition, when taken together, the two medications can often achieve better pain relief at lower doses.

HOW IT WORKS
Acetaminophen appears to interfere with the action of prostaglandins, naturally occurring substances in the body that cause inflammation and make nerves more sensitive to pain impulses. This medication also relieves fever, probably by acting on the heat-regulating center of the brain. Unlike aspirin, however, acetaminophen does not reduce inflammation. Codeine, a narcotic analgesic, is believed to relieve pain by acting on specific areas in the spinal cord and in the brain that together process pain signals from nerves throughout the body.

▼ DOSAGE GUIDELINES

RANGE AND FREQUENCY
Adults—Capsules or tablets: 1 or 2 capsules containing 15 or 30 mg of codeine with acetaminophen or 1 capsule containing 60 mg of codeine with acetaminophen every 4 hours as needed. Oral solution or suspension: 1 tablespoon every 4 hours as needed. Children—Oral solution or suspension: Ages 3 to 6 years: 1 teaspoon 3 or 4 times a day as needed. Ages 7 to 12 years: 2 teaspoons 3 or 4 times a day as needed.

ONSET OF EFFECT
Acetaminophen: Rapid. Codeine: Within 2 hours.

DURATION OF ACTION
Up to 4 hours.

DIETARY ADVICE
Take this with meals or milk to avoid stomach upset, unless your doctor directs you to do otherwise.

STORAGE
Store in a tightly sealed container away from moisture, heat, and direct light. Keep liquid forms from freezing.

MISSED DOSE
If you are taking acetaminophen with codeine on a fixed schedule, take it as soon as you remember. If it is near the time for the next dose, skip the missed dose and resume your regular dosage schedule. Do not double the next dose.

STOPPING THE DRUG
You should take the medication as prescribed for the full treatment period, but you may stop taking it if you are feeling better before the scheduled end of therapy. This drug should never be stopped abruptly after long-term regular use.

PROLONGED USE
Narcotic drugs such as codeine may cause physical dependence. Taking too much acetaminophen may cause liver damage. Therapy with acetaminophen and codeine should not continue for more than 2 weeks and may actually cease to be effective before then.

▼ PRECAUTIONS

Over 60: Adverse reactions may be more likely and more severe in older patients.

Driving and Hazardous Work: Acetaminophen with codeine can cause dizziness or drowsiness; pay attention and proceed with caution.

Alcohol: Avoid alcohol. The combination of alcohol and this drug may increase the depressant effects of the medicine. Drinking alcoholic beverages while taking acetaminophen greatly increases your risk of developing liver damage.

Pregnancy: Use of this drug during pregnancy can cause fetal addiction and may cause breathing problems in the newborn infant if taken during or just before delivery. Consult your doctor for specific guidelines and advice and discuss the relative risks and benefits of using this drug while pregnant.

Breast Feeding: Acetaminophen with codeine passes into breast milk; avoid or discontinue nursing while taking this drug.

Infants and Children: This medicine should not be given to infants. The drug may be used by children over the age of 3 years, but only with extreme caution and under the careful supervision of your doctor. Children are generally prescribed the oral solution or suspension instead of the capsule or tablet.

Special Concerns: Taking a narcotic such as codeine for an extended period of time can lead to physical dependence. When discontinuing the drug after using it for an extended period, it is important to decrease the dosage gradually under the supervision of your doctor to reduce the risk of suffering from

▼ SIDE EFFECTS

SERIOUS
See Overdose and Special Concerns.

COMMON
Dizziness, lightheadedness, nausea or vomiting, drowsiness, constipation, unusual fatigue.

LESS COMMON
Stomach pain, allergic reaction, false sense of well-being (euphoria), depression, loss of appetite, blurring or change in vision, nightmares or unusual dreams, dry mouth, general feeling of illness, headache, nervousness, insomnia.

(continued) **45**

ACETAMINOPHEN WITH CODEINE PHOSPHATE (continued)

withdrawal symptoms. Call your doctor if you notice these symptoms after discontinuing the drug: shivering or trembling; insomnia; goose bumps; nausea or vomiting; body aches; loss of appetite; stomach cramps; weakness; diarrhea; restlessness, nervousness, or irritability; rapid heartbeat; sneezing, runny nose, or fever; increased yawning; or increased sweating. Overuse of acetaminophen with codeine may also lead to anemia, liver problems, or central nervous system disorders. Contact your doctor as soon as possible if you experience any of the following symptoms during or after the use of this drug: bloody, dark, or cloudy urine; severe pain in your lower back or side; frequent urge to urinate; painful or difficult urination; sudden decrease in urine output; pale or black, tarry stools; yellow discoloration of the eyes or skin (jaundice); hallucinations; unusual bleeding or bruising; skin rash, hives, or itching; pinpoint red spots on skin; sore throat and fever; unusual excitability; trembling or uncontrolled muscle movements; or redness, flushing, or swelling of the face.

OVERDOSE

Symptoms: Severe dizziness or drowsiness; cold, clammy skin; difficult or slow breathing or shortness of breath; severe confusion; seizures; stomach cramps or pain; diarrhea; low blood pressure; increased sweating; nausea or vomiting; constricted pupils; irregular heartbeat; severe weakness.

What to Do: Call your doctor, emergency medical services (EMS), or the nearest poison control center immediately.

▼ INTERACTIONS

DRUG INTERACTIONS

Some drugs may interact with acetaminophen and codeine. Consult your doctor for specific advice if you are taking any prescription or over-the-counter drugs, especially if they contain acetaminophen; central nervous system depressants such as antihistamines or medicine for hay fever, allergies, or colds; barbiturates; seizure medicine; muscle relaxants; anesthetics; or tranquilizers, sedatives, or sleep medications.

FOOD INTERACTIONS

No significant food interactions have been reported.

DISEASE INTERACTIONS

Consult your doctor if you have a head injury or brain disease, an underactive thyroid, an enlarged prostate, seizures, kidney or liver disease, gallbladder problems, a blood disorder, or a history of alcohol or drug abuse. Any of these medical conditions may increase the likelihood of developing side effects from acetaminophen and codeine.

ACYCLOVIR

BRAND NAME

Zovirax

Available in: Capsules, tablets, liquid, ointment, injection
Available OTC? No   **As Generic?** Yes
Drug Class: Antiviral

▼ USAGE INFORMATION

WHY IT'S PRESCRIBED
To treat herpes virus infections such as genital herpes, shingles, herpes simplex, and chicken pox.

HOW IT WORKS
Acyclovir interferes with the activity of enzymes needed for the replication of viral DNA in cells. This prevents the virus from multiplying.

▼ DOSAGE GUIDELINES

RANGE AND FREQUENCY
Oral forms—For genital herpes: Up to 1,200 mg a day in evenly distributed doses every 4 or 8 hours. For shingles: Up to 4,000 mg a day in evenly distributed doses every 4 hours. For chicken pox: Up to 800 mg 4 times a day, not to exceed 3,200 mg a day. Topical form—To relieve herpes symptoms: Apply a small amount to lesions every 3 hours (6 times a day) for 7 days. Use a glove or finger cot when applying medication.

ONSET OF EFFECT
2 hours or more.

DURATION OF ACTION
Up to 5 hours following the final dose.

DIETARY ADVICE
Capsule, tablet, and liquid forms should all be taken with food and with a full (8-oz.) glass of water.

STORAGE
Store in a dry place at room temperature, away from direct sunlight. Refrigerate any liquid form of acyclovir but do not allow it to freeze.

MISSED DOSE
If you miss a tablet, capsule, or liquid dose, take it as soon as you remember, up to 2 hours late. If more than 2 hours, wait for the next scheduled dose. Do not double the next dose. For ointment, apply dose as soon as you remember, then return to your regular dosing schedule.

STOPPING THE DRUG
Take the drug as prescribed for the full treatment period, even if you begin to feel better before the scheduled end of therapy. Do not take it for longer than the recommended period.

PROLONGED USE
Women with genital herpes are at increased risk of developing cervical cancer; annual Pap smears are recommended for these patients.

▼ PRECAUTIONS

Over 60: Adverse reactions and side effects may be more common in older persons. Such effects can be minimized by drinking at least 2 to 3 quarts of liquid per day.

Driving and Hazardous Work: The use of acyclovir should not impair your ability to perform such tasks safely.

Alcohol: Alcohol may accentuate the side effects of lightheadedness and dizziness.

Pregnancy: Acyclovir has been used by pregnant women, and no birth defects or other related problems have been reported; however, studies in humans have been limited and inconclusive. Consult your doctor about using acyclovir if you are pregnant or plan to become pregnant.

Breast Feeding: Acyclovir may pass into breast milk. Breast feeding should be avoided while taking any oral form of the drug. No problems are expected with the topical form.

Infants and Children: Acyclovir should not be used for children under 2 years of age. Its use for children under age 12 should be carefully supervised by a physician.

Special Concerns: Be sure to tell your doctor if you have ever had any unusual or allergic reaction to acyclovir. It is important to remember that the use of acyclovir is not a cure and will not help prevent you from spreading herpes infections to others. Avoid using this medication in or near the eyes. If it does get into your eyes, consult your doctor.

OVERDOSE
Symptoms: No specific ones have been reported.

What to Do: An overdose of acyclovir is unlikely to be life-threatening. However, if someone takes a much larger dose than prescribed, call your doctor, emergency medical services (EMS), or the nearest poison control center right away for advice. Prolonged overdose may lead to kidney damage.

▼ INTERACTIONS

DRUG INTERACTIONS
Consult your doctor for specific advice if you are taking cyclosporine, probenecid, meperidine, or zidovudine.

FOOD INTERACTIONS
No significant food interactions have been reported.

DISEASE INTERACTIONS
Use of acyclovir may cause complications in patients with liver or kidney disease, because these organs work together to remove the medication from the body.

≡ SIDE EFFECTS ≡

SERIOUS
No serious side effects have been reported.

COMMON
Rash, nausea, and vomiting. Ointment can cause pain, burning, or itching at the site where it is applied. Should such adverse symptoms persist, notify your doctor. Injection can cause inflammation of the vein (phlebitis); call your doctor if this occurs.

LESS COMMON
Diarrhea, stomach pain, lightheadedness, dizziness, confusion, tremor. In rare cases, kidney function may be altered when the drug is given by injection, causing such symptoms as decreased urine output.

ALBUTEROL

BRAND NAMES

Airet, Proventil, Ventolin, Volmax

Available in: Inhaler, solution, capsules, tablets, syrup
Available OTC? No   **As Generic?** Yes
Drug Class: Bronchodilator/sympathomimetic

▼ USAGE INFORMATION

WHY IT'S PRESCRIBED
To dilate air passages in the lungs that have become narrowed as a result of disease or inflammation. It is used in the treatment of asthma and chronic obstructive pulmonary disease (COPD).

HOW IT WORKS
Albuterol widens constricted airways by relaxing the smooth muscles that surround the bronchial passages in the lungs.

▼ DOSAGE GUIDELINES

RANGE AND FREQUENCY
Use it when needed to relieve breathing difficulty. For bronchospasm: 1 to 2 puffs of aerosol inhaler every 4 to 6 hours, 2.5 mg of solution delivered via nebulizer 3 to 4 times a day, 200 micrograms (µg) of capsules for inhalation using Rotahaler every 4 to 6 hours, or 2 to 4 mg of tablets 3 or 4 times a day, not to exceed 32 mg per day.

Children may require a smaller dose. For prevention of exercise-induced asthma: 1 or 2 inhalations (at least 1 full minute apart) 15 minutes prior to exercise.

ONSET OF EFFECT
Inhalant: Within 5 minutes. Oral forms: Within 15 to 30 minutes.

DURATION OF ACTION
Inhalant: 3 to 6 hours. Oral forms: 8 hours.

DIETARY ADVICE
Albuterol can be taken on an empty stomach or with food or milk.

STORAGE
Contents of aerosol canisters are under pressure; be careful not to puncture the container. Store canister away from heat, open flame, and direct light.

MISSED DOSE
Skip the missed dose and resume your regular dosage schedule. Do not double the next dose.

STOPPING THE DRUG
It may not be necessary to finish the recommended course of therapy. Consult your doctor.

PROLONGED USE
Therapy may require months or years. Excessive use may result in temporary loss of effectiveness.

▼ PRECAUTIONS

Over 60: Adverse reactions may be more likely and more severe in older patients.

Driving and Hazardous Work: Do not drive or engage in hazardous work until you determine how the medicine affects you.

Alcohol: No special warnings.

Pregnancy: Albuterol may cause birth defects in mice when given in extremely large doses. Consult your doctor.

Breast Feeding: Albuterol may pass into breast milk; caution is advised.

Infants and Children: Not recommended for use by children under 2 years.

Special Concerns: Tell your doctor if you have ever had any unusual or allergic reaction to albuterol. Prime the inhaler prior to the first use and when it has not been used for more than 4 days. Prime it by releasing four test sprays before first use (and two test sprays when not used for a period of at least 4 days) in the air away from the face. You should wash your Rotahaler (biweekly) and inhaler (weekly) to prevent

drug buildup and blockage. Wash the two halves of the Rotahaler or the mouthpiece of the inhaler (with the canister removed) with warm water and shake to remove excess water. Both the Rotahaler and the inhaler should be air-dried thoroughly.

OVERDOSE
Symptoms: Confusion, delirium, severe anxiety, seizures, nervousness, headache, nausea, dry mouth, dizziness, insomnia, chest pain, muscle tremors, profound weakness, rapid and irregular pulse.

What to Do: Call your doctor, emergency medical services (EMS), or hospital immediately.

▼ INTERACTIONS

DRUG INTERACTIONS
Albuterol should not be used within 14 days of using an MAO inhibitor or tricyclic antidepressants. Consult your doctor if you are taking beta-blockers, loop or thiazide diuretics, antihypertensives, digitalis drugs, epinephrine, ergot, finasteride, furazolidone, guanadrel, guanethidine, maprotiline, methyldopa, any nitrate, a phenothiazine, products containing pseudoephedrine, rauwolfia alkaloids, terazosin, other asthma medications, or thyroid hormone.

FOOD INTERACTIONS
No known food interactions.

DISEASE INTERACTIONS
Consult your doctor if you have an overactive thyroid, diabetes mellitus, a history of seizures, heart problems, high blood pressure, or blood vessel disease.

≡ SIDE EFFECTS ≡

SERIOUS
Inhaled form: May become ineffective if used too often, resulting in more-severe breathing difficulty that does not improve. Signs include persistent wheezing, coughing, or shortness of breath; confusion; bluish color of lips or fingernails; inability to speak. Ingested form: Chest pain or heaviness; irregular, racing, fluttering, or pounding heartbeat; lightheadedness; fainting; severe weakness; severe headache.

COMMON
Nervousness, tremor, dizziness, headache, insomnia.

LESS COMMON
Dryness and irritation of the nose, mouth, and throat; heartburn; nausea; muscle cramps.

ALENDRONATE SODIUM

Available in: Tablets
Available OTC? No   **As Generic?** No
Drug Class: Bisphosphonate inhibitor of bone resorption

▼ USAGE INFORMATION

WHY IT'S PRESCRIBED
To prevent and treat osteoporosis in postmenopausal women and to treat osteoporosis in men by increasing bone mass. Alendronate also treats glucocorticoid-induced osteoporosis in those receiving corticosteroids in a daily dosage equivalent to 7.5 mg or greater of prednisone and who have low bone mineral density. Also used for Paget's disease, a disorder characterized by rapid breakdown and reformation of bone, which can lead to fragility and malformation of bones.

HOW IT WORKS
Healthy bones are continuously remodeled (broken down and then reformed); the minerals and other components of bones are reabsorbed by one set of cells (osteoclasts) and replaced by another set of cells to form new bone. Alendronate suppresses the activity of osteoclasts; consequently, the breakdown of bone tissue occurs more slowly than the laying down of new bone. This preserves bone density and strength.

▼ DOSAGE GUIDELINES

RANGE AND FREQUENCY
For prevention of osteoporosis: 5 mg a day or 35 mg once a week. For treatment of osteoporosis: 10 mg a day or 70 mg once a week. For glucocorticoid-induced osteoporosis in men and women: 5 mg a day; postmenopausal women not receiving estrogen should take 10 mg a day. For Paget's disease: 40 mg a day. The dose is taken in the morning. Swallow tablets whole; do not suck or chew them. Do not lie down for 30 minutes after taking your dose. The tablet must be taken with an 8-oz glass of water at least 30 minutes before any food or other drug.

ONSET OF EFFECT
Within 2 hours.

DURATION OF ACTION
24 hours to 7 days.

DIETARY ADVICE
Take alendronate with a full glass of water at least 30 minutes before your first food or beverage of the day. Some patients may be advised to take calcium or vitamin C supplements to aid in the formation of new bone tissue.

STORAGE
Store in a tightly sealed container away from moisture, heat, and direct light.

MISSED DOSE
Take it as soon as you remember. If it is near the time for the next dose, skip the missed dose and resume your regular dosage schedule. Do not double the next dose.

STOPPING THE DRUG
The decision to stop taking the drug should be made by your doctor. In most cases, patients with Paget's disease are treated for 6 months; the drug is then stopped. Retreatment may be necessary if such patients show signs of relapse after a subsequent 6-month observation period.

PROLONGED USE
No special precautions.

▼ PRECAUTIONS

Over 60: No special problems are expected.

Driving and Hazardous Work: No special precautions.

Alcohol: Alcohol should be restricted for high-risk women because it is a risk factor for developing osteoporosis.

Pregnancy: The drug should not be given to pregnant women because animal studies have shown adverse effects in the fetus.

Breast Feeding: Alendronate may pass into breast milk. Consult your doctor for advice.

Infants and Children: Use is not recommended for children.

Special Concerns: Patients taking alendronate are encouraged to engage in regular weight-bearing exercise and should avoid cigarettes and limit alcohol, which inhibit healthy bone production.

OVERDOSE
Symptoms: Severe heartburn, stomach cramps, or throat irritation might occur if an overdose of alendronate disturbs the body's normal mineral (electrolyte) balance.

What to Do: Few cases have been reported; however, if someone takes a much larger dose than prescribed, call your doctor or the nearest poison control center.

▼ INTERACTIONS

DRUG INTERACTIONS
Consult your doctor for specific advice if you are taking antacids, calcium supplements, aspirin or other nonsteroidal antiinflammatory drugs (NSAIDs), or hormone replacement therapy. Wait at least 30 minutes after taking alendronate before taking any other drugs.

FOOD INTERACTIONS
Any food eaten within 30 minutes of taking alendronate decreases its effect. Mineral water, coffee, tea, and fruit juice can interfere with the absorption of alendronate.

DISEASE INTERACTIONS
Kidney impairment or a gastrointestinal disease may increase the risk of side effects. Low blood calcium levels and vitamin D deficiency must be treated before using alendronate.

 SIDE EFFECTS

SERIOUS
No serious side effects have been reported.

COMMON
Abdominal pain or bloating (persistent pain should be reported to your doctor), indigestion, heartburn, nausea.

LESS COMMON
Headache, constipation, diarrhea, gas, difficulty swallowing, throat irritation, abdominal swelling or tightness, muscle or bone pain, changes in taste perception.

ALLOPURINOL

BRAND NAMES

Lopurin, Purinol, Zyloprim

Available in: Tablets
Available OTC? No   **As Generic?** Yes
Drug Class: Antigout drug

▼ USAGE INFORMATION

WHY IT'S PRESCRIBED
To treat chronic gout or the excessive uric acid buildup caused by kidney disorders, cancer, or the use of chemotherapy drugs for cancer. Also prescribed to prevent recurrence of uric acid kidney stones. Allopurinol should not be used for treating acute gout attacks in progress.

HOW IT WORKS
Allopurinol blocks the enzyme xanthine oxidase, which is required for the production of uric acid, thus reducing blood levels of uric acid.

▼ DOSAGE GUIDELINES

RANGE AND FREQUENCY
Adults: Initially, 100 mg per day, increased by 100 mg per week to a maximum of 800 mg per day. 100-mg doses are administered once a day; doses of 300 mg or more are taken in 2 or 3 evenly divided portions throughout the day. Children ages 6 to 10 years: 300 mg per day for certain types of cancer. Children age 6 years and under: 50 mg a day in 3 evenly divided portions.

ONSET OF EFFECT
Reduces uric acid levels in 2 to 3 days; may take 6 months for full effect to occur.

DURATION OF ACTION
1 to 2 weeks.

DIETARY ADVICE
Take it with food or milk to avoid stomach irritation. Drink 10 to 12 glasses (8 oz each) of water a day while on this medication.

STORAGE
Store in a tightly sealed container away from heat and direct light.

MISSED DOSE
Take the medicine as soon as you remember. However, if it is near the time for you to take your next dose, skip the missed dose and resume your regular dosage schedule. Do not double the next dose.

STOPPING THE DRUG
Take allopurinol as prescribed for the full treatment period, even if you begin to feel better before the scheduled end of therapy.

PROLONGED USE
Consult your doctor about the need for tests of liver function, kidney function, blood counts, and blood and urine levels of uric acid.

▼ PRECAUTIONS

Over 60: Adverse reactions may be more likely and more severe in older patients.

Driving and Hazardous Work: Allopurinol may cause drowsiness. If possible, avoid driving and hazardous work.

Alcohol: No special precautions are necessary.

Pregnancy: Caution is advised; consult your doctor about whether the benefits outweigh potential risks to the unborn child.

Breast Feeding: Allopurinol passes into breast milk; avoid or discontinue use while breast feeding.

Infants and Children: Follow your doctor's instructions carefully for children.

OVERDOSE
Symptoms: No specific symptoms have been reported.

What to Do: An overdose of allopurinol is unlikely to be life-threatening; however, if someone takes a much larger dose than prescribed, contact your doctor, poison control center, or local emergency room for instructions.

▼ INTERACTIONS

DRUG INTERACTIONS
Consult your doctor for specific advice if you are taking an antibiotic (such as amoxicillin, ampicillin, or bacampicillin), an anticoagulant drug (warfarin, dicumarol), an anticancer (chemotherapy) drug, chlorpropamide, a diuretic, or theophylline.

FOOD INTERACTIONS
None are likely, but a low-purine diet is recommended to reduce the risk of gout attacks. Foods high in purines include anchovies, sardines, legumes, poultry, sweetbreads, liver, kidneys, and other organ meats.

DISEASE INTERACTIONS
Caution is advised when taking allopurinol. Consult your doctor if you have high blood pressure, diabetes mellitus, kidney disease, or impaired iron metabolism.

≡ SIDE EFFECTS ≡

SERIOUS
Anemia or other blood or bone marrow disorders that may produce fatigue, bleeding, or bruising; yellowish tinge to eyes or skin (signifying hepatitis or liver damage); severe skin reactions (marked by rashes, skin ulcers, hives, and intense itching); chest tightness; weakness. Call your doctor immediately if such symptoms occur.

COMMON
Mild rash, drowsiness, nausea, diarrhea. The frequency of gout attacks may increase during the first weeks of use.

LESS COMMON
Headache, abdominal pain, boils on face, chills or fever, vomiting, hair loss.

ALPRAZOLAM

BRAND NAME

Xanax

Available in: Tablets, oral solution
Available OTC? No   **As Generic?** Yes
Drug Class: Benzodiazepine tranquilizer; antianxiety agent

▼ USAGE INFORMATION

WHY IT'S PRESCRIBED
To treat anxiety and panic disorder.

HOW IT WORKS
In general, alprazolam produces mild sedation by depressing activity in the central nervous system. In particular, alprazolam appears to enhance the effect of gamma-aminobutyric acid (GABA), a natural chemical that inhibits the firing of neurons and dampens the transmission of nerve signals, thus decreasing nervous excitation.

▼ DOSAGE GUIDELINES

RANGE AND FREQUENCY
Adults: Initial dose is 1.5 mg a day taken in 3 divided doses; may be gradually increased to a maximum dose of 4 mg a day. Older adults: Initial dose is 0.5 to 0.75 mg a day taken in 2 or 3 divided doses; may be gradually increased to a maximum dose of 2 mg a day. Children: Not usually prescribed.

ONSET OF EFFECT
2 hours.

DURATION OF ACTION
Up to 6 hours.

DIETARY ADVICE
Alprazolam can be taken on an empty stomach or with food or milk.

STORAGE
Store in a tightly sealed container away from heat and direct light.

MISSED DOSE
If you miss a dose, take it if you remember within 1 hour. Otherwise, skip the missed dose and take the next one at the regular time. Do not double the next dose.

STOPPING THE DRUG
Never stop taking the drug abruptly; this can cause withdrawal symptoms (seizures, sleep disruption, nervousness, irritability, diarrhea, abdominal cramps, muscle aches, memory impairment). Dosage should be reduced gradually as directed by your doctor.

PROLONGED USE
Short-term therapy (8 weeks or less) is typical; do not take it for a longer period unless so advised by your doctor.

▼ PRECAUTIONS

Over 60:
Use with caution; side effects such as drowsiness and dizziness may be more pronounced in older patients.

Driving and Hazardous Work:
Alprazolam can impair mental alertness and physical coordination. Adjust your activities accordingly.

Alcohol:
Alcohol intake should be extremely moderate or stopped altogether while taking alprazolam.

Pregnancy:
Use of this drug during pregnancy should be avoided if possible. Be sure to tell your doctor if you are pregnant or if you plan to become pregnant.

Breast Feeding:
Alprazolam passes into breast milk; do not take it while nursing.

Infants and Children:
Safety and effectiveness have not been established for children under age 18.

Special Concerns:
Use of this drug can lead to psychological or physical dependence. Short-term therapy (8 weeks or less) is typical; patients should not take the drug for a longer period unless so advised by their doctor. Never take more than the prescribed daily dose.

OVERDOSE
Symptoms: Extreme drowsiness, confusion, slurred speech, slow reflexes, poor coordination, staggering gait, tremor, slowed breathing, loss of consciousness.

What to Do: Call your doctor, emergency medical services (EMS), or the nearest poison control center immediately.

▼ INTERACTIONS

DRUG INTERACTIONS
Other drugs may interact with alprazolam. Consult your doctor for specific advice if you are taking any drugs that depress the central nervous system; these include antihistamines, antidepressants (including nefazodone) or other psychiatric medications, barbiturates, sedatives, cough medicines, decongestants, and painkillers. Be sure your doctor knows about any over-the-counter medication you may take.

FOOD INTERACTIONS
None reported.

DISEASE INTERACTIONS
Consult your doctor if you have a history of alcohol or drug abuse, stroke or other brain disease, any chronic lung disease, hyperactivity, depression or other mental illness, myasthenia gravis, sleep apnea, epilepsy, porphyria, kidney disease, or liver disease.

 ## ▼ SIDE EFFECTS

SERIOUS
Difficulty concentrating, outbursts of anger, other behavior problems, depression, hallucinations, low blood pressure (causing faintness or confusion), memory impairment, muscle weakness, skin rash or itching, sore throat, fever and chills, sores or ulcers in throat or mouth, unusual bruising or bleeding, extreme fatigue, yellowish tinge to eyes or skin. Call your doctor immediately.

COMMON
Drowsiness, loss of coordination, unsteady gait, dizziness, lightheadedness, slurred speech.

LESS COMMON
Change in sexual desire or ability, constipation, false sense of well-being (euphoria), nausea and vomiting, urinary problems, unusual fatigue.

ALPROSTADIL INJECTION

Available in: Injection
Available OTC? No **As Generic?** Yes
Drug Class: Vasodilator

▼ USAGE INFORMATION

WHY IT'S PRESCRIBED
To treat erectile dysfunction (impotence) in men; also to help maintain an adequate blood flow in infants during heart surgery.

HOW IT WORKS
Alprostadil causes dilation of blood vessels, thereby increasing blood flow to the tissues supplied by the vessels affected by the drug. When injected into the penis, alprostadil causes the penile arteries to dilate, thus promoting erection.

▼ DOSAGE GUIDELINES

RANGE AND FREQUENCY
For adult men: Injection of 0.001 to 0.04 mg self-administered at the base of the penis as needed. It should not be administered more than once a day. For infants: Injection of 0.005 to 0.01 mg before surgery.

ONSET OF EFFECT
5 to 10 minutes.

DURATION OF ACTION
30 minutes to 3 hours.

DIETARY ADVICE
Diet is not significant in alprostadil therapy.

STORAGE
Keep the liquid form of alprostadil refrigerated but do not allow it to freeze.

MISSED DOSE
Not applicable; the drug is taken only when the patient chooses to take it.

STOPPING THE DRUG
Consult your doctor if you wish to discontinue therapy or if you feel that alprostadil is losing its effectiveness.

PROLONGED USE
Alprostadil should not be used more frequently than a physician recommends, which generally is not more than 3 times a week, with at least 24 hours between each dose. Patients who self-administer alprostadil should visit their doctor every 3 months for evaluation; dosage adjustments or the decision to stop using the drug will be made

at these times. Never increase the dosage without consulting your doctor.

▼ PRECAUTIONS

Over 60: Information about use specifically in older persons is not available, but elderly patients are more likely to suffer from circulatory problems and thus may be less responsive to the drug than their younger counterparts. Your doctor may need to adjust the dosage.

Driving and Hazardous Work: No special precautions.

Alcohol: No special precautions are necessary.

Pregnancy: Not applicable; the drug is used only by men and for infants. No problems have been reported in women who became pregnant by partners using alprostadil.

Breast Feeding: Not applicable; the drug is used only by men or for infants.

Infants and Children: Prostin VR Pediatric should be used for infants only in a hospital setting.

Special Concerns: A doctor should instruct you about administering the injection before you attempt to do it yourself. Only men who have been diagnosed with and are being medically treated for erectile dysfunction should use this drug as a sexual aid.

OVERDOSE
Symptoms: Painful erection or an erection that persists for more than 4 hours.

What to Do: Call your doctor, emergency medical services (EMS), or your local hospital right away. Prolonged erection may result in permanent damage to the tissues of the penis and the inability to achieve subsequent erections.

▼ INTERACTIONS

DRUG INTERACTIONS
None reported in infants. Adults should notify their doctor if they are taking any other drugs.

FOOD INTERACTIONS
No significant interactions have been reported.

DISEASE INTERACTIONS
An adult who has a blood coagulation defect, liver disease, sickle cell disease, or a history of priapism (erections lasting more than 4 hours) should inform his physician before using alprostadil.

SIDE EFFECTS

SERIOUS
Painful or prolonged erection (lasting more than 4 hours), usually as a result of excessive dosage. If erection does not resolve on its own in a reasonable amount of time, seek medical help promptly. If erection does resolve on its own, subsequent doses should be reduced; consult your doctor for specific guidelines.

COMMON
Pain, itching, or burning at site of injection.

LESS COMMON
Bruising or bleeding at site of injection.

AMITRIPTYLINE HYDROCHLORIDE

Available in: Tablets
Available OTC? No   **As Generic?** Yes
Drug Class: Tricyclic antidepressant; antimanic agent

▼ USAGE INFORMATION

WHY IT'S PRESCRIBED
To relieve symptoms of major depression and chronic pain.

HOW IT WORKS
Amitriptyline affects levels of certain brain chemicals (serotonin, norepinephrine, and acetylcholine) thought to be linked to mood, emotions, and mental state.

▼ DOSAGE GUIDELINES

RANGE AND FREQUENCY
Adults: To start, 25 mg 2 to 4 times a day; may be increased to 150 mg a day. Teenagers: 10 mg 3 times a day and 20 mg at bedtime. Children ages 6 to 12 years: 10 to 30 mg a day. Older adults: To start, 25 mg a day at bedtime; may be increased to 100 mg a day.

ONSET OF EFFECT
1 to 6 weeks.

DURATION OF ACTION
Unknown.

DIETARY ADVICE
To lessen stomach upset, take with food, unless your doctor instructs otherwise. Increase your intake of fiber and fluids.

STORAGE
Store in a tightly sealed container away from moisture, heat, and direct light.

MISSED DOSE
If you take once-daily bedtime dose, do not take the missed dose in the morning; it may cause drowsiness. Call your doctor. If you take more than 1 dose a day, take the missed dose as soon as you remember. If it is near the time for the next dose, skip the missed dose and resume your regular dosage schedule. Do not double the next dose.

STOPPING THE DRUG
Take it as prescribed for the full treatment period, even if you feel better before the scheduled end of therapy. The decision to stop taking the drug should be made in consultation with your doctor. The dosage should be gradually tapered over 5 to 7 days when stopping.

PROLONGED USE
The usual course of therapy lasts 6 months to 1 year; some patients may benefit from additional therapy.

▼ PRECAUTIONS

Over 60: Adverse reactions are more likely and more severe in older patients. Amitriptyline is generally not recommended, because there are safer alternatives for older patients. A lower dose may be necessary.

Driving and Hazardous Work: Use caution when driving and engaging in hazardous work until you determine how the medicine affects you. Drowsiness or lightheadedness can occur.

Alcohol: Avoid alcohol.

Pregnancy: Adequate human studies have not been done on pregnant women. Consult your doctor for advice.

Breast Feeding: Amitriptyline passes into breast milk; do not use it while nursing.

Infants and Children: Not prescribed for children under the age of 6 years.

Special Concerns: This is a potentially dangerous drug, especially if taken in excess. Tricyclic antidepressants should not be within easy reach of suicidal patients. If dry mouth occurs, use sugar-free gum or candy.

OVERDOSE
Symptoms: Breathing difficulty, fever, severe fatigue, impaired concentration, mental confusion, hallucinations, dilated pupils, irregular heartbeat or palpitations, and seizures.

What to Do: Call your doctor, emergency medical services (EMS), or the nearest poison control center immediately.

▼ INTERACTIONS

DRUG INTERACTIONS
Consult your doctor for specific advice if you are taking antithyroid agents, cimetidine, cisapride, clonidine, guanadrel, guanethidine, metrizamide, appetite suppressants, isoproterenol, ephedrine, epinephrine, amphetamines, phenylephrine, antipsychotic drugs, pimozide, methyldopa, metyrosine, metoclopramide, pemoline, promethazine, trimeprazine, rauwolfia alkaloids, MAO inhibitors, or any drugs that depress the central nervous system.

FOOD INTERACTIONS
No known food interactions.

DISEASE INTERACTIONS
Consult your doctor if you have any of the following: a history of alcohol abuse, difficulty urinating, asthma, bipolar disorder, high blood pressure, stomach or intestinal problems, glaucoma, an overactive thyroid, enlarged prostate, schizophrenia, seizures, a blood disorder, or kidney, heart, or liver disease.

 ## SIDE EFFECTS

SERIOUS
Confusion, heartbeat irregularities, hallucinations, seizures, extreme fatigue or drowsiness, blurred or altered vision, breathing difficulty, constipation, impaired concentration, difficult urination, fever, extreme and persistent restlessness, loss of coordination and balance, difficulty swallowing or speaking, dilated pupils, eye pain, fainting. Also trembling, shaking, weakness, and stiffness in the extremities and shuffling gait. Call your doctor immediately.

COMMON
Drowsiness, dizziness, or lightheadedness; headache; dry mouth or unpleasant taste; fatigue; heightened sensitivity to light; unusual weight gain; increased appetite; nausea.

LESS COMMON
Heartburn, insomnia, diarrhea, increased sweating, vomiting.

AMLODIPINE

Available in: Tablets, capsules
Available OTC? No   **As Generic?** No
Drug Class: Calcium channel blocker

▼ USAGE INFORMATION

WHY IT'S PRESCRIBED
To relieve angina (chest pain associated with heart disease) and to treat hypertension.

HOW IT WORKS
Amlodipine interferes with calcium's movement into cells of the heart muscle and cells of the smooth muscle in artery walls. This relaxes blood vessels (causing them to widen), which lowers blood pressure, increases the heart's blood supply, and decreases the heart's overall workload.

▼ DOSAGE GUIDELINES

RANGE AND FREQUENCY
2.5 to 10 mg a day in one daily dose (usually in the morning with breakfast).

ONSET OF EFFECT
1 to 2 hours.

DURATION OF ACTION
24 hours.

DIETARY ADVICE
It can be taken with or after meals to minimize stomach irritation. Be sure to follow a low-sodium, low-fat diet if your doctor so advises.

STORAGE
Store in a tightly sealed container away from heat and direct light.

MISSED DOSE
If you miss a dose, take it as soon as you remember, unless the next dose is less than 4 hours away. In that case, skip the missed dose and go back to your regular schedule. Do not double the next dose.

STOPPING THE DRUG
Take as prescribed for the full treatment period. Do not stop taking this drug suddenly; this may cause potentially serious health problems. If therapy is to be discontinued, dosage should be reduced gradually, according to your doctor's instructions.

PROLONGED USE
In some cases, amlodipine therapy may be required for years or even a lifetime. Consult your doctor about the need for medical or laboratory tests of heart activity, blood pressure, kidney function, and liver function.

▼ PRECAUTIONS

Over 60: Adverse reactions may be more likely and more severe in older patients. Smaller doses (2.5 mg a day) are generally prescribed.

Driving and Hazardous Work: Avoid driving or engaging in hazardous work until you determine how this medication affects you. Be cautious if it causes dizziness.

Alcohol: Alcohol should be used with caution because it may increase the effect of the drug and cause an excessive drop in blood pressure.

Pregnancy: Amlodipine should not be taken during the first 3 months of pregnancy and should be used in the last 6 months only if your doctor so advises.

Breast Feeding: Amlodipine should not be taken by nursing mothers.

Infants and Children: Amlodipine is not usually prescribed for patients under the age of 12 years.

Special Concerns: The drug should not be taken by anyone who has had a adverse reaction to it in the past. When taking amlodipine, try to avoid abrupt changes in position, especially standing up too quickly after sitting or lying down; such movements may cause dizziness.

OVERDOSE
Symptoms: Severe drop in blood pressure resulting in weakness, dizziness, drowsiness, confusion, or slurred speech.

What to Do: Call your doctor, emergency medical services (EMS), or your local hospital immediately.

▼ INTERACTIONS

DRUG INTERACTIONS
Other heart drugs taken with amlodipine can cause heart rate and rhythm problems. In general, consult your doctor if you are taking any other prescription or OTC drugs.

FOOD INTERACTIONS
Avoid excessive intake of foods high in sodium.

DISEASE INTERACTIONS
Consult your doctor if you have kidney disease, liver disease, high blood pressure, or any heart disease other than coronary artery disease.

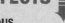

≡ SIDE EFFECTS ≡

SERIOUS
Increased angina attacks, dizziness when rising from a sitting or lying position, shortness of breath, weakness, very slow heartbeat. Call your doctor immediately.

COMMON
Headache, flushing in the face and body, water retention causing decreased urination, swelling of the feet and ankles, weight gain.

LESS COMMON
Fatigue, dizziness, drowsiness, palpitations, nausea, abdominal pain.

AMOXICILLIN

Available in: Capsules, oral suspension, chewable tablets, liquid drops
Available OTC? No   **As Generic?** Yes
Drug Class: Penicillin antibiotic

▼ USAGE INFORMATION

WHY IT'S PRESCRIBED
To treat bacterial infections of the ear, nose, and throat; genitourinary tract; skin and soft tissues; and lower respiratory tract. It is used, often with other drugs, to treat uncomplicated gonorrhea. It is also prescribed preventively before surgery or dental work to patients at risk for endocarditis (infection of the interior lining of the heart). It is also used to treat some stages of Lyme disease and, along with other drugs, to treat *H. pylori* infection (the cause of stomach ulcers).

HOW IT WORKS
Amoxicillin blocks the formation of bacterial cell walls, rendering bacteria unable to multiply and spread.

▼ DOSAGE GUIDELINES

RANGE AND FREQUENCY
For infections—Adults: 250 to 500 mg every 8 hours (3 doses a day). Children: 3 to 6 mg per lb of body weight every 8 hours (3 doses a day). To treat gonorrhea— 3 g in a single oral dose.

ONSET OF EFFECT
Rapid; within 2 hours.

DURATION OF ACTION
8 hours.

DIETARY ADVICE
It is best taken on an empty stomach but may be taken with food to minimize stomach irritation or diarrhea.

STORAGE
Store in a tightly sealed container away from heat and direct light. Keep any liquid form refrigerated, but do not allow it to freeze, and discard after 14 days.

MISSED DOSE
Take it as soon as you remember. If it is near the time for the next dose, skip the missed dose and resume your regular dosage schedule. Do not double the next dose.

STOPPING THE DRUG
Take as prescribed for the full treatment period, even if you begin to feel better before the scheduled end of therapy. Stopping the medication prematurely may slow your recovery or lead to a rebound infection, also known as superinfection, in which the heartier strains of bacteria survive and multiply, leading to a more serious and drug-resistant infection.

PROLONGED USE
Prolonged use of any antibiotic increases the risk of developing a superinfection; caution is advised.

▼ PRECAUTIONS

Over 60: No special problems are expected.

Driving and Hazardous Work: The use of amoxicillin should not impair your ability to perform such tasks safely.

Alcohol: No special precautions are necessary.

Pregnancy: Adequate studies of the use of this drug during pregnancy have not been done; however, no problems have been reported.

Breast Feeding: Amoxicillin passes into breast milk and may cause diarrhea, fungal infections, and allergic reactions in nursing infants; avoid use while nursing.

Infants and Children: No special problems are expected.

Special Concerns: Amoxicillin can cause false results on some urine sugar tests for diabetics. Those who are prone to asthma, hay fever, hives, or allergies may be more likely to have an allergic reaction to a penicillin antibiotic. Oral contraceptives may not be effective while you are taking amoxicillin; use other methods of contraception to avoid unplanned pregnancy.

OVERDOSE
Symptoms: Severe nausea, vomiting, diarrhea, muscle spasticity, seizures.

What to Do: Call your doctor, emergency medical services (EMS), or the nearest poison control center immediately.

▼ INTERACTIONS

DRUG INTERACTIONS
Consult your doctor for specific advice if you are taking: aminoglycosides, ACE (angiotensin-converting enzyme) inhibitors, diuretics, potassium supplements or medications containing potassium, anticoagulants or other anticlotting drugs, nonsteroidal antiinflammatory drugs (NSAIDS), sulfinpyrazone, cholestyramine, colestipol, oral contraceptives, methotrexate, probenecid, allopurinol, or rifampin.

FOOD INTERACTIONS
No known food interactions.

DISEASE INTERACTIONS
Consult your doctor if you have a history of allergies, asthma, congestive heart failure, gastrointestinal disorders (especially colitis associated with the use of antibiotics), or impaired kidney function.

≡ SIDE EFFECTS ≡

SERIOUS
Irregular, rapid, or labored breathing; lightheadedness or sudden fainting; joint pain; fever; severe abdominal pain and cramping with watery or bloody stools; severe allergic reaction (marked by sudden swelling of the lips, tongue, face, or throat; breathing difficulty; and skin rash, itching, or hives); unusual bleeding or bruising; yellowish tinge to eyes or skin. Call your doctor immediately.

COMMON
Rash, mild diarrhea, nausea, vomiting, headache, vaginal discharge and itching, pain or white patches in the mouth or on the tongue.

LESS COMMON
Diminished urine output, chills, weakness, fatigue.

AMOXICILLIN/POTASSIUM CLAVULANATE

BRAND NAME

Augmentin

Available in: Tablets, chewable tablets, oral suspension
Available OTC? No   **As Generic?** No
Drug Class: Penicillin antibiotic combination

▼ USAGE INFORMATION

WHY IT'S PRESCRIBED
To treat a variety of bacterial infections, including those of the sinuses and middle ear, skin and soft tissues, genitourinary tract, and respiratory tract. The medication is effective only against infections caused by bacteria, not against infections caused by viruses, fungi, or other microorganisms.

HOW IT WORKS
Amoxicillin blocks the formation of bacterial cell walls, rendering the bacteria unable to multiply and spread. Clavulanate enhances the overall effectiveness of amoxicillin by inhibiting the activity of a specific enzyme (beta-lactamase) produced by certain drug-resistant strains of bacteria.

▼ DOSAGE GUIDELINES

RANGE AND FREQUENCY
Tablets—Adults and children more than 88 lb: 250 to 500 mg of amoxicillin with 125 mg of clavulanate every 8 hours. Children up to 88 lb: 6.7 to 13.3 mg of amoxicillin with 1.7 to 3.3 mg of clavulanate per 2.2 lb (1 kg) of body weight every 8 hours. Chewable tablets and oral suspension—Adults and children more than 88 lb: 250 to 500 mg of amoxicillin with 62.5 to 125 mg of clavulanate every 8 hours. Children up to 88 lb: 6.7 to 13.3 mg of amoxicillin with 1.7 to 3.3 mg of clavulanate per 2.2 lb (1 kg) of body weight every 8 hours. Newer dosage for adults: 875 mg of amoxicillin with 125 mg of clavulanate twice a day.

ONSET OF EFFECT
1 to 2 hours.

DURATION OF ACTION
6 to 8 hours.

DIETARY ADVICE
It is best taken on an empty stomach but may be taken with food to minimize stomach irritation or diarrhea.

STORAGE
Store in a tightly sealed container away from heat and direct light. Keep the liquid form refrigerated but do not allow it to freeze.

MISSED DOSE
Take it as soon as you remember, unless it is almost time for the next dose. In that case, skip the missed dose and take the next one. Do not double the next dose.

STOPPING THE DRUG
Take this medication as prescribed for the full treatment period, even if you begin to feel better before the scheduled end of therapy.

PROLONGED USE
Prolonged use can make you more susceptible to bacterial or fungal infections (such as yeast infections).

▼ PRECAUTIONS

Over 60: No special problems are expected.

Driving and Hazardous Work: Do not drive or engage in hazardous work until you determine how the medicine affects you.

Alcohol: No special warnings.

Pregnancy: Limited studies have found no evidence of birth defects. Consult your doctor if you are pregnant or plan to become pregnant.

Breast Feeding: Amoxicillin/clavulanate may pass into breast milk and cause problems in the nursing infant; avoid use while breast feeding.

Infants and Children: No special problems are expected.

Special Concerns: Those who are prone to asthma, hay fever, hives, or allergies may be more likely to have an allergic reaction to a penicillin antibiotic. If severe diarrhea occurs as a side effect of this drug, do not take antidiarrheal medications; call your doctor for advice instead. This drug can cause false results on some urine sugar tests for patients who have diabetes.

OVERDOSE
Symptoms: Severe diarrhea, nausea, unusual excitability, seizures, or vomiting.

What to Do: Call your doctor, emergency medical services (EMS), or the nearest poison control center immediately.

▼ INTERACTIONS

DRUG INTERACTIONS
Consult your doctor for advice if you are taking erythromycins, disulfiram, anticoagulants, tetracyclines, oral contraceptives, or gout drugs.

FOOD INTERACTIONS
None expected.

DISEASE INTERACTIONS
Consult your doctor if you have a history of allergies, asthma, congestive heart failure, gastrointestinal disorders (especially colitis associated with the use of antibiotics), or impaired kidney function.

SIDE EFFECTS

SERIOUS
Irregular, rapid, or labored breathing; lightheadedness or sudden fainting; seizures; joint pain; fever; severe abdominal pain and cramping with watery or bloody stools; severe allergic reaction (marked by sudden swelling of the lips, tongue, face, or throat; breathing difficulty; and skin rash, itching, or hives); unusual bleeding or bruising; yellowish tinge to eyes or skin. Call your doctor immediately.

COMMON
Rash, mild diarrhea, nausea, vomiting, headache, vaginal discharge and itching, pain or white patches in the mouth or on the tongue.

LESS COMMON
Weakness, fatigue.

AMPHETAMINE/DEXTROAMPHETAMINE

Available in: Tablets
Available OTC? No   **As Generic?** No
Drug Class: Central nervous system stimulant/amphetamine

▼ USAGE INFORMATION

WHY IT'S PRESCRIBED
To treat narcolepsy and attention-deficit hyperactivity disorder (ADHD).

HOW IT WORKS
Amphetamine and dextroamphetamine activate nerve cells in the brain and spinal cord to increase motor activity and alertness and also to lessen fatigue and drowsiness. In hyperactivity disorders and narcolepsy, amphetamines improve mental focus, as well as the ability to stay awake or concentrate.

▼ DOSAGE GUIDELINES

RANGE AND FREQUENCY
For narcolepsy—Adults: 5 to 60 mg a day 1 to 3 times a day; not to exceed 60 mg a day. Teenagers: To start, 10 mg a day. Children ages 6 to 12 years: To start, 5 mg a day. For ADHD—Children age 6 years and older: To start, 5 mg 1 or 2 times a day. Children ages 3 to 6 years: To start, 2.5 mg a day.

ONSET OF EFFECT
Within 30 to 45 minutes.

DURATION OF ACTION
Adults: 8 to 12 hours.
Children: 6 to 10 hours.

DIETARY ADVICE
Take it with liquid 30 to 45 minutes before meals. Avoid caffeinated beverages, acidic foods rich in vitamin C, and vitamin C tablets.

STORAGE
Store in a tightly sealed container away from moisture, heat, and direct light.

MISSED DOSE
If dosage is once daily, take your missed dose as soon as you remember, unless your bedtime is within 6 hours. If so, do not take the missed dose. Take your next dose at the proper time and resume your regular schedule. Do not double the next dose. If dosage is more than once daily, take your missed dose as soon as you remember, unless the time for your next scheduled dose is within the next 2 hours. If so, do not take the missed dose. Take your next dose at the proper time and resume your regular schedule. Do not double the next dose.

STOPPING THE DRUG
Take it as prescribed for the full treatment period, even if you begin to feel better before the scheduled end of therapy. The decision to stop taking the drug should be made by your doctor. The doctor may taper your dosage gradually to reduce the risk of withdrawal symptoms.

PROLONGED USE
Prolonged use may increase the risk of dependency.

▼ PRECAUTIONS

Over 60: Adverse reactions may be more likely and more severe in older patients.

Driving and Hazardous Work: Do not drive or engage in hazardous work until you determine how the medicine affects you.

Alcohol: Avoid alcohol.

Pregnancy: Amphetamines taken during pregnancy may cause premature delivery, low birth weight, and birth defects. Discuss with your doctor the relative risks and benefits of using this drug while pregnant.

Breast Feeding: Amphetamine passes into breast milk; avoid or discontinue use while nursing.

Infants and Children: Not recommended for use by children under age 3 years.

Special Concerns: Take only as directed and do not increase the dose on your own. Fatigue, excessive drowsiness, or depression that occurs while taking stimulants may mean an emergency situation is developing. Difficulty sleeping may be improved by taking the last scheduled dose several hours before bedtime.

OVERDOSE
Symptoms: Extreme restlessness, agitation, or bizarre behavior; panic; rapid breathing; confusion; high fever; hallucinations; seizures; coma.

What to Do: Call your doctor, emergency medical services (EMS), or the nearest poison control center immediately.

▼ INTERACTIONS

DRUG INTERACTIONS
Consult your doctor for specific advice if you are taking tricyclic antidepressants, caffeine, beta-blockers, digitalis drugs, central nervous system stimulants, meperidine, MAO inhibitors, sympathomimetic agents (such as ephedrine, phenylephrine, and diethylpropion), or thyroid hormones.

FOOD INTERACTIONS
Citrus juices and caffeine may interact with this drug.

DISEASE INTERACTIONS
Consult your doctor if you have any of the following: heart disease, advanced blood vessel disease, hyperthyroidism, high blood pressure, severe anxiety, Tourette's syndrome, glaucoma, or a history of drug abuse.

 SIDE EFFECTS

SERIOUS
Irregular heartbeat, chest pain, increased blood pressure, skin rash, uncontrollable movements of arms and legs, mental changes, unusual weakness, very high fever. Call your doctor immediately.

COMMON
Mood changes, insomnia, drowsiness, restlessness.

LESS COMMON
Blurred vision, constipation, diarrhea, loss of appetite, headache, increased sweating, stomach cramps or pain, nausea or vomiting, changes in sexual desire or decreased sexual ability.

ATENOLOL

BRAND NAME

Tenormin

Available in: Tablets
Available OTC? No   **As Generic?** Yes
Drug Class: Beta-blocker

▼ USAGE INFORMATION

WHY IT'S PRESCRIBED
To treat mild to moderate high blood pressure and to treat angina; also used to prevent or control heartbeat irregularities (cardiac arrhythmias). The injectable form is used in hospitals to treat heart attack.

HOW IT WORKS
Atenolol slows the rate and force of contraction of the heart by blocking certain nerve impulses, thus reducing blood pressure. By modifying nerve impulses to the heart, the drug also helps stabilize heart rhythm.

▼ DOSAGE GUIDELINES

RANGE AND FREQUENCY
50 to 100 mg once a day. Smaller doses may be recommended for elderly patients or for those with impaired kidney function.

ONSET OF EFFECT
Oral: 1 to 2 hours; the full therapeutic effect may take 1 to 2 weeks.

DURATION OF ACTION
Up to 24 hours.

DIETARY ADVICE
Take atenolol on an empty stomach. Avoid alcohol and caffeine.

STORAGE
Store in a tightly sealed container away from heat and direct light.

MISSED DOSE
Take it as soon as you remember. If it is within 4 hours of the next scheduled dose, skip the missed dose and resume your regular schedule. Do not double the next dose.

STOPPING THE DRUG
Suddenly stopping atenolol may cause serious health problems. Slow reduction of the dose over a period of 2 to 3 weeks under doctor's careful supervision is advised.

PROLONGED USE
Therapy with atenolol may be lifelong; prolonged use may be associated with increased risks of side effects.

▼ PRECAUTIONS

Over 60: Adverse reactions may be more likely and more severe in older patients; a reduction in dosage may be warranted.

Driving and Hazardous Work: In rare cases, atenolol may impair your ability to drive or operate machinery safely or perform hazardous work. Use caution, especially soon after beginning therapy.

Alcohol: Drink in careful moderation, if at all. Alcohol may interact with the drug and cause a dangerous drop in blood pressure.

Pregnancy: Discuss with your doctor the relative risks and benefits of using this drug while pregnant.

Breast Feeding: Avoid or discontinue the use of atenolol while nursing.

Infants and Children: A proper dose will be determined by your pediatrician.

Special Concerns: Use of the drug should be considered one element of a comprehensive therapeutic program that includes weight control, smoking cessation, regular exercise, and a healthy low-salt, low-fat diet.

OVERDOSE
Symptoms: Slow heartbeat; severe dizziness, lightheadedness or fainting; rapid or irregular heartbeat; difficulty breathing; extreme weakness; seizures; confusion; coma.

What to Do: Call your doctor, emergency medical services (EMS), or the nearest poison control center immediately.

▼ INTERACTIONS

DRUG INTERACTIONS
Consult your doctor if you are taking amphetamines, oral antidiabetic agents, asthma medication (such as aminophylline or theophylline), calcium channel blockers, clonidine, guanabenz, insulin, halothane, allergy shots, MAO inhibitors, reserpine, or other beta-blockers.

FOOD INTERACTIONS
None known.

DISEASE INTERACTIONS
Atenolol should be used with caution in people with diabetes, especially insulin-dependent diabetes, because the drug may mask symptoms of hypoglycemia. Consult your doctor for specific advice if you have allergies or asthma, heart or blood vessel disease (including congestive heart failure and peripheral vascular disease), irregular (slow) heartbeat, hyperthyroidism, myasthenia gravis, psoriasis, respiratory problems such as bronchitis or emphysema, kidney or liver disease, or a history of mental depression.

≡ SIDE EFFECTS ≡

SERIOUS
Depression, shortness of breath, wheezing, slow heartbeat (especially less than 50 beats per minute), chest pain or tightness, swelling of the ankles, feet, and lower legs. If you experience such symptoms, stop taking atenolol and call your doctor immediately.

COMMON
Decreased sexual ability; decreased ability to engage in usual physical activities or exercise; dizziness or lightheadedness, especially when rising suddenly from a sitting or lying position; drowsiness, fatigue, or weakness; insomnia.

LESS COMMON
Anxiety; irritability; constipation; diarrhea; dry eyes; itching; nausea or vomiting; nightmares or intensely vivid dreams; numbness, tingling, or other unusual sensations in the fingers and toes; abdominal pain; nasal congestion.

ATORVASTATIN

Available in: Tablets
Available OTC? No   **As Generic?** No
Drug Class: Antilipidemic (cholesterol-lowering agent)

▼ USAGE INFORMATION

WHY IT'S PRESCRIBED
To treat high cholesterol. Usually prescribed after the first lines of treatment—including diet changes, weight loss, and exercise—fail to reduce to acceptable levels the amounts of total and low-density lipoprotein (LDL) cholesterol in the blood.

HOW IT WORKS
Atorvastatin blocks the action of an enzyme required for the manufacture of cholesterol, thereby interfering with its formation. By lowering the amount of cholesterol in the liver cells, atorvastatin increases the formation of receptors for LDL and thereby reduces blood levels of total and LDL cholesterol. In addition to lowering LDL cholesterol, atorvastatin modestly reduces triglyceride levels and raises HDL (the so-called "good") cholesterol.

▼ DOSAGE GUIDELINES

RANGE AND FREQUENCY
Initial dose is 10 mg a day taken once daily. It may be increased by your doctor as needed up to a maximum dose of 80 mg per day. Unlike other "statin" (cholesterol-lowering) drugs, atorvastatin does not have to be taken in the evening to be maximally effective.

ONSET OF EFFECT
2 to 4 weeks.

DURATION OF ACTION
The effect persists for the duration of therapy.

DIETARY ADVICE
Cholesterol-lowering drugs are only one part of a total program that should include regular exercise and a healthy low-fat, low-cholesterol, high-fiber diet.

STORAGE
Store in a tightly sealed container in a dry place away from heat and direct light.

MISSED DOSE
Take it as soon as you remember that you skipped a dose. Take your next scheduled dose at the proper time and resume your regular dosage schedule. Do not double your next dose.

STOPPING THE DRUG
The decision to stop taking the drug should be made in consultation with your doctor. Once the medication is discontinued, blood cholesterol is likely to return to original elevated levels.

PROLONGED USE
Side effects are more likely with prolonged use. As you continue to take atorvastatin, your doctor will periodically order blood tests to evaluate liver function.

▼ PRECAUTIONS

Over 60: No special problems are expected in older patients.

Driving and Hazardous Work: The use of atorvastatin should not impair your ability to perform such tasks safely.

Alcohol: No special precautions are necessary.

Pregnancy: Should not be used during pregnancy or by women who plan to become pregnant in the near future.

Breast Feeding: This drug is not recommended for women who are nursing.

Infants and Children: Safety and effectiveness are not known; this drug is rarely used for children. Consult your pediatrician.

Special Concerns: Important elements of high cholesterol treatment include proper diet, weight loss, regular moderate exercise, and avoidance of certain medications that may increase cholesterol levels.

Because atorvastatin has potential side effects, it is important that you maintain a recommended healthy diet and cooperate with other treatments that your doctor suggests.

OVERDOSE
Symptoms: An overdose of atorvastatin is unlikely.

What to Do: Emergency instructions not applicable.

▼ INTERACTIONS

DRUG INTERACTIONS
Consult your doctor if you are taking cyclosporine; gemfibrozil; niacin; antibiotics, especially erythromycin; or medications for fungus infections. All of these drugs may increase the risk of myositis (muscle inflammation) when taken with atorvastatin and may lead to kidney failure.

FOOD INTERACTIONS
No known food interactions.

DISEASE INTERACTIONS
Consult your doctor if you have any of the following problems: liver, kidney, or muscle disease or a medical history involving organ transplantation or recent surgery.

 ≡ SIDE EFFECTS ≡

SERIOUS
Fever, chest pain, unusual or unexplained muscle aches and tenderness. Call your doctor immediately.

COMMON
Side effects occur in only 1% to 2% of patients. These side effects include constipation or diarrhea, dizziness or lightheadedness, bloating or gas, heartburn, nausea, allergic reaction, stomach pain, increase in liver enzymes.

LESS COMMON
Sleeping difficulty, skin rash.

AZITHROMYCIN

Available in: Capsules, tablets, powder, injection
Available OTC? No   **As Generic?** No
Drug Class: Azalide antibiotic

▼ USAGE INFORMATION

WHY IT'S PRESCRIBED
To treat various bacterial infections, particularly of the sinuses, throat, and respiratory tract (such as bronchitis and pneumonia); infections of the ear; venereal disease caused by chlamydial and chancroid infection; skin infections; and diarrhea associated with campylobacter and other bacteria that cause food poisoning. Also used to prevent and treat a tuberculosis-like disease known as *Mycobacterium avium* complex (MAC), which is common in people with advanced AIDS.

HOW IT WORKS
Azithromycin prevents bacterial cells from manufacturing specific proteins necessary for their survival.

▼ DOSAGE GUIDELINES

RANGE AND FREQUENCY
For bronchitis, strep throat, pneumonia, and skin infections: 500 mg (2 pills) taken in a single dose on the first day of treatment, then 250 mg (1 pill) a day on days 2 through 5. For chlamydia and chancroid: 1,000 mg (4 pills) taken in a single one-time dose. To prevent MAC: 1,200 mg weekly. To treat MAC: 500 mg twice a day.

ONSET OF EFFECT
Unknown.

DURATION OF ACTION
Unknown.

DIETARY ADVICE
Take capsules on an empty stomach at least 1 hour before or 2 hours after eating. Tablets may be taken with or without food. Drink plenty of fluids (at least 2 to 3 quarts of water per day).

STORAGE
Store in a sealed container away from heat and light.

MISSED DOSE
Take it as soon as you remember. If you miss a day entirely, skip the missed dose and resume your regular dosage schedule the next day. Do not double the next dose.

STOPPING THE DRUG
It is very important to take this drug as prescribed for the full treatment period, even if you begin to feel better before the scheduled end of therapy.

PROLONGED USE
For acute infections, treatment is usually complete after 5 days with capsules and after 1 day with the powdered form. For MAC prevention and treatment, therapy may be lifelong. Prolonged use may be associated with an increased risk of side effects.

▼ PRECAUTIONS

Over 60: Adverse reactions may be more likely and more severe in this age group.

Driving and Hazardous Work: The use of the drug should not impair your ability to perform such tasks safely.

Alcohol: Avoid alcohol while taking this drug.

Pregnancy: Adequate studies of the use of azithromycin during pregnancy have not been done; consult your doctor for advice.

Breast Feeding: It is not known if azithromycin passes into breast milk; consult your doctor for advice.

Infants and Children: The safety and effectiveness of azithromycin use in patients under 16 years of age have not been established, although no special problems are expected.

Special Concerns: Before taking any antibiotic, make sure you tell your doctor about allergies that you might have. If you are allergic to erythromycin, you are likely to be allergic to azithromycin. Azithromycin is useful only against bacteria that are susceptible to its effects. Therefore, it is important to tell your doctor if your condition has not improved, or instead has worsened, within a few days of starting the drug. The particular bacteria causing your illness may be resistant to azithromycin.

OVERDOSE
Symptoms: No cases of overdose have been reported.

What to Do: Emergency instructions not applicable.

▼ INTERACTIONS

DRUG INTERACTIONS
Other drugs may interact with azithromycin. Consult your doctor for specific advice if you are taking anticoagulants (such as warfarin), anticonvulsants (such as phenytoin and carbamazepine), antihistamines (especially terfenadine), and theophylline. Antacids that contain aluminum or magnesium can interfere with the absorption of azithromycin; separate the use of azithromycin and an antacid by at least 2 hours.

FOOD INTERACTIONS
Azithromycin capsules should be taken on an empty stomach.

DISEASE INTERACTIONS
Consult your doctor if you have a medical history that includes liver disease.

SIDE EFFECTS

SERIOUS
Breathing difficulty; fever; hives; itching; skin rash; swelling of face, mouth, lips, throat, or tongue; sweating; yellowish discoloration of the eyes or skin. These may be signs of a rare but potentially serious allergic reaction. Seek medical assistance immediately.

COMMON
No common side effects have been reported.

LESS COMMON
Nausea and vomiting, abdominal discomfort, diarrhea (generally mild), headache, dizziness.

BECLOMETHASONE INHALANT AND NASAL

BRAND NAMES

Beclovent, Beconase AQ
Nasal Spray, Beconase
Nasal Inhaler, Vancenase
AQ Nasal Spray,
Vancenase Nasal Inhaler,
Vanceril

Available in: Nasal inhaler, oral inhalation
Available OTC? No   **As Generic?** No
Drug Class: Respiratory corticosteroid

▼ USAGE INFORMATION

WHY IT'S PRESCRIBED
To treat bronchial asthma, to treat allergic rhinitis (seasonal and perennial allergies such as hay fever), and to prevent recurrence of nasal polyps after they have been removed surgically.

HOW IT WORKS
Respiratory corticosteroids such as beclomethasone primarily reduce or prevent chronic inflammation of the lining of the airways (the underlying cause of asthma), reduce the allergic response to inhaled allergens, and inhibit secretion of mucus within airways.

▼ DOSAGE GUIDELINES

RANGE AND FREQUENCY
Adults and teenagers—Nasal inhaler: 1 or 2 inhalations in each nostril 1 or 2 times a day. Oral inhalation: 2 inhalations 3 or 4 times a day. For severe asthma: 12 to 16 inhalations daily (maximum of 20 inhalations a day). Children ages 6 to 12 years—Nasal inhaler: 1 inhalation in each nostril 1 to 3 times a day. Oral inhalation: 1 to 2 inhalations 3 or 4 times a day. Maximum of 10 inhalations per day.

ONSET OF EFFECT
Within 5 to 7 days; it may take 3 weeks for the full effect to occur.

DURATION OF ACTION
6 hours or more.

DIETARY ADVICE
Use it before or after meals.

STORAGE
Store away from fire and direct light.

MISSED DOSE
Take it as soon as you remember. However, if it is near the time for the next dose, skip the missed dose and resume your regular dosage schedule. Do not double the next dose.

STOPPING THE DRUG
Take the medication as your doctor has prescribed for the full treatment period, even if you begin to feel better before the scheduled end of the therapy.

PROLONGED USE
Consult your doctor about the need for periodic medical examinations and laboratory tests if you must take this drug for a prolonged period.

▼ PRECAUTIONS

Over 60: No special problems are expected.

Driving and Hazardous Work: The use of beclomethasone should not impair your ability to perform such tasks safely.

Alcohol: No special precautions are necessary.

Pregnancy: Nasal or inhaled steroids have not been reported to cause birth defects if taken during pregnancy. Before using such drugs, tell your doctor if you are pregnant or plan to become pregnant.

Breast Feeding: Beclomethasone may pass into breast milk; caution is advised. Consult your doctor for advice.

Infants and Children: It has not been established whether beclomethasone is safe and effective in young children.

Special Concerns: Inhaled steroids will not help an asthma attack in progress. Inhaled steroids can lower resistance to yeast infections of the mouth, throat, or voice box. To prevent yeast infections, gargle or rinse your mouth with water after each use. Do not swallow the water. Know how to use the inhaler effectively; read and follow the directions that come with the device. Before you have surgery, tell the doctor or dentist that you are using a steroid.

OVERDOSE
Symptoms: No specific symptoms have been reported.

What to Do: An overdose of beclomethasone is unlikely to be life-threatening. However, if someone takes a much larger dose than prescribed, call your doctor, emergency medical services (EMS), or the nearest poison control center immediately.

▼ INTERACTIONS

DRUG INTERACTIONS
Consult your doctor for specific advice if you are taking systemic corticosteroids, other inhaled corticosteroids, or any drugs that suppress the immune system.

FOOD INTERACTIONS
No known food interactions.

DISEASE INTERACTIONS
Consult your doctor if you have any of the following: a lung disease such as tuberculosis; an infection of the mouth, nose, sinuses, throat, or lungs; a herpes infection of the eye; or any other untreated infection.

≣ SIDE EFFECTS ≣

SERIOUS
No serious side effects are associated with the use of beclomethasone.

COMMON
Nasal form: Nosebleeds or bloody nasal secretions, nasal burning or irritation, sore throat. Oral inhalation: Sore throat, white patches in the mouth or throat, hoarseness.

LESS COMMON
Eye pain, watering eyes, gradual decrease of vision, stomach pain and digestive disturbances.

BENAZEPRIL HYDROCHLORIDE

Lotensin

Available in: Tablets
Available OTC? No   **As Generic?** No
Drug Class: Angiotensin-converting enzyme (ACE) inhibitor

▼ USAGE INFORMATION

WHY IT'S PRESCRIBED
To control high blood pressure, to treat congestive heart failure, to treat patients with left ventricular dysfunction (damage to the pumping chamber of the heart), and to minimize additional kidney damage in diabetics with mild kidney disease.

HOW IT WORKS
Angiotensin-converting enzyme (ACE) inhibitors block an enzyme that produces angiotensin, a naturally occurring substance that causes blood vessels to constrict and stimulates the production of the adrenal hormone, aldosterone, which promotes sodium retention in the body. As a result, ACE inhibitors relax blood vessels (causing them to widen) and they also reduce sodium retention. Both of these actions lower blood pressure levels and thus decrease the overall workload of the heart.

▼ DOSAGE GUIDELINES

RANGE AND FREQUENCY
If you are not also taking a diuretic ("water pill"), 10 mg a day to start, increased to 20 to 80 mg a day in 1 or 2 doses. If you are taking a diuretic, 5 mg a day.

ONSET OF EFFECT
60 to 90 minutes.

DURATION OF ACTION
Up to 24 hours.

DIETARY ADVICE
Take it on an empty stomach about 1 hour before mealtime. Follow your doctor's dietary advice (such as low-salt or low-cholesterol restrictions) to improve control over high blood pressure and heart disease. Avoid high-potassium foods, unless you are also taking drugs that lower potassium levels, such as diuretics.

STORAGE
Store in a tightly sealed container away from heat and direct light.

MISSED DOSE
Take it as soon as you remember. If it is near the time for the next dose, skip the missed dose and resume your regular dosage schedule. Do not double the next dose.

STOPPING THE DRUG
Do not stop taking this drug abruptly; this may cause potentially serious health problems. Dosage should be reduced gradually according to your doctor's instructions.

PROLONGED USE
See your doctor regularly for examinations and tests if you must take this drug for a prolonged period. Benazepril helps control hypertension but does not cure it. Lifelong therapy may be necessary.

▼ PRECAUTIONS

Over 60: Adverse reactions may be more likely and more severe in older patients.

Driving and Hazardous Work: Avoid such activities until you determine how the medication affects you.

Alcohol: Consume alcohol only in moderation because it may increase the effect of the drug and cause an excessive drop in blood pressure.

Pregnancy: Tell your doctor before taking this medication if you are pregnant or plan to become pregnant. Use of this drug during the last 6 months of pregnancy may cause severe defects in or even death of the fetus.

Breast Feeding: Benazepril does pass into breast milk;

if possible, avoid using the drug while nursing.

Infants and Children: Benazepril is generally not prescribed for children; benefits must be weighed against risks. Consult your pediatrician.

OVERDOSE
Symptoms: None reported.

What to Do: Overdose is unlikely, but call your doctor, emergency medical services (EMS), or the nearest poison control center immediately if you suspect that someone has taken a much larger dose than prescribed.

▼ INTERACTIONS

DRUG INTERACTIONS
Consult your doctor if you are taking diuretics (especially potassium-sparing diuretics), potassium supplements or drugs containing potassium (check ingredient labels), lithium, anticoagulant drugs, indomethacin or other anti-inflammatory drugs, or any over-the-counter drugs (especially cold remedies and diet pills).

FOOD INTERACTIONS
Avoid low-salt milk and salt substitutes. Many of these products contain potassium.

DISEASE INTERACTIONS
Consult your doctor if you have lupus or if you have had a prior allergic reaction to ACE inhibitors. This drug should be used with caution by patients with severe kidney disease or renal artery stenosis (narrowing of one or both of the arteries that supply blood to the kidneys).

≡ SIDE EFFECTS ≡

SERIOUS
Fever and chills; sore throat and hoarseness; sudden difficulty breathing or swallowing; swelling of the face, mouth, or extremities; impaired kidney function (ankle swelling, decreased urination); confusion; yellow discoloration of the eyes or skin (indicating liver disorder); intense itching, chest pain or palpitations; abdominal pain. Serious side effects are very rare; contact your doctor immediately.

COMMON
Dry, persistent cough.

LESS COMMON
Dizziness or fainting; skin rash; numbness or tingling in the hands, feet, or lips; unusual fatigue or muscle weakness; nausea; drowsiness; loss of taste; headache.

BETAMETHASONE/CLOTRIMAZOLE

Available in: Cream
Available OTC? No **As Generic?** Yes
Drug Class: Topical antifungal

▼ USAGE INFORMATION

WHY IT'S PRESCRIBED
To treat fungal infections of the skin.

HOW IT WORKS
Clotrimazole prevents fungal organisms from producing the vital proteins they require for growth and function. Betamethasone dipropionate is a steroid; it interferes with the formation of natural substances within the body that are directly responsible for the process of inflammation, which produces swelling, redness, and pain. The use of these two effective medications in combination for skin infections appears to hasten recovery more than use of clotrimazole alone. This medication is only effective for infections caused by fungal organisms. It will not work for bacterial or viral infections.

▼ DOSAGE GUIDELINES

RANGE AND FREQUENCY
Adults and children older than 12 years of age: Apply and massage a sufficient amount of cream into the affected site twice daily for 2 to 4 weeks. This combination drug contains a high-potency topical steroid that should not be used in skin creases or with bandages (occlusive dressing) unless closely supervised by your doctor.

ONSET OF EFFECT
Clotrimazole begins killing susceptible fungi shortly after contact. The effects may not be noticeable for several days or weeks.

DURATION OF ACTION
Unknown.

DIETARY ADVICE
Drink plenty of fluids.

STORAGE
Store in a tightly sealed container away from heat and direct light. Keep away from moisture and extremes in temperature.

MISSED DOSE
Apply it as soon as you remember. If it is near the time for the next dose, skip the missed dose and resume your regular dosage schedule. Do not double the next dose or apply an excessively thick layer of topical medication to try to compensate for a missed dose.

STOPPING THE DRUG
Apply as prescribed for the full treatment period, even if the fungal infection appears to be eradicated before the scheduled end of therapy. Unfortunately, it can be difficult to assess when the drug has achieved its desired effect because it suppresses redness and inflammation of the skin before the infection is completely clear; recurrence of fungal infection caused by inadequate length of therapy is a significant risk.

PROLONGED USE
Therapy with this medication should not exceed 4 weeks.

▼ PRECAUTIONS

Over 60: Adverse reactions may be more likely and more severe in older patients.

Driving and Hazardous Work: No special precautions are necessary.

Alcohol: No special precautions are necessary.

Pregnancy: Not recommended during pregnancy.

Breast Feeding: Betamethasone dipropionate/clotrimazole may pass into breast milk; caution is advised. Consult your doctor for advice.

Infants and Children: Not recommended for use by children under age 12 years.

Special Concerns: Avoid contact with eyes. Wash hands thoroughly after application. Tell your doctor if your condition has not improved within a few days of starting the medication. As with any other antifungal, betamethasone dipropionate/clotrimazole is useful only against organisms that are vulnerable to its effects. Therefore, it is important to tell your doctor if your condition has not improved, or has worsened, within a few days of starting betamethasone dipropionate/clotrimazole. The specific organism causing your illness may be resistant to this medication.

OVERDOSE
Symptoms: No specific symptoms have been reported.

What to Do: An overdose is unlikely to be life-threatening. However, if someone applies a much larger dose than prescribed or ingests the medication, call your doctor, emergency medical services (EMS), or the nearest poison control center immediately.

▼ INTERACTIONS

DRUG INTERACTIONS
No specific drug interactions have been documented.

FOOD INTERACTIONS
No known food interactions.

DISEASE INTERACTIONS
Consult your doctor if you have ever experienced an allergic reaction to any topical medication or undesirable reactions to any steroid or preparation containing steroids.

≡ SIDE EFFECTS ≡

SERIOUS
Blistering or ulceration of the skin; blistering of the lips, nose, and mouth.

COMMON
Brief burning or irritation after application; peeling.

LESS COMMON
Severe burning, itching, swelling, increased redness, or any increased discomfort at the application site that was not present before therapy; dry skin; pus or inflammation at base of hair follicles; change in skin color at site of application; acne.

BISOPROLOL FUMARATE/HYDROCHLOROTHIAZIDE

BRAND NAME

Ziac

Available in: Tablets
Available OTC? No   **As Generic?** Yes
Drug Class: Beta-blocker/thiazide diuretic

▼ USAGE INFORMATION

WHY IT'S PRESCRIBED
To control hypertension (high blood pressure).

HOW IT WORKS
Bisoprolol, a beta-blocker, blocks certain nerve impulses to various parts of the body, which accounts for its many effects. For example, it reduces the rate and force of the heart's contractions (which helps lower blood pressure), decreases the heart's oxygen requirement (which helps prevent angina) and helps stabilize heart rhythm. Hydrochlorothiazide (HCTZ), a diuretic, increases the excretion of salt and water in the urine. By reducing the overall amount of fluid in the body, diuretics reduce pressure within the blood vessels.

▼ DOSAGE GUIDELINES

RANGE AND FREQUENCY
Tablets contain 6.25 mg HCTZ and 2.5, 5, or 10 mg bisoprolol. Therapy is initiated with the lowest dose and may be increased at 1 week intervals to 2 tablets with 10 mg bisoprolol once a day.

ONSET OF EFFECT
Within 1 to 4 hours.

DURATION OF ACTION
Up to 24 hours.

DIETARY ADVICE
No special restrictions.

STORAGE
Store in a tightly sealed container away from moisture, heat, and direct light.

MISSED DOSE
If you miss a dose on one day, resume your regular dosage schedule the next day. Do not double the next dose.

STOPPING THE DRUG
The decision to stop taking the drug should be made in consultation with a physician. Do not stop taking this drug abruptly; your doctor will gradually decrease the dose before stopping it completely.

PROLONGED USE
Bisoprolol/hydrochlorothiazide can control high blood pressure but cannot cure it. Lifelong therapy may be necessary. See your doctor regularly for tests and examinations if you must take this drug for a prolonged period of time.

▼ PRECAUTIONS

Over 60: Adverse reactions, especially dizziness, lightheadedness, and reduced tolerance to cold, may be more likely and more severe in older patients.

Driving and Hazardous Work: Do not drive or engage in hazardous work until you determine how the medicine affects you.

Alcohol: Drink in careful moderation if at all. Alcohol may interact with the bisoprolol component and cause a dangerous drop in blood pressure.

Pregnancy: Beta-blockers and thiazide diuretics may cause problems during pregnancy. Before taking this medication, tell your doctor if you are pregnant or plan to become pregnant.

Breast Feeding: This drug passes into breast milk; caution is advised. Consult your doctor for specific advice.

Infants and Children: Adequate studies have not been done on the use of this drug in children. No special problems are expected. Consult your pediatrician for advice.

Special Concerns: In addition to taking this medicine, follow your doctor's instructions on weight control and diet for reduction of blood pressure.

OVERDOSE
Symptoms: Slow heartbeat, severe dizziness or fainting, difficulty breathing, bluish-colored fingernails or palms, seizures.

What to Do: Call your doctor, emergency medical services (EMS), or the nearest poison control center immediately.

▼ INTERACTIONS

DRUG INTERACTIONS
Do not take with other beta-blockers. Consult your doctor for specific advice if you are taking any other antihypertensive medications, insulin, oral diabetes medications, digitalis drugs, cholestyramine, colestipol, clonidine, lithium, nonsteroidal antiinflammatory drugs, MAO inhibitors, rifampin, narcotic analgesics, or skeletal muscle relaxants.

FOOD INTERACTIONS
Avoid foods high in sodium.

DISEASE INTERACTIONS
Do not use if you have a history of bronchospasm. Consult your doctor if you have any of the following: bronchial asthma, emphysema, slow heartbeat, heart or blood vessel disease, diabetes mellitus, congestive heart failure, gout, kidney disease, liver disease, depression, parathyroid disease, or an overactive thyroid (hyperthyroidism).

≣ SIDE EFFECTS ≣

SERIOUS
Slow heartbeat, difficulty breathing, mental depression, cold hands and feet, swelling of ankles, feet, or lower legs. Call your doctor immediately.

COMMON
Dizziness or lightheadedness, decreased sexual ability, drowsiness, insomnia, fatigue, diarrhea.

LESS COMMON
Anxiety, loss of appetite, upset stomach, nervousness or excitability, constipation, numbness and tingling in the fingers and toes, stuffy nose.

BRIMONIDINE TARTRATE

Available in: Ophthalmic solution
Available OTC? No   **As Generic?** No
Drug Class: Antiglaucoma agent

▼ USAGE INFORMATION

WHY IT'S PRESCRIBED
To treat glaucoma.

HOW IT WORKS
Glaucoma, a sight-threatening disorder, occurs when aqueous humor (fluid inside the eye) cannot drain properly, causing increased pressure within the eyeball (intraocular pressure). Increased eye pressure can damage the optic nerve and lead to a gradually progressive loss of vision. Brimonidine decreases the production of aqueous humor and promotes its outflow, thereby reducing intraocular pressure.

▼ DOSAGE GUIDELINES

RANGE AND FREQUENCY
1 drop of brimonidine in each eye 3 times a day at 8-hour intervals.

ONSET OF EFFECT
Within 60 minutes.

DURATION OF ACTION
8 hours or more.

DIETARY ADVICE
No special restrictions.

STORAGE
Store in a tightly sealed container away from moisture, heat, and direct light. Do not allow the medication to freeze.

MISSED DOSE
Apply it as soon as you remember. If it is near the time for the next dose, skip the missed dose and resume your regular dosage schedule. Do not double the next dose.

STOPPING THE DRUG
The decision to stop using the drug should be made by your doctor.

PROLONGED USE
You should see your doctor regularly for examinations and tests as part of a glaucoma follow-up if you take this drug for a prolonged period.

▼ PRECAUTIONS

Over 60: Adverse reactions may be more likely and more severe in older patients.

Driving and Hazardous Work: Do not drive or engage in hazardous work until you determine how the drug affects your vision.

Alcohol: Use alcohol with caution.

Pregnancy: In animal studies, brimonidine caused impaired fetal circulation. Human studies have not been done. Before you take brimonidine, tell your doctor if you are pregnant or are planning to become pregnant.

Breast Feeding: Brimonidine may pass into breast milk; caution is advised. Consult your doctor for advice.

Infants and Children: The safety and effectiveness of brimonidine in children have not been established.

Special Concerns: To use the eye drops, first wash your hands. Tilt your head back. Gently apply pressure to the inside corner of the eyelid and with the index finger of the same hand, pull downward on the lower eyelid to make a space. Drop the medicine into this space and close your eye. Apply pressure for 1 or 2 minutes while keeping the eye closed without blinking. Then wash your hands again. Make sure the tip of the dropper does not touch your eye, finger, or any other surface. Bromonidine may make your eyes more sensitive to sunlight. If this occurs, wear sunglasses or avoid bright light as comfort dictates.

OVERDOSE
Symptoms: No specific symptoms have been reported.

What to Do: An overdose of brimonidine is unlikely to be life-threatening. However, if someone takes a much larger dose than prescribed or accidentally ingests the medicine, call your doctor, emergency medical services (EMS), or the nearest poison control center immediately.

▼ INTERACTIONS

DRUG INTERACTIONS
Consult your doctor for advice if you are taking MAO inhibitors, tricyclic antidepressants, central nervous system depressants, beta-blockers, antihypertensives, or digitalis drugs (such as digoxin).

FOOD INTERACTIONS
No known food interactions.

DISEASE INTERACTIONS
Caution is advised when taking brimonidine. Consult your doctor if you have cardiovascular disease, cerebral or coronary insufficiency, kidney disease, liver disease, depression, Raynaud's phenomenon, orthostatic hypotension, or thromboangiitis obliterans.

SIDE EFFECTS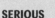

SERIOUS
Fainting: Call your doctor immediately.

COMMON
Burning or stinging of the eyes, fatigue, dry mouth, eye discomfort, drowsiness.

LESS COMMON
Excess tear production, redness of eyes or inner lining of the eyelids, headache, swelling of eye or eyelid, eye ache or pain, blurring or other changes in vision, dizziness, mental depression, insomnia, muscle pain or weakness, nausea, increased blood pressure, vomiting, anxiety, pounding heartbeat, change in taste, crusting in corner of eye or on eyelid, discoloration of eyeball, paleness of inner lining of eyelid, dry eyes, sensitivity of eyes to light.

BUPROPION HYDROCHLORIDE

Available in: Tablets, extended-release tablets
Available OTC? No   **As Generic?** Yes (immediate-release form only)
Drug Class: Antidepressant/smoking deterrent

▼ USAGE INFORMATION

WHY IT'S PRESCRIBED
To relieve symptoms of major depression. Bupropion is also used as a nicotine-free agent to help stop smoking. It should be used as a part of a comprehensive smoking cessation program carried out under the supervision of your doctor.

HOW IT WORKS
The exact mechanism of action of bupropion is not known. It appears to help balance the levels of neurotransmitters (brain chemicals) that are thought to be linked to mood, emotions, and mental state. Unlike other smoking cessation medications, bupropion does not contain nicotine. It is believed that bupropion's effects on the chemistry of the brain help curb the desire for nicotine and enhance the patient's ability to abstain from smoking.

▼ DOSAGE GUIDELINES

RANGE AND FREQUENCY
For depression—Adults: To start, 100 mg twice a day. Dosage may be increased to 450 mg a day. No more than 150 mg should be taken within 4 hours. Older adults: To start, 75 or 100 mg twice a day. Children: Dosages must be determined by your doctor. For smoking cessation—Adults: For the first 3 days of treatment, 150 mg a day. Dosage may then be increased to 150 mg 2 times a day. The doses should be taken at least 8 hours apart. Do not take more than 300 mg a day. You should not stop smoking until you have been taking Zyban for 1 week. Treatment generally lasts 7 to 12 weeks.

ONSET OF EFFECT
1 to 3 weeks.

DURATION OF ACTION
Unknown.

DIETARY ADVICE
Bupropion can be taken with food to reduce stomach irritation. The tablet should be swallowed whole, because it has a bitter taste and can produce an unpleasant numbing sensation inside of the mouth.

STORAGE
Store in a tightly sealed container away from moisture, heat, and direct light.

MISSED DOSE
Take it as soon as you remember, unless your next scheduled dose is within the next 4 hours (8 hours for smoking cessation). If so, do not take the missed dose. Take your next scheduled dose at the proper time and resume your regular dosage schedule. Do not double the next dose.

STOPPING THE DRUG
Depression: Take it as prescribed for the full treatment period, even if you begin to feel better before the scheduled end of therapy. Discontinuing the drug abruptly may produce unpleasant withdrawal symptoms. Dosage should be reduced gradually according to your doctor's instructions. The decision to stop taking the drug should be made in consultation with your doctor. Smoking cessation: If you have not made significant progress toward abstinence by the end of the seventh week of treatment, consult your doctor. Treatment should probably be discontinued. You do not need to gradually decrease the dose before stopping.

PROLONGED USE
Depression: The usual course of therapy lasts 6 months to 1 year; some patients benefit from additional therapy. Smoking cessation: Treatment generally lasts 7 to 12 weeks.

▼ PRECAUTIONS

Over 60: Dosage may be decreased because of age-related decline in liver or kidney function.

Driving and Hazardous Work: Use caution until you determine how the medication affects you. Drowsiness or lightheadedness can occur.

Alcohol: Alcohol increases the risk of seizures. It is recommended to abstain from alcohol or to drink very little while taking bupropion. If you regularly drink a lot of alcohol and then suddenly stop, this may increase your chance of having a seizure; gradual tapering of alcohol intake is recommended.

Pregnancy: Bupropion has not caused birth defects in animals. Adequate human studies have not been done. The drug is not recommended while you are pregnant. Before taking it, tell your doctor if you are pregnant or plan to become pregnant.

Breast Feeding: Bupropion passes into breast milk; avoid or discontinue using the drug while nursing.

Infants and Children: Adequate studies in children have not been done. Bupropion is not recommended for use by children under age 18 years.

▼ SIDE EFFECTS

SERIOUS
When treating depression: Hallucinations, heartbeat irregularities, confusion, skin rash, insomnia, severe headache, excitement or agitation, seizures. Call your doctor immediately. Smoking cessation: None reported.

COMMON
When treating depression: Nausea or vomiting, constipation, unusual weight loss, dry mouth, loss of appetite, dizziness, increased sweating, trembling or shaking. Smoking cessation: Dry mouth, insomnia.

LESS COMMON
When treating depression: Fever or chills, concentration difficulties, drowsiness, fatigue, change in or blurred vision, unusual feeling of euphoria, hostility or anger. Smoking cessation: Mild rash, tremor.

Special Concerns: This is a potentially dangerous drug, especially if taken in excess. Antidepressants should not be within easy reach of suicidal patients. To prevent insomnia, take the last dose several hours before bedtime. When taking bupropion for smoking cessation, it is advisable to continue smoking through the first week of treatment. Set a target date to stop smoking no later than the second week of therapy. Continuing to smoke beyond the designated date reduces your chances of successfully quitting. You may use a nicotine transdermal patch (see Nicotine) while taking Zyban, but consult your doctor before initiating such therapy. The combination of nicotine and bupropion increases the risk of hypertension; blood pressure should be monitored regularly throughout treatment. Zyban should be seen as just one small part of a comprehensive treatment program that includes counseling, social support, and regular contact with your doctor. The goal of therapy with Zyban is complete abstinence from cigarettes. Do not chew, divide, or crush the tablets or extended-release tablets.

OVERDOSE

Symptoms: Hallucinations, seizures, rapid heartbeat, chest pain, breathing difficulty, loss of consciousness. A few cases of overdose associated with treatment for smoking cessation have been reported. Some of the symptoms experienced include vomiting, blurred vision, lightheadedness, confusion, lethargy, nausea, jitteriness, hallucinations, drowsiness, and seizures.

What to Do: Call your doctor, emergency medical services (EMS), or the nearest poison control center immediately.

▼ INTERACTIONS

DRUG INTERACTIONS

Bupropion should not be used if you are taking other medicines containing bupropion or within 14 days of taking an MAO inhibitor. Consult your doctor if you are currently taking loxapine, tricyclic antidepressants, phenothiazines, clozapine, molindone, fluoxetine, lithium, thioxanthenes, haloperidol, trazodone, maprotiline, levodopa, or theophylline.

FOOD INTERACTIONS

No known food interactions.

DISEASE INTERACTIONS

Bupropion should not be taken if you have a history of seizures, anorexia nervosa, or bulimia. Caution is advised when taking bupropion. Consult your doctor if you have any of the following: a tumor of the brain or spinal cord, heart disease, or head injury. Because the liver and kidneys work together to remove bupropion from the body, a lower dose may be prescribed for patients with impaired liver or kidney function.

BUSPIRONE HYDROCHLORIDE

Available in: Tablets
Available OTC? No   **As Generic?** Yes
Drug Class: Antianxiety drug

▼ USAGE INFORMATION

WHY IT'S PRESCRIBED
To treat anxiety.

HOW IT WORKS
Buspirone affects the activity of specific brain chemicals (dopamine and especially serotonin) that are profoundly linked to mood, emotions, and mental state. Unlike many other medications used to treat anxiety disorders, buspirone has no muscle relaxant or sedative effects and does not appear to lead to physical dependence.

▼ DOSAGE GUIDELINES

RANGE AND FREQUENCY
To start, 5 mg 3 times a day (for a total of 15 mg a day). Can be increased to 60 mg a day, taken in divided doses every 6 to 8 hours.

ONSET OF EFFECT
May take 1 to 2 weeks to attain the full therapeutic benefit of buspirone.

DURATION OF ACTION
8 hours or more.

DIETARY ADVICE
No special restrictions.

STORAGE
Store in a tightly sealed container away from moisture, heat, and direct light.

MISSED DOSE
If you miss a dose, take it as soon as you remember. If it is near the time for your next dose, skip the missed dose and resume your regular dosage schedule. Do not double the next dose.

STOPPING THE DRUG
The decision to stop taking buspirone should be made in consultation with your doctor.

PROLONGED USE
No known problems.

▼ PRECAUTIONS

Over 60: Adverse side effects and reactions may be more common and more severe in older patients.

Driving and Hazardous Work: The use of buspirone may impair your ability to drive or perform hazardous tasks safely. The danger increases if you drink alcohol or take other medications that can affect alertness, such as antihistamines, painkillers, or mind-altering drugs.

Alcohol: Avoid alcohol while using this medication.

Pregnancy: No problems are expected, but adequate studies of buspirone use during pregnancy have not been done. Consult your doctor if you are pregnant or plan to become pregnant.

Breast Feeding: Buspirone can pass into breast milk. Avoid taking it if possible or refrain from breast feeding.

Infants and Children: The safety and effectiveness of buspirone have not been established for anyone under the age of 18 years.

Special Concerns: Be sure to notify the surgeon that you are taking buspirone before you undergo surgery that requires anesthesia.

OVERDOSE
Symptoms: Severe drowsiness, dizziness, nausea and vomiting, constricted (pinpoint) pupils.

What to Do: Call your doctor, emergency medical services (EMS), or the nearest poison control center immediately.

▼ INTERACTIONS

DRUG INTERACTIONS
Other drugs may interact with buspirone. Consult your doctor for specific advice if you take any of the following: antihistamines, barbiturates, MAO inhibitors, muscle relaxants, narcotics, sedatives, or other tranquilizers.

FOOD INTERACTIONS
None expected.

DISEASE INTERACTIONS
Use of buspirone may cause complications in patients with liver or kidney disease, because these organs work together to remove the medication from the body.

≣ SIDE EFFECTS ≣

SERIOUS
No serious side effects have been directly associated with the use of buspirone.

COMMON
Dizziness or lightheadedness, nausea, paradoxical increase in nervousness or excitability, restlessness, headache.

LESS COMMON
Blurred vision; impaired ability to concentrate; drowsiness; dry mouth; difficulty sleeping; muscle cramps or spasms; fatigue or weakness; ringing in the ears; unusual, disturbing, or vivid dreams.

BUTALBITAL/ASPIRIN/CAFFEINE

BRAND NAMES

B-A-C, Butalgen, Fiorgen, Fiorinal, Fiormor, Fortabs, Isobutal, Isobutyl, Isolin, Isollyl, Laniroif, Lanorinal, Marnal, Vibutal

Available in: Capsules, tablets
Available OTC? No   **As Generic?** Yes
Drug Class: Nonnarcotic analgesic

▼ USAGE INFORMATION

WHY IT'S PRESCRIBED
To treat headaches or migraines.

HOW IT WORKS
Butalbital, a barbiturate, acts on the central nervous system to cause sedation. Aspirin appears to interfere with the action of prostaglandins, naturally occurring substances in the body that cause inflammation and make nerves more sensitive to pain impulses. Caffeine is believed to enhance the effectiveness of pain relievers.

▼ DOSAGE GUIDELINES

RANGE AND FREQUENCY
1 or 2 capsules or tablets every 4 hours. Do not take more than 6 pills a day.

ONSET OF EFFECT
Within 1 hour.

DURATION OF ACTION
4 hours.

DIETARY ADVICE
Take this drug with food or a full glass of water to avoid stomach irritation.

STORAGE
Store in a tightly sealed container away from heat, moisture, and direct light.

MISSED DOSE
If your doctor has directed you to take this drug on a regular schedule, take it as soon as you remember. If it is near the time for the next dose, skip the missed dose and resume your regular dosage schedule. Do not double the next dose.

STOPPING THE DRUG
Take it as prescribed for the full treatment period, but you may stop taking the drug if you are feeling better before the scheduled end of therapy. This drug should never be stopped abruptly after long-term regular use.

PROLONGED USE
Prolonged use may result in physical dependence and may cause kidney damage. Periodic kidney function tests are recommended. Prolonged use may make exposure to cold weather more hazardous.

▼ PRECAUTIONS

Over 60: Adverse reactions may be more likely and more severe in older patients.

Driving and Hazardous Work: Do not drive or engage in hazardous work until you determine how the medicine affects you.

Alcohol: Avoid alcohol.

Pregnancy: Taking this medicine late in pregnancy may cause drug dependence in the unborn child. Before you take it, tell your doctor if you are pregnant or are planning to become pregnant.

Breast Feeding: Butalbital and aspirin pass into breast milk; avoid or discontinue use while nursing.

Infants and Children: Consult your doctor before giving this medicine to anyone under age 18 who has a viral illness, especially chicken pox or influenza. The aspirin may cause a serious illness called Reye's syndrome.

Special Concerns: Tell any doctor or dentist with whom you consult that you are taking this medicine. It works best if taken at the first sign of a headache. Tell your doctor if you begin having headaches more frequently than before you started using it or if the drug stops working as well as it did at the outset of therapy. This may be a sign of drug dependence. Do not try to get better pain relief by increasing the dose. Do not take the drug if it has a strong vinegar odor.

OVERDOSE
Symptoms: Deep sleep, weak pulse, ringing in the ears, nausea, vomiting, dizziness, deep and rapid breathing, convulsions, loss of consciousness.

What to Do: Call your doctor, emergency medical services (EMS), or the nearest poison control center immediately.

▼ INTERACTIONS

DRUG INTERACTIONS
Consult your doctor for advice if you are taking acetazolamide, gout medicines, beta-blockers, anticoagulants, methotrexate, narcotic pain relievers, nonsteroidal anti-inflammatory drugs, oral contraceptives, oral diabetes medicines, steroid medicines, tranquilizers, or valproic acid.

FOOD INTERACTIONS
No known food interactions.

DISEASE INTERACTIONS
Consult your doctor if you have any of the following: stomach or duodenal ulcers, asthma, epilepsy, anemia, gout, or a history of alcohol or drug abuse. Use of this drug may cause complications in patients with liver or kidney disease, because these organs work together to remove the medication from the body.

≡ SIDE EFFECTS ≡

SERIOUS
Difficulty breathing, tightness in chest, coughing, or wheezing; sores or white spots in mouth; bluish discoloration, flushing, or redness of skin; stuffy nose; pinpoint pupils; fever; swollen eyelids, face, lips, or tongue; difficulty swallowing; crusting or bleeding sores on lips; sore throat; burning, tenderness, or peeling of skin. Call your physician immediately.

COMMON
Drowsiness, dizziness, heartburn.

LESS COMMON
Insomnia, nightmares, headache, constipation, increased sweating, unusual fatigue.

CALCITONIN—SALMON

BRAND NAMES
Calcimar, Miacalcin

Available in: Injection, nasal spray
Available OTC? No   **As Generic?** No
Drug Class: Hormone/bone resorption inhibitor

▼ USAGE INFORMATION

WHY IT'S PRESCRIBED
To treat Paget's disease, a disorder in which bone tissue is broken down and restored too rapidly, resulting in bone fragility and in some cases malformation; to prevent bone loss in women with postmenopausal osteoporosis; to treat abnormally high blood calcium levels; to treat osteoporosis resulting from hormonal disturbances, drug therapy, and immobilization; and to relieve compression of nerves that may occur with Paget's disease of bone.

HOW IT WORKS
Calcitonin blocks the bone mineral absorbing activity of the osteoclasts (bone cells), increases calcium excretion by the kidneys, and slows bone resorption (the speed at which bone is broken down before it is replaced).

▼ DOSAGE GUIDELINES

RANGE AND FREQUENCY
Injection—For Paget's disease: 100 international units (IU) injected under the skin once a day to start. The dosage may be reduced depending on results. To prevent postmenopausal bone loss: 100 IU injected into muscle or under the skin once a day, once every other day, or 3 times a week. For excessive blood calcium: 1.8 IU per lb of body weight injected every 12 hours to start. Dose may be increased or decreased by your doctor. Nasal spray—200 IU (1 spray) a day delivered in alternating nostrils.

ONSET OF EFFECT
Within 15 minutes.

DURATION OF ACTION
8 to 24 hours.

DIETARY ADVICE
If you are using this drug to lower blood calcium, your doctor may want you to follow a low-calcium diet. An injection is best administered at bedtime.

STORAGE
Store in a tightly sealed container away from heat and direct light.

MISSED DOSE
If you take 2 doses a day: Take the missed dose if you remember within 2 hours; if not, skip the missed dose and resume your regular dosage schedule. If you take 1 dose a day: Take the missed dose if you remember it the same day, then resume your regular dosage schedule. If you remember the next day, skip the missed dose and resume your regular dosage schedule. If you take one dose every other day: Take the missed dose if you remember the same day. Otherwise, take the dose the next day, skip a day and resume your regular dosage schedule. If you take 1 dose 3 times a week: Take the missed dose the next day, set each dose back a day for the rest of the week, then resume your regular dosage schedule. In no case should you double the next dose.

STOPPING THE DRUG
The decision to stop taking the drug should be made by your doctor.

PROLONGED USE
Development of antibodies to the medicine may diminish its effectiveness over time.

▼ PRECAUTIONS

Over 60: Fluid balance should be monitored if the drug is given to reduce blood levels of calcium.

Driving and Hazardous Work: The use of calcitonin should not impair your ability to perform such tasks safely.

Alcohol: Avoid alcohol.

Pregnancy: In animal studies, large doses of calcitonin reduced birth weight. Before you take calcitonin, tell your doctor if you are pregnant or plan to become pregnant.

Breast Feeding: Calcitonin may pass into breast milk; caution is advised. Consult your doctor for advice.

Infants and Children: Studies of calcitonin use in infants and children have not been done. Consult your doctor for specific advice.

Special Concerns: You should not take calcitonin if you have a recently healed bone fracture.

OVERDOSE
Symptoms: No specific symptoms have been reported.

What to Do: An overdose of calcitonin is unlikely to be life-threatening; however, if someone takes a much larger dose than prescribed, call your doctor, emergency medical services (EMS), or the nearest poison control center.

▼ INTERACTIONS

DRUG INTERACTIONS
There are no known drug interactions.

FOOD INTERACTIONS
No known food interactions.

DISEASE INTERACTIONS
Caution is advised when taking calcitonin. Consult your doctor for specific advice if you have a kidney problem or a history of allergies.

≣ SIDE EFFECTS ≣

SERIOUS
Skin rash or hives. Call your doctor immediately.

COMMON
Diarrhea, loss of appetite, nausea or vomiting, stomach pain, pain and redness at injection site, flushing or redness of face, ears, hands, or feet.

LESS COMMON
Increased output of urine, headache, dizziness, pressure in the chest, breathing difficulty, stuffy nose, nasal bleeding or crusting, tingling of hands or feet, weakness, back pain, joint pain, chills.

CAPTOPRIL

Available in: Tablets
Available OTC? No   **As Generic?** Yes
Drug Class: Angiotensin-converting enzyme (ACE) inhibitor

▼ USAGE INFORMATION

WHY IT'S PRESCRIBED
To control high blood pressure; to treat congestive heart failure (CHF); to treat patients with left ventricular dysfunction (damage to the pumping chamber of the heart); and to minimize further kidney damage in people with diabetes who have mild kidney disease.

HOW IT WORKS
Angiotensin-converting enzyme (ACE) inhibitors block an enzyme that produces angiotensin, a naturally occurring substance that causes blood vessels to constrict and stimulates production of the adrenal hormone aldosterone, which promotes sodium retention in the body. As a result, ACE inhibitors relax blood vessels (causing them to widen) and reduces sodium retention, which lowers blood pressure and thus decreases the workload of the heart.

▼ DOSAGE GUIDELINES

RANGE AND FREQUENCY
Adults— For high blood pressure: 12.5 to 150 mg 2 or 3 times a day. For CHF: 6.25 to 100 mg 2 or 3 times a day. For left ventricular dysfunction: 6.25 to 50 mg 3 times a day. For kidney problems associated with diabetes: 25 mg 3 times a day. Children— Consult your pediatrician.

ONSET OF EFFECT
15 to 60 minutes.

DURATION OF ACTION
6 to 12 hours.

DIETARY ADVICE
Take it on an empty stomach about 1 hour before mealtime. Follow your doctor's dietary advice (such as low-salt or low-cholesterol restrictions) to improve control over high blood pressure and heart disease. Avoid high-potassium foods like bananas and citrus fruits and juices unless you are also taking medications, that lower potassium levels.

STORAGE
Store in a tightly sealed container away from heat and direct light.

MISSED DOSE
Take it as soon as you remember. If it is near the time for the next dose, skip the missed dose and resume your regular dosage schedule. Do not double the next dose.

STOPPING THE DRUG
Do not stop taking this drug abruptly; this may cause potentially serious health problems. Dosage should be reduced gradually according to your doctor's instructions.

PROLONGED USE
See your doctor regularly for examinations and tests if you must take this medicine for a prolonged period. Remember that captopril helps control high blood pressure but does not cure it. Lifelong therapy may be necessary.

▼ PRECAUTIONS

Over 60: Adverse reactions may be more likely and more severe in older patients.

Driving and Hazardous Work: Avoid such activities until you determine how the medication affects you.

Alcohol: Alcohol may increase the effect of the drug and cause an excessive drop in blood pressure. Consult your doctor for advice.

Pregnancy: Captopril should not be used during the final 6 months of pregnancy. Notify your doctor immediately if you become pregnant.

Breast Feeding: If possible, avoid using captopril while nursing.

Infants and Children: Captopril is only prescribed for children when other means of controlling hypertension fail; benefits must be weighed against risks.

OVERDOSE
Symptoms: Dizziness or fainting; weak, rapid pulse; nausea, or vomiting; chest pain.

What to Do: Call your doctor, emergency medical services (EMS), or the nearest poison control center immediately.

▼ INTERACTIONS

DRUG INTERACTIONS
Consult your doctor if you are taking diuretics (especially potassium-sparing diuretics), potassium supplements or drugs containing potassium, lithium, anticoagulants, anti-inflammatory drugs, or over-the-counter drugs (especially cold remedies and diet pills).

FOOD INTERACTIONS
Avoid low-salt milk and salt substitutes. Many of these products contain potassium.

DISEASE INTERACTIONS
Consult your doctor if you have systemic lupus erythematosus or if you have had an allergic reaction to angiotensin-converting enzyme (ACE) inhibitors in the past. This medication should be used with caution by patients with severe kidney disease or renal artery stenosis (narrowing of one or both of the arteries that supply blood to the kidneys).

 SIDE EFFECTS

SERIOUS
Fever and chills; sore throat and hoarseness; sudden difficulty breathing or swallowing; swelling of the face, mouth, or extremities; impaired kidney function (ankle swelling, decreased urination); confusion; yellow discoloration of the eyes or skin (indicating liver disorder); intense itching; chest pain or palpitations; abdominal pain. Serious side effects are very rare; contact your doctor immediately.

COMMON
Dry, persistent cough.

LESS COMMON
Dizziness or fainting; skin rash; numbness or tingling in the hands, feet, or lips; unusual fatigue or muscle weakness; nausea; drowsiness; loss of taste; headache.

CARBAMAZEPINE

Available in: Oral suspension, tablets, extended-release tablets and capsules
Available OTC? No   **As Generic?** Yes
Drug Class: Anticonvulsant/analgesic

▼ USAGE INFORMATION

WHY IT'S PRESCRIBED
To control certain types of seizures caused by epilepsy. Also to treat facial pain in those with trigeminal neuralgia (tic douloureux).

HOW IT WORKS
Carbamazepine appears to inhibit neurons from firing repeatedly and uncontrollably (which causes seizures).

▼ DOSAGE GUIDELINES

RANGE AND FREQUENCY
Adults: 600 to 2,000 mg a day in 3 or 4 divided doses. Children: 9 to 18 mg per lb of body weight in 3 or 4 divided doses. Some patients require higher doses. A low dose should be used initially, then gradually increased if needed. The extended-release forms may be given twice a day.

ONSET OF EFFECT
Several hours or longer.

DURATION OF ACTION
Maximum effectiveness: 12 hours or longer; the drug's effectiveness then gradually decreases.

DIETARY ADVICE
Take with food to lessen the chance of stomach upset.

STORAGE
Store in a tightly sealed container away from moisture, heat, and direct light.

MISSED DOSE
Take the medication as soon as you remember. If it is near the time for the next dose, skip the missed dose and resume your regular dosage schedule. Do not double the next dose, unless advised to do so by your doctor. Call your doctor if you miss more than a full day's amount of the drug.

STOPPING THE DRUG
Never stop this drug abruptly; seizures may occur. Your doctor will taper the dose over many weeks.

PROLONGED USE
Therapy may last several years or more. Some side effects may diminish after a few weeks of therapy.

▼ PRECAUTIONS

Over 60: Older patients may require lower doses to minimize side effects.

Driving and Hazardous Work: Avoid such tasks until you determine how the medication affects you.

Alcohol: May contribute to excessive drowsiness.

Pregnancy: This drug increases the risk of birth defects. However, seizures during pregnancy also increase the risks to the fetus. Discuss potential risks and benefits with your doctor. Folate supplementation is advised starting 1 to 2 months before conception and continuing throughout pregnancy. Vitamin K_1 may be needed during the last 4 weeks of pregnancy.

Breast Feeding: This drug passes into breast milk, although at low levels. Consult your doctor for advice.

Infants and Children: Behavioral side effects are more likely to be seen in children.

Special Concerns: The generic form is not recommended. Do not change the brand you are taking without consulting your doctor. Your doctor may suggest that you carry an ID card or wear a bracelet saying that you take this drug.

OVERDOSE
Symptoms: Confusion, double vision, seizures, extreme drowsiness, spasms, loss of consciousness, poor muscle control, tremors, walking difficulty, abnormal heartbeat, slow or irregular breathing.

What to Do: Seek medical assistance immediately.

▼ INTERACTIONS

DRUG INTERACTIONS
Carbamazepine may interact with many drugs, including other anticonvulsants (clonazepam, ethosuximide, primidone, phenobarbital, valproic acid, and phenytoin), anticoagulants, certain anti-infectives (erythromycin, doxycycline, troleandomycin, isoniazid), oral contraceptives, cimetidine, corticosteroids, danazol, diltiazem, lithium, nicotinamide, propoxyphene, theophylline, thyroid hormones, and verapamil.

FOOD INTERACTIONS
No known food interactions.

DISEASE INTERACTIONS
Special caution is advised in those with lupus; heart, kidney, or liver disease; diabetes; or glaucoma.

SIDE EFFECTS

SERIOUS
Fever, sore throat, swollen glands, pointlike rash, blistering or peeling, easy bruising, pallor, weakness, confusion, lethargy, or seizures may be a sign of a potentially fatal blood reaction (aplastic anemia). Call your doctor at once.

COMMON
Drowsiness, rash, itching, increased sensitivity of the skin to sunlight, dizziness, blurred vision, incoordination, nausea, vomiting, stomach pain or upset, diarrhea, constipation, loss of appetite, dry or inflamed mouth.

LESS COMMON
Impaired speech; involuntary movements of the face, limbs, or tongue; tingling or numbness in the extremities; depression; agitation; psychosis; talkativeness; abnormal eye movements; ringing in the ears; heart rhythm abnormalities; impotence; hair loss, excessive hair growth. There are numerous additional potential side effects.

CARISOPRODOL

BRAND NAMES
Rela, Soma, Vanadom

Available in: Tablets
Available OTC? No **As Generic?** Yes
Drug Class: Muscle relaxant

▼ USAGE INFORMATION

WHY IT'S PRESCRIBED
Skeletal muscle relaxants are used to relieve stiffness and discomfort caused by severe sprains and strains, muscle spasms, or other muscle problems. They may be prescribed in conjunction with other treatment methods, such as physical therapy.

HOW IT WORKS
Muscle relaxants such as carisoprodol depress activity in the central nervous system, which in turn interferes with the transmission of nerve impulses from the spinal cord to the muscles.

▼ DOSAGE GUIDELINES

RANGE AND FREQUENCY
Adults and teenagers: 350 mg 3 to 4 times a day. Children ages 5 to 12 years: 6.25 mg per 2.2 lb (1 kg) of body weight 4 times a day.

ONSET OF EFFECT
30 minutes.

DURATION OF ACTION
4 to 6 hours.

DIETARY ADVICE
Eat a well-balanced diet; the healing of injured tissue increases the body's protein and calorie requirements. To avoid dry mouth, maintain adequate fluid intake and suck on ice chips.

STORAGE
Store in a tightly sealed container in a dry place away from heat and direct light.

MISSED DOSE
Take it as soon as you remember. If it is within 2 hours of the next dose, skip the missed dose and resume your regular dosage schedule. Do not double the next dose.

STOPPING THE DRUG
This medication should be taken as prescribed for the full treatment period. Do not stop taking carisoprodol abruptly.

PROLONGED USE
Therapy with carisoprodol ranges from several days to weeks. Prolonged use may be associated with an increased risk of side effects.

▼ PRECAUTIONS

Over 60: Adverse reactions to medications such as carisoprodol may be more likely and more severe in older patients.

Driving and Hazardous Work: Carisoprodol may impair your ability to drive or perform hazardous work.

Alcohol: Avoid alcohol while taking this medication because it may compound the sedative effect and may cause liver damage.

Pregnancy: Adequate studies of carisoprodol during pregnancy have not been done; discuss the relative risks and benefits with your doctor.

Breast Feeding: Breast feeding is not recommended during therapy.

Infants and Children: No special problems have been documented; consult your pediatrician for advice.

Special Concerns: Carisoprodol will intensify the effect that alcohol, sedatives, and other central nervous system depressants have on the brain. It is not a substitute for other safe, nonmedical therapies for muscle stiffness,

including rest, gentle guided exercise, and physical therapy.

OVERDOSE
Symptoms: Excessive drowsiness or difficulty awakening, even when being shaken or pinched; confusion; weakness; slowed breathing; coma.

What to Do: Call emergency medical services (EMS) or the nearest poison control center immediately.

▼ INTERACTIONS

DRUG INTERACTIONS
Consult your doctor for specific advice if you are taking antihistamines and decongestants, antidepressants, sleep aids, sedatives, tranquilizers, pain medication, barbiturates, or seizure medication.

FOOD INTERACTIONS
No known food interactions.

DISEASE INTERACTIONS
Caution is advised when taking carisoprodol. Consult your doctor if you have a history of any of the following medical conditions: allergies, drug abuse or dependence, kidney disease, liver disease, porphyria, epilepsy, or any other seizure disorder.

☰ SIDE EFFECTS ☰

SERIOUS
Fainting; palpitations or rapid heartbeat; fever; hives or severe swelling of face, lips or tongue along with shortness of breath, chest tightness, or wheezing (indicating a potentially life-threatening allergic reaction); depression. Seek medical help immediately.

COMMON
Drowsiness, dizziness, dry mouth.

LESS COMMON
Inability to pass urine; sores on lips; ulcers in mouth; abdominal cramps or pain; clumsiness; unsteady gait; confusion; constipation; diarrhea; excitability, nervousness, restlessness, or irritability; flushing or redness of face; headache; heartburn; hiccups; muscle weakness; nausea and vomiting; trembling; insomnia or fitful sleep; burning, red eyes; stuffy nose.

CEFPROZIL

Available in: Oral suspension, tablets
Available OTC? No   **As Generic?** No
Drug Class: Cephalosporin antibiotic

▼ USAGE INFORMATION

WHY IT'S PRESCRIBED
To treat a variety of bacterial infections, including those of the ear, nose, tonsils, and throat; skin and soft tissues; and the respiratory tract. The drug cefprozil is effective only against infections caused by bacteria; it is ineffective against infections caused by viruses, fungi, or other microorganisms.

HOW IT WORKS
Cefprozil prevents bacteria from forming protective cell walls that are necessary for its survival.

▼ DOSAGE GUIDELINES

RANGE AND FREQUENCY
Adults and teenagers: 250 to 500 mg every 12 to 24 hours. Children ages 2 to 12 years: 7.5 mg per 2.2 lb (1 kg) of body weight every 12 hours. Children 6 months to 12 years: 15 mg per 2.2 lb every 12 hours.

ONSET OF EFFECT
Approximately 90 minutes.

DURATION OF ACTION
Unknown.

DIETARY ADVICE
It may be taken with food to reduce stomach irritation.

STORAGE
Store in a tightly sealed container away from moisture, heat, and direct light. Keep the liquid form refrigerated but do not allow it to freeze.

MISSED DOSE
Take it as soon as you remember. This will help keep a constant level of medication in your system. If it is near the time for the next dose, skip the missed dose and resume your regular dosage schedule. Do not double the next dose.

STOPPING THE DRUG
Take it as prescribed for the full treatment period, even if you begin to feel better before the scheduled end of therapy. Stopping cefprozil prematurely may slow your recovery or lead to a rebound infection, also known as superinfection, in which the heartier strains of bacteria survive and multiply, leading to a more serious and drug-resistant infection. When taking this drug to treat a streptococcal (strep) infection, it is particularly important to take it for the entire treatment period. Serious heart and kidney problems can develop later if the drug is discontinued prematurely.

PROLONGED USE
Cefprozil is generally prescribed for short-term therapy (10 to 14 days). Use of cefprozil beyond this period increases risks of adverse effects and superinfection.

▼ PRECAUTIONS

Over 60: Adverse reactions may be more likely and more severe in older patients.

Driving and Hazardous Work: Do not drive or engage in hazardous work until you determine how the medicine affects you.

Alcohol: Avoid alcohol.

Pregnancy: Adequate studies of cephalosporin use in pregnant women have not been done. Before taking cefprozil, tell your doctor if you are pregnant or are planning to become pregnant.

Breast Feeding: Cefprozil passes into breast milk; caution is advised. Consult your doctor for specific advice.

Infants and Children: Cefprozil may be used by children 6 months and older. Consult your pediatrician for specific advice.

Special Concerns: People who are allergic to penicillin may have equally serious allergic reactions to cephalosporin antibiotics such as cefprozil. This drug is useful only against bacteria that are susceptible to its effects, not against colds, the flu, or other viral infections. If your condition does not improve after a few days of taking cefprozil or instead has worsened, tell your doctor.

OVERDOSE
Symptoms: Seizures, severe abdominal pain, bloody diarrhea, vomiting.

What to Do: Call your doctor, emergency medical services (EMS), or the nearest poison control center immediately.

▼ INTERACTIONS

DRUG INTERACTIONS
Consult your doctor for specific advice if you are getting a carbenicillin injection or are taking heparin, divalproex, anticoagulants, dipyridamole, sulfinpyrazone, pentoxifylline, plicamycin, ticarcillin, probenecid, or valproic acid.

FOOD INTERACTIONS
No known food interactions.

DISEASE INTERACTIONS
Caution is advised when taking cefprozil. Consult your doctor if you have a history of kidney disease, phenylketonuria, or colitis.

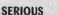

≡ SIDE EFFECTS ≡

SERIOUS
Severe allergic reaction (breathing difficulties, confusion, lightheadedness, itching, hives, swelling of the face or throat, unusual sweating), severe stomach pain and cramps, fever, severe, sometimes bloody diarrhea. Call your doctor immediately.

COMMON
Mild diarrhea or stomach cramps, sore mouth or tongue, nausea and vomiting.

LESS COMMON
Vaginal itching or unusual discharge, decreased white blood cell count causing increased susceptibility to infection, decreased blood platelets causing increased risk of bleeding problems.

CEFUROXIME

BRAND NAMES

Ceftin, Kefurox, Zinacef

Available in: Tablets, injection, oral suspension
Available OTC? No   **As Generic?** Yes
Drug Class: Cephalosporin antibiotic

▼ USAGE INFORMATION

WHY IT'S PRESCRIBED
To treat a variety of bacterial infections, including those of the brain, ear, nose, tonsils, and throat; skin and soft tissues; genitourinary tract; respiratory tract; blood; bones; joints; and other organs. Cefuroxime also is used to treat gonorrhea and is given before some surgeries to prevent infection. It is effective only against susceptible infections caused by bacteria.

HOW IT WORKS
Cefuroxime prevents bacteria from forming cell walls.

▼ DOSAGE GUIDELINES

RANGE AND FREQUENCY
Adults and teenagers—
Tablets: 125 to 500 mg every 12 hours for 5 to 10 days. Injection: 750 to 1,500 mg every 6 to 8 hours into a vein or muscle. Children 3 months to 12 years—Tablets: 125 mg every 12 hours for 10 days. Injection: 16.7 to 33.3 mg per 2.2 lb (1 kg) of body weight every 8 hours into a vein or muscle. Oral suspension: 10 to 15 mg per 2.2 lb every 12 hours for 10 days. Gonorrhea is treated with a one-time tablet dose of 1,000 mg or a one-time injected dose of 1,500 mg into a muscle. The injected dose is divided and administered at two sites on the body, along with a single 1,000-mg oral dose of probenecid.

ONSET OF EFFECT
Into a vein: Immediate. Into a muscle: 15 to 60 minutes. Oral forms: Unknown.

DURATION OF ACTION
5 to 8 hours.

DIETARY ADVICE
Tablets can be taken without regard to meals. Take the oral suspension with food to increase the absorption of the drug by the body. Maintain normal fluid intake.

STORAGE
Store in a tightly sealed container away from moisture, heat, and direct light. Keep liquid form refrigerated, but do not allow it to freeze.

MISSED DOSE
Take it as soon as you remember. If it is near the time for the next dose, skip the missed dose and resume your regular dosage schedule. Do not double the next dose.

STOPPING THE DRUG
Take it as prescribed for the full treatment period. Stopping prematurely may slow your recovery or lead to a rebound infection, also known as superinfection, in which the heartier strains of bacteria survive and multiply, leading to a more serious and drug-resistant infection. When taking this drug to treat a streptococcal (strep) infection, it is particularly important to take it for the entire treatment period. Serious heart and kidney problems can develop later if the drug is discontinued prematurely.

PROLONGED USE
Cefuroxime is generally prescribed for short-term therapy (5 to 10 days). Using the drug beyond this period increases the risks of adverse effects and superinfection.

▼ PRECAUTIONS

Over 60: Adverse reactions may be more likely and more severe in older patients.

Driving and Hazardous Work: Do not drive or engage in hazardous work until you determine how the medicine affects you.

Alcohol: Avoid alcohol.

Pregnancy: Adequate studies of use during pregnancy have not been done. Consult your doctor for advice.

Breast Feeding: Cefuroxime passes into breast milk; caution is advised. Consult your doctor for advice.

Infants and Children: May be used by children 3 months and older. Consult your pediatrician for advice.

Special Concerns: Those who are allergic to penicillin may have equally serious allergic reactions to cephalosporin antibiotics. If your condition has not improved within a few days or instead has worsened, tell your doctor. The tablets and the oral suspension cannot be equally substituted for each other.

OVERDOSE
Symptoms: Seizures, severe abdominal pain, bloody diarrhea, vomiting.

What to Do: Seek medical assistance immediately.

▼ INTERACTIONS

DRUG INTERACTIONS
Consult your doctor if you are taking carbenicillin injection, divalproex, anticoagulants, sulfinpyrazone, dipyridamole, pentoxifylline, plicamycin, ticarcillin, probenecid, or valproic acid.

FOOD INTERACTIONS
No known food interactions.

DISEASE INTERACTIONS
Consult your doctor if you have a history of kidney disease or colitis.

SIDE EFFECTS

SERIOUS
Severe allergic reaction (breathing difficulties, confusion, hives, swelling of the face or throat, lightheadedness), severe stomach pain and cramps, fever, severe, sometimes bloody diarrhea. Call your doctor immediately.

COMMON
Mild diarrhea or stomach cramps, sore mouth or tongue, nausea and vomiting.

LESS COMMON
Vaginal itching or discharge, pain at site of injection, rash, decreased white blood cell count causing increased susceptibility to infection, decreased blood platelets causing increased risk of bleeding problems.

CELECOXIB

Available in: Capsules
Available OTC? No   **As Generic?** No
Drug Class: Nonsteroidal antiinflammatory drug (NSAID)/COX-2 inhibitor

▼ USAGE INFORMATION

WHY IT'S PRESCRIBED
To relieve pain, inflammation, and stiffness of osteoarthritis and rheumatoid arthritis.

HOW IT WORKS
By inhibiting the activity of the enzyme cyclooxygenase-2 (COX-2), celecoxib reduces the synthesis of prostaglandins that play a role in causing arthritis pain and inflammation. It does not inhibit the activity of COX-1, the enzyme involved in the synthesis of prostaglandins that help protect against stomach ulcers and other health problems.

▼ DOSAGE GUIDELINES

RANGE AND FREQUENCY
For osteoarthritis: 200 mg a day. For rheumatoid arthritis: 100 to 200 mg twice a day. To minimize potential gastrointestinal side effects, the lowest effective dose should be used for the shortest possible time.

ONSET OF EFFECT
Within 24 to 48 hours.

DURATION OF ACTION
Unknown.

DIETARY ADVICE
Celecoxib may be taken with or without food.

STORAGE
Store in a tightly sealed container away from moisture, heat, and direct light.

MISSED DOSE
Take it as soon as you remember. If it is near the time for the next dose, skip the missed dose and resume your regular dosage schedule. Do not double the next dose.

STOPPING THE DRUG
The decision to stop taking this prescription medication should be made in consultation with your doctor.

PROLONGED USE
The risk of gastrointestinal side effects may increase with extended use.

▼ PRECAUTIONS

Over 60: Adverse reactions may be more likely and more severe in older patients.

Driving and Hazardous Work: No special problems are expected.

Alcohol: Avoid alcohol when using this medication because it increases the risk of stomach irritation.

Pregnancy: Discuss with your doctor the relative risks and benefits of using this drug while pregnant. Do not use celecoxib during the last trimester.

Breast Feeding: Celecoxib may pass into breast milk; caution is advised. Consult your doctor for advice on whether to discontinue nursing or discontinue the drug.

Infants and Children: The safety and effectiveness of this medication have not been established for children under the age of 18 years.

OVERDOSE
Symptoms: No cases of overdose have been reported. Symptoms may include nausea; lethargy; drowsiness; vomiting; abdominal pain; black, tarry stools; breathing difficulty; and coma.

What to Do: If you suspect an overdose or if someone takes a much larger dose than prescribed, call your doctor, emergency medical services (EMS), or the nearest poison control center immediately.

▼ INTERACTIONS

DRUG INTERACTIONS
Do not take this drug with aspirin or any other NSAIDs without your doctor's approval. Consult your doctor if you are taking furosemide, ACE (angiotensin-converting enzyme) inhibitors, fluconazole, lithium, or warfarin.

FOOD INTERACTIONS
No known food interactions.

DISEASE INTERACTIONS
Celecoxib should not be taken by people who have experienced asthma, hives, or allergic-type reactions after taking aspirin or other NSAIDs. Consult your doctor if you have any of the following: bleeding problems, inflammation or ulcers of the stomach and intestines, asthma, high blood pressure, or heart failure. Use of celecoxib may cause complications in patients with liver or kidney disease, because these organs work together to remove the medication from the body.

 SIDE EFFECTS

SERIOUS
Stomach ulcers. Black, tarry stools may signal stomach bleeding. Symptoms of liver disease (nausea, fatigue, lethargy, itching, yellowish discoloration of the eyes or skin, fluid retention). Call your doctor immediately.

COMMON
Indigestion, diarrhea, and mild abdominal pain.

LESS COMMON
Flatulence, mild swelling, sore throat, upper respiratory tract infection.

CEPHALEXIN

Available in: Capsules, oral suspension, tablets
Available OTC? No   **As Generic?** Yes
Drug Class: Cephalosporin antibiotic

▼ USAGE INFORMATION

WHY IT'S PRESCRIBED
To treat a variety of bacterial infections, including those of the ear, nose, tonsils, and throat; bones; joints; skin and soft tissues; genitourinary tract; and respiratory tract. It is effective only against infections caused by bacteria; it is ineffective against those caused by viruses, fungi, or other microorganisms.

HOW IT WORKS
Cephalexin prevents bacteria from forming cell walls.

▼ DOSAGE GUIDELINES

RANGE AND FREQUENCY
Adults and teenagers: 250 to 500 mg every 6 to 12 hours. Children: 6.25 to 25 mg per 2.2 lb (1 kg) of body weight every 6 hours or 12.5 to 50 mg per 2.2 lb every 12 hours.

ONSET OF EFFECT
1 hour.

DURATION OF ACTION
Unknown.

DIETARY ADVICE
Cephalexin may be taken on a full or empty stomach, but taking it with food will reduce stomach irritation.

STORAGE
Store in a tightly sealed container away from moisture, heat, and direct light. Keep liquid form refrigerated, but do not allow it to freeze.

MISSED DOSE
Take it as soon as you remember. This will help keep a constant level of medication in your system. If it is near the time for the next dose, skip the missed dose and resume your regular dosage schedule. Do not double the next dose.

STOPPING THE DRUG
Take it as prescribed for the full treatment period, even if you begin to feel better before the scheduled end of therapy. Stopping cephalexin prematurely may slow your recovery or lead to a rebound infection, also known as superinfection, in which the heartier strains of bacteria survive and multiply, leading to a more serious and drug-resistant infection. When taking this drug to treat a streptococcal (strep) infection, it is particularly important to take it for the entire treatment period. Serious heart and kidney problems can develop later if it is discontinued prematurely.

PROLONGED USE
Cephalexin is generally prescribed for short-term therapy (10 to 14 days). Further use increases the risk of adverse effects and superinfection.

▼ PRECAUTIONS

Over 60: Adverse reactions may be more likely and more severe in older patients.

Driving and Hazardous Work: Do not drive or engage in hazardous work until you determine how the medicine affects you.

Alcohol: Avoid alcohol.

Pregnancy: Adequate studies of cephalosporin use in pregnant women have not been done. Before you take cephalexin, tell your doctor if you are pregnant or plan to become pregnant.

Breast Feeding: Cephalexin passes into breast milk; caution is advised. Consult your doctor for specific advice.

Infants and Children: Adequate studies of cephalexin use in children have not been done to date. Consult your pediatrician.

Special Concerns: People who are allergic to penicillin may have equally serious allergic reactions to cephalosporin antibiotics such as cephalexin. This drug is useful only against bacteria that are susceptible to its effects, not against colds, the flu, or other viral infections. If your condition has not improved within a few days of starting the medicine or instead has worsened, tell your doctor.

OVERDOSE
Symptoms: Seizures, severe abdominal pain, bloody diarrhea, vomiting.

What to Do: Call your doctor, emergency medical services (EMS), or the nearest poison control center immediately.

▼ INTERACTIONS

DRUG INTERACTIONS
Consult your doctor for specific advice if you are taking carbenicillin injections, heparin, divalproex, anticoagulants, sulfinpyrazone, dipyridamole, pentoxifylline, plicamycin, ticarcillin, probenecid, or valproic acid.

FOOD INTERACTIONS
No known food interactions.

DISEASE INTERACTIONS
Caution is advised when taking cephalexin. Consult your doctor if you have a history of kidney disease or colitis.

≡ SIDE EFFECTS ≡

SERIOUS
Severe allergic reaction (breathing difficulties, confusion, hives, itching, swelling of the face or throat, unusual sweating, lightheadedness), severe stomach pain and cramps, fever, severe, sometimes bloody diarrhea. Call your doctor immediately.

COMMON
Mild diarrhea or stomach cramps, sore mouth or tongue, nausea and vomiting.

LESS COMMON
Vaginal itching or unusual discharge, rash, decreased white blood cell count causing increased susceptibility to infection, decreased blood platelets causing increased risk of bleeding problems.

CEPHRADINE

BRAND NAME

Velosef

Available in: Oral suspension, capsules
Available OTC? No   **As Generic?** Yes
Drug Class: Cephalosporin antibiotic

▼ USAGE INFORMATION

WHY IT'S PRESCRIBED
To treat a variety of bacterial infections, including those of the ear, nose, tonsils, and throat; skin and soft tissues; genitourinary tract; and respiratory tract. Cephradine is effective only against infections caused by bacteria; it is ineffective against those caused by viruses, fungi, or other microorganisms.

HOW IT WORKS
Cephradine prevents bacteria from forming cell walls.

▼ DOSAGE GUIDELINES

RANGE AND FREQUENCY
Oral suspension and capsules—Adults and teenagers: 250 to 500 mg every 6 hours or 500 to 1,000 mg every 12 hours. Children: 6.25 to 25 mg every 6 hours.

ONSET OF EFFECT
1 hour.

DURATION OF ACTION
Unknown.

DIETARY ADVICE
Cephradine may be taken on a full or empty stomach, but taking it with food will reduce stomach irritation.

STORAGE
Store in a tightly sealed container away from moisture, heat, and direct light. Keep liquid form refrigerated, but do not allow it to freeze.

MISSED DOSE
Take it as soon as you remember. This will help keep a constant level of medication in your system. If it is near the time for the next dose, skip the missed dose and resume your regular dosage schedule. Do not double the next dose.

STOPPING THE DRUG
Take it as prescribed for the full treatment period, even if you begin to feel better before the scheduled end of therapy. Stopping cephradine prematurely may slow your recovery or lead to a rebound infection, also known as superinfection, in which the heartier strains of bacteria survive and multiply, leading to a more serious and drug-resistant infection. When taking this drug to treat a streptococcal (strep) infection, it is particularly important to take it for the entire treatment period. Serious heart and kidney problems can develop later if it is discontinued prematurely.

PROLONGED USE
Cephradine is generally prescribed for short-term therapy (10 to 14 days). Use of this antibiotic beyond this time frame increases the risk of adverse effects and superinfection.

▼ PRECAUTIONS

Over 60: Adverse reactions may be more likely and more severe in older patients.

Driving and Hazardous Work: Do not drive or engage in hazardous work until you determine how the medicine affects you.

Alcohol: Avoid alcohol.

Pregnancy: Adequate studies of cephalosporin use during pregnancy have not been done. Consult your doctor for specific advice about using the medication.

Breast Feeding: Cephradine passes into breast milk; caution is advised. Consult your doctor for specific advice.

Infants and Children: Cephradine may be used by children age 1 and older. Consult your pediatrician for specific advice about using the medication.

Special Concerns: People who are allergic to penicillin may have equally serious reactions to cephalosporin antibiotics such as cephradine. This drug is useful only against bacteria that are susceptible to its effects, not against colds, the flu, or other viral infections. If your condition has not improved within a few days of starting to take cephradine or instead has worsened, tell your doctor.

OVERDOSE
Symptoms: Seizures, severe abdominal pain, bloody diarrhea, vomiting.

What to Do: Call your doctor, emergency medical services (EMS), or the nearest poison control center immediately.

▼ INTERACTIONS

DRUG INTERACTIONS
Consult your doctor for specific advice if you are taking carbenicillin injection, heparin, divalproex, anticoagulants, sulfinpyrazone, dipyridamole, pentoxifylline, plicamycin, ticarcillin, probenecid, or valproic acid.

FOOD INTERACTIONS
No known food interactions.

DISEASE INTERACTIONS
Caution is advised when taking cephradine. Consult your doctor if you have a history of kidney disease or colitis.

 SIDE EFFECTS

SERIOUS
Severe allergic reaction (breathing difficulties, confusion, hives, itching, swelling of the face or throat, sweating, lightheadedness), severe stomach pain and cramps, fever, severe, sometimes bloody diarrhea. Call your doctor immediately.

COMMON
Mild diarrhea or stomach cramps, sore mouth or tongue, nausea and vomiting.

LESS COMMON
Vaginal itching or discharge.

CETIRIZINE

BRAND NAME

Zyrtec

Available in: Tablets, syrup
Available OTC? No   **As Generic?** No
Drug Class: Histamine (H1) blocker

▼ USAGE INFORMATION

WHY IT'S PRESCRIBED
For symptomatic relief of perennial and seasonal allergies (including hay fever), itchy skin, and chronic hives.

HOW IT WORKS
Cetirizine blocks the effects of histamine, a naturally occurring substance in the body that causes swelling, itching, sneezing, watery eyes, hives, and other symptoms of allergic reaction.

▼ DOSAGE GUIDELINES

RANGE AND FREQUENCY
Adults and teenagers: 5 to 10 mg once a day. Do not increase the dose to obtain quicker relief of symptoms. A lower dose (no more than 5 mg a day) is recommended for patients with impaired kidney or liver function.

ONSET OF EFFECT
Within 20 to 40 minutes.

DURATION OF ACTION
Approximately 24 hours.

DIETARY ADVICE
Cetirizine can be taken without regard to diet.

STORAGE
Store in a tightly sealed container away from moisture, heat, and direct light. Do not allow the syrup to freeze.

MISSED DOSE
This drug is prescribed to be taken once a day. If you miss a day, skip the missed dose and resume your regular dosage schedule. Do not double the next dose.

STOPPING THE DRUG
Take it as prescribed for the full treatment period, even if you feel better before the scheduled end of therapy.

PROLONGED USE
Safety and effectiveness during prolonged use have yet to be established.

▼ PRECAUTIONS

Over 60:
The dosage may need to be reduced in elderly patients, especially for those individuals who have impaired kidney function.

Driving and Hazardous Work:
Do not drive or engage in hazardous work until you determine how the medication affects you.

Alcohol: Avoid alcohol while taking this medication, because it can magnify side effects such as drowsiness and fatigue.

Pregnancy: Adequate human studies of the use of this drug during pregnancy have not been done; caution is advised. Before taking cetirizine, tell your doctor if you are pregnant or if you plan to become pregnant.

Breast Feeding: Cetirizine passes into breast milk; avoid or discontinue use of this drug while nursing.

Infants and Children: The safety and effectiveness of cetirizine use by children under the age of 12 years have not been established.

Special Concerns: If cetirizine causes dry mouth as a side effect, use sugar-free gum, sugar-free sour hard candy, or ice chips for relief.

OVERDOSE
Symptoms: No cases of overdose have been reported.

What to Do: An overdose of cetirizine is unlikely to be life-threatening. However, if someone takes a much larger dose than prescribed, call your doctor, emergency medical services (EMS), or the nearest poison control center immediately.

▼ INTERACTIONS

DRUG INTERACTIONS
No significant drug interactions have been reported. Cetirizine may, however, increase the depressant effects of alcohol, sedatives, tranquilizers, painkillers, barbiturates, or other antihistamines on the central nervous system. Consult your doctor for specific advice.

FOOD INTERACTIONS
No food interactions have been reported.

DISEASE INTERACTIONS
Cetirizine blood levels may increase in patients with liver or kidney disease, because these organs work together to remove the medication from the body. Reduced doses may be required for such persons.

⯯ SIDE EFFECTS ⯯

SERIOUS
No serious side effects are associated with the use of cetirizine.

COMMON
Drowsiness, fatigue, headache, dry mouth.

LESS COMMON
Nausea and vomiting.

CIMETIDINE

Available in: Tablets, oral solution, oral suspension
Available OTC? Yes   **As Generic?** Yes
Drug Class: Histamine (H2) blocker

▼ USAGE INFORMATION

WHY IT'S PRESCRIBED
To treat ulcers of the stomach and duodenum, as well as other conditions, such as esophagitis (chronic inflammation of the esophagus), and gastroesophageal reflux (backwash of stomach acid into the esophagus, resulting in heartburn).

HOW IT WORKS
Cimetidine blocks the action of histamine (a compound produced in the body's cells), which in turn decreases the stomach's secretion of hydrochloric acid. Once stomach acid production is decreased, the body is better able to heal itself.

▼ DOSAGE GUIDELINES

RANGE AND FREQUENCY
For treatment of acute (symptomatic, bothersome) duodenal or gastric ulcers— Adults and teenagers: Various dosage schedules are used, including 300 mg 4 times a day (with meals and at bedtime), 400 or 600 mg 2 times a day, or 800 mg taken once daily at bedtime. For prevention of duodenal ulcers— Adults and teenagers: Usual dose is 300 mg 2 times a day; another common dosage schedule is 400 mg taken once daily at bedtime. For treatment as needed of heartburn and acid indigestion— Adults and teenagers: 200 mg with water when symptoms start; another 200 mg may be taken within the next 24 hours for a maximum of 400 mg in a 24-hour period. For treatment of gastroesophageal reflux disease— Adults: 800 to 1,600 mg a day in 2 to 4 divided doses for approximately 12 weeks.

ONSET OF EFFECT
Within 1 hour.

DURATION OF ACTION
At least 4 to 5 hours.

DIETARY ADVICE
Avoid foods that cause stomach irritation.

STORAGE
Store away from heat and direct light. Keep the liquid form from freezing.

MISSED DOSE
Take it as soon as you remember. If it is near the time for the next dose, skip the missed dose and resume your regular dosage schedule. Do not double the next dose.

STOPPING THE DRUG
Prescription-strength: Take it for the full treatment period, even if you begin to feel better before the scheduled end of therapy. Nonprescription-strength: Take as needed.

PROLONGED USE
Do not take nonprescription-strength cimetidine for more than 2 weeks unless told to do so by your physician.

▼ PRECAUTIONS

Over 60: Adverse reactions may be more likely and more severe in older patients.

Driving and Hazardous Work: Do not drive or engage in hazardous work until you determine how the medicine affects you.

Alcohol: Avoid alcohol.

Pregnancy: Avoid or discontinue use if you are pregnant or trying to become pregnant.

Breast Feeding: Cimetidine passes into breast milk; avoid or discontinue use while breast feeding.

Infants and Children: Not recommended for use by children under age 16.

Special Concerns: Avoid cigarette smoking because it may increase stomach acid secretion and thus worsen the disease. Do not take cimetidine if you have ever had an allergic reaction to a histamine (H2) blocker. If stomach pain becomes worse while you are using the drug, tell your doctor immediately.

OVERDOSE
Symptoms: No symptoms have been reported.

What to Do: An overdose is unlikely to be life-threatening; however, if someone takes a much larger dose than directed, seek medical assistance immediately.

▼ INTERACTIONS

DRUG INTERACTIONS
Consult your doctor for specific advice if you are taking aminophylline, anticoagulants, caffeine, metoprolol, oxtriphylline, phenytoin, propranolol, theophylline, tricyclic antidepressants, itraconazole, ketoconazole, or metronidazole.

FOOD INTERACTIONS
Carbonated drinks, citrus fruits and juices, beverages containing caffeine, and other acidic foods or liquids may irritate the stomach or interfere with the therapeutic action of cimetidine.

DISEASE INTERACTIONS
Patients with kidney or liver disease or weakened immune systems should not use cimetidine or should use it in smaller, limited doses under careful medical supervision.

▼ SIDE EFFECTS ▼

SERIOUS
Irregular heart rhythm (palpitations), slowed heartbeat, severe blood problems resulting in unusual bleeding, bruising, fever, chills, and increased susceptibility to infection. Call your doctor immediately.

COMMON
Headache, fatigue, drowsiness, dizziness, nausea, vomiting, abdominal pain, diarrhea.

LESS COMMON
Blurred vision, decreased sexual desire or function, swelling of breasts in males or females, temporary hair loss, hallucinations, depression, insomnia, skin rash, hives, or redness.

CIPROFLOXACIN SYSTEMIC

Available in: Tablets, oral suspension
Available OTC? No   **As Generic?** No
Drug Class: Fluoroquinolone antibiotic

▼ USAGE INFORMATION

WHY IT'S PRESCRIBED
To treat mild to severe bacterial infections, including those of the urinary tract, lower respiratory tract, bones and joints, and skin. It is also used to treat certain sexually transmitted diseases (such as chancroid and gonorrhea) and diarrhea caused by a bacterial infection.

HOW IT WORKS
Ciprofloxacin inhibits the activity of a bacterial enzyme (gyrase) that is necessary for proper DNA formation and replication. This fights infection by preventing bacteria cells from reproducing.

▼ DOSAGE GUIDELINES

RANGE AND FREQUENCY
250 to 750 mg every 12 hours (2 times a day) for 5 to 14 days, depending on kidney function and the infection being treated. Gonorrhea is usually treated with a one-time dose of 250 mg.

ONSET OF EFFECT
Varies depending on the infection being treated.

DURATION OF ACTION
Unknown.

DIETARY ADVICE
Be sure to drink plenty of fluids, but avoid milk and dairy derivatives.

STORAGE
Store in a tightly sealed container away from heat and direct light.

MISSED DOSE
Take it as soon as you remember. If it is near the time for the next dose, skip the missed dose and resume your regular dosage schedule. Do not double the next dose.

STOPPING THE DRUG
Take the drug as prescribed for the full treatment period, even if you begin to feel better before the scheduled end of therapy.

PROLONGED USE
See your doctor regularly for tests and examinations if you must take this medicine for a prolonged period.

▼ PRECAUTIONS

Over 60: No special problems are expected.

Driving and Hazardous Work: Do not drive or engage in hazardous work until you determine how the medicine affects you.

Alcohol: It is advisable to abstain from alcohol when fighting an infection.

Pregnancy: In some animal tests, ciprofloxacin has caused birth defects. Adequate studies in humans have not been done. The drug should be used during pregnancy only if potential benefits clearly justify the risks. Before you take ciprofloxacin, tell your doctor if you are pregnant or plan to become pregnant.

Breast Feeding: Ciprofloxacin passes into breast milk and may cause serious side effects in the nursing infant; use of the drug is discouraged when nursing.

Infants and Children: Ciprofloxacin is not recommended for use by persons under the age of 18 years, because it has been shown to interfere with bone development.

Special Concerns: If ciprofloxacin causes sensitivity to sunlight, stop taking the drug and try to avoid exposure to sunlight for the next 5 days; also wear protective clothing and use a sunblock. Ciprofloxacin should not be taken by patients whose work makes it impossible to avoid exposure to sunlight. It is important to drink plenty of fluids while taking this drug.

OVERDOSE
Symptoms: No specific symptoms have been reported.

What to Do: If you have any reason to suspect an overdose, call your doctor, emergency medical services (EMS), or the nearest poison control center.

▼ INTERACTIONS

DRUG INTERACTIONS
Consult your doctor for specific advice if you are taking aminophylline, antacids, didanosine, iron supplements, oxtriphylline, sucralfate, theophylline, warfarin, or zinc salts. Also tell your doctor if you are taking any other prescription or over-the-counter medication.

FOOD INTERACTIONS
The effects of caffeine may be magnified by this drug. Milk and dairy products can reduce blood levels of ciprofloxacin by as much as half.

DISEASE INTERACTIONS
Caution is advised when taking ciprofloxacin. Consult your doctor if you have any other medical condition. Use of ciprofloxacin can cause complications in patients with kidney disease, because this organ works to remove the medication from the body.

SIDE EFFECTS

SERIOUS
Serious reactions to ciprofloxacin are rare and include seizures, mental confusion, hallucinations, agitation, nightmares, depression, shortness of breath, unusual swelling in the face or extremities, and loss of consciousness. Also skin burning, redness, blisters, rash, or itching on exposure to sunlight. Call your doctor immediately.

COMMON
Increased sensitivity to sunlight (and increased risk of sunburn) for days following therapy.

LESS COMMON
Diarrhea, nausea and vomiting, stomach pain and upset, gas, headache, dizziness, insomnia, changes in taste perception, drowsiness, itching, dry mouth, unusual body aches or pains.

CITALOPRAM HYDROBROMIDE

BRAND NAME

Celexa

Available in: Tablet, oral solution
Available OTC? No   **As Generic?** No
Drug Class: Selective serotonin reuptake inhibitor (SSRI) antidepressant

▼ USAGE INFORMATION

WHY IT'S PRESCRIBED
To treat symptoms of major depression.

HOW IT WORKS
Citalopram increases brain levels of serotonin, a chemical that is thought to be linked to mood, emotions, and mental state.

▼ DOSAGE GUIDELINES

RANGE AND FREQUENCY
To start, 20 mg once a day taken in the morning or evening; dose may be gradually increased by your doctor to 40 mg a day.

ONSET OF EFFECT
Unknown.

DURATION OF ACTION
Unknown.

DIETARY ADVICE
No special restrictions.

STORAGE
Store in a tightly sealed container away from moisture, heat, and direct light.

MISSED DOSE
If you miss a dose on one day, do not double the dose the next day.

STOPPING THE DRUG
Take the drug as prescribed for the full treatment period, even if you notice improvement. When it is time to stop therapy, your dosage will be lowered gradually by your doctor.

PROLONGED USE
Usual course of therapy for depression lasts 6 months to 1 year; some patients may benefit from additional therapy with this drug.

▼ PRECAUTIONS

Over 60: Adverse reactions may be more likely and more severe in older patients. A lower dose may be warranted.

Driving and Hazardous Work: Use caution when driving or engaging in hazardous work until you determine how the medicine affects you.

Alcohol: Avoid alcohol.

Pregnancy: Citalopram should be used during pregnancy only if the potential benefit justifies the potential risk to the fetus. Before you take this medicine, tell your doctor if you are pregnant or plan to become pregnant.

Breast Feeding: Citalopram passes into breast milk; caution is advised. Consult your doctor for specific advice.

Infants and Children: The safety and effectiveness of the use of citalopram in children under age 18 years have not been established.

OVERDOSE
Symptoms: Dizziness, nausea, sweating, vomiting, trembling, drowsiness, rapid heartbeat.

What to Do: Call your doctor, emergency medical services (EMS), or the nearest poison control center immediately.

▼ INTERACTIONS

DRUG INTERACTIONS
Citalopram and MAO inhibitors should not be used within 14 days of each other. Very serious side effects such as myoclonus (uncontrolled muscle spasms), hyperthermia (excessive rise in body temperature), and extreme stiffness may result. The following drugs may also interact with citalopram; consult your doctor for advice if you are taking cimetidine, warfarin, lithium, carbamazepine, antifungals (such as ketoconazole, itraconazole, and fluconazole), erythromycin antibiotics, omeprazole, tricyclic antidepressants, or any prescription or over-the-counter drugs that depress the central nervous system (this includes antihistamine medications, barbiturates, sedatives, cough medicines, and decongestants).

FOOD INTERACTIONS
No known food interactions.

DISEASE INTERACTIONS
Caution is advised when taking citalopram, especially if you have heart disease or a seizure disorder. Use of citalopram may cause complications in patients with liver or kidney disease.

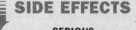
≡ SIDE EFFECTS ≡

SERIOUS
Chest pain, rapid or irregular heartbeat, lightheadedness or fainting. Call your doctor immediately.

COMMON
Delayed ejaculation (males); dry mouth; increased sweating; nausea; trembling; diarrhea; drowsiness; numbness, tingling, or prickling sensations.

LESS COMMON
Fatigue, fever, loss of appetite, agitation, nasal congestion, sinus infection, erectile dysfunction.

CLARITHROMYCIN

BRAND NAME

Biaxin

Available in: Tablets, oral suspension
Available OTC? No **As Generic?** No
Drug Class: Macrolide antibiotic

▼ USAGE INFORMATION

WHY IT'S PRESCRIBED
To treat various bacterial infections, including those of the sinuses, tonsils, and respiratory tract (such as bronchitis and pneumonia); ear infections; and venereal disease caused by chlamydial infection. Clarithromycin may also be used to treat certain skin infections, Legionnaires' disease, Lyme disease, and peptic ulcers caused by the bacterium *Helicobacter pylori*. Also used to prevent and, when taken with other drugs, treat a tuberculosis-like disease known as *Mycobacterium avium* complex (MAC), which is common in people with advanced acquired immunodeficiency syndrome (AIDS).

HOW IT WORKS
Clarithromycin prevents bacterial cells from manufacturing the specific proteins that are necessary for their survival.

▼ DOSAGE GUIDELINES

RANGE AND FREQUENCY
For bacterial infections—Usual adult dose: 250 to 500 mg every 12 hours for 7 to 14 days. Children 6 months of age or older: 3.4 mg per lb of body weight, up to 500 mg every 12 hours for 10 days. To prevent MAC—500 mg 2 times a day. To treat MAC—500 mg 2 times a day in combination with other medications.

ONSET OF EFFECT
Within 2 hours; full effect may take 2 to 5 days to occur.

DURATION OF ACTION
Unknown.

DIETARY ADVICE
Clarithromycin may be taken with or without food. Drink plenty of liquids.

STORAGE
Store in a tightly sealed container away from moisture, heat, and direct light.

MISSED DOSE
Take it as soon as you remember. If it is near the time for the next dose, skip the missed dose and resume your regular dosing schedule. Do not double the next dose. If you are taking 2 doses a day, wait 5 to 6 hours before taking the next dose.

STOPPING THE DRUG
For acute infections, take it exactly as prescribed for the full treatment period, even if you feel better before the scheduled end of therapy. Therapy for prevention of MAC should be lifelong.

PROLONGED USE
You may become susceptible to infections caused by germs that are not responsive to clarithromycin. Also, severe drug-induced gastrointestinal problems may result from long-term use.

▼ PRECAUTIONS

Over 60: Older patients, especially those with kidney disease, may require a decrease in dose.

Driving and Hazardous Work: No special precautions are necessary.

Alcohol: No special precautions are necessary.

Pregnancy: Adequate studies of the use of this drug during pregnancy have not been done; discuss potential risks and benefits with your doctor.

Breast Feeding: It is not known if clarithromycin passes into breast milk; consult your doctor for advice.

Infants and Children: No special problems are expected.

OVERDOSE
Symptoms: Severe nausea, vomiting, diarrhea, abdominal discomfort.

What to Do: Call your doctor, emergency medical services (EMS), or the nearest poison control center immediately.

▼ INTERACTIONS

DRUG INTERACTIONS
This drug should not be taken by patients known to have had allergic reactions to erythromycins or other macrolide antibiotics in the past. Do not take clarithromycin if you are taking astemizole, pimozide, or cisapride. Also, alert your doctor if you are taking any of the following drugs: carbamazepine, digoxin, theophylline, warfarin, rifabutin, rifampin, or zidovudine.

FOOD INTERACTIONS
No known food interactions.

DISEASE INTERACTIONS
Consult your doctor if you have a history of a blood disorder, liver disease, or any allergy.

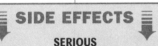

≣ SIDE EFFECTS ≣

SERIOUS
Colitis (inflammation of the lower gastrointestinal tract, with symptoms including severe abdominal pain, watery or bloody stools, severe diarrhea, and fever); liver toxicity (causing fever, nausea, vomiting, and yellowish tinge to eyes or skin); allergic reaction (swelling of the lips, tongue, face, and throat; breathing difficulty; skin rash or hives); blood clotting disorders (causing unusual bleeding and bruising); confusion or change in behavior; heartbeat irregularities in patients with predisposing heart conditions. Such side effects are rare, but if they do occur, stop taking the drug and seek medical assistance immediately.

COMMON
No common side effects.

LESS COMMON
Changes in taste perception; mild abdominal pain or discomfort; mild diarrhea; mild nausea or vomiting; headache; oral thrush (fungal infections of the mouth or throat).

CLINDAMYCIN

BRAND NAMES

Cleocin, Cleocin Pediatric, Cleocin T Gel, Cleocin T Topical Solution, Cleocin Vaginal Ovules, Clinda-Derm

Available in: Capsules, oral solution, injection, topical forms, vaginal suppositories
Available OTC? No   **As Generic?** Yes
Drug Class: Antibiotic

▼ USAGE INFORMATION

WHY IT'S PRESCRIBED
Clindamycin is used orally and by injection to treat serious bacterial infections. It is used topically to treat acne and vaginal infections.

HOW IT WORKS
Clindamycin inhibits the synthesis of protein in bacterial organisms.

▼ DOSAGE GUIDELINES

RANGE AND FREQUENCY
For systemic infections (oral forms)– Adults and teenagers: 150 to 300 mg 4 times a day. Children 1 month and older: See your pediatrician. For systemic infections (injection)– Your doctor will determine the appropriate dose. For acne (gel, solution, or suspension)– Adults and teenagers: Apply 2 times a day. Use and dose for children under 12 years must be determined by your doctor. For vaginal infections (vaginal cream)– Nonpregnant adults and teenagers: 100 mg inserted in vagina once daily at bedtime for 3 or 7 days (7-day therapy is prescribed for pregnant patients). Dose for children must be determined by your doctor. For bacterial vaginal infections (vaginal suppositories)– Nonpregnant adults and teenagers: 1 suppository (containing 100 mg) inserted in vagina once daily at bedtime for 3 days.

ONSET OF EFFECT
Unknown.

DURATION OF ACTION
Unknown.

DIETARY ADVICE
Take the oral forms with food to minimize stomach upset. Take the capsule with water.

STORAGE
Store in a tightly sealed container away from heat, moisture, and direct light. Do not refrigerate the liquid forms, cream, or suppositories.

MISSED DOSE
Take it as soon as you remember. If it is near the time for the next dose, skip the missed dose and resume your regular dosage schedule. Do not double the next dose.

STOPPING THE DRUG
Take it as prescribed for the full treatment period.

PROLONGED USE
See your doctor regularly for tests and examinations if you must take this medicine for a prolonged period.

▼ PRECAUTIONS

Over 60: No special problems are expected.

Driving and Hazardous Work: No special problems are expected.

Alcohol: It is advisable to abstain from alcohol when fighting an infection.

Pregnancy: Consult your doctor before taking it during pregnancy.

Breast Feeding: Clindamycin may pass into breast milk; consult your doctor for specific advice.

Infants and Children: Adequate studies of clindamycin use by children have not been done, although no special problems are expected.

Special Concerns: Wash and dry the skin thoroughly before applying the gel, topical solution, or suspension. When using vaginal cream or suppository, avoid sexual intercourse. Clindamycin may weaken latex or rubber products, such as condoms and vaginal contraceptive diaphragms; use of such products is not recommended within 72 hours of the application of these forms. Do not use other vaginal products, such as tampons or douches, when using the suppositories.

OVERDOSE
Symptoms: None reported.

What to Do: If you have reason to suspect an overdose, call your doctor, emergency medical services (EMS), or the nearest poison control.

▼ INTERACTIONS

DRUG INTERACTIONS
Consult your doctor for advice if you are taking chloramphenicol, erythromycin, or any diarrhea medicine containing kaopectate or attapulgite.

FOOD INTERACTIONS
No known food interactions.

DISEASE INTERACTIONS
Consult your doctor if you have a history of kidney disease, liver disease, or intestinal or stomach disease, especially colitis. The vaginal suppositories should not be used if you have a history of enteritis, ulcerative colitis, or "antibiotic-associated" colitis.

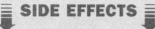
▼ SIDE EFFECTS ▼

SERIOUS
For oral forms, injection, gel, solution, and suspension: Severe stomach or abdominal pains and cramps, weight loss, severe diarrhea, fever, sore throat, skin rash, itching, and redness, unusual bleeding or bruising. For vaginal cream and suppositories: Itching of genital area, pain during intercourse, whitish vaginal discharge, diarrhea, dizziness, headache, nausea, vomiting, stomach cramps or pain. Call your doctor immediately.

COMMON
For oral forms: Mild diarrhea, nausea, vomiting, stomach pain. For gel, topical solution, and suspension: Dry, peeling, or scaly skin.

LESS COMMON
For oral forms: Itching of rectal or genital regions. For topical forms: Stomach pain, mild diarrhea, irritated or oily skin, stinging or burning skin, dizziness (cream and suppository), headache (cream and suppository).

CLONAZEPAM

Available in: Tablets, wafer
Available OTC? No   **As Generic?** Yes
Drug Class: Benzodiazepine tranquilizer; antianxiety agent

▼ USAGE INFORMATION

WHY IT'S PRESCRIBED
To control seizures; for relief of anxiety and panic attacks.

HOW IT WORKS
In general, clonazepam produces mild sedation by depressing activity in the central nervous system (the brain and spinal cord). In particular, clonazepam appears to enhance the effect of gamma-aminobutyric acid (GABA), a natural chemical that inhibits firing of neurons and dampens transmission of nerve signals, thus decreasing nervous excitation.

▼ DOSAGE GUIDELINES

RANGE AND FREQUENCY
Adults: Initial dose of 0.5 mg 3 times a day. Patients with seizures may require significantly higher doses. Your doctor will determine the optimal dose. Maximum dose rarely exceeds 20 mg a day.

Children: Dose is based on age and body weight.

ONSET OF EFFECT
Within 1 to 2 hours.

DURATION OF ACTION
Less than 24 hours.

DIETARY ADVICE
No special restrictions.

STORAGE
Store in a tightly sealed container away from moisture, heat, and direct light.

MISSED DOSE
Take it as soon as you remember, unless your next scheduled dose is within the next 2 hours. If so, do not take the missed dose. Take your next scheduled dose at the proper time and resume your regular dosage schedule. Do not double the next dose.

STOPPING THE DRUG
Discontinuing the drug abruptly may produce withdrawal symptoms (sleep disruption, nervousness, irritability, diarrhea, abdominal cramps, muscle aches, memory impairment). Dosage should be reduced gradually according to your doctor's instructions.

PROLONGED USE
Short-term therapy (8 weeks or less) is typical; do not take it for a longer period unless so advised by your doctor.

▼ PRECAUTIONS

Over 60: Adverse reactions are more likely and more severe in older patients.

Driving and Hazardous Work: Clonazepam can impair mental alertness and physical coordination. Adjust your activities accordingly.

Alcohol: Alcohol must be avoided while taking this medication.

Pregnancy: Taking clonazepam during pregnancy is not recommended.

Breast Feeding: Clonazepam passes into breast milk and may be harmful to the infant; do not take it while nursing.

Infants and Children: This drug is rarely prescribed for young patients.

Special Concerns: Clonazepam use can lead to psychological or physical dependence. Never take more than the prescribed daily dose.

OVERDOSE
Symptoms: Extreme drowsiness, confusion, slurred speech, slow reflexes, poor coordination, staggering gait, tremor, slowed breathing, loss of consciousness.

What to Do: Call your doctor, emergency medical services (EMS), or the nearest poison control center immediately.

▼ INTERACTIONS

DRUG INTERACTIONS
Other drugs may interact with clonazepam. Consult your doctor for specific advice if you are taking any drugs that depress the central nervous system; these include antihistamines, antidepressants or other psychiatric medications, barbiturates, sedatives, cough medicines, decongestants, and painkillers. Be sure your doctor knows about any over-the-counter medication you may take.

FOOD INTERACTIONS
None reported.

DISEASE INTERACTIONS
Caution is advised when taking clonazepam. Consult your doctor if you have a history of alcohol or drug abuse, stroke or other brain disease, any chronic lung disease, hyperactivity, depression or other mental illness, sleep apnea, myasthenia gravis, epilepsy, porphyria, kidney disease, or liver disease.

 SIDE EFFECTS

SERIOUS
Difficulty concentrating, outbursts of anger, other behavior problems, depression, hallucinations, low blood pressure (causing faintness or confusion), memory impairment, muscle weakness, skin rash or itching, sore throat, fever and chills, sores or ulcers in throat or mouth, unusual bruising or bleeding, extreme fatigue, yellowish tinge to eyes or skin. Call your doctor immediately.

COMMON
Drowsiness, loss of coordination, unsteady gait, dizziness, lightheadedness, slurred speech.

LESS COMMON
Change in sexual desire or ability, constipation, false sense of well-being (euphoria), nausea and vomiting, urinary problems, unusual fatigue.

CLONIDINE HYDROCHLORIDE

BRAND NAMES

Catapres, Catapres-TTS

Available in: Tablets, skin patch
Available OTC? No   **As Generic?** Yes
Drug Class: Centrally acting antihypertensive

▼ USAGE INFORMATION

WHY IT'S PRESCRIBED
To treat high blood pressure (hypertension).

HOW IT WORKS
Clonidine acts on certain areas of the central nervous system (the brain and spinal cord) that regulate the activity of the heart and the smooth muscle tissue surrounding the arteries. It causes the blood vessels to relax and widen, which lowers blood pressure.

▼ DOSAGE GUIDELINES

RANGE AND FREQUENCY
Tablets—Adults: Initial dose is 0.1 mg 2 times a day. Your doctor may increase this to 0.3 mg 2 times a day. Most patients achieve adequate blood pressure control with 1 mg or less a day; maximum daily dose is 2.4 mg. Children: Pediatrician will determine proper dosage. Skin patch—The starting dose is one TTS-1 patch per week. Doses higher than two TTS-3 patches per week are usually not effective. The patch should be applied to a hairless area of skin, ideally on the chest or on the upper arm. The skin must be free of rashes, blisters, or any form of skin disease.

ONSET OF EFFECT
Tablets: 30 to 60 minutes. Skin patch: 2 to 3 days.

DURATION OF ACTION
Tablets: Up to 8 hours. Skin patch: 7 days per patch if patch is left in place as directed; otherwise, up to 8 hours from the time the patch is removed.

DIETARY ADVICE
Follow a healthy diet (low-salt, low-fat, low-cholesterol) as advised by your doctor to help control blood pressure and prevent heart disease.

STORAGE
Store in a tightly sealed container away from moisture, heat, and direct light.

MISSED DOSE
Take your missed dose as soon as you remember, unless the time for your next scheduled dose is within the next 2 hours. If so, do not take the missed dose. Take your next dose at the proper time and resume your regular dosage schedule. Do not take a double dose. If you miss more than 1 day of clonidine, inform your doctor.

STOPPING THE DRUG
Stopping clonidine abruptly can lead to a dangerous increase in blood pressure. Do not stop taking clonidine on your own, even if you are feeling better. Your doctor will gradually decrease your dose if necessary.

PROLONGED USE
Long-term use may be necessary and may lead to an increased risk of side effects.

▼ PRECAUTIONS

Over 60: Adverse reactions may be more likely and more severe in older patients.

Driving and Hazardous Work: This medication may cause drowsiness and dizziness; avoid potentially dangerous activities until you know how it affects you.

Alcohol: Avoid alcohol while taking this drug.

Pregnancy: Clonidine use is not recommended during pregnancy.

Breast Feeding: Clonidine passes into breast milk; consult your doctor for advice.

Infants and Children: This drug is not recommended for young patients.

Special Concerns: Blood pressure may rise significantly after missing a few doses.

Signs of dangerously high blood pressure are chest pain, dizziness, headache, blurred vision, confusion, restlessness, trembling of hands and fingers, anxiety, stomach pains, nausea, and vomiting. Make sure you have enough clonidine to last through weekends, vacations, or extended trips. Apply each skin patch to a different area of the chest or upper arm.

OVERDOSE
Symptoms: Low blood pressure; slow heartbeat; difficulty breathing; severe dizziness; confusion; weakness or faintness; tiny, constricted pupils.

What to Do: Call your doctor, emergency medical services (EMS), or the nearest poison control center immediately.

▼ INTERACTIONS

DRUG INTERACTIONS
Consult your doctor if you are taking beta-blockers or tricyclic antidepressants.

FOOD INTERACTIONS
No known food interactions.

DISEASE INTERACTIONS
Tell your doctor if you have any of the following problems: heart or blood vessel disease, including strokes and cardiac arrhythmias; skin disease, such as scleroderma (a concern with the skin patch only); kidney disease; mental depression; Raynaud's syndrome; or systemic lupus erythematosus.

≣ SIDE EFFECTS ≣

SERIOUS
Serious side effects are less likely when clonidine is used as directed.

COMMON
Dry mouth, reduced saliva, drowsiness, dizziness, constipation. Also itching or skin irritation (with skin patch only).

LESS COMMON
Mental depression, swelling of feet and lower legs, pale or cold fingertips and toes, vivid dreams or nightmares. Also darkening of skin (skin patch only).

CLOPIDOGREL BISULFATE

Available in: Tablets
Available OTC? No   **As Generic?** No
Drug Class: Antiplatelet drug

▼ USAGE INFORMATION

WHY IT'S PRESCRIBED
To reduce the risk of recurrence of heart attack or stroke in patients diagnosed with severe arterial disease (atherosclerosis).

HOW IT WORKS
Heart attacks and strokes occur when a blood clot that forms in a narrowed portion of an artery blocks blood flow and thus cuts off the supply of oxygen and nutrients to the tissue that lies beyond the site of the clot. Clopidogrel can prevent heart attacks and strokes by preventing the aggregation (clumping) of platelets, a type of blood cell that initiates clot formation.

▼ DOSAGE GUIDELINES

RANGE AND FREQUENCY
75 mg once a day.

ONSET OF EFFECT
2 hours or more.

DURATION OF ACTION
Unknown.

DIETARY ADVICE
Clopidogrel can be taken with or without food.

STORAGE
Store in a tightly sealed container away from moisture, heat, and direct light.

MISSED DOSE
If you miss a dose on one day, do not double the dose the next day. Instead, resume your regular dosage schedule.

STOPPING THE DRUG
Take it as prescribed for the full treatment period.

PROLONGED USE
Side effects are more likely with prolonged use.

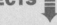

≡ SIDE EFFECTS ≡

SERIOUS
Gastrointestinal bleeding, fainting, palpitations, extreme fatigue, shortness of breath, chest pain. Call your doctor immediately. In rare instances, the drug can block production of white blood cells (a major component of the immune system), leading to potentially severe infections. Seek medical attention promptly at the first signs of infection, especially a high fever.

COMMON
Stomach pain, indigestion, diarrhea, skin rash, itching, flu-like symptoms, body aches or pain, headache, dizziness, joint pain, back pain, increased risk of upper respiratory infection.

LESS COMMON
General weakness, hernia, leg cramps, tingling and numbness in the limbs, vomiting, gout, arthritis, anxiety, insomnia, anemia, dermatitis and skin eruptions, bladder infection, cataract, conjunctivitis.

▼ PRECAUTIONS

Over 60: No special problems are expected.

Driving and Hazardous Work: The use of this drug should not impair your ability to perform such tasks safely.

Alcohol: No special precautions are necessary.

Pregnancy: Adequate human studies have not been done. Before taking clopidogrel, be sure to tell your doctor if you are pregnant or are planning to become pregnant.

Breast Feeding: Clopidogrel passes into breast milk; extreme caution is advised. Consult your doctor for specific advice.

Infants and Children: The safety and effectiveness of clopidogrel use in infants and children have not been established.

Special Concerns: Tell the surgeon or dentist that you are taking this drug before you schedule surgery.

OVERDOSE
Symptoms: No overdose symptoms have been reported.

What to Do: If a greatly excessive dose is taken, call your doctor, emergency medical services (EMS), or the nearest poison control center.

▼ INTERACTIONS

DRUG INTERACTIONS
Consult your doctor for specific advice if you are taking any of the following drugs that may interact with clopidogrel: aspirin or any other nonsteroidal antiinflammatory drugs (NSAIDs), phenytoin, tamoxifen, tolbutamide, torsemide, fluvastatin, or warfarin.

FOOD INTERACTIONS
No known food interactions.

DISEASE INTERACTIONS
This drug should not be used if you have a peptic ulcer or a history of brain hemorrhage. Caution is advised when taking clopidogrel. Consult your doctor if you have a history of bleeding problems or if you develop bleeding problems while taking this drug. Use of clopidogrel may cause complications in patients with liver disease, because the liver inactivates the drug.

CODEINE

BRAND NAMES

Codeine is available in generic form only.

Available in: Tablets, oral solution
Available OTC? No   **As Generic?** Yes
Drug Class: Opioid (narcotic) analgesic

▼ USAGE INFORMATION

WHY IT'S PRESCRIBED
To treat mild to moderate pain or to control a severe cough.

HOW IT WORKS
Narcotics such as codeine relieve pain by acting on specific areas of the spinal cord and brain that process pain signals from nerves throughout the body. Codeine dulls the cough reflex, which is why it may be used to treat certain coughs.

▼ DOSAGE GUIDELINES

RANGE AND FREQUENCY
Adults—For pain: 15 to 60 mg every 3 to 6 hours as needed; usual dose is 30 mg. For cough: 10 to 20 mg every 3 to 6 hours as needed. Children—Oral solution: For pain: 0.5 mg per 2.2 lb (1 kg) of body weight every 4 to 6 hours as needed. For cough: Age 2 years: 3 mg every 4 to 6 hours. Take no more than 12 mg a day. Age 3 years: 3.5 mg every 4 to 6 hours. Take no more than 14 mg a day. Age 4 years: 4 mg every 4 to 6 hours, no more than 16 mg a day. Age 5 years: 4.5 mg every 4 to 6 hours, no more than 18 mg a day. Ages 6 to 12 years: 5 to 10 mg every 4 to 6 hours, no more than 60 mg per day.

ONSET OF EFFECT
30 to 45 minutes.

DURATION OF ACTION
4 to 6 hours.

DIETARY ADVICE
Codeine is constipating; make sure your diet contains adequate amounts of fiber and vegetables.

STORAGE
Store in a tightly sealed container away from moisture, heat, and direct light.

MISSED DOSE
Take it as soon as you remember. If it is near the time for the next dose, skip the missed dose and resume your regular dosage schedule. Do not double the next dose.

STOPPING THE DRUG
You should take the drug as prescribed for the full treatment period, but you may stop taking the drug if you are feeling better before the scheduled end of therapy.

PROLONGED USE
Therapy varies, depending on the cause of the pain. Some patients require long-term narcotic therapy. Side effects may be more likely with prolonged use.

▼ PRECAUTIONS

Over 60: Adverse reactions may be more likely and more severe in older patients.

Driving and Hazardous Work: The use of codeine may impair your ability to perform such tasks safely.

Alcohol: Avoid alcohol.

Pregnancy: Adequate human studies have not been completed. Before taking codeine, tell your physician if you are pregnant or plan to become pregnant.

Breast Feeding: Codeine passes into breast milk; caution is advised. Consult your doctor for specific advice.

Infants and Children: Adverse reactions may be more likely and more severe in children.

Special Concerns: Codeine can cause physical dependence. Some patients may experience withdrawal symptoms when the medication is discontinued. These may include body aches, abdominal pain, stomach cramps, diarrhea, runny nose, goose bumps, nervousness, agita-tion, sweating, yawning, loss of appetite, shivering, insomnia, dilated pupils, and weakness. Do not exceed recommended doses or increase the dose on your own.

OVERDOSE
Symptoms: Confusion; sleepiness; slurred speech; unconsciousness; small, pinpoint pupils; cold, clammy skin; slow breathing; seizures; severe drowsiness, weakness, or dizziness.

What to Do: Call your doctor, emergency medical services (EMS), or the nearest poison control center immediately.

▼ INTERACTIONS

DRUG INTERACTIONS
Consult your doctor for specific advice if you are taking carbamazepine or other medicine for seizures, barbiturates, sedatives, cough medicines, decongestants, antidepressants, other prescription pain medications, MAO inhibitors, naltrexone, rifampin, or zidovudine.

FOOD INTERACTIONS
None known.

DISEASE INTERACTIONS
Consult your doctor if you have any of the following: emotional illness; brain disorders or head injury; seizures; lung disease; prostate problems or other problems with urination; gallstones; colitis; heart, kidney, liver, or thyroid disease; or a history of alcohol or drug abuse.

⬇ SIDE EFFECTS ⬇

SERIOUS
Serious side effects of codeine are indistinguishable from those of overdose: Confusion; sleepiness; slurred speech; unconsciousness; small, pinpoint pupils; cold, clammy skin; slow breathing; seizures; and severe drowsiness, weakness, or dizziness.

COMMON
Mild dizziness or lightheadedness, nausea or vomiting, constipation, drowsiness, itching.

LESS COMMON
Headache, sweating, false sense of well-being (euphoria).

CONTRACEPTIVES, ORAL (COMBINATION PRODUCTS)

Available in: Tablets
Available OTC? No **As Generic?** Yes
Drug Class: Hormones, estrogen with progestins

BRAND NAMES

Brevicon, Demulen, Desogen, Genora, Intercon, Jenest, Levlen, Levora, Lo/Ovral, Loestrin, Mircette, ModiCon, N.E.E., Necon, Nelova, Nordette, Norethin, Norinyl, Ortho Tri-Cyclen, Ortho-Cept, Ortho-Cyclen, Ortho-Novum, Ovcon, Ovral, Tri-Levlen, Tri-Norinyl, Triphasil, Trivora-21, Trivora-28, Zovia

▼ USAGE INFORMATION

WHY IT'S PRESCRIBED
To prevent pregnancy.

HOW IT WORKS
Such products stop a woman's egg from fully developing each month.

▼ DOSAGE GUIDELINES

RANGE AND FREQUENCY
For 21-day cycle: 1 tablet a day for 21 days. Skip 7 days; repeat the cycle. For 28-day cycle: 1 tablet a day for 28 days. Repeat cycle. Each package of pills has 21 active tablets only or 21 active tablets and 7 placebos. When taking placebos or no tablets, menstruation should occur.

ONSET OF EFFECT
At least 7 days.

DURATION OF ACTION
As long as tablets are taken.

DIETARY ADVICE
Take it with food if stomach upset occurs.

STORAGE
Store in a tightly sealed container away from heat and direct light.

MISSED DOSE
If you miss the first tablet of a new cycle or 1 tablet during the cycle, take the missed tablet as soon as you remember and take the next tablet at the usual time. If you miss 2 tablets in a row in the first or second week, take 2 tablets the day you remember and 2 the next day, then resume normal dosage schedule and use another birth control method until the next cycle begins. If you miss 2 tablets during the third week or 3 tablets at any time, begin a new cycle on its scheduled starting day, but use another birth control method for 7 days into the new cycle.

STOPPING THE DRUG
You may stop at any time you choose after completing a full 21-day cycle of tablets.

PROLONGED USE
See your doctor at least every 6 months.

▼ PRECAUTIONS

Over 60: Generally not used by older persons.

Driving and Hazardous Work: No special precautions are necessary.

Alcohol: No special precautions are necessary.

Pregnancy: Discontinue use if you become pregnant or suspect that you might be pregnant.

Breast Feeding: Oral contraceptive hormones pass into breast milk; avoid or discontinue use while nursing.

Infants and Children: No special problems have been found in teenagers who use oral contraception.

Special Concerns: Limit your exposure to sunlight until you determine how this medication affects you. Smoking can reduce the effectiveness of oral contraceptives and can increase the risk of potentially dangerous blood clots.

OVERDOSE
Symptoms: Unexplained vaginal bleeding.

What to Do: An overdose is unlikely to be life-threatening; however, if someone takes a much larger dose than prescribed, call your doctor, emergency medical services (EMS), or the nearest poison control center immediately.

▼ INTERACTIONS

DRUG INTERACTIONS
Consult your doctor for advice if you are taking amiodarone, anabolic steroids, corticosteroids, androgens, antiinfectives, barbiturates, carbamazepine, carmustine, dantrolene, daunorubicin, disulfiram, divalproex, estrogens, etretinate, gold salts, griseofulvin, hydroxychloroquine, mercaptopurine, methotrexate, naltrexone, phenothiazines, phenylbutazone, phenytoin, plicamycin, primidone, rifabutin, rifampin, troleandomycin, theophylline, cyclosporine, or ritonavir.

FOOD INTERACTIONS
No known food interactions.

DISEASE INTERACTIONS
Consult your doctor if you have any of the following: endometriosis, fibroid tumors of the uterus, heart or circulation disease, a history of stroke, breast disease, cancer, gallbladder disease, diabetes, high blood cholesterol, liver disease, mental depression, epilepsy, or migraines.

≡ SIDE EFFECTS ≡

SERIOUS
Sudden, severe, or continuing stomach pain; sudden or severe headache or migraine; loss of coordination; loss of or change in vision; pains in chest, groin, or leg; sudden slurring of speech; weakness, numbness, or pain in an arm or leg; changes in uterine bleeding pattern; prolonged bleeding at menses; vaginal infection. Call your doctor immediately.

COMMON
Abdominal cramps or bloating; acne; breast pain, tenderness, or swelling; dizziness; nausea; swelling of ankles or feet; unusual fatigue; vomiting; absence of normal menstruation. Call your doctor if you do not have your period at the end of the cycle and before you start a new cycle.

LESS COMMON
Blotchy spots on skin, gain or loss of hair, increased sensitivity to sunlight, changes in sexual interest.

CYCLOBENZAPRINE

Available in: Tablets
Available OTC? No   **As Generic?** Yes
Drug Class: Muscle relaxant

▼ USAGE INFORMATION

WHY IT'S PRESCRIBED
To relieve painful, temporary muscle stiffness and spasms. It is not used for stiffness and spasms caused by serious chronic illnesses of the nervous system and muscles, such as spinal cord injury or cerebral palsy.

HOW IT WORKS
Cyclobenzaprine appears to work by decreasing nerve impulses from the brain and spinal cord that lead to tensing or tightening of muscles.

▼ DOSAGE GUIDELINES

RANGE AND FREQUENCY
Adults and teenagers 15 years of age and older: Usual dose is 10 mg 3 times a day, which may be increased by your doctor to a maximum total dose of no more than 60 mg per day. Children and teenagers up to 15 years of age: Consult pediatrician.

ONSET OF EFFECT
Within 1 hour. The maximum effect may require 1 to 2 weeks of therapy.

DURATION OF ACTION
12 to 24 hours following a single dose.

DIETARY ADVICE
Dry mouth is a common complaint with muscle relaxants; maintain adequate fluid intake and suck on ice chips if desired.

STORAGE
Store in a tightly sealed container away from heat and direct light. Keep it away from moisture and extremes in temperature.

MISSED DOSE
Take it as soon as you remember. If it is near the time for the next dose, skip the missed dose and resume your regular dosage schedule. Do not double the next dose.

STOPPING THE DRUG
You should take it as prescribed for the full treatment period, but you may stop if you are feeling better before the scheduled end of therapy.

PROLONGED USE
Therapy with cyclobenzaprine is usually completed within 14 to 21 days. Do not take cyclobenzaprine for a longer period without your doctor's approval. Muscle pain and stiffness that do not improve within 14 to 21 days may require a more thorough evaluation.

▼ PRECAUTIONS

Over 60: Adverse reactions may be more likely and more severe in older patients.

Driving and Hazardous Work: The use of cyclobenzaprine may impair your ability to perform such tasks safely; use caution.

Alcohol: Avoid alcohol.

Pregnancy: Adequate studies of cyclobenzaprine use during pregnancy have not been done; discuss the relative risks and benefits of taking the drug with your doctor.

Breast Feeding: Cyclobenzaprine may pass into breast milk; caution is advised. Consult your doctor for advice.

Infants and Children: Cyclobenzaprine is not recommended for use by children under the age of 15 years.

Special Concerns: Cyclobenzaprine is not meant to be used as the only treatment for sore or stiff muscles. It should be accompanied by bed rest, physical therapy, and other measures to relieve discomfort, such as the application of heat or ice packs (as suggested by your physician).

OVERDOSE
Symptoms: Severe mental confusion, agitation, impaired concentration, difficulty walking or standing, dilated pupils, severe drowsiness, coma.

What to Do: Call emergency medical services (EMS), your doctor, or the nearest poison control center immediately.

▼ INTERACTIONS

DRUG INTERACTIONS
Consult your doctor for specific advice if you are taking sedatives, tranquilizers, or other medications that cause drowsiness (including alcohol); tricyclic antidepressants; or MAO inhibitors.

FOOD INTERACTIONS
No known food interactions.

DISEASE INTERACTIONS
Consult your doctor if you have a history of any of the following conditions: glaucoma, difficult urination, prostate problems, heart disease, or overactive thyroid.

 SIDE EFFECTS

SERIOUS
Unusual heartbeat (racing, pounding, or fluttering), confusion, seizures, hallucinations.

COMMON
Drowsiness, dry mouth, dizziness.

LESS COMMON
Fatigue or excessive tiredness, weakness, nausea, heartburn, constipation, unpleasant bitter or metallic taste in mouth, vision problems, headache, restlessness, nervousness, difficulty urinating, unusual bleeding or bruising.

DEXAMETHASONE SYSTEMIC

Available in: Elixir, oral solution, tablets, injection
Available OTC? No   **As Generic?** Yes
Drug Class: Corticosteroid

▼ USAGE INFORMATION

WHY IT'S PRESCRIBED
To treat numerous conditions that involve inflammation (a response by body tissues, producing redness, warmth, swelling, and pain). Such conditions include arthritis, allergic reactions, asthma, some skin diseases, multiple sclerosis flare-ups, and other autoimmune diseases. Also prescribed to treat deficiency of natural steroid hormones.

HOW IT WORKS
This hormone mimics the effects of the body's natural corticosteroids. It depresses the synthesis, release, and activity of inflammation-producing body chemicals. It also suppresses the activity of the immune system.

▼ DOSAGE GUIDELINES

RANGE AND FREQUENCY
Adults and teenagers—Oral dosage: 25 to 300 mg a day, depending on condition, in 1 or several doses. Injection: 20 to 300 mg once a day, depending on condition. Children—Consult your doctor.

ONSET OF EFFECT
Within 2 hours of oral form, 1 hour of injection.

DURATION OF ACTION
More than 2 days for oral form; 6 days after injection.

DIETARY ADVICE
It can be taken with food or milk to minimize any stomach upset. Your doctor may recommend a low-salt, high-potassium, high-protein diet.

STORAGE
Store in a tightly sealed container away from moisture, heat, and direct light.

MISSED DOSE
Take it as soon as you remember. If you take several doses a day and it is close to the next dose, double the next dose. If you take 1 dose a day and you do not remember until the next day, skip the missed dose and do not double the next dose.

STOPPING THE DRUG
With long-term therapy, do not stop taking the drug abruptly; the dosage should be decreased gradually.

PROLONGED USE
See your doctor regularly for tests and examinations. Long-term use of the drug may lead to cataracts, diabetes, hypertension, or osteoporosis.

▼ PRECAUTIONS

Over 60: Adverse reactions may be more likely and more severe in older patients.

Driving and Hazardous Work: Do not drive or engage in hazardous work until you determine how the medicine affects you.

Alcohol: May cause stomach problems; avoid alcohol unless your physician approves occasional moderate drinking.

Pregnancy: Overuse during pregnancy can retard the child's growth and cause other developmental problems. Consult your physician.

Breast Feeding: Do not use while nursing.

Infants and Children: Dexamethasone may retard the normal growth and development of bone and other tissues. Consult your doctor.

Special Concerns: Avoid immunizations with live vaccines if possible. Remember that this drug can lower your resistance to infection. Those undergoing long-term therapy should wear a medical-alert bracelet. Call your doctor if you develop a fever.

OVERDOSE

Symptoms: Fever, muscle or joint pain, nausea, dizziness, fainting, difficulty breathing. Prolonged overuse: Moon face, obesity, unusual hair growth, acne, loss of sexual function, muscle wasting.

What to Do: Call your doctor, emergency medical services (EMS), or the nearest poison control center immediately.

▼ INTERACTIONS

DRUG INTERACTIONS
Consult your doctor for specific advice if you are taking aminoglutethimide, antacids, barbiturates, carbamazepine, griseofulvin, mitotane, phenylbutazone, phenytoin, primidone, rifampin, injectable amphotericin B, oral antidiabetes agents, insulin, digitalis drugs, diuretics, or medications containing potassium or sodium.

FOOD INTERACTIONS
Avoid excess sodium.

DISEASE INTERACTIONS
Consult your doctor if you have a history of bone disease, chicken pox, measles, gastrointestinal disorders, diabetes, recent serious infection, tuberculosis, glaucoma, heart disease, hypertension, liver or kidney disorders, high blood cholesterol, overactive or underactive thyroid, myasthenia gravis, or lupus.

 SIDE EFFECTS

SERIOUS
Vision problems, frequent urination, increased thirst, rectal bleeding, blistering skin, confusion, hallucinations, paranoia, euphoria, depression, mood swings, redness and swelling at injection site. Call your doctor immediately.

COMMON
Increased appetite, indigestion, nervousness, insomnia, greater susceptibility to infections, increased blood pressure, slow healing of wounds, weight gain, easy bruising, fluid retention.

LESS COMMON
Change in skin color, dizziness, headache, increased sweating, unusual growth of body or facial hair, increased blood sugar, peptic ulcers, adrenal insufficiency, muscle weakness, cataracts, glaucoma, osteoporosis.

DIAZEPAM

Available in: Tablets, capsules, injection, rectal gel
Available OTC? No   **As Generic?** Yes
Drug Class: Benzodiazepine tranquilizer; antianxiety agent/muscle relaxant

▼ USAGE INFORMATION

WHY IT'S PRESCRIBED
To treat anxiety, panic attacks, and muscle spasms; also used in acute treatment of seizures.

HOW IT WORKS
Diazepam generally produces mild sedation by depressing activity in the central nervous system. This medication appears to enhance the effect of gamma-aminobutyric acid (GABA), a natural chemical produced by the body that inhibits the firing of neurons and dampens the transmission of nerve signals, thus decreasing nervous excitation.

▼ DOSAGE GUIDELINES

RANGE AND FREQUENCY
For anxiety—Adults: 2 to 10 mg 4 times a day. Children: 1 to 2.5 mg 3 or 4 times a day. For muscle spasms—2 to 10 mg 2 to 4 times a day. For treatment of seizures—Injection and rectal gel: Your doctor will determine the correct dosage.

ONSET OF EFFECT
30 minutes.

DURATION OF ACTION
Up to 48 hours.

DIETARY ADVICE
No special restrictions.

STORAGE
Store in a tightly sealed container away from moisture, heat, and direct light.

MISSED DOSE
Take the missed dose if you remember within 2 hours. If more than 2 hours, skip the missed dose and return to your regular schedule. Do not double the next dose.

STOPPING THE DRUG
Discontinuing the drug abruptly may produce withdrawal symptoms (seizures, sleep disruption, nervousness, irritability, diarrhea, abdominal cramps, muscle aches, memory impairment). Dosage should be reduced gradually according to your physician's instructions.

PROLONGED USE
Diazepam may slowly lose its effectiveness with prolonged use. You should see your doctor for periodic evaluation if you must take it for an extended time.

▼ PRECAUTIONS

Over 60: Dosage is often reduced because adverse reactions are more likely and may be more severe in older patients.

Driving and Hazardous Work: Diazepam can impair mental alertness and physical coordination. Adjust your activities accordingly.

Alcohol: Alcohol intake should be extremely moderate or stopped altogether while taking this drug.

Pregnancy: Use during pregnancy should be avoided if possible. Be sure to tell your doctor if you are pregnant or plan to become pregnant.

Breast Feeding: Diazepam passes into breast milk; do not take it while nursing.

Infants and Children: Diazepam should be used by children only under close medical supervision.

Special Concerns: Diazepam use can lead to psychological or physical dependence. Never take more than the prescribed daily dose. Your physician will teach you how to determine when it is appropriate and how to properly administer the rectal gel.

OVERDOSE
Symptoms: Extreme drowsiness, confusion, slurred speech, slow reflexes, poor coordination, staggering gait, tremor, slowed breathing, loss of consciousness.

What to Do: Call your doctor, emergency medical services (EMS), or the nearest poison control center immediately.

▼ INTERACTIONS

DRUG INTERACTIONS
Other drugs may interact with diazepam. Consult your doctor for advice if you are taking any drugs that depress the central nervous system; these include antihistamines, antidepressants or other psychiatric medications, barbiturates, sedatives, cough medicines, decongestants, and painkillers. Be sure your doctor knows about any over-the-counter drug you may take.

FOOD INTERACTIONS
None reported.

DISEASE INTERACTIONS
Do not take diazepam if you have acute narrow-angle glaucoma. Consult your doctor if you have a history of alcohol or drug abuse, stroke or other brain disease, any chronic lung disease, hyperactivity, depression or other mental illness, myasthenia gravis, sleep apnea, epilepsy, porphyria, kidney disease, or liver disease.

 SIDE EFFECTS

SERIOUS
Difficulty concentrating, outbursts of anger, other behavior problems, depression, hallucinations, low blood pressure (causing faintness or confusion), memory impairment, muscle weakness, skin rash or itching, sore throat, fever and chills, sores or ulcers in throat or mouth, unusual bruising or bleeding, extreme fatigue, yellowish tinge to eyes or skin. Call your doctor immediately.

COMMON
Drowsiness, loss of coordination, unsteady gait, dizziness, lightheadedness, slurred speech.

LESS COMMON
Change in sexual desire or ability, constipation, false sense of well-being (euphoria), nausea and vomiting, urinary problems, unusual fatigue.

DICLOFENAC/MISOPROSTOL

Available in: Tablets
Available OTC? No   **As Generic?** No
Drug Class: Antirheumatic

▼ USAGE INFORMATION

WHY IT'S PRESCRIBED
To relieve the symptoms of osteoarthritis or rheumatoid arthritis in patients at high risk of developing peptic ulcers as a result of NSAID therapy.

HOW IT WORKS
Diclofenac, a nonsteroidal antiinflammatory drug (NSAID), works by interfering with the formation of prostaglandins, substances that cause pain and inflammation. Ongoing NSAID therapy can irritate and damage the stomach lining, increasing the risk of peptic ulcers. Misoprostol, a synthetic prostaglandin, helps prevent ulcers and promotes healing by increasing the production of protective mucus and inhibiting the secretion of stomach acid.

▼ DOSAGE GUIDELINES

RANGE AND FREQUENCY
Osteoarthritis: 1 tablet of Arthrotec 50 (50 mg diclofenac/200 micrograms [µg] misoprostol) 3 times a day. Rheumatoid arthritis: 1 tablet of Arthrotec 75 (75 mg diclofenac/200 µg misoprostol) 3 to 4 times a day. Different doses may be necessary in some patients.

ONSET OF EFFECT
Unknown.

DURATION OF ACTION
Unknown.

DIETARY ADVICE
The drug should be taken with food to minimize stomach upset and diarrhea.

STORAGE
Store in a tightly sealed container away from moisture, heat, and direct light.

MISSED DOSE
Take it as soon as you remember you missed a dose. If it is near the time for the next dose, skip the missed dose and resume your regular dosage schedule. Do not double the next dose.

STOPPING THE DRUG
Take it as prescribed for the full treatment period.

PROLONGED USE
Side effects are more likely with prolonged use; regular follow-up visits with your doctor are important. To minimize the risk of an adverse effect, take the lowest effective dose for the shortest possible duration (misoprostol is generally not prescribed for longer than 4 weeks).

▼ PRECAUTIONS

Over 60: No special problems are expected.

Driving and Hazardous Work: Do not drive or engage in hazardous work until you determine how the medicine affects you.

Alcohol: Avoid alcohol; it may increase the risk of stomach irritation.

Pregnancy: This drug combination should not be used during pregnancy. The misoprostol component can cause miscarriage and induce abortion. Before the drug can be prescribed, female patients are required to have had a negative pregnancy test within the previous 2 weeks. Therapy then begins only on the second or third day of the following menstrual period. An effective method of birth control should be used while taking this drug. If you suspect you are pregnant, stop taking the drug immediately and consult your doctor.

Breast Feeding: Avoid use while nursing.

Infants and Children: Not recommended for use by children under 18 years.

OVERDOSE
Symptoms: Nausea, vomiting, severe headache, confusion, seizures, tremors, sleepiness, difficulty breathing, stomach pain, severe diarrhea, fever, palpitations, dizziness or fainting, slow heartbeat.

What to Do: Call your doctor, emergency medical services (EMS), or the nearest poison control center immediately.

▼ INTERACTIONS

DRUG INTERACTIONS
The following drugs may interact with this drug: aspirin, digoxin, blood pressure medication, warfarin, methotrexate, cyclosporine, oral diabetes drugs, lithium, antacids, diuretics, or any over-the-counter drugs. Consult your doctor. To minimize the risk of diarrhea, avoid the use of antacids containing magnesium.

FOOD INTERACTIONS
No known food interactions.

DISEASE INTERACTIONS
You should not take this drug if you have ever experienced breathing difficulty; hives; swelling of the face, tongue, or throat; or any other allergic reactions after taking aspirin or other NSAIDs. Caution is advised if you have a history of high blood pressure or asthma. Use of this drug combination may cause complications in patients with liver or kidney disease, because these organs work together to remove the medications from the body.

SIDE EFFECTS

SERIOUS
Irregular heartbeat, fainting, coma, seizures, yellowish tinge to eyes or skin, or pain or tenderness in the upper right abdomen. Call your doctor immediately.

COMMON
Stomach pain or upset, diarrhea, indigestion, nausea, gas.

LESS COMMON
Fatigue, fever, tremor, dizziness, loss of appetite, breathing difficulty, persistent but unproductive urge to urinate or defecate, hemorrhoids, breast pain, painful menstruation, menstrual irregularities, hives, impotence, unexpected changes in weight, muscle and joint pain, mental depression, sleeping difficulty, nightmares or unusually vivid dreams, hallucinations, irritability, nervousness, bruising, skin rash, blurred or abnormal vision.

DIGOXIN

BRAND NAMES
Lanoxicaps, Lanoxin

Available in: Tablets, capsules, elixir
Available OTC? No   **As Generic?** Yes
Drug Class: Digitalis drug (cardiac glycoside)

▼ USAGE INFORMATION

WHY IT'S PRESCRIBED
To treat congestive heart failure and atrial arrhythmias (irregularities in the rhythm of the heartbeat).

HOW IT WORKS
Digitalis drugs such as digoxin enhance and strengthen the force of the heart's contractions, and help regulate the rate and rhythm of the heartbeat.

▼ DOSAGE GUIDELINES

RANGE AND FREQUENCY
Adults: Initial dose is 0.5 mg. Maintenance dosage, starting the next day, ranges from 0.125 to 0.25 mg a day (rarely more) taken once a day. Periodic blood tests are necessary to determine the proper dose. Children: Consult your doctor.

ONSET OF EFFECT
30 minutes to 2 hours.

DURATION OF ACTION
3 to 4 days.

DIETARY ADVICE
Take it on an empty stomach, at the same time every day. Taking digoxin with food can decrease the absorption rate and the peak concentration.

STORAGE
Store in a tightly sealed container away from moisture, heat, and direct light.

MISSED DOSE
Take it as soon as you remember. If it is within 12 hours of the next scheduled dose, skip the missed dose and resume your regular dosage schedule. Do not double the next dose.

STOPPING THE DRUG
Do not stop taking it unless a doctor advises otherwise. Abrupt discontinuation can cause serious heart problems. Most patients take digoxin for an extended period or for the rest of their lives.

PROLONGED USE
Prolonged use requires a doctor's supervision and periodic assessments of the continued need to take the drug. Blood levels of digoxin must be measured at regular intervals to ensure proper dosing.

▼ PRECAUTIONS

Over 60: Underweight or frail older persons may require a lower maintenance dose.

Driving and Hazardous Work: Digoxin may cause drowsiness or vision changes. Do not drive or engage in hazardous work until you determine how it affects you.

Alcohol: No interactions are expected.

Pregnancy: Human studies have not been done. In animal studies, no birth defects have been reported. Digoxin should be used during pregnancy only if your doctor decides it is clearly needed.

Breast Feeding: Digoxin passes into breast milk. The nursing infant should be monitored carefully. Stop using the drug or discontinue breast feeding if adverse effects develop.

Infants and Children: The dosage for infants and children must be determined by your pediatrician.

Special Concerns: You should carry a card that says you are taking digoxin. Do not take over-the-counter antacids or cold or allergy remedies without consulting your doctor. Digoxin causes

impotence and enlarged breasts in a third of the men who take it. Mental changes induced by the drug may be mistaken for psychosis or senility.

OVERDOSE
Symptoms: Heart palpitations, abdominal pain, diarrhea, nausea, vomiting, very slow pulse.

What to Do: Call your doctor, emergency medical services (EMS), or the nearest poison control center immediately.

▼ INTERACTIONS

DRUG INTERACTIONS
Numerous drugs interact with digoxin and may alter blood levels of the drug, leading to toxicity. Consult your doctor for specific advice if you are taking any medications, especially antiarrhythmic drugs, such as quinidine or procainamide, airway-opening drugs (bronchodilators), antacids, antibiotics such as neomycin or tetracycline, anticholinergic drugs such as atropine, cholesterol-lowering drugs, diuretics (water pills), steroids, indomethacin, or any other heart drug.

FOOD INTERACTIONS
Ask your doctor about the advisability of eating high-potassium foods.

DISEASE INTERACTIONS
Tell your doctor if you have any other medical condition, especially lung disease, kidney disease, or poor thyroid function.

SIDE EFFECTS

SERIOUS
Heartbeat irregularities causing dizziness, palpitations, shortness of breath, sweating, or fainting. Other serious side effects include hallucinations, confusion, and mental changes; extreme drowsiness; visual disturbances such as double vision or seeing colored halos around objects; weakness, fatigue, blurred vision; nausea; and agitation. Call your doctor immediately.

COMMON
Erectile dysfunction, male breast enlargement. Notify your doctor if such symptoms occur.

LESS COMMON
Headache, vertigo, numbness or tingling sensation, overall feeling of illness, sensitivity of eyes to light, diarrhea, vomiting. Call your doctor if such symptoms persist.

DILTIAZEM HYDROCHLORIDE

Available in: Tablets, extended-release capsules, injection
Available OTC? No   **As Generic?** Yes
Drug Class: Calcium channel blocker

▼ USAGE INFORMATION

WHY IT'S PRESCRIBED
To relieve and control angina (chest pain associated with heart disease), to reduce high blood pressure, and to correct heartbeat irregularities (cardiac arrhythmia).

HOW IT WORKS
Diltiazem interferes with the movement of calcium into heart muscle cells and the smooth muscle cells in the walls of the arteries. This action relaxes blood vessels (causing them to widen), which lowers blood pressure, increases the blood supply to the heart, and decreases the heart's overall workload.

▼ DOSAGE GUIDELINES

RANGE AND FREQUENCY
Tablets (for chest pain): 30 mg 3 or 4 times a day to start, increased to 40 to 60 mg 3 or 4 times a day. Extended-release capsules (for high blood pressure): 120 to 240 mg a day taken in 1 or 2 divided doses. (For heartbeat irregularities, diltiazem is administered by injection by a health-care professional.)

ONSET OF EFFECT
Tablets: 30 to 60 minutes. Extended-release capsules: 2 to 3 hours.

DURATION OF ACTION
Tablets: 6 to 8 hours. Extended-release capsules: 10 to 14 hours.

DIETARY ADVICE
Diltiazem is best taken before meals or at bedtime.

STORAGE
Store tablets and capsules in a tightly sealed container away from heat, moisture, and direct light.

MISSED DOSE
Take it as soon as you remember. However, if it is near the time for the next dose, skip the missed dose and resume your regular dosage schedule. Do not double the next dose.

STOPPING THE DRUG
Do not stop taking this drug suddenly; this may cause potentially serious health problems. If therapy is to be discontinued, dosage should be reduced gradually according to doctor's instructions.

PROLONGED USE
No unusual side effects are expected with prolonged use.

▼ PRECAUTIONS

Over 60: Weakness, dizziness, and fainting are more likely in older persons.

Driving and Hazardous Work: Diltiazem can cause dizziness or drowsiness. Do not drive or engage in hazardous work until you determine how the medicine affects you.

Alcohol: Use alcohol with caution because it may increase the effect of the drug and cause an excessive drop in blood pressure.

Pregnancy: Birth defects have occurred in animal studies. Adequate human studies have not been done. Avoid this drug during the first 3 months of pregnancy and take it during the last 6 months only if your doctor says it is clearly needed.

Breast Feeding: Diltiazem passes into breast milk; avoid or discontinue use while breast feeding.

Infants and Children: Usually not prescribed; the safety and effectiveness of diltiazem for children under the age of 12 years have not been established.

Special Concerns: It is important to brush and floss your teeth and see your dentist regularly, because using diltiazem may promote dental problems. This medication may make you sensitive to sunlight.

OVERDOSE
Symptoms: Heart block causing unusual shortness of breath; fatigue; excessive dizziness; fainting.

What to Do: Call your doctor, emergency medical services (EMS), or the nearest poison control center immediately.

▼ INTERACTIONS

DRUG INTERACTIONS
Consult your doctor for specific advice if you are taking aspirin, beta-blockers, digitalis preparations, carbamazepine, cyclosporine, digoxin, lithium, oral diabetes agents, phenytoin, rifampin, cimetidine, fluvoxamine, or ranitidine.

FOOD INTERACTIONS
Avoid excessive salt intake.

DISEASE INTERACTIONS
Consult your doctor if you have any of the following: kidney disease, liver disease, high blood pressure, or any kind of heart or blood vessel disease.

≣ SIDE EFFECTS ≣

SERIOUS
Irregular or slow heartbeat, shortness of breath, fatigue caused by heart failure. Call your doctor immediately.

COMMON
Headache, drowsiness, swelling of feet and ankles, constipation, nausea, sudden weight gain, fatigue.

LESS COMMON
Dizziness, weakness, depression, nervousness, insomnia, confusion, slow pulse, vomiting, diarrhea, excessive urination, itch, sensitivity to sunlight, yellowish tinge to eyes or skin caused by liver failure, skin rash, overgrowth of the gums.

DONEPEZIL

BRAND NAME
Aricept

Available in: Tablets
Available OTC? No   **As Generic?** No
Drug Class: Acetylcholinesterase inhibitor

▼ USAGE INFORMATION

WHY IT'S PRESCRIBED
To treat mild to moderate Alzheimer's disease.

HOW IT WORKS
Donepezil prevents the breakdown of acetylcholine, a brain chemical crucial to memory. Acetylcholine deficiency is thought to result in memory loss associated with Alzheimer's disease.

▼ DOSAGE GUIDELINES

RANGE AND FREQUENCY
To start, 5 mg at bedtime. The dose may be increased after 4 to 6 weeks to 10 mg at bedtime.

ONSET OF EFFECT
Unknown.

DURATION OF ACTION
Unknown.

DIETARY ADVICE
No special restrictions.

STORAGE
Store in a tightly sealed container away from moisture, heat, and direct light.

MISSED DOSE
Skip the missed dose and resume your regular dosage schedule. Do not double the next dose.

STOPPING THE DRUG
The decision to stop taking the drug should be made by your doctor.

PROLONGED USE
No problems are expected with long-term use.

▼ PRECAUTIONS

Over 60: No special problems are expected.

Driving and Hazardous Work: Do not drive or engage in hazardous work until you determine how the medicine affects you.

Alcohol: Avoid alcohol while using this medication.

Pregnancy: In some animal studies, large doses of donepezil were shown to cause problems. Before you take donepezil, tell your doctor if you are pregnant or plan to become pregnant.

Breast Feeding: It is not known whether donepezil passes into breast milk; caution is advised. Consult your doctor for specific advice.

Infants and Children: Donepezil is not intended for use in children.

Special Concerns: Before you have any surgery or dental or emergency treatment, tell the doctor or dentist in charge that you are taking donepezil. Donepezil will not cure Alzheimer's disease and will not stop the disease from getting worse, but it will improve cognitive ability of some patients.

OVERDOSE
Symptoms: Seizures, severe nausea, slow heartbeat, increased muscle weakness, vomiting, greatly increased sweating, greatly increased watering of the mouth, weak pulse, irregular breathing, enlargement of the pupils of the eyes.

What to Do: Call your doctor, emergency medical services (EMS), or the nearest poison control center immediately.

▼ INTERACTIONS

DRUG INTERACTIONS
The following drugs may interact with donepezil. Consult your doctor for specific advice if you are taking carbamazepine, dexamethasone, ketoconazole, phenobarbital, phenytoin, quinidine, or rifampin. Also tell your doctor if you are taking any other prescription or over-the-counter medication.

FOOD INTERACTIONS
No known food interactions.

DISEASE INTERACTIONS
Caution is advised when taking donepezil. Consult your doctor if you have any of the following conditions: asthma, chronic obstructive pulmonary disease (COPD), urinary difficulties, heart disease, liver disease, a seizure disorder, stomach ulcers, or a blockage of the urinary tract.

≡ SIDE EFFECTS ≡

SERIOUS
No serious side effects are associated with the use of donepezil.

COMMON
Nausea, vomiting, diarrhea, headache, dizziness, fatigue, insomnia.

LESS COMMON
Vivid or unusual dreams, drowsiness, depression, loss of appetite, unusual bleeding or bruising, fainting, muscle cramps, frequent urination, joint pain, stiffness, or swelling.

DOXAZOSIN MESYLATE

BRAND NAME

Cardura

Available in: Tablets
Available OTC? No **As Generic?** Yes
Drug Class: Antihypertensive; BPH (benign prostatic hyperplasia) therapy agent

▼ USAGE INFORMATION

WHY IT'S PRESCRIBED
To treat mild to moderate high blood pressure and to ease urinary tract symptoms caused by benign prostatic hyperplasia (BPH)—that is, noncancerous enlargement of the prostate gland, which is extremely common among men over the age of 50. Note: Findings from a major clinical trial indicate that doxazosin is associated with an unacceptably high incidence of cardiovascular complications. The American Academy of Cardiology has since recommended that physicians reconsider the use of doxazosin in the treatment of their hypertensive patients on a case-by-case basis.

HOW IT WORKS
For high blood pressure, the drug relaxes and widens blood vessels so blood passes through them more easily. For prostate enlargement, it relaxes muscles in the prostate and the opening of the bladder. Note that doxazosin will not shrink the prostate; symptoms may worsen and surgery may be required eventually.

▼ DOSAGE GUIDELINES

RANGE AND FREQUENCY
For high blood pressure: Initial dose is 1 mg taken once a day. It can be increased gradually to a maximum of 16 mg a day. For prostate enlargement: Initial dose is 1 mg taken once a day, which may be gradually increased to a maximum of 12 mg a day.

ONSET OF EFFECT
For high blood pressure: 1 to 2 hours. For prostate enlargement: 1 to 2 weeks.

DURATION OF ACTION
For high blood pressure: 24 hours. For prostate enlargement: Unknown.

DIETARY ADVICE
No special restrictions.

STORAGE
Store in a tightly sealed container in a dry place away from heat and direct light.

MISSED DOSE
Take it as soon as you remember. If it is near the time for the next dose, skip the missed dose and resume your regular dosage schedule. Do not double the next dose.

STOPPING THE DRUG
Take it as prescribed for the full treatment period, even if you feel better before the scheduled end of therapy.

PROLONGED USE
Consult your doctor about the need for follow-up medical examinations and laboratory studies if you must take doxazosin for a prolonged period.

▼ PRECAUTIONS

Over 60: Adverse reactions may be more likely and more severe in older patients. Dose should be increased slowly in patients over 60.

Driving and Hazardous Work: Do not drive or engage in hazardous work until you determine how the medicine affects you.

Alcohol: Alcohol should be avoided while taking this medicine because it may cause an excessive drop in blood pressure.

Pregnancy: In animal studies, very high doses of doxazosin damaged the fetus. Before taking this medicine, tell your doctor if you are pregnant or plan to become pregnant.

Breast Feeding: Doxazosin may pass into breast milk; caution is advised. Consult your doctor for advice.

Infants and Children: This drug is not recommended for use by children.

Special Concerns: The first dose is likely to cause dizziness or lightheadedness. Take the drug at night and get out of bed slowly the next day. Be cautious while exercising and during hot weather. Tell your doctor whether you will have surgery requiring general anesthesia, including dental surgery, within the next 2 months.

OVERDOSE
Symptoms: Cold, sweaty skin, rapid pulse, weakness, loss of consciousness.

What to Do: Call your doctor, emergency medical services (EMS), or the nearest poison control center immediately.

▼ INTERACTIONS

DRUG INTERACTIONS
Consult your doctor for specific advice if you are taking amphetamines, other antihypertensive drugs, nonsteroidal antiinflammatory drugs (NSAIDs), estrogen, or sympathomimetic drugs.

FOOD INTERACTIONS
No known food interactions.

DISEASE INTERACTIONS
Use of doxazosin may cause complications in patients with liver or kidney disease, because these organs work together to remove the medication from the body. Also, consult your doctor if you have coronary artery disease, impaired blood circulation to the brain, or mental depression.

 SIDE EFFECTS

SERIOUS
Irregular heartbeat. Call your doctor immediately. Another serious but rare side effect is priapism, a condition characterized by a prolonged or painful erection (lasting more than 4 hours).

COMMON
Dizziness, drowsiness.

LESS COMMON
Headache, weakness, palpitations, rapid pulse, pain and tingling sensations in the fingers or toes, diarrhea or constipation, runny nose, rash or itchy skin, muscle or joint pain, headache, mental depression.

ENALAPRIL MALEATE

Available in: Tablets
Available OTC? No **As Generic?** Yes
Drug Class: Angiotensin-converting enzyme (ACE) inhibitor

BRAND NAME

Vasotec

▼ USAGE INFORMATION

WHY IT'S PRESCRIBED
To control high blood pressure, to treat congestive heart failure, to treat patients with left ventricular dysfunction (damage to the pumping chamber of the heart), and to minimize further kidney damage in diabetic patients with mild kidney disease.

HOW IT WORKS
Angiotensin-converting enzyme (ACE) inhibitors block an enzyme that produces angiotensin, a naturally occurring substance that causes blood vessels to constrict and stimulates production of the adrenal hormone, aldosterone, which promotes sodium retention in the body. As a result, ACE inhibitor medications relax blood vessels (causing them to widen) and reduce sodium retention, which in turn lowers blood pressure and so decreases the workload of the heart.

▼ DOSAGE GUIDELINES

RANGE AND FREQUENCY
Adults: 2.5 to 40 mg a day taken 1 or 2 times a day. Children ages 1 month to 16 years (for high blood pressure): To start, 0.08 mg per 2.2 lb (1 kg)) once a day, up to 5 mg a day. Your doctor may gradually increase the dose up to 40 mg a day.

ONSET OF EFFECT
Within 1 hour.

DURATION OF ACTION
Up to 24 hours.

DIETARY ADVICE
Take it on an empty stomach about 1 hour before mealtime. Follow your doctor's dietary advice (such as low-salt or low-cholesterol restrictions) to improve control over hypertension and heart disease. Avoid high-potassium foods such as bananas and citrus fruits and juices unless you are also taking drugs that lower potassium levels, such as diuretics.

STORAGE
Keep in a tightly sealed container in a cool, dry place.

MISSED DOSE
Take it as soon as you remember. If it is near the time for the next dose, skip the missed dose and resume your regular dosage schedule. Do not double the next dose.

STOPPING THE DRUG
Do not stop taking this drug abruptly; this may cause potentially serious health problems. Dosage should be reduced gradually, according to your doctor's instructions.

PROLONGED USE
See your doctor regularly for exams and tests if you must take this drug for a prolonged period. Enalapril helps control high blood pressure but does not cure it. Lifelong therapy may be necessary.

▼ PRECAUTIONS

Over 60: Smaller doses may be warranted.

Driving and Hazardous Work: Do not drive or engage in hazardous work until you determine how the medicine affects you.

Alcohol: Consume alcoholic beverages only in moderation because they may increase the effect of the medicine and cause an excessive drop in blood pressure.

Pregnancy: Enalapril use is not recommended, especially during the final 6 months of pregnancy. If you become pregnant, notify your doctor as soon as possible.

Breast Feeding: Although trace amounts of enalapril can be found in breast milk, adverse effects in infants have not been documented. Consult your doctor.

Infants and Children: Consult your pediatrician for specific advice.

OVERDOSE
Symptoms: No specific symptoms have been reported.

What to Do: Overdose is unlikely, but call your doctor, emergency medical services (EMS), or the nearest poison control center immediately if you suspect that someone has taken a much larger dose than prescribed.

▼ INTERACTIONS

DRUG INTERACTIONS
Consult your doctor if you are taking diuretics (especially potassium-sparing diuretics), potassium supplements or drugs containing potassium, lithium, anticoagulants, anti-inflammatory drugs, or over-the-counter drugs (especially cold remedies and diet pills).

FOOD INTERACTIONS
Avoid low-salt milk and salt substitutes. Many of these products contain potassium.

DISEASE INTERACTIONS
Consult your doctor if you have lupus or if you have had a prior allergic reaction to ACE inhibitors. This drug should be used with caution by patients with severe kidney disease or renal artery stenosis (narrowing of one or both of the arteries that supply blood to the kidneys).

 SIDE EFFECTS

SERIOUS
Fever and chills; sore throat and hoarseness; sudden difficulty breathing or swallowing; swelling of the face, mouth, or extremities; impaired kidney function (ankle swelling, decreased urination); confusion; yellow discoloration of the eyes or skin (indicating liver disorder); intense itching; chest pain or palpitations; abdominal pain. Serious side effects are very rare; contact your doctor immediately.

COMMON
Dry, persistent cough.

LESS COMMON
Dizziness or fainting; skin rash; numbness or tingling in the hands, feet; or lips; unusual fatigue or muscle weakness; nausea; drowsiness; loss of taste; headache; unusual dreams.

ERYTHROMYCIN SYSTEMIC

Available in: Capsules, tablets, oral suspension, injection
Available OTC? No   **As Generic?** Yes
Drug Class: Erythromycin antibiotic

▼ USAGE INFORMATION

WHY IT'S PRESCRIBED
To treat bacterial infections, including throat infections, pneumonia, Legionnaires' disease, chlamydia, and diphtheria. It is also prescribed to prevent strep infections that may damage heart valves in susceptible patients (those with a history of rheumatic fever or heart valve replacement, for example) who are allergic to penicillin.

HOW IT WORKS
Erythromycin prevents bacterial cells from manufacturing specific proteins necessary for their survival.

▼ DOSAGE GUIDELINES

RANGE AND FREQUENCY
To treat infections—Adults and teenagers: 250 to 800 mg 2 to 4 times a day. Children: 3.4 to 12.5 mg per lb of body weight 2 to 4 times a day. To prevent strep infections—Adults and teenagers: 1 to 1.6 g before a dental appointment or surgery and 500 to 800 mg 6 hours later. Children: 1.7 to 11.4 mg per lb of body weight before dental appointment or surgery and 4.5 mg per lb of body weight 6 hours later.

ONSET OF EFFECT
Immediate after injection; unknown for oral forms.

DURATION OF ACTION
Unknown.

DIETARY ADVICE
This drug is best taken on an empty stomach at least 1 hour before or 2 hours after meals, with a full glass of water. If it causes stomach upset, it can be taken with food or milk.

STORAGE
Store in a tightly sealed container away from heat and direct light. Refrigerate the liquid form but do not freeze it.

MISSED DOSE
Take it as soon as you remember. If it is near the time for the next dose, skip the missed dose and resume your regular dosage schedule. Do not double the next dose.

STOPPING THE DRUG
Take it as prescribed for the full treatment period.

PROLONGED USE
You should see your doctor regularly for tests and examinations, including those to evaluate liver function, if this medicine is taken for a prolonged period.

▼ PRECAUTIONS

Over 60: Older patients may be at higher risk of experiencing hearing loss as a side effect of the drug.

Driving and Hazardous Work: No special precautions are necessary.

Alcohol: No special warnings.

Pregnancy: Erythromycin has been shown to cause liver damage in some pregnant women. It has not been shown to cause birth defects or other problems in babies. Before taking erythromycin, tell your doctor if you are pregnant or if you plan to become pregnant.

Breast Feeding: Erythromycin passes into breast milk; caution is advised. Consult your doctor for specific advice.

Infants and Children: No special problems expected.

Special Concerns: Consult your doctor if your symptoms do not improve or instead become worse after a few days of therapy.

OVERDOSE
Symptoms: Severe nausea, vomiting, abdominal pain, diarrhea, dizziness, loss of hearing.

What to Do: Call your doctor, emergency medical services (EMS), or the nearest poison control center immediately.

▼ INTERACTIONS

DRUG INTERACTIONS
Do not use erythromycin if you are taking astemizole or cisapride. Consult your doctor for specific advice if you are taking acetaminophen, amiodarone, anabolic steroids, androgens, antibiotics, azithromycin, carbamazepine, carmustine, chloramphenicol, chloroquine, clarithromycin, cyclosporine, dantrolene, daunorubicin, disulfiram, divalproex, estrogens, etretinate, gold salts, hydroxychloroquine, lincomycin, methotrexate, mercaptopurine, methyldopa, naltrexone, oral contraceptives, phenothiazines, phenytoin, plicamycin, theophylline, valproic acid, warfarin, tacrolimus, disopyramide, lovastatin, or bromocriptine.

FOOD INTERACTIONS
No known food interactions.

DISEASE INTERACTIONS
Use of this medication is not advised for patients who have a history of heart rhythm disorders, kidney disease, liver disease, or hearing problems. Consult your doctor.

⋚ SIDE EFFECTS ⋚

SERIOUS
Fever, nausea, skin reddening or itching, severe stomach pain, yellow discoloration of the eyes or skin, fainting, slow or irregular heartbeat in patients with predisposing heart conditions, breathing difficulty, persistent or severe diarrhea, abdominal pain, temporary deafness. Also pain, swelling, or redness at injection site. Although serious side effects are rare, call your doctor immediately.

COMMON
Stomach cramps and abdominal discomfort, diarrhea, nausea, vomiting.

LESS COMMON
Soreness of mouth or tongue, vaginal itching or discharge.

ESTRADIOL

Available in: Tablets, skin patch, vaginal cream, injection
Available OTC? No   **As Generic?** Yes
Drug Class: Female sex hormone

▼ USAGE INFORMATION

WHY IT'S PRESCRIBED
To provide estrogen when the body does not produce enough; to treat carefully selected cases of advanced breast cancer; to reduce risk of osteoporosis after menopause; to ease unpleasant symptoms of menopause, including vaginal dryness; to prevent breast engorgement following childbirth; and to ease symptoms of advanced prostate cancer.

HOW IT WORKS
In women, estradiol replaces deficient natural levels of estrogen in the body. In men, the hormone inhibits growth of cells in the prostate gland.

▼ DOSAGE GUIDELINES

RANGE AND FREQUENCY
To treat breast cancer: 10 mg 3 times a day. For post-menopausal vaginal dryness or prevention of osteoporosis: 1 to 2 mg a day of oral form, 10 to 20 mg injected every 4 weeks, or 1 Estraderm, Alora, or Vivelle patch (0.05 mg) 2 times a week or 1 Climara patch weekly. A progestin should also be taken for 10 to 14 days in each month of use, except by women who have had a hysterectomy. To relieve postmenopausal vaginal dryness using intravaginal estrogen creams: To start, ½ to 1 applicatorful daily and tapered to 1 applicatorful 1 to 3 times weekly. To treat menopausal symptoms: 1 to 5 mg injected every 3 to 4 weeks. To prevent breast engorgement after childbirth: 10 to 25 mg injected in a muscle at the time of delivery. To treat prostate cancer: 1 to 2 mg 3 times daily.

ONSET OF EFFECT
Within 1 hour.

DURATION OF ACTION
Up to 24 hours.

DIETARY ADVICE
No special restrictions.

STORAGE
Keep in a tightly sealed container away from heat and direct light.

MISSED DOSE
Take the missed dose as soon as you remember. If it is near time for the next dose, skip the missed dose and resume your regular dosage schedule. Do not double the next dose.

STOPPING THE DRUG
The decision to stop taking the drug should be made in consultation with your doctor.

PROLONGED USE
May increase the risk of endometrial cancer and perhaps breast cancer. Consult your doctor about periodic examinations and other measures to help prevent these diseases.

▼ PRECAUTIONS

Over 60: No special problems are expected.

Driving and Hazardous Work: Do not drive or engage in hazardous work until you determine how the medicine affects you.

Alcohol: No special warnings.

Pregnancy: Not recommended during pregnancy; estrogens have been shown to cause birth defects in animals and humans.

Breast Feeding: Do not use estradiol while nursing.

Infants and Children: Not recommended for use by young patients in whom bone growth is not complete.

Special Concerns: Swelling or bleeding of gums may occur; see your dentist regularly. Do not apply a patch to the same site more than once a week.

OVERDOSE
Symptoms: Nausea, unexpected vaginal bleeding.

What to Do: An overdose is unlikely to occur. However, if someone takes a much larger dose than prescribed, seek immediate medical assistance.

▼ INTERACTIONS

DRUG INTERACTIONS
Consult your doctor for specific advice if you are taking acetaminophen, amiodarone, anticonvulsants, antiinfective drugs, antithyroid agents, carmustine, chloroquine, dantrolene, daunorubicin, gold salts, divalproex, etretinate, hydroxychloroquine, mercaptopurine, methotrexate, oral contraceptives, methyldopa, naltrexone, phenothiazines, plicamycin, steroids, bromocriptine, or cyclosporine.

FOOD INTERACTIONS
No known food interactions.

DISEASE INTERACTIONS
You should not take estradiol if you have blood clot disorders, breast cancer, any hormone-dependent cancer, or abnormal genital bleeding.

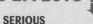

SIDE EFFECTS

SERIOUS
For women: breast pain or enlargement, swelling of legs and feet, rapid weight gain. For men being treated for prostate cancer: sudden or severe headache, loss of coordination; sudden changes in vision; pains in chest, groin, or leg; shortness of breath; slurring of speech; weakness or numbness in arm or leg. Call your doctor immediately.

COMMON
Abdominal bloating, stomach cramps, loss of appetite, skin irritation at site of patch.

LESS COMMON
Diarrhea, dizziness, headaches, discomfort when wearing contact lenses, increased sexual desire in women, decreased sexual desire in men, vomiting.

ESTROGENS, CONJUGATED

Available in: Tablets, injection, vaginal cream
Available OTC? No   **As Generic?** Yes
Drug Class: Female sex hormone

▼ USAGE INFORMATION

WHY IT'S PRESCRIBED
To provide estrogen after menopause, when the body produces too little; to treat carefully selected cases of advanced breast cancer; to ease unpleasant symptoms of menopause, including vaginal dryness; to prevent breast engorgement following childbirth; and to ease symptoms of advanced prostate cancer.

HOW IT WORKS
In women, conjugated estrogens replace deficient natural levels of estrogen in the body. In men, estrogens inhibit growth of cells in the prostate gland.

▼ DOSAGE GUIDELINES

RANGE AND FREQUENCY
Usual adult dose is taken in cycles, with no dosing on certain days of the month. Except those who have had a hysterectomy (and may take estrogen daily), women must also take a progestin 10 to 14 days in each month of use. To treat breast cancer in men or postmenopausal women: 10 mg 3 times a day for 3 months or more. To prevent bone loss from osteoporosis: 0.3 to 1.25 mg a day. To ease symptoms of menopause: 0.625 to 1.25 mg a day. To treat prostate cancer: 1.25 to 2.5 mg a day.

ONSET OF EFFECT
Unknown.

DURATION OF ACTION
Unknown.

DIETARY ADVICE
Conjugated estrogens may be taken with food to reduce stomach upset.

STORAGE
Store in a tightly sealed container away from moisture, heat, and direct light. Keep it away from extremes in temperature. Keep the liquid form refrigerated, but do not allow the medication to freeze.

MISSED DOSE
Take it as soon as you remember. If it is near the time for the next dose, skip the missed dose and resume your regular dosage schedule. Do not double the next dose.

STOPPING THE DRUG
The decision to stop taking the drug should be made by your doctor.

PROLONGED USE
Prolonged use of estrogens has been reported to increase the risk of endometrial cancer and perhaps of breast cancer. Consult your doctor about the need for periodic examinations and other measures to screen for these diseases.

▼ PRECAUTIONS

Over 60: No special problems are expected.

Driving and Hazardous Work: Use of this hormone should not impair your ability to perform such tasks safely.

Alcohol: No special warnings.

Pregnancy: Do not use if you are pregnant. Estrogen use in pregnant women has been associated with birth defects.

Breast Feeding: Talk to your doctor about whether the benefits of the therapy outweigh the potential harm to the nursing infant.

Infants and Children: Should be used with caution by children, because the drug may interfere with bone growth.

OVERDOSE
Symptoms: Nausea, unexpected vaginal bleeding.

What to Do: An overdose of estrogen is unlikely to be life-threatening; however, if someone takes a much larger dose than prescribed, call your doctor, emergency medical services (EMS), or the nearest poison control center immediately.

▼ INTERACTIONS

DRUG INTERACTIONS
Other drugs may interact with estrogens. Consult a doctor if you are taking anticoagulants, anticonvulsants, antidiabetic drugs, thyroid hormones, tricyclic antidepressants, barbiturates, tranquilizers, cyclosporine, corticosteroids, corticotropin, tamoxifen, rifampin, carbamazepine, or bromocriptine.

FOOD INTERACTIONS
Calcium supplements used with estrogen may increase calcium absorption. Vitamin C may increase the effects of estrogen.

DISEASE INTERACTIONS
You should not take conjugated estrogens if you have thrombophlebitis, thromboembolitis, breast cancer, any hormone-dependent cancer, or abnormal genital bleeding. Consult your doctor if you have any of the following: a history of liver disease, heart attack, stroke, a blood clotting disorder, or gallbladder disease or gallstones, or if you smoke tobacco heavily.

SIDE EFFECTS

SERIOUS
For women: breast pain or enlargement, swelling of legs and feet, rapid weight gain. For men being treated for prostate cancer: sudden or severe headache; loss of coordination; sudden changes in vision; pains in chest, groin, or leg; sudden shortness of breath; slurred speech; weakness or numbness in arm or leg. Call your doctor immediately.

COMMON
Abdominal bloating or cramps, loss of appetite, breast tenderness.

LESS COMMON
Diarrhea, dizziness, headaches, discomfort when wearing contact lenses, decreased sexual desire in men, increased sexual desire in women, vomiting.

ESTROGENS, CONJUGATED/ MEDROXYPROGESTERONE ACETATE

Available in: Tablets
Available OTC? No   **As Generic?** No
Drug Class: Female sex hormones

▼ USAGE INFORMATION

WHY IT'S PRESCRIBED
To provide estrogen after menopause, when the body produces too little; to ease unpleasant symptoms of menopause, including hot flashes and vaginal dryness; and to treat atrophy (wasting) of the vulva or vagina. Estrogen also protects women from developing coronary artery disease.

HOW IT WORKS
Estrogen protects against osteoporosis by diminishing the loss of bone that results from estrogen deficiency. Conjugated estrogens replace deficient levels of natural estrogen in women. When given alone to menopausal women, estrogen increases the risk of excessive growth of the uterine lining, which can lead to endometrial cancer. Medroxyprogesterone (a type of progestin) given in conjunction with estrogen nearly eliminates this risk.

▼ DOSAGE GUIDELINES

RANGE AND FREQUENCY
1 tablet taken once a day. Prempro contains 0.45 mg of conjugated estrogen (Premarin) and 1.5 mg of medroxyprogesterone (MPA). Premphase contains 0.625 mg Premarin and 5 mg of MPA.

ONSET OF EFFECT
Unknown.

DURATION OF ACTION
As long as the medication is taken.

DIETARY ADVICE
Take it with food to reduce stomach upset.

STORAGE
Store in a sealed container away from moisture, heat, and direct light. Keep it away from temperature extremes.

MISSED DOSE
If you miss a dose on one day, do not double the dose the next day. Resume your regular dosage schedule.

STOPPING THE DRUG
The decision to stop taking this hormone combination should be made in consultation with your doctor.

PROLONGED USE
You should be reevaluated at 3-month to 6-month intervals by your doctor to determine whether or not continued treatment is necessary.

▼ PRECAUTIONS

Over 60: No special problems are expected.

Driving and Hazardous Work: Use of this hormone combination should not impair your ability to perform such tasks safely.

Alcohol: No special warnings.

Pregnancy: Do not use this hormone combination if you are or are planning to become pregnant. Estrogen use in pregnant women has been associated with birth defects in the fetus.

Breast Feeding: Do not use this hormone combination if you are nursing.

Infants and Children: Not recommended for use by children.

Special Concerns: When this hormone combination is being used in the management or prevention of osteoporosis, regular weight-bearing exercise and good nutrition are important.

OVERDOSE
Symptoms: No serious ill effects have been reported following an overdose; however, nausea, vomiting, and withdrawal bleeding may occur when extremely large doses are ingested.

What to Do: An overdose is unlikely, but if someone takes a much larger dose than prescribed, seek medical attention.

▼ INTERACTIONS

DRUG INTERACTIONS
Other drugs may interact with this hormone combination. Consult your doctor if you are taking anticoagulants, anticonvulsants, antidiabetic drugs, thyroid hormones, tricyclic antidepressants, barbiturates, tranquilizers, cyclosporine, corticosteroids, corticotropin, tamoxifen, rifampin, carbamazepine, or bromocriptine.

FOOD INTERACTIONS
Estrogen may increase calcium absorption from calcium supplements. Vitamin C may increase the effects of estrogen.

DISEASE INTERACTIONS
You should not take this hormone combination drug if you have thrombophlebitis, breast cancer, any hormone-dependent cancer, or abnormal vaginal bleeding. Consult a doctor if you have a history of any of the following: liver disease, heart attack, diabetes mellitus, stroke, a blood clotting disorder, thromboembolic disease, gallbladder disease or gallstones, or liver disease, or if you are a heavy smoker of cigarettes.

 SIDE EFFECTS

SERIOUS
The most serious side effect is a modest increase in the incidence of breast cancer among women taking estrogen, especially for a long time (10 years or longer). Other side effects requiring your doctor's attention include swelling of legs and feet, rapid weight gain, abnormal menstrual bleeding, mental depression, and skin rash.

COMMON
Nausea, breast tenderness, headache, abdominal pain.

LESS COMMON
Change in appetite, vomiting, stomach cramps or bloating, change in blood pressure, dizziness, nervousness, insomnia, sleepiness, increase or decrease in weight, fatigue, backache.

FELODIPINE

BRAND NAME

Plendil

Available in: Tablets, extended-release tablets
Available OTC? No **As Generic?** No
Drug Class: Calcium channel blocker

▼ USAGE INFORMATION

WHY IT'S PRESCRIBED
To control high blood pressure (hypertension).

HOW IT WORKS
Felodipine interferes with the movement of calcium into heart muscle cells and the smooth muscle cells in the walls of the arteries. This action relaxes blood vessels (causing them to widen), which lowers blood pressure, increases the blood supply to the heart, and decreases the heart's overall workload.

▼ DOSAGE GUIDELINES

RANGE AND FREQUENCY
To start, 5 to 10 mg once a day. The dose may be increased to a maximum of 20 mg once a day. For patients over 65, starting dose is 2.5 mg per day and a maximum of 10 mg per day.

ONSET OF EFFECT
Within 2 to 5 hours.

DURATION OF ACTION
24 hours.

DIETARY ADVICE
Felodipine should be taken either on an empty stomach or with a light meal. Do not crush or chew tablets.

STORAGE
Store in a tightly sealed container away from moisture, heat, and direct light.

MISSED DOSE
Take it as soon as you remember. However, if it is near the time for the next dose, skip the missed dose and resume your regular dosage schedule. Do not double the next dose.

STOPPING THE DRUG
Do not stop taking felodipine suddenly; this may cause potentially serious health problems. If therapy is to be discontinued, the dosage should be reduced gradually, according to your doctor's instructions.

PROLONGED USE
Consult your doctor about the need for medical examinations or laboratory tests to check liver function, kidney function, and heart function.

▼ PRECAUTIONS

Over 60: Older patients are prescribed lower starting doses, which may be gradually increased until the doctor determines the appropriate individual maintenance dose.

Driving and Hazardous Work: Do not drive or engage in hazardous work until you determine how felodipine affects you.

Alcohol: Avoid alcohol while taking this medication because it may cause an excessive drop in blood pressure.

Pregnancy: Consult your physician to determine whether the benefits of felodipine outweigh its possible risks during pregnancy.

Breast Feeding: Felodipine may pass into breast milk; caution is advised. Consult your doctor for advice.

Infants and Children: Felodipine is generally not prescribed for children.

Special Concerns: Tell all of your health-care providers that you are taking felodipine and carry a note that says you take this medicine. Felodipine can cause erectile dysfunction in some men. Nicotine can reduce the effectiveness of the medicine. Hot environments can also exaggerate the drug's blood pressure lowering effect.

OVERDOSE
Symptoms: Weakness, light-headedness, rapid pulse, shortness of breath, tremors, flushed skin, fainting, and slurred speech.

What to Do: Call your doctor, emergency medical services (EMS), or the nearest poison control center immediately.

▼ INTERACTIONS

DRUG INTERACTIONS
Consult your doctor for advice if you are taking anti-convulsants, beta-blockers, digitalis drugs, carbamazepine, cyclosporine, digoxin, disopyramide, magnesium, phenobarbital, phenytoin, quinidine, rifampin, cimetidine, or erythromycin.

FOOD INTERACTIONS
Grapefruit juice should be avoided because it can amplify the effect of the drug and cause a serious drop in blood pressure. Avoid excessive salt intake.

DISEASE INTERACTIONS
Caution is advised when taking felodipine. Consult your doctor if you have any of the following: congestive heart failure, a history of heart attack or stroke, heart rhythm disturbances, or impaired liver or kidney function.

 SIDE EFFECTS

SERIOUS
Irregular or slow heartbeat, low blood pressure (causing dizziness or faintness).

COMMON
Flushing or skin rash, headache, swelling of the lower legs or feet.

LESS COMMON
Dizziness, numbness or tingling sensation, chest pain, palpitations, weakness, runny nose, rapid pulse, sore throat, abdominal discomfort, nausea, constipation or diarrhea, cough, muscle cramps, back pain, overgrowth of the gums.

FEXOFENADINE

Available in: Capsules
Available OTC? No   **As Generic?** No
Drug Class: Antihistamine

▼ USAGE INFORMATION

WHY IT'S PRESCRIBED
To prevent or relieve symptoms of hay fever and other allergies, and to treat itchy skin and hives.

HOW IT WORKS
Fexofenadine blocks the effects of histamine, a naturally occurring substance within the body that causes swelling, itching, sneezing, watery eyes, hives, and other symptoms of allergic reaction.

▼ DOSAGE GUIDELINES

RANGE AND FREQUENCY
For adults and children age 12 years and over: 60 mg 2 times a day. Also available as 180 mg; take once daily. For patients with decreased kidney function, a starting dose of 60 mg once a day is recommended. Children under age 12 years: Safety and effectiveness of fexofenadine in this age group have not been established.

ONSET OF EFFECT
Within 1 to 2 hours.

DURATION OF ACTION
12 hours or longer.

DIETARY ADVICE
This drug can be taken without regard to food or drink.

STORAGE
Store in a tightly sealed container in a dry place away from heat and direct light at room temperature.

MISSED DOSE
Take it as soon as you remember. If it is near the time for the next dose, skip the missed dose and resume your regular dosage schedule. Do not double the next dose.

STOPPING THE DRUG
You should take it as prescribed for the full treatment period, but you may stop if you are feeling better before the scheduled end of therapy. Fexofenadine can be used as needed to relieve symptoms of hay fever or other allergies.

PROLONGED USE
Tolerance, or decreased responsiveness to the drug, generally does not develop with prolonged use of fexofenadine; if it does, consult your physician. No special problems are expected with long-term use.

▼ PRECAUTIONS

Over 60: No special problems are expected.

Driving and Hazardous Work: In rare cases, fexofenadine may cause drowsiness and fatigue. Do not drive or engage in hazardous work until you determine how the medicine affects you.

Alcohol: No special precautions are necessary.

Pregnancy: Adequate and well-controlled studies in humans have not been done. Consult your doctor about taking fexofenadine if you are pregnant or are planning to become pregnant.

Breast Feeding: Fexofenadine may pass into breast milk; caution is advised. Consult your doctor for specific advice about the use of fexofenadine while nursing.

Infants and Children: Side effects are not expected to be any different in children ages 12 to 18 years than those in patients 18 years and older. The safety and effectiveness of fexofenadine for children up to 12 years of age have not been established.

OVERDOSE
Symptoms: Extreme drowsiness or fatigue.

What to Do: An overdose of fexofenadine is unlikely to be life-threatening. However, if someone takes a much larger dose than prescribed, call your doctor, emergency medical services (EMS), or local poison control right away.

▼ INTERACTIONS

DRUG INTERACTIONS
There are no known interactions between fexofenadine and other drugs.

FOOD INTERACTIONS
No known food interactions.

DISEASE INTERACTIONS
Consult your physician before taking if you have impaired kidney function.

▣ SIDE EFFECTS ▣

SERIOUS
No serious side effects are associated with the use of fexofenadine.

COMMON
No common side effects are associated with the use of fexofenadine.

LESS COMMON
Drowsiness, fatigue, stomach upset, painful menstrual bleeding.

FEXOFENADINE/PSEUDOEPHEDRINE

Available in: Extended-release tablets
Available OTC? No **As Generic?** No
Drug Class: Antihistamine/decongestant

▼ USAGE INFORMATION

WHY IT'S PRESCRIBED
To prevent or relieve symptoms of seasonal allergies such as hay fever.

HOW IT WORKS
Fexofenadine blocks the effects of histamine, a naturally occurring substance within the body that causes swelling, itching, sneezing, watery eyes, hives, and other symptoms of allergic reaction. Pseudoephedrine narrows and constricts blood vessels to decrease the blood flow to swollen nasal passages and other tissues, which in turn reduces nasal secretions, shrinks swollen nasal mucous membranes, and improves airflow in nasal passages.

▼ DOSAGE GUIDELINES

RANGE AND FREQUENCY
Adults and teenagers: 1 tablet (60 mg fexofenadine/120 mg pseudoephedrine) twice a day.

ONSET OF EFFECT
Within 1 to 2 hours.

DURATION OF ACTION
12 hours or longer.

DIETARY ADVICE
This medication should be taken at least 1 hour before or 2 hours after a meal. Taking it with food delays the onset of the drug's effects. The tablet should be swallowed whole.

STORAGE
Store in a tightly sealed container away from moisture, heat, and direct light.

MISSED DOSE
Take it as soon as you remember. If it is near the time for the next dose, skip the missed dose and resume your regular dosage schedule. Do not double the next dose.

STOPPING THE DRUG
You may stop taking it before the scheduled end of therapy if you are feeling better.

PROLONGED USE
Consult your doctor about taking this drug for more than 5 to 7 days.

▼ PRECAUTIONS

Over 60: Adverse reactions may be more likely and more severe in older patients.

Driving and Hazardous Work: Do not drive or engage in hazardous work until you determine how the medicine affects you.

Alcohol: No special warnings.

Pregnancy: Adequate human studies have not been done. Before taking this drug, tell your doctor if you are pregnant or are planning to become pregnant. Discuss with your doctor the relative risks and benefits of using this drug while pregnant.

Breast Feeding: The pseudoephedrine component of this drug passes into breast milk; avoid or discontinue this drug while breast feeding.

Infants and Children: Not recommended for use by children under age 12 years.

Special Concerns: If your symptoms do not improve within 7 days, check with your doctor. To help prevent insomnia, take the last dose of the day at least 2 hours before your bedtime.

OVERDOSE
Symptoms: No cases of overdose have been reported.

What to Do: An overdose is unlikely; however, if you have reason to suspect an overdose has occurred, call emergency medical services (EMS) for evaluation and treatment.

▼ INTERACTIONS

DRUG INTERACTIONS
This drug and MAO inhibitors should not be used within 14 days of each other. Consult your doctor for advice if you are taking antihypertensives or digitalis drugs.

FOOD INTERACTIONS
No known food interactions.

DISEASE INTERACTIONS
You should not take this medication if you have a history of narrow-angle glaucoma, urinary retention, severe high blood pressure, or severe coronary artery disease. Caution is advised if you have mild to moderate high blood pressure, diabetes mellitus, a history of angina or heart attack, an overactive thyroid gland, impaired kidney function, or an enlarged prostate.

≡ SIDE EFFECTS ≡

SERIOUS
Palpitations, shortness of breath, breathing difficulty. Stop taking the medication and call your doctor right away.

COMMON
Headache, insomnia, nausea.

LESS COMMON
Dry mouth, indigestion, throat irritation, dizziness, agitation, back pain, anxiety, nervousness, stomach pain, upper respiratory infection.

FINASTERIDE

BRAND NAMES

Propecia, Proscar

Available in: Tablets
Available OTC? No   **As Generic?** No
Drug Class: 5-alpha reductase inhibitor

▼ USAGE INFORMATION

WHY IT'S PRESCRIBED
To treat benign prostatic hyperplasia (BPH)–that is, noncancerous enlargement of the prostate gland, which is extremely common among men over 50. Also used to treat male pattern hair loss.

HOW IT WORKS
Finasteride halts or reverses enlargement of the prostate by blocking the action of the enzyme 5-alpha reductase, which the body needs to produce dihydrotestosterone (DHT), a chemical involved in the mechanism that enlarges the prostate. DHT is also integral to the process of male pattern hair loss; by decreasing DHT concentrations in the scalp, finasteride may slow or reverse this process.

▼ DOSAGE GUIDELINES

RANGE AND FREQUENCY
For BPH: 5 mg once a day. For male pattern hair loss: 1 mg once a day.

ONSET OF EFFECT
Unknown.

DURATION OF ACTION
For BPH: 24 hours for a single dose; up to 2 weeks after standard therapy is ended. For hair loss: New hair that results from finasteride treatments will probably regress after treatment ends.

DIETARY ADVICE
Finasteride can be taken without regard to diet. If you have trouble swallowing the tablet whole, you can crush it and take it with liquid or food.

STORAGE
Store in a tightly sealed container away from moisture, heat, and direct light.

MISSED DOSE
If you miss a dose on one day, do not double the dose the next day.

STOPPING THE DRUG
The decision to stop taking the drug should be made by your doctor.

PROLONGED USE
If you take this drug for a prolonged period for BPH, see your doctor regularly so that changes in prostate size can be monitored. For hair loss, continued use is usually recommended to sustain the drug's benefits.

▼ PRECAUTIONS

Over 60: No special problems are expected.

Driving and Hazardous Work: The use of finasteride should not impair your ability to perform such tasks safely.

Alcohol: No special precautions are necessary.

Pregnancy: Although finasteride is not prescribed for women, those who are pregnant or planning to become pregnant should not handle the medication, especially if it is crushed or broken, because it can have an adverse effect on a male fetus. Men who take finasteride should use a barrier method of birth control (such as a condom), which prevents the female sexual partner from being exposed to small quantities of the drug present in semen.

Breast Feeding: Women who are nursing should avoid contact with finasteride or the sperm of a man who is taking the drug.

Infants and Children: Finasteride is not prescribed for children.

Special Concerns: Before taking this medicine for BPH, you should have a digital rectal examination and other tests for prostate cancer. Note that finasteride may affect the results of the prostate-specific antigen (PSA) test for prostate cancer; be sure any doctor you see for treatment, including your dentist, knows that you are taking this drug.

OVERDOSE
Symptoms: No specific symptoms have been reported.

What to Do: An overdose of finasteride is unlikely to be life-threatening. However, if someone takes a much larger dose than prescribed, call your doctor, emergency medical services (EMS), or the nearest poison control center.

▼ INTERACTIONS

DRUG INTERACTIONS
Consult your doctor for specific advice if you are taking amantadine, amphetamines, antihistamines, antidepressants, antidyskinetics (medications for Parkinson's disease or similar conditions), antipsychotics, appetite suppressants, anticholinergics (drugs for stomach spasms or cramps), bronchodilators, decongestants, ephedrine, phenylpropanolamine, or pseudoephedrine.

FOOD INTERACTIONS
No known food interactions.

DISEASE INTERACTIONS
Caution is advised when taking finasteride. Before you start, consult your doctor if you have liver disease, which may magnify the effects of the medication.

≣ SIDE EFFECTS ≣
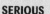

SERIOUS
No serious side effects are associated with the use of finasteride.

COMMON
No common side effects are associated with the use of finasteride.

LESS COMMON
Reduced sex drive, erectile dysfunction (impotence), decreased quantity of ejaculate. It should be noted that this decrease is not a sign of reduced fertility.

FLUCONAZOLE

BRAND NAME

Diflucan

Available in: Tablets, oral suspension, injection
Available OTC? No   **As Generic?** No
Drug Class: Antifungal

▼ USAGE INFORMATION

WHY IT'S PRESCRIBED
To treat fungal infections of the mouth and throat (thrush), of the vagina (yeast infection), or throughout the body, as well as meningitis (inflammation of the protective membranes surrounding the brain). Often used to treat AIDS-related fungal infections. May also be used to prevent recurring fungal infections in susceptible patients weakened by AIDS or by chemotherapy or radiation treatment.

HOW IT WORKS
Fluconazole prevents fungal organisms from manufacturing vital substances required for their growth and function. This drug is effective only for infections caused by fungal organisms. It will not work for bacterial or viral infections.

▼ DOSAGE GUIDELINES

RANGE AND FREQUENCY
Adults and teenagers—For fungal infections: 200 to 400 mg on the first day, then 100 to 400 mg once a day using oral forms or injection.

Injections are into a vein. For vaginal yeast infection: 1 dose of 150 mg as tablet or oral suspension.

ONSET OF EFFECT
Oral forms: Unknown.
Injection: Immediate.

DURATION OF ACTION
Unknown.

DIETARY ADVICE
Swallow tablets with liquid. The oral suspension should be shaken and carefully measured out before you take it. This drug can be taken without regard to diet.

STORAGE
Store fluconazole in a tightly sealed container away from moisture, heat, and direct light. Keep any liquid form of the drug refrigerated but do not allow it to freeze.

MISSED DOSE
Take it as soon as you remember. This will help keep a constant level of medication in your system. If it is near the time for the next dose, skip the missed dose and resume your regular dosage schedule. Do not double the next dose.

STOPPING THE DRUG
Take it as prescribed for the full treatment period, even if you begin to feel better before the scheduled end of therapy. The decision to stop taking the drug should be made by your doctor. Gradual reduction of the dose may be necessary if you have been taking this medicine for a long time.

PROLONGED USE
Notify your doctor if your condition does not improve or instead becomes worse within a few weeks of the beginning of treatment.

▼ PRECAUTIONS

Over 60: Dosage may need to be reduced in older patients who have impaired kidney function.

Driving and Hazardous Work: The use of fluconazole should not impair your ability to perform such tasks safely.

Alcohol: No special precautions are necessary.

Pregnancy: Adequate studies of fluconazole use during pregnancy have not been done. Consult your doctor for specific advice if you are currently pregnant or plan to become pregnant.

Breast Feeding: Fluconazole may pass into breast milk; caution is advised. Consult your doctor for advice.

Infants and Children: Fluconazole is not generally prescribed for children under 14 years.

Special Concerns: A doctor should monitor your kidney function while you take fluconazole. Tell any doctor or dentist whom you consult that you are taking this medicine. Be sure to shake the oral suspension well before taking it.

OVERDOSE
Symptoms: An overdose with fluconazole is unlikely.

What to Do: Emergency instructions not applicable.

▼ INTERACTIONS

DRUG INTERACTIONS
Do not take cisapride with fluconazole. Other drugs may interact with fluconazole. Consult your doctor for specific advice if you are taking oral antidiabetic medications, cyclosporine, rifampin, phenytoin, rifabutin, tacrolimus, astemizole, or warfarin.

FOOD INTERACTIONS
No food interactions have been reported.

DISEASE INTERACTIONS
Caution is advised when taking fluconazole. Consult your doctor if you have a history of alcohol abuse (and associated liver problems), or any type of liver or kidney disease, because these organs work together to remove the medication from the body.

⬇ SIDE EFFECTS ⬇

SERIOUS
Skin rash or itching, fever or chills. Call your doctor right away.

COMMON
No common side effects have been reported with the use of fluconazole.

LESS COMMON
Diarrhea, nausea, vomiting, constipation, dizziness, headache, redness or flushing of skin.

FLUOXETINE HYDROCHLORIDE

Available in: Capsules, oral solution
Available OTC? No   **As Generic?** Yes
Drug Class: Selective serotonin reuptake inhibitor (SSRI) antidepressant

▼ USAGE INFORMATION

WHY IT'S PRESCRIBED
To treat major depression, obsessive-compulsive disorder (OCD), panic disorder, chronic pain, and premenstrual dysphoric disorder (PMDD).

HOW IT WORKS
Fluoxetine affects levels of serotonin, a brain chemical that is thought to be linked to mood, emotions, and mental state.

▼ DOSAGE GUIDELINES

RANGE AND FREQUENCY
To start, 20 mg a day taken in the morning. Your doctor may increase the dose gradually to a maximum of 80 mg a day. Older adults: To start, 10 to 20 mg a day. This dosage may be increased gradually by your doctor to a maximum of 40 to 60 mg a day.

ONSET OF EFFECT
1 to 4 weeks.

DURATION OF ACTION
Unknown.

DIETARY ADVICE
Taking the drug with liquid or food can lessen stomach irritation. Capsules may be opened and mixed with food or juice to aid swallowing.

STORAGE
Store fluoxetine in a tightly sealed container away from moisture, heat, and direct light. Keep the liquid form refrigerated but do not allow it to freeze.

MISSED DOSE
Take it as soon as you remember. If it is near the time for the next dose, skip the missed dose and resume your regular dosage schedule. Do not double the next dose.

STOPPING THE DRUG
Take it as prescribed for the full treatment period, even if you begin to feel better before the scheduled end of therapy. Discontinuing the drug abruptly may produce unpleasant withdrawal symptoms. Dosage should be reduced gradually according to your doctor's specific instructions.

PROLONGED USE
The usual course of therapy lasts 6 months to 1 year; some patients may benefit from additional therapy. For obsessive-compulsive disorder, the usual course of therapy lasts 1 year or more.

▼ PRECAUTIONS

Over 60: Adverse reactions may be more likely and more severe in older patients, because their metabolisms are slower. A lower dose may be necessary.

Driving and Hazardous Work: Use caution when driving or engaging in hazardous work until you determine how the medicine affects you.

Alcohol: Avoid alcohol.

Pregnancy: Fluoxetine should be used during pregnancy only if the potential benefit justifies the potential risk to the fetus. Before you take this medicine, tell your doctor if you are pregnant or plan to become pregnant.

Breast Feeding: Fluoxetine may pass into breast milk; caution is advised. Consult your doctor for advice.

Infants and Children: Not recommended for use by children under age 12 years.

Special Concerns: Take it at least 6 hours before bedtime to prevent insomnia, unless the drug causes drowsiness.

OVERDOSE
Symptoms: Agitation, excitement, severe nausea and vomiting, seizures.

What to Do: Call your doctor, emergency medical services (EMS), or the nearest poison control center immediately.

▼ INTERACTIONS

DRUG INTERACTIONS
Fluoxetine should not be used within 5 weeks of taking MAO (monoamine oxidase) inhibitors or thioridazine. The following drugs may interact with fluoxetine. Be sure to consult your doctor for specific advice if you are taking nortriptyline, caffeine, oral anticoagulants, central nervous system depressants, digitalis preparations, lithium, loratadine, dextromethorphan, ketorolac, buspirone, phenytoin, trazodone, tryptophan, sumatriptan, naratriptan, or zolmitriptan.

FOOD INTERACTIONS
No known food interactions.

DISEASE INTERACTIONS
Use of fluoxetine may cause complications in patients with liver or kidney disease, because these organs work together to remove the medication from the body. Use of the drug may make diabetes or seizures worse.

⬇ SIDE EFFECTS ⬇

SERIOUS
Agitation, shaking, difficulty breathing, rash, hives, itching, joint or muscle pain, chills or fever. If such symptoms occur, call your doctor immediately.

COMMON
Nervousness, drowsiness, anxiety, insomnia, headache, diarrhea, excessive sweating, nausea, decreased appetite, decreased initiative.

LESS COMMON
Nasal congestion, unusual or vivid dreams, cough, increased appetite, chest pain, constipation, vision disturbances, abdominal pain, stomach gas, constipation, vomiting, frequent urination, difficulty concentrating, sexual dysfunction, heartbeat irregularities, trembling, fatigue, dizziness, change in taste, flushing of the skin on the face and neck, dry mouth, menstrual pain.

FLUTICASONE

BRAND NAMES
Flonase, Flovent

Available in: Oral inhalation, nasal spray
Available OTC? No   **As Generic?** No
Drug Class: Respiratory corticosteroid

▼ USAGE INFORMATION

WHY IT'S PRESCRIBED
To prevent bronchial asthma and to treat allergic rhinitis (seasonal or perennial allergies such as hay fever).

HOW IT WORKS
Respiratory corticosteroids such as fluticasone primarily reduce or prevent inflammation of the lining of airways (the underlying cause of asthma), reduce the allergic response to inhaled allergens, and inhibit the secretion of mucus within the airways.

▼ DOSAGE GUIDELINES

RANGE AND FREQUENCY
For asthma—Oral inhalation: 88 to 220 micrograms (µg) a day 2 times per day; not to exceed 440 µg a day. For patients previously treated with oral corticosteroids: 880 µg 2 times a day. Dosage may gradually be reduced after 1 week of therapy. For allergic rhinitis—Nasal spray: Adults: 2 sprays (50 µg each) in each nostril once a day, or 1 spray in each nostril twice a day (in the morning and at night).

Children ages 4 to 17 years: One spray in each nostril once a day. If needed, dose may be increased to 2 sprays in each nostril once a day. Maximum daily dose should not exceed 200 µg. After relief is achieved, the dose may be reduced to 1 spray a day.

ONSET OF EFFECT
Usually within 1 week; it may take 3 weeks for the full effect to occur.

DURATION OF ACTION
Unknown.

DIETARY ADVICE
No special restrictions.

STORAGE
Store the inhaler in a dry place away from heat and light.

MISSED DOSE
Take it as soon as you remember. If it is near the time for the next dose, skip the missed dose and resume your regular dosage schedule. Do not double the next dose.

STOPPING THE DRUG
If you have been using fluticasone for a long period, do not stop taking it suddenly.

Consult your doctor about how to stop.

PROLONGED USE
Consult your doctor about the need for regular medical tests and examinations if you must take this drug for a prolonged period of time.

▼ PRECAUTIONS

Over 60: No special problems are expected.

Driving and Hazardous Work: The use of fluticasone should not impair your ability to perform such tasks safely.

Alcohol: No special precautions are necessary.

Pregnancy: Well-controlled studies of fluticasone use during pregnancy have not been done; it is generally not recommended unless the benefits clearly outweigh the risks. Consult your doctor.

Breast Feeding: Fluticasone may pass into breast milk; caution is advised. Consult your doctor for advice.

Infants and Children: Safety and effectiveness have not been established for children under 4 years old.

Special Concerns: Inhaled steroids will not help an asthma attack in progress. Inhaled steroids can lower resistance to yeast infections of the mouth, throat, or voice box. To prevent yeast infections, gargle or rinse your mouth with water after each use; do not swallow the water. Know how to use the spray properly; read and fol-

low the directions that come with the device. Before you have surgery, tell the doctor or dentist that you are using a steroid.

OVERDOSE
Symptoms: No cases of overdose have been reported.

What to Do: An overdose of fluticasone is unlikely. If you have any reason to suspect an overdose, contact your doctor or seek medical assistance right away.

▼ INTERACTIONS

DRUG INTERACTIONS
Consult your doctor for specific advice if you are taking systemic corticosteroids, other inhaled corticosteroids, or drugs that suppress the immune system.

FOOD INTERACTIONS
No known food interactions.

DISEASE INTERACTIONS
Caution is advised when taking fluticasone. Consult your doctor if you have any of the following: a lung disease such as tuberculosis, a herpes infection of the eye, nasal ulcers or recent nose surgery or injury, or any bacterial, viral, or fungal infection. If you have been exposed to chicken pox or measles, tell your doctor at once.

 SIDE EFFECTS

SERIOUS
No serious side effects are associated with the use of fluticasone.

COMMON
Oral inhalation: Sore throat, white patches in mouth or throat, hoarseness. Nasal spray: Nosebleeds or bloody nasal secretions, nasal burning or irritation, sore throat.

LESS COMMON
Eye pain, watering eyes, gradual decrease of vision, stomach pain and digestive disturbances.

FLUVASTATIN

Available in: Capsules
Available OTC? No   **As Generic?** No
Drug Class: Antilipidemic (cholesterol-lowering agent)

▼ USAGE INFORMATION

WHY IT'S PRESCRIBED
To treat high cholesterol. Usually prescribed after first lines of treatment—including diet, weight loss, and exercise—fail to reduce total and low-density lipoprotein (LDL) cholesterol to acceptable levels.

HOW IT WORKS
Fluvastatin blocks the action of an enzyme required for the manufacture of cholesterol, thereby interfering with its formation. By lowering the amount of cholesterol in the liver cells, fluvastatin then increases the formation of receptors for LDL, and thus reduces blood levels of total and LDL cholesterol. In addition to lowering LDL cholesterol, fluvastatin modestly reduces triglyceride levels and raises levels of HDL (the so-called "good" cholesterol).

▼ DOSAGE GUIDELINES

RANGE AND FREQUENCY
Initial dose is 20 mg, taken once a day in the evening. Dose may be increased by your doctor to 40 mg taken once a day in the evening.

ONSET OF EFFECT
Within 2 to 4 weeks after starting therapy.

DURATION OF ACTION
The effect persists for the duration of therapy.

DIETARY ADVICE
Cholesterol-lowering drugs are only one part of a total lifestyle program that should include regular exercise and a healthy diet. The American Heart Association publishes a "Healthy Heart" diet, which is widely recommended for reducing cholesterol levels.

STORAGE
Store in a tightly sealed container away from heat and direct light. Keep away from moisture and extremes in temperature.

MISSED DOSE
Take it as soon as you remember. Take your next dose at the proper time and resume your regular dosage schedule. Do not double the next dose.

STOPPING THE DRUG
The decision to stop taking the drug should be made in consultation with your doctor. Once the medication is discontinued, blood cholesterol is likely to return to original elevated levels.

PROLONGED USE
Side effects are more likely with prolonged use. As you continue with fluvastatin, your doctor will periodically order blood tests to evaluate liver function.

▼ PRECAUTIONS

Over 60: No special problems are expected in older patients.

Driving and Hazardous Work: The use of fluvastatin should not impair your ability to perform such tasks safely.

Alcohol: No special precautions are necessary.

Pregnancy: Should not be used during pregnancy or by women who plan to become pregnant in the near future.

Breast Feeding: Fluvastatin passes into breast milk and is not recommended while breast feeding.

Infants and Children: Rarely used in children.

Special Concerns: Important elements for treating high cholesterol include proper diet, weight loss, regular moderate exercise, and the avoidance of certain medications that may increase your cholesterol levels. Because fluvastatin has potential side effects, it is important that you maintain a recommended healthy diet and cooperate with other treatments your physician may suggest.

OVERDOSE
Symptoms: An overdose of fluvastatin is unlikely.

What to Do: Emergency instructions not applicable.

▼ INTERACTIONS

DRUG INTERACTIONS
Consult your doctor if you are taking cyclosporine; gemfibrozil; niacin; antibiotics, especially erythromycin; or medications for fungus infections. All of these drugs may increase the risk of myositis (muscle inflammation) when taken with fluvastatin and may lead to kidney failure.

FOOD INTERACTIONS
No known food interactions.

DISEASE INTERACTIONS
Consult your doctor if you have any of the following problems: liver, kidney, or muscle disease or a medical history involving organ transplantation or recent surgery.

≡ SIDE EFFECTS ≡

SERIOUS
Fever, unusual or unexplained muscle aches and tenderness. Call your doctor immediately.

COMMON
Side effects occur in only 1% to 2% of patients. These include constipation or diarrhea, dizziness or lightheadedness, bloating or gas, heartburn, nausea, skin rash, stomach pain, increase in liver enzymes.

LESS COMMON
Sleeping difficulty.

FOLIC ACID (FOLACIN; FOLATE)

BRAND NAME

BRAND NAME

Folvite

Available in: Tablets, injectable form (for use in hospitals)
Available OTC? Yes   **As Generic?** Yes
Drug Class: Vitamin

▼ USAGE INFORMATION

WHY IT'S PRESCRIBED
The vitamin folic acid (also known as folacin and folate) is prescribed for treatment or prevention of certain types of anemia that result from folic acid deficiency. Such deficiencies may be caused by insufficient intake of folic acid (the result of a poor diet or malnutrition), an inability to absorb the vitamin (such as occurs in gastrointestinal disease), impaired ability to utilize the vitamin (caused by excessive alcohol intake or phenytoin use), or as a result of medical conditions requiring increased amounts of folic acid (such as with pregnancy, breast feeding, hemodialysis, hemolytic anemia, and bone marrow failure).

HOW IT WORKS
Folic acid, which is one of the B vitamins, enhances chemical reactions that contribute to the production of red blood cells, the manufacture of DNA needed for cell replication, and the metabolism of amino acids (compounds necessary for the manufacture of proteins).

▼ DOSAGE GUIDELINES

RANGE AND FREQUENCY
For severe deficiency—Adults and children regardless of age: 1 mg daily. For daily supplementation after correction of a severe deficiency—Adults and adolescents: 1 mg once daily. During pregnancy: 400 micrograms (µg), once daily. While breast feeding: 260 to 280 µg, once daily. Children, newborn to 3 years of age: 25 to 50 µg, once daily; children 4 to 6 years of age: 75 µg, once daily; children 7 to 10 years of age: 100 µg, once daily.

ONSET OF EFFECT
Folic acid is used immediately by the body for a number of vital chemical functions.

DURATION OF ACTION
Folic acid is required by your body on a daily basis throughout your lifetime.

DIETARY ADVICE
Maintain your usual food and fluid intake. Increase fluids if you have a fever or diarrhea, in hot weather, or during exercise. Follow your doctor's dietary advice (such as low-cholesterol, low-fat, or low-salt restrictions) to improve control over high blood pressure and heart disease.

STORAGE
Store this medication in a tightly sealed container away from heat and direct light. Keep container away from moisture and extremes in temperature.

MISSED DOSE
Take it as soon as you remember. If it is near the time for the next dose, skip the missed dose and resume your regular dosage schedule. Do not double the next dose.

STOPPING THE DRUG
The decision to stop taking the drug should be made by your doctor.

PROLONGED USE
Therapy with folacin may require weeks or months.

▼ PRECAUTIONS

Over 60: No special problems are expected in older individuals.

Driving and Hazardous Work: The use of folic acid should not impair your ability to perform such tasks safely.

Alcohol: Alcohol impairs the body's utilization of folic acid; avoid it completely if you are taking folic acid.

Pregnancy: Folic acid supplementation is recommended during pregnancy.

Breast Feeding: Folic acid supplementation is recommended while nursing.

Infants and Children: Folic acid may be used regardless of age.

Special Concerns: Folic acid ingestion can mask vitamin B_{12} deficiency and lead to irreversible neurological damage; therefore, folic acid should be taken only on the recommendation of your doctor. Folic acid deficiency should not occur and supplementation is not necessary in healthy individuals who consume a normal balanced diet.

OVERDOSE
Symptoms: No specific symptoms have been reported.

What to Do: A folic acid overdose is not life-threatening. No emergency procedures are necessary.

▼ INTERACTIONS

DRUG INTERACTIONS
Consult your doctor for advice if you are taking pain relievers, antibiotics, anticonvulsants, epoetin, estrogens, oral contraceptives, methotrexate, pyrimethamine, triamterene, sulfasalazine, or zinc supplements.

FOOD INTERACTIONS
No known food interactions.

DISEASE INTERACTIONS
Consult your doctor if you have pernicious anemia.

 SIDE EFFECTS

SERIOUS
Wheezing, breathing difficulty, chest pain, swelling, tightness in throat or chest, dizziness, rash, itching. Such symptoms may indicate a serious allergic reaction, although this is extremely rare.

COMMON
The are no known common side effects associated with the use of folic acid.

LESS COMMON
Mild allergic reactions.

FOSINOPRIL SODIUM

Monopril

Available in: Tablets
Available OTC? No   **As Generic?** Yes
Drug Class: Angiotensin-converting enzyme (ACE) inhibitor

▼ USAGE INFORMATION

WHY IT'S PRESCRIBED
To control high blood pressure, to treat congestive heart failure, to treat patients with left ventricular dysfunction (damage to the pumping chamber of the heart), and to minimize further kidney damage in diabetics with mild kidney disease.

HOW IT WORKS
Angiotensin-converting enzyme (ACE) inhibitors block an enzyme that produces angiotensin, a naturally occurring substance that causes blood vessels to constrict and stimulates production of the adrenal hormone, aldosterone, which promotes sodium retention in the body. As a result, ACE inhibitor medications relax blood vessels (causing them to widen) and reduce sodium retention, which in turn lowers blood pressure and so decreases the workload of the heart.

▼ DOSAGE GUIDELINES

RANGE AND FREQUENCY
Initial dose: 10 mg once a day. Maintenance dose: 20 to 80 mg a day in 1 or 2 doses.

ONSET OF EFFECT
Within 1 hour.

DURATION OF ACTION
24 hours.

DIETARY ADVICE
Take fosinopril on an empty stomach about 1 hour before mealtime. Follow your doctor's dietary advice to improve control over high blood pressure and heart disease. Avoid high-potassium foods (such as bananas and citrus fruits and juices) unless you are also taking specific medications that lower potassium levels, such as diuretics.

STORAGE
Store this in a sealed container away from heat and light. Keep away from moisture and extremes in temperature.

MISSED DOSE
Take it as soon as you remember. If it is near the time for the next dose, skip the missed dose and resume your regular dosage schedule. Do not double the next dose.

STOPPING THE DRUG
Do not stop taking this drug abruptly; this may cause potentially serious health problems. Dosage should be reduced gradually, according to your doctor's instructions.

PROLONGED USE
Therapy with this medication may require months or years. Prolonged use may increase the risk of adverse effects.

▼ PRECAUTIONS

Over 60: Adverse reactions may be more likely and more severe.

Driving and Hazardous Work: Avoid such activities until you determine how this medication affects you.

Alcohol: Consume alcohol only in moderation because it may increase the effect of the drug and cause an excessive drop in blood pressure. Consult your doctor for advice.

Pregnancy: Do not use fosinopril if you are pregnant or trying to become pregnant. Use of this drug during the last 6 months of pregnancy may cause severe defects in or even death of the fetus.

Breast Feeding: Fosinopril passes into breast milk and may be harmful to the infant; avoid using the drug while you are nursing.

Infants and Children: Fosinopril is generally not recommended for children.

OVERDOSE
Symptoms: No specific symptoms have been reported.

What to Do: Although overdose is unlikely, call your doctor, emergency medical services (EMS), or the nearest poison control center immediately if you suspect that someone has taken a much larger dose than prescribed.

▼ INTERACTIONS

DRUG INTERACTIONS
Consult your doctor if you are taking diuretics (especially potassium-sparing diuretics), potassium supplements or drugs containing potassium (check ingredient labels), lithium, anticoagulants (such as warfarin), indomethacin or other antiinflammatory drugs, antacids, allopurinol, or any over-the-counter medications (especially cold remedies and diet pills).

FOOD INTERACTIONS
Avoid low-salt milk and salt substitutes. Many brands have high amounts of potassium. Avoid high-potassium foods such as bananas and citrus fruits and juices.

DISEASE INTERACTIONS
Consult your doctor if you have lupus or if you have had a prior allergic reaction to ACE inhibitors. This medicine should be used with caution by patients with severe kidney disease or renal artery stenosis (narrowing of one or both of the arteries that supply blood to the kidneys).

≡ SIDE EFFECTS ≡

SERIOUS
Fever and chills; sore throat and hoarseness; sudden difficulty breathing or swallowing; swelling of the face, mouth, or extremities; impaired kidney function (ankle swelling, decreased urination); confusion; yellow discoloration of the eyes or skin (indicating liver disorder); intense itching; chest pain or palpitations; abdominal pain. Serious side effects are very rare; contact your doctor immediately.

COMMON
Dry, persistent cough.

LESS COMMON
Dizziness or fainting; skin rash; numbness or tingling in the hands, feet, or lips; unusual fatigue or muscle weakness; nausea; drowsiness; loss of taste; headache.

FUROSEMIDE

Available in: Tablets, oral solution, injection
Available OTC? No **As Generic?** Yes
Drug Class: Loop diuretic

▼ USAGE INFORMATION

WHY IT'S PRESCRIBED
To reduce the fluid (salt and water) accumulation that can lead to edema (swelling) and breathlessness in patients who have heart disease, cirrhosis of the liver, and kidney disease. Furosemide is sometimes used to help control high blood pressure levels.

HOW IT WORKS
Loop diuretics work on a specific portion of the kidney (the loop of Henle) to increase the excretion of water and sodium in urine.

▼ DOSAGE GUIDELINES

RANGE AND FREQUENCY
20 to 600 mg a day. Tablets and solution: dosage is given in 1, 2, or 3 divided doses daily. Injection (given in a hospital setting only): dosage is given in divided doses every 2 to 3 hours or as a continuous infusion.

ONSET OF EFFECT
20 to 60 minutes.

DURATION OF ACTION
Tablets and solution: 6 to 8 hours. Injection: 2 hours.

DIETARY ADVICE
Take with food to reduce stomach irritation.

STORAGE
Keep it in refrigerator in a light-resistant container. Do not allow liquid forms to freeze.

MISSED DOSE
Take it as soon as you remember. If it is near the time for the next dose, skip the missed dose and resume your regular dosage schedule. Do not double the next dose.

STOPPING THE DRUG
The decision to stop taking the drug should be made by your doctor.

PROLONGED USE
There are no apparent problems. Regular doctor examinations are advised.

▼ PRECAUTIONS

Over 60: No special problems are expected.

Driving and Hazardous Work: No special precautions are required.

Alcohol: No special precautions are required.

Pregnancy: Diuretics are not useful for relieving the normal fluid retention that occurs during pregnancy. In patients who do need diuretic therapy, furosemide is generally preferred but should be taken only after careful consultation with your primary care doctor or OB-GYN.

Breast Feeding: Furosemide passes into breast milk; avoid or discontinue use while breast-feeding.

Infants and Children: Use furosemide only under careful supervision by a pediatrician.

Special Concerns: To prevent sleep disruption, avoid taking furosemide in the evening. You may also have to take a potassium supplement or consume foods or fluids high in potassium while you are using this drug. Diabetic patients should monitor their blood sugar levels carefully.

OVERDOSE
Symptoms: Weakness, lethargy, mental confusion, muscle cramps.

What to Do: Call your doctor, emergency medical services (EMS), or the nearest poison control center immediately.

▼ INTERACTIONS

DRUG INTERACTIONS
Consult your doctor about any other drugs you are taking, especially antibiotics, other blood pressure drugs, ACE (angiotensin-converting enzyme) inhibitors, pain relievers, lithium, cortisone-related drugs, digitalis-related drugs, or nonsteroidal antiinflammatory drugs.

FOOD INTERACTIONS
None reported.

DISEASE INTERACTIONS
Caution is advised when taking this medication. Consult your doctor if you have diabetes, gout, or a hearing problem or have had a recent heart attack.

≡ SIDE EFFECTS ≡

SERIOUS
Skin rash, hives, intense itching, swelling of the mouth and throat, breathing difficulty, mood or mental changes, nausea and vomiting, unusual fatigue, black or tarry stools. Call your doctor immediately.

COMMON
Muscle cramps or pain. Potassium depletion may lead to heart palpitations and weakness. Fluid depletion may lead to dizziness, especially on rising from a sitting or lying position, and thirst, dry mouth, and constipation.

LESS COMMON
Buzzing or ringing in ears, loss of hearing (particularly after intravenous treatment), diarrhea, loss of appetite, gout, increased blood sugar (a problem for diabetic patients).

GABAPENTIN

Available in: Capsules, tablets
Available OTC? No **As Generic?** No
Drug Class: Anticonvulsant

▼ USAGE INFORMATION

WHY IT'S PRESCRIBED
To control certain kinds of seizures in the treatment of epilepsy. Gabapentin is often prescribed in combination with another anticonvulsant medication.

HOW IT WORKS
The drug's mechanism of action is not well understood. It is believed that gabapentin inhibits activity in certain parts of the brain and suppresses the abnormal firing of neurons that causes seizures.

▼ DOSAGE GUIDELINES

RANGE AND FREQUENCY
Adults and teenagers: 900 to 3,600 mg a day in 3 or 4 divided doses. Some patients require higher doses. The dose is started low and then gradually increased by your doctor to achieve maximum therapeutic benefit with a minimum of side effects. Children ages 3 to 12 years: To start, 10 to 15 mg per 2.2 lb (1 kg) in 3 divided doses. The dose is started low and then gradually increased by your doctor to achieve maximum therapeutic benefit with a minimum of side effects.

ONSET OF EFFECT
Several hours.

DURATION OF ACTION
Maximum effectiveness lasts 5 to 8 hours or longer; effectiveness then gradually decreases over time.

DIETARY ADVICE
No special restrictions.

STORAGE
Store this medication in a tightly sealed container away from moisture, heat, and direct light. Refrigerate the oral solution, but do not allow it to freeze.

SIDE EFFECTS

SERIOUS
Fever, sore throat, swollen glands, red or purple pointlike rash on the skin or mucous membranes, blistering or peeling skin lesions, mouth sores, easy bruising, paleness, weakness, confusion, lethargy, or seizures may be a sign of a potentially fatal blood disorder (aplastic anemia) or other complication. Call your physician immediately.

COMMON
Fatigue, dizziness, sedation, clumsiness or unsteadiness, unusual eye movements, blurred or altered vision, nausea, vomiting, tremor.

LESS COMMON
Diarrhea, muscle aches or weakness, dry mouth, headache, sleep disturbances, irritability, slurred speech. There are numerous additional side effects associated with the use of this drug; consult your doctor if you are concerned about any adverse or unusual reactions.

MISSED DOSE
Take it as soon as you remember. If your next dose is scheduled within the next 2 hours, take the missed dose and take the next dose 1 to 2 hours later. Resume your regular dosage schedule. Do not double the next dose unless advised to do so by your doctor. Do not wait more than 12 hours between doses.

STOPPING THE DRUG
The decision to stop taking the drug should be made by your doctor. Never stop this drug abruptly; this may cause seizures. The dose is typically tapered over a period of weeks.

PROLONGED USE
Therapy with gabapentin may be required for months or years. Some side effects that are prominent during the first few weeks of therapy may subsequently diminish.

▼ PRECAUTIONS

Over 60: Older persons may require lower doses to minimize side effects.

Driving and Hazardous Work: Avoid such activities until you determine how the medication affects you.

Alcohol: May contribute to excessive drowsiness.

Pregnancy: Adequate human studies have not been done, but the use of other anticonvulsants is associated with an increased risk of birth defects. However, seizures during pregnancy can also increase the risks to the unborn child. Discuss with your doctor the potential risks and benefits of using gabapentin during pregnancy. Folate supplementation is recommended beginning 1 to 2 months before conception and throughout pregnancy.

Breast Feeding: Gabapentin may pass into breast milk, although at low levels. Consult your doctor for advice.

Infants and Children: There are few published studies about the use of gabapentin in children age 12 years and younger, but effectiveness should be similar to that seen in older patients. Safety and effectiveness have not been established for children under the age of 3 years.

Special Concerns: Your doctor may advise you to wear a medical bracelet or carry an identification card saying that you are taking this drug.

OVERDOSE
Symptoms: Few cases of overdose have been reported. Symptoms include double vision, slurred speech, drowsiness, lethargy, and diarrhea.

What to Do: Call your doctor, emergency medical services (EMS), or the nearest poison control center immediately.

▼ INTERACTIONS

DRUG INTERACTIONS
No significant interactions.

FOOD INTERACTIONS
No known food interactions.

DISEASE INTERACTIONS
Gabapentin dosage may need to be lower in patients with kidney disease.

GEMFIBROZIL

BRAND NAME

Lopid

Available in: Tablets
Available OTC? No **As Generic?** Yes
Drug Class: Antilipidemic (triglyceride-lowering agent)

▼ USAGE INFORMATION

WHY IT'S PRESCRIBED
To treat high levels of blood triglyceride. Usually prescribed after other treatments, including diet, weight loss, exercise, and control of diabetes (when present), fail to lower triglyceride levels adequately.

HOW IT WORKS
Gemfibrozil speeds the removal of triglycerides from the lipoprotein known as very-low-density lipoprotein (VLDL), which is converted to low-density lipoprotein (LDL). In some people, total and LDL cholesterol levels may rise while triglycerides fall.

▼ DOSAGE GUIDELINES

RANGE AND FREQUENCY
Adults: 600 mg 2 times a day, usually taken 30 to 60 minutes before morning and evening meals.

ONSET OF EFFECT
Begins in about 1 week and is noticeable in about 4 weeks.

DURATION OF ACTION
Blood triglyceride levels increase within a few weeks of stopping gemfibrozil.

DIETARY ADVICE
Follow your doctor's dietary advice to improve control over high blood pressure and help prevent heart disease. The American Heart Association publishes a "Healthy Heart" diet; discuss this with your doctor. Limit your intake of alcohol, which can raise triglyceride levels.

STORAGE
Store in a tightly sealed container away from heat and direct light.

MISSED DOSE
Take your missed dose as soon as you remember that you skipped it, unless the time for your next scheduled dose is within the next 2 hours. If so, do not take the missed dose. Take your next scheduled dose at the proper time and resume your regular dosage schedule. Do not double the next dose.

STOPPING THE DRUG
Do not stop taking gemfibrozil on your own; the level of triglycerides in your blood will increase.

PROLONGED USE
Gemfibrozil is often taken for long periods of time. If your blood triglycerides do not decrease, your physician may stop the medication.

▼ PRECAUTIONS

Over 60: Adverse reactions may be more likely and more severe in older patients.

Driving and Hazardous Work: The use of gemfibrozil should not impair your ability to perform such tasks safely.

Alcohol: Alcohol intake should be limited because it can raise triglyceride levels.

Pregnancy: Do not take gemfibrozil while pregnant unless your doctor indicates that the risks of stopping the drug are too great. Triglycerides increase substantially during pregnancy, and extremely high triglycerides can trigger an attack of acute pancreatitis.

Breast Feeding: Avoid or discontinue use while nursing.

Infants and Children: Rarely used in infants and children.

Special Concerns: The most important treatments for high levels of blood triglycerides are a proper diet, weight loss, regular moderate exercise, the avoidance of certain medications, and the control of diabetes. Because gemfibrozil has potential side effects, it is important that you maintain a healthy diet and cooperate with other treatment strategies your physician may suggest. Gemfibrozil may increase the chances of gallbladder, liver, and pancreas problems; your physician will order periodic blood tests.

OVERDOSE
Symptoms: No specific symptoms have been reported.

What to Do: Emergency instructions not applicable.

▼ INTERACTIONS

DRUG INTERACTIONS
Certain drugs may interact adversely with gemfibrozil, particularly anticoagulants (blood thinners, such as warfarin), niacin, and any of the group of cholesterol-lowering drugs referred to as "statins." It may be necessary to reduce the dose of warfarin to prevent bleeding. The combination of gemfibrozil with either niacin or a statin drug can cause severe myositis (muscle inflammation), which can release a protein that damages the kidneys. Consult your doctor.

FOOD INTERACTIONS
No known food interactions.

DISEASE INTERACTIONS
Be sure to inform your doctor if you have any of the following problems: gallstones, stomach or intestinal ulcer, muscle disease, or kidney or liver disease. The dose of gemfibrozil must be reduced in those with significant kidney damage.

SIDE EFFECTS

SERIOUS
Muscle aches and tenderness; crampy abdominal pain, especially in the area under the ribs on the right side, with nausea and vomiting (this is an uncommon, serious side effect that may indicate gallbladder disease); decreased urine output.

COMMON
Diarrhea, nausea, gas.

LESS COMMON
Decreased sexual ability (erectile dysfunction) in men; headache; weight gain; feelings similar to the flu, with muscle aches or cramps, weakness, and unusual tiredness; inflammation of mouth and lips; heartburn.

GLIMEPIRIDE

Available in: Tablets
Available OTC? No   **As Generic?** Yes
Drug Class: Antidiabetic agent/sulfonylurea

▼ USAGE INFORMATION

WHY IT'S PRESCRIBED
To treat diabetes (high blood sugar) in patients who require little or no injectable insulin. It is used in conjunction with a special diet and exercise. Some patients may fail to respond initially to or gradually lose their responsiveness to glimepiride. The antidiabetic agent metformin may be used with glimepiride to achieve the desired results.

HOW IT WORKS
Glimepiride stimulates the release of insulin from the pancreas and makes the tissues of your body more responsive to insulin.

▼ DOSAGE GUIDELINES

RANGE AND FREQUENCY
Adults: 1 to 4 mg once daily 30 minutes before breakfast. Children: Not recommended.

ONSET OF EFFECT
2 to 3 hours.

DURATION OF ACTION
12 to 24 hours.

DIETARY ADVICE
Maintain any special diet that your doctor recommends. Restrict excessive intake of snacks containing sugar. Read food labels carefully.

STORAGE
Keep glimepiride away from direct light, moisture, and extremes in temperature.

MISSED DOSE
Take it as soon as you remember. If it is near the time for the next dose, skip the missed dose and resume your regular dosage schedule. Do not double the next dose.

STOPPING THE DRUG
The decision to stop taking glimepiride should be made by your doctor.

PROLONGED USE
Therapy with glimepiride may require months or years. Prolonged use may be associated with an increased risk of side effects.

▼ PRECAUTIONS

Over 60: Adverse reactions from this drug may be more likely and more severe.

Driving and Hazardous Work: Do not drive or engage in hazardous work until you determine how the medicine affects you.

Alcohol: Use only in a moderate, responsible fashion. Consult your doctor.

Pregnancy: It should not be used during pregnancy.

Breast Feeding: It should not be used by nursing mothers.

Infants and Children: Not recommended for children.

Special Concerns: Understand the symptoms of low blood sugar. Always have easy access to sources of simple sugar—juice, candy bars, energy bars, hard candy, honey, sugar cubes, sugar dissolved in water—in case you experience symptoms of hypoglycemia (low blood sugar). Inform your physician promptly about changes in the way you are feeling, changes in your lifestyle and level of activity, medications that you may have been prescribed by other specialists, medications that you have stopped taking, unusually high or low results for any at-home tests you use to check your urine or blood, episodes of low blood sugar, and pregnancy. Wear a special medical ID bracelet. Do not miss meals. Use caution when exercising.

OVERDOSE
Symptoms: Symptoms are similar to serious side effects.

What to Do: Call emergency medical services (EMS), your doctor, or the nearest poison control center immediately.

▼ INTERACTIONS

DRUG INTERACTIONS
Consult your doctor for specific advice if you are taking steroids and nonsteroidal antiinflammatory drugs (such as ibuprofen, aspirin, or drugs containing aspirin); anticoagulants; certain antibiotics; especially for fungal infections; diuretics; lithium; beta-blockers; ulcer medications; ciprofloxacin; cyclosporine; guanethidine; MAO (monoamine oxidase) inhibitors; quinidine; quinine; chloramphenicol; estrogen; isoniazid; thyroid hormones; theophylline; pentamidine phenothiazines; or phenytoin.

FOOD INTERACTIONS
No known food interactions.

DISEASE INTERACTIONS
Consult your doctor if you have diarrhea; persistent vomiting; malabsorption disease; liver, thyroid, kidney, or adrenal gland disease; fever; or infection.

≡ SIDE EFFECTS ≡

SERIOUS
Serious side effects are related to hypoglycemia, or low blood sugar, whose symptoms include perspiration or a cold sweat; restlessness; rapid pulse; anxious feeling; nausea; feelings of dizziness, weakness, or lightheadedness; poor coordination; slurred speech; confusion; sleepiness; seizures or convulsions; weakness of an arm, leg, or an entire side of the body; and fainting. Seek emergency assistance. Administer substances containing sugar only if the patient is conscious and alert. Other serious but less common side effects include low white blood cell count and elevation of liver-associated enzymes; these problems can be detected by your doctor.

COMMON
Dizziness, weakness, nausea, headache.

LESS COMMON
Skin reactions, such as itching, peeling, rashes, and hives; blurred vision; edema (swelling caused by fluid retention) of face or extremities; severe tiredness; abdominal pain.

GLIPIZIDE

Available in: Tablets, extended-release tablets
Available OTC? No   **As Generic?** Yes
Drug Class: Antidiabetic agent/sulfonylurea

▼ USAGE INFORMATION

WHY IT'S PRESCRIBED
To treat diabetes (high blood sugar) in patients who require little or no injectable insulin. It is used in conjunction with a special diet and exercise. Some patients may fail to respond initially or gradually lose their responsiveness to glipizide. Other antidiabetic agents may be used in conjunction with glipizide to achieve the desired results.

HOW IT WORKS
Glipizide stimulates the release of insulin from special cells in the pancreas and therefore helps lower blood glucose levels.

▼ DOSAGE GUIDELINES

RANGE AND FREQUENCY
Usual starting dose: 5 mg a day taken 30 minutes before breakfast. Dosage should be adjusted by 2.5 to 5 mg per day based on blood sugar response. If your dosage is greater than 15 mg a day, it should be divided. In older patients or patients with liver disease, the initial dose should be 2.5 mg a day. Extended-release tablets: 5 to 10 mg, once daily, usually with breakfast.

ONSET OF EFFECT
Within 30 minutes.

DURATION OF ACTION
12 to 24 hours.

DIETARY ADVICE
Maintain a special diet recommended by your doctor, nutritionist, or the American Diabetes Association. Restrict excessive intake of sugary snacks. Read labels carefully when buying food.

STORAGE
Store away from direct light, moisture, and extremes in temperature.

MISSED DOSE
Take it as soon as you remember. If it is near the time for the next dose, skip the missed dose and resume your regular dosage schedule. Do not double the next dose.

STOPPING THE DRUG
The decision to stop taking it should be made by your doctor.

PROLONGED USE
Therapy may require months or years. Prolonged use may be associated with an increased risk of side effects.

▼ PRECAUTIONS

Over 60: Adverse reactions from this drug may be more likely and more severe.

Driving and Hazardous Work: Do not drive or engage in hazardous work until you determine how the medication affects you.

Alcohol: Drink in moderation.

Pregnancy: Insulin is the treatment of choice for pregnant women with diabetes.

Breast Feeding: This drug passes into breast milk, although it is uncertain whether the drug is harmful to nursing infants.

Infants and Children: Not recommended for children.

Special Concerns: Keep simple sugars—juice, candy bars, hard candy—on hand in the event of hypoglycemia. Inform your doctor promptly of changes in how you feel, unusually high or low results for any at-home tests, episodes of low blood sugar, or pregnancy. Wear a medical ID bracelet. Do not miss meals. Use caution when exercising.

OVERDOSE
Symptoms: Symptoms similar to serious side effects.

What to Do: Call emergency medical services (EMS), your doctor, or the nearest poison control center immediately.

▼ INTERACTIONS

DRUG INTERACTIONS
Consult your doctor for specific advice if you are taking anticoagulants, antibiotics (especially antibiotics containing sulfa or those used to treat fungal infections), steroids, diuretics, seizure medications, beta-blockers (which may include eye drops for glaucoma) or other blood pressure medications, lithium, ulcer drugs, guanethidine, MAO (monoamine oxidase) inhibitors, quinidine, quinine, salicylates, chloramphenicol, estrogens, isoniazid, thyroid hormones, theophylline, or pentamidine.

FOOD INTERACTIONS
Food delays the absorption of immediate-release tablets.

DISEASE INTERACTIONS
Consult your doctor if you have diarrhea; persistent vomiting; malabsorption disease; liver, thyroid, kidney, or adrenal gland disease; fever; infection; or impending or recent surgery.

≡ SIDE EFFECTS ≡

SERIOUS
Serious side effects are related to hypoglycemia, or low blood sugar, whose symptoms include perspiration or a cold sweat; restlessness; rapid pulse; anxious feeling; nausea; feelings of dizziness, weakness, or lightheadedness; poor coordination; slurred speech; confusion; drowsiness; seizures; weakness of an arm, leg, or an entire side of the body; and fainting. Seek emergency assistance. Administer substances containing sugar only if the patient is conscious and alert. Other serious but less common side effects include low white blood cell count and elevation of liver-associated enzymes; these can be detected by your doctor.

COMMON
Dizziness, constipation, nausea, heartburn, unusual or changed taste of food, or unusual taste in the mouth.

LESS COMMON
Peeling, red, bruised, or itching skin; pale skin; edema (swelling) of face or extremities; reduced ability to exercise; headache; fever.

GLYBURIDE

Available in: Tablets
Available OTC? No **As Generic?** Yes
Drug Class: Antidiabetic agent/sulfonylurea

▼ USAGE INFORMATION

WHY IT'S PRESCRIBED
To help control adult-onset (non-insulin-dependent, or type 2) diabetes. Glyburide is sometimes used in conjunction with metformin (another oral antidiabetic).

HOW IT WORKS
Glyburide stimulates the release of insulin by the pancreas and decreases sugar production in the liver.

▼ DOSAGE GUIDELINES

RANGE AND FREQUENCY
Starting dose is 2.5 to 5 mg daily 30 minutes before breakfast. It can be increased by your doctor in increments of 2.5 mg to a maximum of 20 mg per day or decreased if needed. Older patients or those with kidney or liver dysfunction should receive an initial dose of 1.25 mg per day. If the daily maintenance dose is increased to 10 mg or more, the total dose should be divided equally between breakfast and dinner.

ONSET OF EFFECT
1 hour.

DURATION OF ACTION
24 hours.

DIETARY ADVICE
It is usually taken 30 minutes before breakfast.

STORAGE
Store glyburide in a tightly sealed container away from heat and direct light.

MISSED DOSE
Take it as soon as you remember. If it is near the time for the next dose, skip the missed dose and resume your regular dosage schedule. Do not double the next dose.

STOPPING THE DRUG
The decision to stop taking the drug should be made by your doctor. You may need to take glyburide for the rest of your life.

PROLONGED USE
Periodic blood tests should be done to determine how prolonged use affects blood sugar levels.

▼ PRECAUTIONS

Over 60: Treatment should start with lower doses, which should be increased slowly as determined by periodic tests. Adverse reactions may be more likely and more severe in older patients.

Driving and Hazardous Work: Do not drive or engage in hazardous work until you determine how the medication affects you.

Alcohol: Avoid alcohol.

Pregnancy: Having uncontrolled blood sugar levels during pregnancy is associated with an increased risk of birth defects, so many experts recommend a switch to insulin during pregnancy.

Breast Feeding: Glyburide may pass into breast milk; caution is advised. Consult your doctor for advice.

Infants and Children: Glyburide does not work for juvenile-onset, insulin-dependent diabetes.

Special Concerns: Carry medical identification that says you have diabetes. If you are under stress because of an infection, fever, injury, or surgery, you may need insulin therapy in addition to or instead of glyburide.

OVERDOSE
Symptoms: Symptoms are similar to serious side effects.

What to Do: An overdose of glyburide is unlikely to be life-threatening. However, if someone takes a much larger dose than prescribed, call your doctor, emergency medical services (EMS), or the nearest poison control center.

▼ INTERACTIONS

DRUG INTERACTIONS
Consult your doctor for specific advice if you are taking anabolic steroids, aspirin or other salicylates, cimetidine, gemfibrozil, fenfluramine, MAO (monoamine oxidase) inhibitors, phenylbutazone, ranitidine, sulfa drugs, beta-blockers, bumetanide, diazoxide, ethacrynic acid, furosemide, phenytoin, rifampin, thiazide diuretics, thyroid hormone, antacids, antifungal agents, enalapril, steroids, or warfarin.

FOOD INTERACTIONS
Glyburide is just part of the treatment for diabetes; be sure to follow the diet recommended by your doctor.

DISEASE INTERACTIONS
Use of this medication may cause complications in patients with liver or kidney disease, because these organs work together to remove the drug from the body.

SIDE EFFECTS

SERIOUS
Serious side effects are related to hypoglycemia, or low blood sugar, whose symptoms include perspiration or a cold sweat; restlessness; rapid pulse; anxious feeling; nausea; feelings of dizziness, weakness, or lightheadedness; poor coordination; slurred speech; confusion; sleepiness; seizures; weakness of an arm, leg, or an entire side of the body; and fainting. Seek emergency assistance. Administer substances containing sugar only if the patient is conscious and alert. Other serious but less common side effects include bone marrow suppression, hemolytic anemia, and elevation of liver-associated enzymes; these problems can be detected by your doctor.

COMMON
Bloating, heartburn, nausea, indigestion.

LESS COMMON
Blurred vision, changes in taste, itching, hives, joint or muscle pain.

GUAIFENESIN

Available in: Capsules, tablets, oral solution, syrup, extended-release forms
Available OTC? Yes   **As Generic?** Yes
Drug Class: Expectorant

▼ USAGE INFORMATION

WHY IT'S PRESCRIBED
Guaifenesin is classified as an expectorant; that is, it is designed to reduce the thickness of mucus and phlegm, making it easier to cough up and out of the lungs and so improve breathing. It is used to treat minor upper respiratory infections and related conditions, such as bronchitis, colds, and sinus or throat infections. Guaifenesin is not a cough suppressant, and despite its popularity and its FDA approval as an expectorant, there is little scientific evidence that it is truly effective at reducing the thickness of mucous.

HOW IT WORKS
Guaifenesin supposedly increases the production of fluids in the respiratory tract and helps liquefy and thin mucus secretions.

▼ DOSAGE GUIDELINES

RANGE AND FREQUENCY
Adults—Capsules, tablets, oral solution, syrup: 200 to 400 mg every 4 hours to a maximum of 2,400 mg a day. Extended-release capsules and tablets: 600 to 1,200 mg every 12 hours to a maximum of 2,400 mg a day. Children 2 to 12 years of age: Consult your doctor.

ONSET OF EFFECT
Usually within several hours.

DURATION OF ACTION
The exact duration of action is not known.

DIETARY ADVICE
Maintain your usual food and fluid intake. Increase fluids if you have a fever or diarrhea. Coughing also increases your daily fluid requirements.

STORAGE
Store in a tightly sealed container away from heat and direct light. Keep liquid forms of guaifenesin refrigerated, but do not allow it to freeze. Keep away from moisture and extremes in temperature.

MISSED DOSE
Take it as soon as you remember. If it is near the time for the next dose, skip the missed dose and resume your regular dosage schedule. Do not double the next dose.

STOPPING THE DRUG
You may stop taking guaifenesin before the scheduled end of therapy if you are feeling better; otherwise, take it as prescribed for the full treatment period.

PROLONGED USE
Therapy with guaifenesin is usually completed within 7 to 10 days. Persistent cough may require special evaluation. Do not take nonprescription guaifenesin for more than 7 days without your doctor's approval.

▼ PRECAUTIONS

Over 60: Adverse reactions may be more likely and more severe.

Driving and Hazardous Work: Do not drive or engage in hazardous work until you determine how the medicine affects you.

Alcohol: No special warnings.

Pregnancy: Thorough studies have not been done, although no serious problems have been reported; consult your doctor for advice.

Breast Feeding: Guaifenesin may pass into breast milk, although no problems have been documented. Consult your doctor for advice.

Infants and Children: Generally, it should not be given to children under 2 unless directed otherwise by a pediatrician; children under 12 who have a persistent cough should be examined by a doctor before they are given guaifenesin.

Special Concerns: Guaifenesin is present in numerous nonprescription cough and cold remedies, so ask your pharmacist if you are unsure whether a product you are buying contains it. Do not treat a persistent cough on your own for more than a week or so without seeking medical advice. When treating young children, avoid capsules or tablets, because it is difficult to rely on children to swallow these dosage forms in one piece. Capsules and tablets should not be chewed.

OVERDOSE
Symptoms: No specific ones have been reported.

What to Do: An overdose of guaifenesin is unlikely to be life-threatening. However, if someone takes a much larger dose than prescribed, call your doctor, emergency medical services (EMS), or the nearest poison control center.

▼ INTERACTIONS

DRUG INTERACTIONS
None reported.

FOOD INTERACTIONS
None reported.

DISEASE INTERACTIONS
None reported.

SIDE EFFECTS

SERIOUS
No serious side effects are associated with guaifenesin.

COMMON
No common side effects are associated with guaifenesin.

LESS COMMON
Diarrhea; dizziness; headache; abdominal pain, nausea, or vomiting; skin rash; itching; hives.

HALOPERIDOL

Available in: Tablets, liquid, injection
Available OTC? No   **As Generic?** Yes
Drug Class: Neuroleptic; antipsychotic

▼ USAGE INFORMATION

WHY IT'S PRESCRIBED
To treat moderate to severe psychiatric conditions including schizophrenia, manic states, and drug-induced psychosis. It is also used to treat extreme behavior problems in children (including infantile autism), to ease the symptoms of Tourette's syndrome, and to reduce nausea and vomiting associated with chemotherapy for cancer.

HOW IT WORKS
Haloperidol blocks receptors of dopamine (a chemical that aids in the transmission of nerve impulses) in the central nervous system. Presumably, this produces a tranquilizing or antipsychotic effect.

▼ DOSAGE GUIDELINES

RANGE AND FREQUENCY
For psychotic disorders—
Adults: Initial dose is 0.5 to 5 mg 2 or 3 times a day; maximum dose is 100 mg a day. Children ages 3 to 12 years: 0.05 to 0.15 mg for every 2.2 lb (1 kg) of body weight. For Tourette's syndrome—Adults: 0.5 to 5 mg 2 or 3 times a day. Children ages 3 to 12 years: 0.075 mg for every 2.2 lb daily.

ONSET OF EFFECT
Sedation may occur within minutes, but onset of antipsychotic effect may take hours or may not occur until days or weeks after the beginning of therapy.

DURATION OF ACTION
12 to 24 hours, but effects may persist for several days.

DIETARY ADVICE
Take haloperidol with food or a full glass of milk or water. To prevent stomach irritation, the oral solution can be diluted in beverages such as orange, apple, or tomato juice or cola.

SIDE EFFECTS

SERIOUS
Rapid heartbeat, profuse sweating, seizures, difficulty breathing, neck stiffness, swelling of the tongue, difficulty swallowing. Also a rare condition can develop called neuroleptic malignant syndrome, characterized by stiffness or spasms of the muscles, high fever, and confusion or disorientation. Call your doctor immediately.

COMMON
Nausea, reduced sweating, dry mouth, blurred vision, drowsiness, shaking of hands, stiffness, stooped posture.

LESS COMMON
Difficult urination, menstrual irregularities, breast pain or swelling, unexpected weight gain, uncontrolled movements of the tongue, fever, chills, sore throat, unusual bruising or bleeding, heart palpitations, skin rash, itching, increased sensitivity of the skin to sunlight.

STORAGE
Store haloperidol in a tightly sealed container away from heat and direct light.

MISSED DOSE
Take it as soon as you remember. Do not double the next dose. Space any remaining doses for that day at regular intervals. Return to your regular schedule the next day.

STOPPING THE DRUG
The decision to stop taking the drug should be made in consultation with your doctor. Gradual reduction of doses may be required if you have taken it for a long period.

PROLONGED USE
Prolonged use may lead to tardive dyskinesia (involuntary movements of the jaw, lips, tongue, and, in rare cases, the arms, legs, hands, or body). Consult your doctor about the need for periodic evaluation and lab tests.

▼ PRECAUTIONS

Over 60: Adverse reactions are more likely and more severe in older patients.

Driving and Hazardous Work: Exercise caution until you determine how the medication affects you.

Alcohol: Avoid alcohol.

Pregnancy: Before taking haloperidol, be sure to tell your doctor if you are or plan to become pregnant.

Breast Feeding: Haloperidol passes into breast milk and may be harmful to the child; do not use it while nursing.

Infants and Children: Not recommended for children under age 3 or those weighing less than 33 lb.

Special Concerns: Avoid prolonged exposure to high temperatures or hot climates. Drink plenty of fluids and stay cool in the summertime. Avoid overexposure to sunlight until you determine if the drug heightens your skin's sensitivity to ultraviolet light.

OVERDOSE
Symptoms: Shallow, slow breathing, weak or rapid pulse, muscle weakness or tremor, dizziness, confusion, seizures, deep sleep, coma.

What to Do: Call your doctor, emergency medical services (EMS), or the nearest poison control center immediately.

▼ INTERACTIONS

DRUG INTERACTIONS
Consult your doctor for specific advice if you are taking anticholinergics, anticonvulsants, antidepressants, antihistamines, antihypertensives, bupropion, central nervous system depressants such as barbiturates, clozapine, dronabinol, ethinamate, fluoxetine, guanethidine, guanfacine, lithium, methyldopa, carbamazepine, rifampin, or trihexyphenidyl.

FOOD INTERACTIONS
No known food interactions.

DISEASE INTERACTIONS
Consult your doctor if you have Parkinson's disease or any movement disorder, glaucoma, epilepsy, or liver or kidney disease.

HYDROCHLOROTHIAZIDE/TRIAMTERENE

BRAND NAMES
Dyazide, Maxzide

Available in: Capsules, tablets
Available OTC? No   **As Generic?** Yes
Drug Class: Thiazide diuretic

▼ USAGE INFORMATION

WHY IT'S PRESCRIBED
To treat high blood pressure (hypertension) and conditions that cause edema (swelling of body tissues resulting from excess salt and water retention).

HOW IT WORKS
This drug combines a thiazide diuretic (hydrochlorothiazide) and a potassium-sparing diuretic (triamterene). Diuretics increase the excretion of salt and water in the urine. By reducing the overall fluid volume in the body, these drugs reduce blood volume and so reduce pressure within the blood vessels.

▼ DOSAGE GUIDELINES

RANGE AND FREQUENCY
Adults: 1 or 2 capsules or tablets once a day. Children: The dose must be determined by your doctor.

ONSET OF EFFECT
Within 2 hours.

DURATION OF ACTION
6 to 12 hours.

DIETARY ADVICE
This medication should be taken in the morning after breakfast.

STORAGE
Store in a tightly sealed container away from heat and direct light.

MISSED DOSE
Take this medication as soon as you remember. If it is near the time for the next dose, skip the missed dose and resume your regular dosage schedule. Do not double the next dose.

STOPPING THE DRUG
The decision to stop taking this prescription medication should be made by your doctor.

PROLONGED USE
See your doctor regularly for physical examinations and appropriate laboratory tests if you must take this medicine for an extended period.

▼ PRECAUTIONS

Over 60: Adverse reactions may be more likely and more severe in this age group.

Driving and Hazardous Work: No special precautions are necessary.

Alcohol: No special precautions are necessary.

Pregnancy: This drug should not be taken during pregnancy unless recommended by your doctor. Other diuretics are generally preferred.

Breast Feeding: This drug passes into breast milk; avoid or discontinue use while breast feeding.

Infants and Children: No unusual side effects are expected in children. The dose must be determined by a pediatrician.

Special Concerns: To prevent hydrochlorothiazide from interfering with sleep, take it in the morning. If you are taking it for high blood pressure, follow the diet and weight control measures that are recommended by your doctor. Avoid exposure to sunlight, use a sunblock, or wear protective clothing.

OVERDOSE
Symptoms: Dehydration, muscle weakness, cramps, heart arrhythmias.

What to Do: Call your doctor, emergency medical services (EMS), or the nearest poison control center immediately.

▼ INTERACTIONS

DRUG INTERACTIONS
Consult your doctor for specific advice if you are taking ACE (angiotensin-converting enzyme) inhibitors, cyclosporine, cholestyramine, colestipol, digitalis drugs, lithium, any over-the-counter medication, or medications or dietary supplements that contain potassium.

FOOD INTERACTIONS
The triamterene in this combination diuretic drug reduces excess loss of potassium in the body. For this reason, patients are usually advised not to consume large servings of potassium-rich foods. These include bananas, citrus fruits and juices, melons, prunes (and most fruits in general), avocados, potatoes, nuts, baked beans, brussels sprouts, and skim milk.

DISEASE INTERACTIONS
Caution is advised when taking this medicine. Consult your doctor if you have diabetes, gout, kidney stones, lupus erythematosus, heart disease, pancreatitis, blood vessel disease, menstrual problems, liver disease, or kidney disease.

SIDE EFFECTS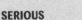

SERIOUS
Skin rash, hives, intense itching, swelling of the mouth and throat, breathing difficulty, heart rhythm irregularities or palpitations, lightheadedness or dizziness, unusual bleeding or bruising. Call your doctor immediately.

COMMON
Fluid depletion may lead to dizziness, especially on rising from a sitting or lying position, as well as thirst, dry mouth, and constipation.

LESS COMMON
Decreased sexual ability, increased sensitivity to sunlight, loss of appetite, gout, increased blood sugar (a problem for diabetic patients).

HYDROCHLOROTHIAZIDE (HCTZ)

Available in: Tablets, oral suspension
Available OTC? No   **As Generic?** Yes
Drug Class: Thiazide diuretic

▼ USAGE INFORMATION

WHY IT'S PRESCRIBED
To treat high blood pressure (hypertension) and conditions that cause edema (swelling of body tissues resulting from excess salt and water retention).

HOW IT WORKS
Diuretics increase the excretion of salt and water in the urine. By reducing the overall fluid volume in the body, these drugs reduce pressure within the blood vessels.

▼ DOSAGE GUIDELINES

RANGE AND FREQUENCY
Adults—To reduce excess body water: 25 to 100 mg 1 or 2 times a day. Your doctor may change the frequency to every other day or 3 to 5 days a week. For high blood pressure: 25 to 100 mg a day. Children—to reduce body water: Ages 2 to 12 years: 37.5 to 100 mg a day in 2 doses. Ages 6 months to 2 years: 12.5 to 37.5 mg a day in 2 doses. Infants under 6 months: Up to 3.3 mg per 2.2 lb (1 kg) of body weight in 2 doses.

ONSET OF EFFECT
Within 2 hours.

DURATION OF ACTION
6 to 12 hours.

DIETARY ADVICE
It can be be taken with food to avoid stomach upset.

STORAGE
Store in a tightly sealed container away from heat and direct light. Keep the liquid form from freezing.

MISSED DOSE
Take it as soon as you remember. If it is near the time for the next dose, skip the missed dose and resume your regular dosage schedule. Do not double the next dose.

STOPPING THE DRUG
The decision to stop taking the drug should be made by your doctor.

PROLONGED USE
See your doctor regularly for examinations and tests if you must take this medicine for an extended period.

▼ PRECAUTIONS

Over 60: Adverse reactions may be more likely and more severe in older patients.

Driving and Hazardous Work: No special precautions are necessary.

Alcohol: No special precautions are necessary.

Pregnancy: Hydrochlorothiazide has caused birth defects in animals. Human studies have not been done. This medicine should not be taken during pregnancy unless recommended by your doctor; other diuretics are generally preferred for pregnant women.

Breast Feeding: Hydrochlorothiazide passes into breast milk; avoid or discontinue use during the first month of nursing.

Infants and Children: No unusual side effects are expected in children. The dose must be determined by a pediatrician.

Special Concerns: Hydrochlorothiazide is usually prescribed to be taken once a day. To prevent it from interfering with sleep, take it in the morning. If you are taking this drug for high blood pressure, follow the diet and weight control measures recommended by your doctor. Avoid exposure to sunlight, use a sunblock, or wear protective clothing. This medicine may cause your body to lose potassium. Follow your doctor's instructions about eating potassium-rich foods or taking a potassium supplement.

OVERDOSE
Symptoms: Fainting, lethargy, dizziness, drowsiness, confusion, gastrointestinal irritation.

What to Do: Call your doctor, emergency medical services (EMS), or the nearest poison control center immediately.

▼ INTERACTIONS

DRUG INTERACTIONS
Consult your doctor for specific advice if you are taking anticoagulants, cholestyramine, colestipol, drugs for diabetes, nonsteroidal anti-inflammatory drugs, digitalis drugs, or lithium.

FOOD INTERACTIONS
No known food interactions.

DISEASE INTERACTIONS
Caution is advised when taking hydrochlorothiazide. Consult your doctor if you have any of the following: diabetes, gout, lupus erythematosus, pancreatitis, heart disease, blood vessel disease, liver disease, or kidney disease.

≡ SIDE EFFECTS ≡

SERIOUS
Skin rash, hives, intense itching, swelling of the mouth and throat, breathing difficulty, heart rhythm irregularities, light-headedness, unusual bleeding or bruising. Call your doctor immediately.

COMMON
Muscle cramps or pain. Potassium depletion may lead to heart palpitations and weakness. Fluid depletion may lead to dizziness, especially on rising from a sitting or lying position, as well as thirst, dry mouth, and constipation.

LESS COMMON
Decreased sexual ability (erectile dysfunction) in men, increased sensitivity to sunlight, loss of appetite, gout, increased blood sugar, pancreatitis (rare).

HYDROCODONE BITARTRATE/ACETAMINOPHEN

Available in: Capsules, oral solution, tablets
Available OTC? No   **As Generic?** Yes
Drug Class: Opioid (narcotic) analgesic

▼ USAGE INFORMATION

WHY IT'S PRESCRIBED
To relieve moderate to severe pain when nonprescription pain relievers prove inadequate. When taken in combination with acetaminophen, hydrocodone may provide better pain relief at lower doses than either medication does when used alone at higher doses.

HOW IT WORKS
Hydrocodone, a narcotic, is believed to relieve pain by acting on specific areas both in the spinal cord and in the brain that process pain signals from nerves throughout the body. Acetaminophen appears to interfere with the action of prostaglandins, hormonelike chemical substances in the body that cause inflammation and make nerves more sensitive to pain impulses.

▼ DOSAGE GUIDELINES

RANGE AND FREQUENCY
Adults—Capsules: 1 every 4 to 6 hours. Oral solution: 1 to 3 teaspoons every 4 to 6 hours. Tablets: 1 or 2 that contain 2.5 mg of hydrocodone or 1 that contains 5, 7.5, or 10 mg of hydrocodone every 4 to 6 hours.

ONSET OF EFFECT
30 to 60 minutes.

DURATION OF ACTION
4 to 6 hours.

DIETARY ADVICE
This drug can be taken without regard to diet.

STORAGE
Store in a sealed container away from heat and light.

MISSED DOSE
If you are taking this medicine on a fixed schedule, take it as soon as you remember. If it is near the time for the next dose, skip the missed dose and resume your regular dosage schedule. Do not double the next dose.

STOPPING THE DRUG
The decision to stop taking the drug should be made by your doctor.

PROLONGED USE
See your doctor regularly for tests and examinations. Prolonged use can cause mental or physical dependence.

▼ PRECAUTIONS

Over 60: Adverse reactions may be more likely and more severe in older patients.

Driving and Hazardous Work: Do not drive or engage in hazardous work until you determine how the medicine affects you.

Alcohol: Avoid alcohol.

Pregnancy: Overuse during pregnancy can cause drug dependence in the fetus.

Breast Feeding: It is not known whether this drug passes into breast milk; caution is advised. Consult your doctor for specific advice.

Infants and Children: Adverse reactions may be more likely and more severe in children.

Special Concerns: If you feel that the medication is not working properly after a few weeks of use, do not increase the dose on your own. See your doctor for advice.

OVERDOSE

Symptoms: Severe dizziness or drowsiness; cold, clammy skin; slow breathing or shortness of breath; seizures; severe confusion; stomach cramps or pain; diarrhea; sweating; constricted pupils; nausea or vomiting; irregular heartbeat; severe weakness.

What to Do: Call your doctor, emergency medical services (EMS), or the nearest poison control center immediately.

▼ INTERACTIONS

DRUG INTERACTIONS
Consult your doctor for specific advice if you are taking any prescription or over-the-counter medications, especially drugs with acetaminophen or central nervous system depressants such as barbiturates, seizure medicine, muscle relaxants, anesthetics, tranquilizers, or sedatives.

FOOD INTERACTIONS
No known food interactions.

DISEASE INTERACTIONS
Consult your doctor if you have a head injury or brain disease, hypothyroidism, an enlarged prostate, seizures, kidney or liver disease, gallbladder problems, a blood disorder, or a history of alcohol or drug abuse.

⇊ SIDE EFFECTS ⇊

SERIOUS
Bloody, dark, or cloudy urine; severe pain in lower back or side; pale or black, tarry stools; yellow-tinged eyes or skin; hallucinations; frequent urge to urinate; painful or difficult urination; sudden decrease in amount of urine; increased sweating; unusual bleeding or bruising; irregular heartbeat; skin rash, hives, or itching; unusual excitement; irregular breathing or wheezing; ringing or buzzing in ears; pinpoint red spots on skin; sore throat and fever; confusion; trembling or uncontrolled muscle movements; flushing or swelling of face. Call your doctor immediately.

COMMON
Dizziness, lightheadedness, nausea or vomiting, drowsiness, constipation, itching.

LESS COMMON
Stomach pain, allergic reaction, false sense of well-being (euphoria), depression, loss of appetite, blurring or change in vision, feeling of illness, headache, nervousness, insomnia.

HYDROXYZINE

BRAND NAMES

Anxanil, Atarax, Hydroxacen, Hyzine-50, Vistaject-25, Vistaject-50, Vistaril, Vistazine 50

Available in: Tablets, syrup, injection
Available OTC? No   **As Generic?** Yes
Drug Class: Antihistamine/mild sedative

▼ USAGE INFORMATION

WHY IT'S PRESCRIBED
Hydroxyzine is used for several conditions. Its mild sedative effect is useful in treating insomnia and agitation in some patients. It is also used to treat itching, hives, and other allergy symptoms; to control nausea and vomiting; to ease the symptoms of alcohol withdrawal; and to provide mild sedation prior to a dental procedure or to the administration of general anesthesia before surgery.

HOW IT WORKS
Hydroxyzine is an antihistamine; that is, it blocks the effects of histamine, a naturally occurring substance in the body that causes swelling, itching, sneezing, watery eyes, hives, and other symptoms of allergic reactions. In addition to its antihistamine effect, hydroxyzine has a sedative effect and appears to suppress activity in some regions of the central nervous system (the brain and spinal cord) associated with nausea and psychological distress.

▼ DOSAGE GUIDELINES

RANGE AND FREQUENCY
For sedation—Adults: 50 to 100 mg a day. For allergy symptoms—Adults: 25 to 100 mg 3 or 4 times a day, as needed. Children age 6 years and older: 12.5 to 25 mg every 6 hours as needed. Children up to age 6 years: 12.5 mg every 6 hours as needed. For nausea and vomiting—Adults: 25 to 100 mg 3 or 4 times a day. Children: 0.6 mg per 2.2 lb (1 kg) of body weight per day.

ONSET OF EFFECT
15 to 30 minutes.

DURATION OF ACTION
Approximately 6 to 8 hours.

DIETARY ADVICE
Drink plenty of fluids.

STORAGE
Store in a tightly sealed container away from heat and direct light. Keep tablets away from moisture and extremes in temperature. Keep liquid forms refrigerated, but do not allow to them freeze.

MISSED DOSE
Take it as soon as you remember. If it is near the time for the next dose, skip the missed dose and resume your regular dosage schedule. Do not double the next dose.

STOPPING THE DRUG
The decision to stop taking the drug should be made in consultation with your doctor.

PROLONGED USE
Therapy with hydroxyzine may require days or weeks, depending on the condition. Side effects may be more likely with prolonged use.

▼ PRECAUTIONS

Over 60: Adverse reactions may be more likely and more severe in older patients.

Driving and Hazardous Work: Hydroxyzine may impair mental alertness; caution is advised.

Alcohol: Avoid alcohol.

Pregnancy: Adequate studies of hydroxyzine use during pregnancy have not been done; consult your doctor for specific advice.

Breast Feeding: Hydroxyzine may pass into breast milk and cause side effects in the nursing infant, so do not use it while breast feeding.

Infants and Children: Use this drug for children only under close supervision by your pediatrician.

Special Concerns: Antihistamines are widely available without prescription; if you are taking a prescription antihistamine, avoid other cough, cold, flu, sinus, or allergy preparations.

OVERDOSE
Symptoms: Severe dryness in mouth, nose, and throat; extreme drowsiness; loss of coordination; faintness; flushing; tremor; hallucinations; breathing difficulty.

What to Do: Call emergency medical services (EMS), your doctor, or the nearest poison control center immediately.

▼ INTERACTIONS

DRUG INTERACTIONS
Consult your doctor for specific advice if you are taking any drugs that depress the central nervous system, including antidepressants or other psychiatric medications, other antihistamines, barbiturates, sedatives, cough medicines, decongestants, and painkillers. Be sure your doctor knows about any over-the-counter drug you may take.

FOOD INTERACTIONS
None are known.

DISEASE INTERACTIONS
Consult your doctor if you have any of the following: asthma, glaucoma or another eye disorder, thyroid disease, heart or blood vessel disease, high blood pressure, enlarged prostate, or urinary difficulty.

≡ SIDE EFFECTS ≡

SERIOUS
Loss of coordination, seizures, extreme drowsiness, breathing difficulty, inability to urinate.

COMMON
Drowsiness; dryness in the mouth, nasal passages, and other mucous membranes.

LESS COMMON
Difficult urination, dizziness, rash, sore throat, fever, nightmares, restlessness, sleep disruption, irritability, increased skin sensitivity to sunlight, loss of appetite, stomach upset, decreased sexual ability in men.

INDINAVIR

Available in: Capsules
Available OTC? No   **As Generic?** No
Drug Class: Antiviral/protease inhibitor

▼ USAGE INFORMATION

WHY IT'S PRESCRIBED
To treat advanced HIV (human immunodeficiency virus) infection and AIDS (acquired immunodeficiency syndrome), usually in combination with other drugs. Although not a cure for HIV infection, this drug may suppress the replication of the virus and delay the progression of the disease.

HOW IT WORKS
Indinavir blocks the activity of a viral protease, an enzyme that HIV needs to reproduce. Blocking the protease causes HIV to make copies that cannot infect new cells.

▼ DOSAGE GUIDELINES

RANGE AND FREQUENCY
800 mg every 8 hours alone or in combination with other antiviral agents. Higher or lower doses are sometimes prescribed when indinavir is being combined with medications such as nevirapine and delavirdine, which alter indinavir blood levels.

ONSET OF EFFECT
Unknown. With most antiretroviral drugs, an early response can be seen within the first few days of therapy, but the maximum effect may take 12 to 16 weeks.

DURATION OF ACTION
Unknown. Effects of the drug may be prolonged if indinavir is used in combination with other effective drugs and the virus is maximally suppressed.

DIETARY ADVICE
Indinavir should be taken with plenty of water or other liquid, preferably at least 1 hour before or 2 hours after a meal. It may also be taken with a light, nonfat snack. Drink at least 48 ounces of water a day.

STORAGE
Store in a tightly sealed container away from moisture, heat, and direct light.

MISSED DOSE
Take it as soon as you remember. However, if it is near the time for the next dose, skip the missed dose and resume your regular dosage schedule. Do not double the next dose.

STOPPING THE DRUG
The decision to stop taking the drug should be made by your doctor.

PROLONGED USE
See your doctor regularly for tests and examinations.

▼ PRECAUTIONS

Over 60: No special precautions are necessary.

Driving and Hazardous Work: Do not drive or engage in hazardous work until you determine how the medicine affects you.

Alcohol: Avoid alcohol if liver function is impaired.

Pregnancy: Indinavir has been shown to cause birth defects in animals. Human studies have not been done. Nevertheless, indinavir is increasingly used in combination with other antiretroviral drugs to treat pregnant HIV-infected women.

Breast Feeding: Women infected with HIV should not breast-feed to avoid transmitting the virus to an uninfected child.

Infants and Children: Safety and effectiveness of indinavir for children under the age of 16 years have not been established.

Special Concerns: Indinavir should not be taken concurrently with St. John's wort; this herb can increase blood levels of the drug in the body, which may lead to possible resistance to indinavir. It is important to drink at least 48 ounces of water or other liquids every 24 hours to help prevent kidney stones. Indinavir therapy may be interrupted for patients who develop kidney stones. Tell any doctors or dentists treating you that you are taking this medication.

OVERDOSE
Symptoms: Pain in the lower back, blood in the urine, nausea, vomiting, diarrhea.

What to Do: An overdose is unlikely to be life-threatening. However, if someone takes a much larger dose than prescribed, call your doctor, emergency medical services (EMS), or the nearest poison control center immediately.

▼ INTERACTIONS

DRUG INTERACTIONS
Consult your doctor for specific advice if you are taking any other prescription or over-the-counter drug, especially astemizole, cisapride, didanosine, delavirdine, efavirenz, itraconazole, ketoconazole, midazolam, triazolam, rifabutin, rifampin, phenobarbital, phenytoin, carbamazepine, cholesterol-lowering drugs, or dexamethasone.

FOOD INTERACTIONS
Food, especially fatty foods, will decrease absorption of the drug.

DISEASE INTERACTIONS
Use of indinavir may cause complications in patients with liver disease.

 ## SIDE EFFECTS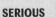

SERIOUS
Blood in urine and sharp back pain caused by kidney stones. High blood sugar (diabetes) has occurred in patients taking drugs of this class, although a cause-and-effect relationship has not been established. Call your doctor if you develop increased thirst or excessive urination.

COMMON
Weakness, abdominal pains, diarrhea, nausea, vomiting, headache, insomnia, changes in taste, dry skin, chapped lips.

LESS COMMON
Dizziness, drowsiness, depression, memory changes, abdominal bloating, muscle wasting.

INSULIN GLARGINE (RDNA ORIGIN)

BRAND NAME

Lantus

Available in: Injection
Available OTC? No   **As Generic?** No
Drug Class: Antidiabetic agent

▼ USAGE INFORMATION

WHY IT'S PRESCRIBED
For long-term treatment of diabetes mellitus. All patients with type 1 diabetes require lifelong insulin treatment. Patients with type 2 diabetes may require insulin if they are unable to control their blood glucose (sugar) levels with diet and oral medications. Insulin glargine is a slightly modified form of human insulin that maintains a relatively constant glucose-lowering effect over a 24-hour period and thus permits dosing once a day.

HOW IT WORKS
Insulin, a hormone secreted by the beta cells of the pancreas, plays an essential role in controlling the metabolism and storage of carbohydrates, fat, and protein. Insulin is secreted in response to a rise in blood sugar (glucose). Insulin lowers blood glucose by increasing its uptake by body cells, especially muscle, and by reducing the release of glucose from the liver between meals.

▼ DOSAGE GUIDELINES

RANGE AND FREQUENCY
Injected under the skin (of the stomach, thigh, or upper arm) once a day at bedtime. Doses are determined by your doctor. The solution should be clear and colorless, without any visible particles. Insulin glargine must not be diluted or mixed with any other insulin or solution.

ONSET OF EFFECT
About 1 to 2 hours.

DURATION OF ACTION
At least 24 hours.

≡ SIDE EFFECTS ≡

SERIOUS
Symptoms of hypoglycemia can be caused by the release of adrenaline or by an inadequate supply of glucose to the brain. With severe hypoglycemia, lack of sufficient glucose to the brain may cause slurred speech, impaired concentration, confusion, seizures, coma, irreversible brain damage, and death. Mild hypoglycemia may cause restless sleep, nightmares, or a cold sweat that awakens patients at night.

COMMON
Symptoms resulting from release of adrenaline are common manifestations of mild to moderate hypoglycemia. They include cold sweats, anxiety, shakiness, hunger, rapid heartbeat, headache, and nervousness. Weight gain is common when taking insulin.

LESS COMMON
Allergic reactions, lipoatrophy (depressions in the skin caused by loss of fat tissue), and lipohypertrophy (excessive accumulation of fat tissue).

DIETARY ADVICE
All patients with diabetes should follow the general dietary recommendations of the American Diabetes Association. Intake of simple sugars is not forbidden, but consuming large amounts of sugary foods at one time may trigger a rapid rise in blood glucose that can increase urination and thirst. In addition, patients who take insulin must remain consistent from day to day in the timing and caloric content of their meals. Depending on the timing, dose, and types of insulin prescribed, snacks may be recommended in the late afternoon, before bedtime, or prior to unusual physical activity. Diabetic patients must always have available juice, food, or tablets that can rapidly raise blood glucose levels to counter an episode of hypoglycemia.

STORAGE
Refrigerate insulin but do not allow it to freeze. If refrigeration is not possible, the 10-milliliter (ml) vial or 3-ml cartridge in use can be kept unrefrigerated for up to 28 days away from direct heat and light, as long as the temperature is not greater than 86°F. Unrefrigerated 10-ml vials and 3-ml cartridges must be used within the 28-day period or they must be discarded. If refrigeration is not possible, the 5-ml vial in use can be kept unrefrigerated for up to 14 days away from direct heat and light, as long as the temperature is not greater than 86°F. Unrefrigerated 5-ml vials must be used within the 14-day period or they must be discarded. If refrigerated, the 5-ml vial in use can be kept for up to 28 days. Once the 3-ml cartridge is placed into an OptiPen One, it should not be put in the refrigerator.

MISSED DOSE
Timing of insulin doses is extremely important. The best approach is to measure blood glucose and add a dose of regular insulin if glucose levels are too high. Otherwise, wait for the next scheduled dose.

STOPPING THE DRUG
Do not stop taking insulin injections unless ordered to do so by your doctor. Patients with diabetes are often given general instructions for modifying their insulin doses based on home blood glucose measurements.

PROLONGED USE
After many years with diabetes, some patients become insensitive to the symptoms of hypoglycemia and are at risk for serious brain complications of prolonged, unrecognized hypoglycemia.

▼ PRECAUTIONS

Over 60: No special warnings. Some older people may, however, have vision problems that may make it difficult for them to draw up the correct dose of insulin.

Driving and Hazardous Work: Patients taking insulin must be very careful to avoid hypoglycemia when driving or engaging in hazardous work.

Alcohol: Moderate alcohol intake, especially when taken with large meals, does not adversely affect control of diabetes or alter the dose of insulin. However, large amounts of alcohol increase the risk of hypoglycemia.

Pregnancy: Strict metabolic control—using insulin injections in most women—must be maintained during pregnancy to reduce the risk of birth defects, fetal complications, or death at the time of delivery. In women who had diabetes before the onset of pregnancy, the dose of insulin is often smaller during the first trimester of pregnancy and then higher during the final two trimesters. When women first develop diabetes during pregnancy (gestational diabetes), insulin requirements drop rapidly after delivery and most do not need to continue with insulin treatment.

Breast Feeding: Insulin requirements tend to be lower during breast feeding. Home glucose monitoring

is important to avoid hypoglycemia. Insulin glargine may pass into breast milk; consult your doctor for advice.

Infants and Children: Treatment with insulin in young patients age 6 years and older is the same as that in older people with diabetes. The safety and effectiveness of insulin glargine in children under the age of 6 years have not been established.

Special Concerns: Inadequate amounts of insulin in type 1 diabetes may lead to the serious complication of diabetic ketoacidosis, characterized by loss of appetite, excessive thirst and urination, nausea, vomiting, deep breathing, fruity breath odor, drowsiness, confusion, and loss of consciousness. Insulin glargine is not the insulin of choice for treating diabetic ketoacidosis. An intravenous short-acting insulin is the preferred treatment.

OVERDOSE

Symptoms: Insulin overdose results in hypoglycemia (see Side Effects for symptoms).

What to Do: For mild to moderate hypoglycemia, ingest drinks or food containing sugar. For more severe hypoglycemia, administer injections of glucagon or call emergency medical services (EMS) immediately.

▼ **INTERACTIONS**

DRUG INTERACTIONS
A large number of drugs can promote either elevated blood glucose levels or hypoglycemia. Be sure that your doctor knows about all of the medications you take and is informed before you start taking any new drugs, either by prescription or over the counter. Corticosteroids in particular are likely to raise blood glucose levels and insulin requirements. Beta-

blockers (commonly prescribed for hypertension) may cause either high blood glucose levels or hypoglycemia; in addition, because these medications may dampen the symptoms of hypoglycemia that are caused by adrenaline release, mild degrees of hypoglycemia may progress unnoticed to more serious hypoglycemia affecting the brain.

FOOD INTERACTIONS
Insulin requirements are increased by the ingestion of large amounts of calories, especially simple sugars and other carbohydrates.

DISEASE INTERACTIONS
Insulin requirements are increased by infections, psychological stress, or an uncontrolled overactive thyroid, and often at a time of surgery. Requirements may diminish with kidney disease or an underactive adrenal or pituitary gland.

INSULIN LISPRO (RDNA ORIGIN)

Available in: Injection
Available OTC? No   **As Generic?** No
Drug Class: Antidiabetic agent

▼ USAGE INFORMATION

WHY IT'S PRESCRIBED
For long-term treatment of diabetes mellitus. All patients with type 1 diabetes require lifelong insulin treatment. Patients with type 2 diabetes may require insulin if they are unable to control their blood glucose (sugar) levels with diet and oral medications.

HOW IT WORKS
Insulin, a hormone secreted by the beta cells of the pancreas, plays an essential role in controlling the metabolism and storage of carbohydrates, fat, and protein. Insulin is secreted in response to a rise in blood sugar (glucose). Insulin lowers blood glucose by increasing its uptake by body cells, especially muscle, and by reducing the release of glucose from the liver between meals.

▼ DOSAGE GUIDELINES

RANGE AND FREQUENCY
It may be taken 1 to 4 times daily, before meals and possibly at bedtime. Doses and frequency are determined by your doctor. Rapid-acting (lispro rDNA origin) insulin should be administered 15 minutes before a meal.

ONSET OF EFFECT
Within 30 to 45 minutes; the peak effect occurs within 1 hour.

DURATION OF ACTION
3 to 4 hours.

DIETARY ADVICE
All patients with diabetes should follow the general dietary recommendations of the American Diabetes Association. Although intake of simple sugars is not forbidden, consuming a large amount of sugary foods at one time may trigger a rapid rise in blood glucose that can increase urination and thirst. In addition, patients who take insulin must remain consistent from day to day in the timing and caloric content of their meals. Depending on the timing, dose, and types of insulin prescribed, snacks may be recommended for the late afternoon, before bedtime, or prior to unusual physical activity. Diabetic patients must always have available juice, food, or tablets that can raise blood glucose levels rapidly to counter an episode of hypoglycemia.

STORAGE
Refrigerate insulin but do not allow it to freeze. Insulin does not have to be kept refrigerated when you're traveling for short periods, but exposure to high temperatures must be avoided.

MISSED DOSE
Timing of insulin doses is extremely important. The best approach is to measure blood glucose and add a dose of regular insulin if your glucose levels are too high. Otherwise, wait for the next scheduled dose.

STOPPING THE DRUG
Do not stop taking insulin injections unless ordered to do so by your doctor. Patients with diabetes are often given general instructions for modifying their insulin doses based on their home blood glucose measurements.

PROLONGED USE
After many years with diabetes, some patients become insensitive to the symptoms of hypoglycemia and are at risk for serious brain complications from prolonged, unrecognized hypoglycemia.

▼ PRECAUTIONS

Over 60: No special warnings. Some older people may, however, have vision problems that may make it difficult for them to draw up the correct dose for them of insulin.

Driving and Hazardous Work: Patients taking insulin must be very careful to avoid hypoglycemia when driving or engaging in hazardous work.

Alcohol: Moderate alcohol intake, especially when taken with large meals, does not adversely affect control of diabetes or alter the dose of insulin. However, large amounts of alcohol increase the risk of hypoglycemia.

Pregnancy: Strict metabolic control—using insulin injections in most women—must be maintained during pregnancy to reduce the risk of birth defects, fetal complications, or death at the time of delivery. In women who had diabetes before the onset of pregnancy, the dose of insulin is often smaller during the first trimester of pregnancy and then higher during the final two trimesters. When women first develop diabetes during pregnancy (gestational diabetes), insulin requirements drop rapidly after delivery and most do not need to continue with insulin treatment.

Breast Feeding: Insulin requirements tend to be

SIDE EFFECTS

SERIOUS
Symptoms of hypoglycemia can be caused by the release of adrenaline or by an inadequate supply of glucose to the brain. With severe hypoglycemia, lack of sufficient glucose to the brain may cause slurred speech, impaired concentration, confusion, seizures, coma, irreversible brain damage, and death. Mild hypoglycemia may cause restless sleep, nightmares, or a cold sweat that awakens patients at night.

COMMON
Symptoms resulting from release of adrenaline are common manifestations of mild to moderate hypoglycemia. They include cold sweats, anxiety, shakiness, hunger, rapid heartbeat, headache, and nervousness. Weight gain is common when taking insulin.

LESS COMMON
Allergic reactions, lipoatrophy (depressions in the skin caused by loss of fat tissue), and lipohypertrophy (excessive accumulation of fat tissue).

lower during breast feeding. Home glucose monitoring is important to avoid hypoglycemia. Insulin is not present in breast milk.

Infants and Children: Treatment with insulin in young patients is the same as that in older people with diabetes.

Special Concerns: Inadequate amounts of insulin in type 1 diabetes may lead to the serious complication of diabetic ketoacidosis, characterized by loss of appetite, excessive thirst and urination, nausea, vomiting, deep breathing, fruity breath odor, drowsiness, confusion, and loss of consciousness.

OVERDOSE

Symptoms: Insulin overdose results in hypoglycemia (see Side Effects for symptoms).

What to Do: For mild to moderate hypoglycemia, ingest drinks or food containing sugar. For more severe hypoglycemia, administer injections of glucagon or call emergency medical services (EMS) immediately.

▼ INTERACTIONS

DRUG INTERACTIONS

A large number of drugs can promote either elevated blood glucose levels or hypoglycemia. Be sure your doctor knows about all of the medications you take and is informed before you start taking any new drugs, either by prescription or over the counter. Corticosteroids in particular are likely to raise blood glucose levels and insulin requirements. Beta-blockers (commonly prescribed for hypertension) may cause either high blood glucose levels or hypoglycemia; in addition, because these medications may dampen the symptoms of hypoglycemia that are caused by adrenaline release, mild degrees of hypoglycemia may progress unnoticed over time to more serious hypoglycemia affecting the brain.

FOOD INTERACTIONS

Insulin requirements are increased when larger amounts of calories are ingested, especially simple sugars and carbohydrates.

DISEASE INTERACTIONS

Insulin requirements are increased by infections, psychological stress, or an uncontrolled overactive thyroid, and often at a time of surgery. Requirements may diminish with kidney disease or an underactive adrenal or pituitary gland.

INTERFERON BETA-1B (RIFN-B)

Available in: Powder for injection
Available OTC? No   **As Generic?** No
Drug Class: Immunomodulator

▼ USAGE INFORMATION

WHY IT'S PRESCRIBED
To treat relapsing-remitting multiple sclerosis (the most common form of MS, in which periods of active disease alternate with periods of remission or reduced severity of symptoms).

HOW IT WORKS
It acts in the same way as the body's natural interferons, which are proteins released by the immune system to fight viruses, cancer cells, and other types of disease. The exact way in which this drug fights MS is unknown, but it appears to interfere with the immune system's attack on healthy tissue.

▼ DOSAGE GUIDELINES

RANGE AND FREQUENCY
8 million units (0.25 mg) by injection every other day.

ONSET OF EFFECT
Unknown.

DURATION OF ACTION
Unknown.

DIETARY ADVICE
Drink plenty of fluids to reduce the risk of excessively low blood pressure.

STORAGE
Keep the liquid form refrigerated but do not allow it to freeze.

MISSED DOSE
If you miss a dose, do not take the missed dose and do not double the next dose. Notify your doctor.

STOPPING THE DRUG
The decision to stop taking the drug should be made by your doctor.

PROLONGED USE
See your doctor regularly for tests and examinations if you must take this drug for a prolonged period.

▼ PRECAUTIONS

Over 60: Adverse reactions may be more likely and more severe in older patients.

Driving and Hazardous Work: Do not drive or engage in hazardous work until you determine how the medicine affects you.

Alcohol: Avoid alcohol.

Pregnancy: Adequate studies have not been done. Consult your doctor for advice.

Breast Feeding: Interferon beta-1b may pass into breast milk; caution is advised. Consult your doctor for advice.

Infants and Children: No special studies have been done on the effects of beta interferon in children.

Special Concerns: Interferon beta-1b should be used with caution in patients with a history of depression, because it has been linked to an increase in suicidal impulses. Try to avoid contact with people with infections, because this drug can lower white blood cell levels temporarily and increase susceptibility to disease. Be careful when using a toothbrush, dental floss, or toothpick. Your doctor or dentist may recommend other ways to clean your teeth. Check with your doctor before having any dental work done. Be careful not to cut yourself when using sharp objects such as a razor. Avoid contact sports or other situations in which bruising could occur. Do not touch your eyes or the inside of your mouth unless you have just washed your hands.

OVERDOSE
Symptoms: No specific symptoms have been reported.

What to Do: Call your doctor or emergency medical services (EMS) immediately if you suspect an overdose.

▼ INTERACTIONS

DRUG INTERACTIONS
Consult your doctor for specific advice if you are taking any prescription or over-the-counter medication.

FOOD INTERACTIONS
None are known.

DISEASE INTERACTIONS
Caution is advised when taking interferon beta-1b. Consult your doctor if you have a history of bleeding or clotting disorders, chicken pox, shingles, psychological or neurological disorders, diabetes, autoimmune disorders, heart disease, kidney disease, liver disease, lung disease, or thyroid disease.

 SIDE EFFECTS

SERIOUS
Seizures, swelling and fluid retention, pelvic pain, pounding in the chest, breast pain, frequent urination, sweating, anxiety, confusion, joint pain, breathing difficulty, depression, suicidal thoughts or impulses. Call your doctor right away.

COMMON
Pain, inflammation, or allergic reaction at injection site (most common side effect); flulike symptoms, including headache, fever, muscle aches, general weakness, and fatigue (these symptoms tend to diminish as the body adjusts to therapy); insomnia; increased susceptibility to infection; nausea and vomiting; diarrhea; abdominal pain; temporary hair loss.

LESS COMMON
Dizziness, dry mouth, dry or itching skin, increased sweating, joint pain, vision or hearing problems. Tissue death at the site of injection has occurred in a few patients.

IPRATROPIUM BROMIDE

BRAND NAME
Atrovent

Available in: Inhalation aerosol, inhalation solution
Available OTC? No   **As Generic?** Yes
Drug Class: Respiratory inhalant

▼ USAGE INFORMATION

WHY IT'S PRESCRIBED
To control the symptoms of lung diseases, such as asthma, chronic bronchitis, and emphysema.

HOW IT WORKS
It inhibits the cough reflex by blocking the activity of acetylcholine, a chemical that, in the lungs, causes the smooth muscles surrounding the airways to constrict. Therefore, when inhaled, ipratropium bromide causes the airways to widen (bronchodilation).

▼ DOSAGE GUIDELINES

RANGE AND FREQUENCY
The drug may be used as needed to relieve respiratory symptoms. For chronic obstructive lung disease such as bronchitis or emphysema–Inhalation aerosol: Adults and children 6 years and over: 2 to 4 inhalations 3 or 4 times a day at regularly spaced intervals. Some patients may need 6 to 8 inhalations a day. Inhalation solution: Adults and children 12 years and over: 250 to 500 micrograms (μg) in a nebulizer 3 or 4 times a day every 6 to 8 hours.

ONSET OF EFFECT
5 to 15 minutes.

DURATION OF ACTION
3 to 4 hours.

DIETARY ADVICE
Sugar-free hard candy or gum can be used to relieve dry mouth.

STORAGE
Store it in a tightly sealed container away from heat and direct light. Open bottles of the solution should be refrigerated but do not allow it to freeze.

MISSED DOSE
Take it as soon as you remember. If it is near the time for the next dose, skip the missed dose and resume your regular dosage schedule. Do not double the next dose.

STOPPING THE DRUG
It may not be necessary to continue using the medication for as long as originally prescribed; consult your doctor.

PROLONGED USE
You should see your doctor regularly if you must take this drug for a prolonged period.

▼ PRECAUTIONS

Over 60: Ipratropium is not expected to cause different problems in older patients than in younger persons.

Driving and Hazardous Work: Do not drive or engage in hazardous work until you determine how the medicine affects you.

Alcohol: No special precautions are necessary.

Pregnancy: Ipratropium has not caused birth defects in animals. Human studies have not been done. Before you take ipratropium, tell your doctor if you are pregnant or plan to become pregnant.

Breast Feeding: It is not known whether ipratropium passes into breast milk; caution is advised. Consult your doctor for specific advice.

Infants and Children: Ipratropium has been tested in children and has not been shown to cause different effects than in adults.

Special Concerns: To test the inhaler, insert the canister into the mouthpiece, take the cap off the mouthpiece, shake the inhaler 3 or 4 times, and spray once into the air. To use the inhaler, hold it upright, with the mouthpiece end down; shake it 3 or 4 times; and then breathe out. Spray into open mouth or with mouth closed over inhaler, as recommended by your doctor. Clean the inhaler, mouthpiece, and spacer at least twice a week. To take the inhalation solution, use a power-operated nebulizer with a face mask or mouthpiece. Get instructions for using the nebulizer from your doctor.

OVERDOSE
Symptoms: No specific symptoms have been reported.

What to Do: An overdose of ipratropium is unlikely to be life-threatening. However, if someone takes a much larger dose than prescribed, call your doctor, emergency medical services (EMS), or the nearest poison control center.

▼ INTERACTIONS

DRUG INTERACTIONS
Before you use ipratropium, tell your doctor if you are using any other prescription or over-the-counter drug.

FOOD INTERACTIONS
No known food interactions.

DISEASE INTERACTIONS
Consult your doctor if you have glaucoma or difficulty urinating.

≣ SIDE EFFECTS ≣

SERIOUS
Persistent constipation, lower abdominal pain or bloating, wheezing or difficulty breathing, tightness in chest, severe eye pain, skin rash or hives, swelling of face, lips, or eyelids. Call your doctor immediately.

COMMON
Dry mouth, cough, unpleasant taste.

LESS COMMON
Blurred vision, other changes in vision, burning eyes, difficult urination, dizziness, headache, nausea, pounding heartbeat, nervousness, sweating, trembling.

IRBESARTAN

BRAND NAME

Avapro

Available in: Tablets
Available OTC? No **As Generic?** No
Drug Class: Antihypertensive/angiotensin II antagonist

▼ USAGE INFORMATION

WHY IT'S PRESCRIBED
To control high blood pressure. This drug appears to have the same benefits as the class of antihypertensive drugs known as ACE (angiotensin-converting enzyme) inhibitors, without producing the common side effect (experienced by as many as 30% of patients) of a dry cough. The drug may be used by itself or in conjunction with other antihypertensive medications.

HOW IT WORKS
Irbesartan blocks the effects of angiotensin II, a naturally occurring substance that causes blood vessels to narrow. Irbesartan causes the blood vessels to dilate, thereby lowering blood pressure and decreasing the workload of the heart.

▼ DOSAGE GUIDELINES

RANGE AND FREQUENCY
To start, 150 mg once a day. It may be increased by your doctor to a maximum dose of 300 mg a day.

ONSET OF EFFECT
Within 2 to 4 hours.

DURATION OF ACTION
More than 24 hours.

DIETARY ADVICE
No special restrictions unless your doctor has advised a low-sodium diet or other dietary modifications to help control your blood pressure.

STORAGE
Store in a tightly sealed container away from moisture, heat, and direct light.

MISSED DOSE
If you miss a dose on one day, do not double the dose the next day. Resume your regular dosage schedule.

STOPPING THE DRUG
Take it as prescribed for the full treatment period. The decision to stop taking the drug should be made in consultation with your physician.

PROLONGED USE
Lifelong therapy may be necessary. However, if you do change certain health habits (for example, losing weight or increasing exercise), a reduced dose may be possible under a doctor's supervision.

▼ PRECAUTIONS

Over 60: Adverse reactions may be more likely and more severe in older patients.

Driving and Hazardous Work: Do not drive or engage in hazardous work until you determine how the medicine affects you.

Alcohol: No special precautions are necessary.

Pregnancy: Irbesartan should not be used by pregnant women. Stop taking the drug as soon as possible when pregnancy is detected and discuss treatment alternatives with your doctor.

Breast Feeding: Irbesartan may pass into breast milk; caution is advised. Consult your doctor for advice.

Infants and Children: The safety and effectiveness of use in children have not been established.

Special Concerns: Irbesartan may cause excessively low blood pressure with dizziness or lightheadedness, which is most noticeable when you change position. This may lead to fainting, falls, and injury. Sit or lie down immediately if you feel dizzy or lightheaded. This side effect may be worsened by alcohol, hot weather, dehydration, salt depletion from diuretic use, fever, prolonged standing, prolonged sitting, or exercise.

▼ OVERDOSE

Symptoms: No cases of overdose have been reported. If you take a much larger dose than your doctor prescribes, however, you may experience extremely low blood pressure or heartbeat irregularities.

What to Do: If you take a much larger dose than prescribed, contact your doctor.

▼ INTERACTIONS

DRUG INTERACTIONS
No drug interactions have been observed with irbesartan. Consult your doctor for specific advice if you are taking any other medication, including other drugs for high blood pressure. Irbesartan can be taken together with diuretics or other medications for high blood pressure if your doctor approves.

FOOD INTERACTIONS
No known food interactions.

DISEASE INTERACTIONS
Patients with liver or kidney disease are advised to exercise caution when they are taking irbesartan.

 SIDE EFFECTS

SERIOUS
No serious side effects are associated with the use of irbesartan. (In clinical trials, the incidence of adverse effects was not significantly greater with the medication than with a placebo.)

COMMON
No common side effects are associated with the use of irbesartan.

LESS COMMON
Diarrhea, indigestion, heartburn, fatigue, muscle pain, edema, sexual dysfunction, low blood pressure.

ISOSORBIDE MONONITRATE

Available in: Tablets, extended-release tablets
Available OTC? No **As Generic?** Yes
Drug Class: Nitrate

▼ USAGE INFORMATION

WHY IT'S PRESCRIBED
To prevent or relieve attacks of angina (chest pain associated with heart disease).

HOW IT WORKS
Isosorbide relaxes the smooth muscle of the blood vessels and increases the supply of blood and oxygen to the heart. It also reduces the heart's workload and demand for oxygen.

▼ DOSAGE GUIDELINES

RANGE AND FREQUENCY
To prevent angina attacks—Tablets: 20 mg 2 times a day, with doses 7 hours apart. Extended-release tablets: 30 to 240 mg once a day.

ONSET OF EFFECT
60 minutes.

DURATION OF ACTION
Unknown.

DIETARY ADVICE
Take tablets on an empty stomach at least 30 minutes before or 1 to 2 hours after a meal.

STORAGE
Store in a tightly sealed container away from heat and direct light.

MISSED DOSE
Take it as soon as you remember. If it is near the time for the next dose, skip the missed dose and resume your regular dosage schedule as prescribed. Do not double the next dose.

STOPPING THE DRUG
The decision to stop taking the drug should be made by your doctor.

PROLONGED USE
You should see your doctor regularly if you take this medicine for an extended period.

▼ PRECAUTIONS

Over 60: Adverse reactions may be more likely and more severe in older patients.

Driving and Hazardous Work: Avoid such activities until you determine how the medicine affects you.

Alcohol: Avoid alcohol.

Pregnancy: Animal tests have shown that the drug has adverse effects on the fetus. Human tests have not been done. Before taking isosorbide, tell your doctor if you are pregnant or if you plan to become pregnant.

Breast Feeding: Isosorbide mononitrate may pass into breast milk; caution is advised. Consult your doctor for specific advice.

Infants and Children: No studies on the use of this medicine in children have been done. Use and dose should be determined by your doctor.

Special Concerns: Do not stop taking this medicine suddenly; this can cause a spasm of the blood vessels in the heart. Consult your doctor about reducing the dose gradually. Use extra care in hot weather, during exercise, or when you must stand for long periods. This medicine may cause headaches at the beginning of therapy. Headaches can be treated with aspirin or acetaminophen and usually stop after your body becomes accustomed to the medication. The dose may be reduced temporarily because of headaches. The effectiveness of the drug may decrease over time; notify your doctor if this occurs.

OVERDOSE
Symptoms: Bluish fingernails, lips, or palms; extreme dizziness or fainting; unusual weakness; fever; weak and fast heartbeat; seizures.

What to Do: Call your doctor, emergency medical services (EMS), or the nearest poison control center immediately.

▼ INTERACTIONS

DRUG INTERACTIONS
Do not take isosorbide mononitrate within 24 hours of taking sildenafil citrate. Sildenafil can enhance the action of nitrates (such as isosorbide), causing potentially dangerous decreases in blood pressure. Consult your doctor for specific advice if you are taking other heart medicines or antihypertensive drugs.

FOOD INTERACTIONS
No known food interactions.

DISEASE INTERACTIONS
Consult your doctor if you have any of the following: anemia, glaucoma, a recent head injury or stroke, an overactive thyroid, or a recent heart attack. Use of isosorbide mononitrate may cause complications in patients with severe liver or kidney disease, because these organs work together to remove the medication from the body.

SIDE EFFECTS

SERIOUS
Blurred vision, dry mouth, severe or prolonged headache. Call your doctor immediately.

COMMON
Dizziness or lightheadedness, especially when rising suddenly to a standing position; flushing of the face and neck; rapid pulse or heartbeat; nausea or vomiting; restlessness.

LESS COMMON
Skin rash.

LANSOPRAZOLE

BRAND NAMES

Prevacid, Prevpac

Available in: Delayed-release capsules
Available OTC? No   **As Generic?** No
Drug Class: Antacid/proton pump inhibitor

▼ USAGE INFORMATION

WHY IT'S PRESCRIBED
To treat stomach and duodenal ulcers, gastroesophageal reflux disease (chronic heartburn caused by the backwash of stomach acid into the esophagus), and conditions that cause increased stomach acid secretion; to treat and prevent stomach ulcers associated with nonsteroidal antiinflammatory drugs (NSAIDs). Lansoprazole is also prescribed in conjunction with the antibiotics amoxicillin and clarithromycin to eradicate the bacterium *H. pylori* and thus prevent the recurrence of duodenal ulcers caused by this bacterium.

HOW IT WORKS
Lansoprazole blocks the action of a specific enzyme in the cells that line the stomach, decreasing the production of stomach acid. Reduction of stomach acid creates a more favorable environment for the eradication of *H. pylori* and promotes ulcer healing.

▼ DOSAGE GUIDELINES

RANGE AND FREQUENCY
Prevacid—To treat duodenal ulcers: Initial dose is 15 mg once a day; it may later be increased. To treat gastroesophageal reflux disease: 15 mg once a day for up to 8 weeks. To treat NSAID-associated stomach ulcers: 30 mg once a day for 8 weeks. To reduce the risk of NSAID-associated stomach ulcer: 15 mg once a day for up to 12 weeks. To treat other conditions: Initial dose is 60 mg once a day; it may be increased. Treatment usually runs 4 to 8 weeks. A second course of treatment may be necessary. Prevpac—To prevent duodenal ulcers: 30 mg lansoprazole, 1 g amoxicillin, and 500 mg clarithromycin every 12 hours for 14 days.

ONSET OF EFFECT
1 to 3 hours.

DURATION OF ACTION
More than 24 hours.

DIETARY ADVICE
The drug is best taken 30 minutes or more before a meal, preferably in the morning before breakfast.

STORAGE
Store in a tightly sealed container away from moisture, heat, and direct light.

MISSED DOSE
Take it as soon as you remember. However, if it is near the time for the next dose, skip the missed dose and resume your regular dosage schedule. Do not double the next dose.

STOPPING THE DRUG
Take as prescribed for the full treatment period, even if your symptoms improve before the scheduled end of therapy.

PROLONGED USE
See your doctor regularly for tests and examinations if you must take this drug for a prolonged period. Lansoprazole should not be used indefinitely as maintenance therapy for esophagitis or a duodenal ulcer; other treatments are recommended.

▼ PRECAUTIONS

Over 60: No special problems are expected.

Driving and Hazardous Work: Do not drive or engage in hazardous activities until you determine how lansoprazole affects you. Taking it may be a disqualification for piloting aircraft.

Alcohol: Avoid alcohol for the duration of therapy.

Pregnancy: Adequate human studies have not been done. Before taking lansoprazole, tell your doctor if you are pregnant or if you plan to become pregnant.

Breast Feeding: Lansoprazole may pass into breast milk; caution is advised. Consult your doctor for advice.

Infants and Children: Use and dose for anyone under 18 years should be determined by your doctor or pediatrician.

Special Concerns: Tell any doctor or dentist you see for treatment that you are taking lansoprazole. Do not chew the capsules. If you have trouble swallowing them, you may open them and sprinkle the contents on 1 tbsp of applesauce, cottage cheese, yogurt, or similar food. If your doctor so directs, you may take an antacid along with lansoprazole.

OVERDOSE
Symptoms: No cases of overdose have been reported.

What to Do: An overdose is unlikely to be life-threatening. However, if someone takes a much larger dose than prescribed, call your doctor, emergency medical services (EMS), or the nearest poison control center immediately.

▼ INTERACTIONS

DRUG INTERACTIONS
Consult your doctor for specific advice if you are taking ampicillin, sucralfate, iron salts or supplements, cyclosporine, diazepam, disulfiram, ketoconazole, phenytoin, or theophylline.

FOOD INTERACTIONS
No significant food interactions have been reported.

DISEASE INTERACTIONS
Caution is advised when taking lansoprazole. Consult your doctor if you have liver disease, because it may increase the risk of side effects.

≡ SIDE EFFECTS ≡

SERIOUS
No serious side effects have been reported.

COMMON
Diarrhea, itching or rash, headache, dizziness.

LESS COMMON
Abdominal or stomach pain, nausea, increase or decrease in appetite, anxiety, flulike symptoms, constipation, coughing, mental depression, muscle pain.

LATANOPROST

Available in: Ophthalmic solution
Available OTC? No   **As Generic?** No
Drug Class: Antiglaucoma agent

▼ USAGE INFORMATION

WHY IT'S PRESCRIBED
To treat glaucoma.

HOW IT WORKS
Glaucoma, a sight-threatening disorder, occurs when the aqueous humor (fluid inside the eye) cannot drain properly, causing increased pressure within the eyeball (intraocular pressure). Increased eye pressure can damage the optic nerve and lead to a gradually progressive loss of vision. Latanoprost promotes outflow of aqueous humor, thereby reducing intraocular pressure.

▼ DOSAGE GUIDELINES

RANGE AND FREQUENCY
1 drop of latanoprost in each eye once daily in the evening.

ONSET OF EFFECT
3 to 4 hours.

DURATION OF ACTION
24 hours or more.

DIETARY ADVICE
This medication can be used without regard to diet.

STORAGE
Store it in a tightly sealed container away from moisture, heat, and direct light. Do not allow the medicine to freeze.

MISSED DOSE
Apply it as soon as you remember. If it is near the time for the next dose, skip the missed dose and resume your regular dosage schedule. Do not double the next dose.

STOPPING THE DRUG
The decision to stop using the drug should be made by your doctor.

PROLONGED USE
See your doctor regularly for tests and examinations if you must take this drug for an extended period.

▼ PRECAUTIONS

Over 60: No special problems are expected.

Driving and Hazardous Work: Do not drive or engage in hazardous work until you determine how the medicine affects your vision.

Alcohol: No special precautions are necessary.

Pregnancy: Latanoprost has not caused birth defects in animals. Human studies have not been done. Before you take latanoprost, tell your doctor if you are pregnant or plan to become pregnant.

Breast Feeding: Latanoprost may pass into breast milk; caution is advised. Consult your doctor for advice.

Infants and Children: The safety and effectiveness of latanoprost in infants and children have not been established.

Special Concerns: To use the eye drops, first wash your hands. Tilt your head back. Gently apply pressure to the inside corner of the eyelid and with the index finger of the same hand, pull downward on the lower eyelid to make a space. Drop the medicine into this space and close your eye. Apply pressure for 1 or 2 minutes while keeping the eye closed without blinking. Then wash your hands again. Make sure the tip of the dropper does not touch your eye, finger, or any other surface. Latanoprost may make your eyes more sensitive to sunlight. If this occurs, wear sunglasses or avoid exposure to bright light as necessary. Latanoprost may change eye color, increasing the brown pigment in the iris over a period of months or years. The color change may be permanent. Latanoprost contains ingredients that may damage contact lenses. Contact lenses should be removed 15 minutes before applying the medication and reinserted 15 minutes or more afterward.

OVERDOSE
Symptoms: No specific symptoms have been reported.

What to Do: An overdose of latanoprost is unlikely to be life-threatening. If a large volume enters the eyes, flush them with water. If someone ingests the medication accidentally, immediately call your doctor, emergency medical services (EMS), or the nearest poison control center.

▼ INTERACTIONS

DRUG INTERACTIONS
Other drugs may interact with latanoprost. Consult your doctor for specific advice if you are taking any other prescription or over-the-counter medication. If you are using other ophthalmic medications to reduce fluid pressure in the eye, administer them at least 5 minutes apart.

FOOD INTERACTIONS
No known food interactions.

DISEASE INTERACTIONS
Use of latanoprost may cause complications in patients with liver or kidney disease, because these organs work together to remove the drug from the body.

SIDE EFFECTS

SERIOUS
Chest pain, difficulty breathing. Call your doctor right away.

COMMON
Blurred vision, burning and stinging of the eye, sensation of something in the eye, increased brown pigmentation of the iris, eye redness.

LESS COMMON
Dry eye, excessive tearing, eye pain, lid crusting, swollen eyelid, eyelid pain or discomfort, sensitivity to light, upper respiratory tract infection, double vision, pain in the chest and back.

LEVODOPA

Available in: Tablets, capsules
Available OTC? No   **As Generic?** Yes
Drug Class: Antiparkinsonism drug

▼ USAGE INFORMATION

WHY IT'S PRESCRIBED
To treat Parkinson's disease and Parkinson-like syndromes. Such syndromes can occur following injury to or infection of the central nervous system, damage to the blood vessels in the brain (after a stroke, for example), or exposure to certain toxins.

HOW IT WORKS
Levodopa replenishes the supply of dopamine in the brain. Dopamine is a chemical in the central nervous system that plays an essential role in the initiation and smooth control of voluntary muscle movement.

▼ DOSAGE GUIDELINES

RANGE AND FREQUENCY
Adults: To start, 0.5 g per day in 2 or more divided doses. The dose is increased gradually (by 0.5 to 0.75 g per day) over the course of 4 to 7 days until the desired therapeutic response is achieved. The onset of adverse side effects may preclude the use of higher doses. The maximum beneficial dose is usually 5 to 6 g per day. Children: Smaller doses are used; consult your pediatrician for specific information.

ONSET OF EFFECT
Within 1 to 2 hours.

DURATION OF ACTION
From 4 to 5 hours.

DIETARY ADVICE
Eating food soon after taking this medication may minimize the chance of stomach upset. Eating food before taking the medicine or at the same time may blunt levodopa's effects.

STORAGE
Store it in a tightly sealed container away from moisture, heat, and direct light.

MISSED DOSE
Take it as soon as you remember. However, if it is near the time for the next dose, skip the missed dose and resume your regular dosage schedule. Do not double the next dose.

STOPPING THE DRUG
Consult your doctor for the best approach to stopping this drug. The dose should be decreased very gradually. Abruptly stopping the drug can cause an acute (sudden-onset) adverse reaction.

PROLONGED USE
Prolonged use of levodopa can result in a less predictable therapeutic response and bothersome involuntary muscle movements.

▼ PRECAUTIONS

Over 60: Adverse reactions to levodopa may be more likely and more severe in older patients. The dose should be increased very gradually in this age group.

Driving and Hazardous Work: Do not drive or engage in hazardous work until the full dose has been attained and you determine how the drug affects you.

Alcohol: Do not consume alcohol. Alcohol can cause pronounced confusion or delirium in patients taking this medication.

Pregnancy: Adequate human studies have not been done, and the effects of levodopa during pregnancy have not been determined, so pregnant women should avoid taking levodopa.

Breast Feeding: Levodopa passes into breast milk; this medication should not be used by nursing mothers.

Infants and Children: Levodopa should be used with caution by infants and children. The dose should be smaller than that for adults and should be determined by your pediatrician.

Special Concerns: Patients taking levodopa should not eat a high-protein diet, because it can reduce the medication's effectiveness.

OVERDOSE
Symptoms: The symptoms of levodopa overdose are unknown.

What to Do: If you have any reason to suspect an overdose, call your doctor, emergency medical services (EMS), or the nearest poison control center.

▼ INTERACTIONS

DRUG INTERACTIONS
Consult your doctor for specific advice if you are taking any of the following drugs: MAO (monoamine oxidase) inhibitor antidepressants (such as phenelzine sulfate or tranylcypromine sulfate) or antihypertensives.

FOOD INTERACTIONS
A high-protein diet can reduce the effectiveness of levodopa. Persons taking levodopa should therefore decrease their protein intake if it is high.

DISEASE INTERACTIONS
Caution is advised when taking levodopa. Consult your doctor if you have any of the following: heart disease or heart rhythm abnormalities, bronchial asthma, glaucoma, malignant melanoma, or changes in mental state.

≡ SIDE EFFECTS ≡

 SERIOUS
Irregular heartbeat, heart rhythm abnormalities, low blood pressure, fainting or near-fainting, hallucinations.

COMMON
Nausea, confusion.

LESS COMMON
Breathing difficulty.

LEVOFLOXACIN

Available in: Tablets, injection
Available OTC? No   **As Generic?** No
Drug Class: Fluoroquinolone antibiotic

▼ USAGE INFORMATION

WHY IT'S PRESCRIBED
To treat pneumonia, chronic bronchitis, and other infections caused by bacteria.

HOW IT WORKS
Levofloxacin inhibits the activity of a bacterial enzyme (gyrase) that is necessary for proper DNA formation and replication. This fights infection by preventing bacteria cells from reproducing.

▼ DOSAGE GUIDELINES

RANGE AND FREQUENCY
Adults: 250 to 500 mg once a day for 7 to 14 days. After an initial dose of 250 to 500 mg, patients with kidney problems receive 250 mg every day for 7 to 14 days.

ONSET OF EFFECT
Varies depending on the infection being treated.

DURATION OF ACTION
Unknown.

DIETARY ADVICE
Drink plenty of fluids.

STORAGE
Store it in a tightly sealed container away from heat and direct light. Do not allow the injection form to freeze.

MISSED DOSE
Take it as soon as you remember. If it is near the time for the next dose, skip the missed dose and resume your regular dosage schedule. Do not double the next dose.

STOPPING THE DRUG
It is very important to take this drug as prescribed for the full treatment period, even if you begin to feel better before the scheduled end of therapy (unless you experience intolerable side effects, including increased sensitivity to sunlight).

PROLONGED USE
See your doctor regularly for tests and examinations if you must take this medicine for an extended period.

▼ PRECAUTIONS

Over 60: No special problems are expected.

Driving and Hazardous Work: Do not drive or engage in hazardous work until you determine how the medicine affects you.

Alcohol: It is advisable to abstain from alcohol when fighting an infection.

Pregnancy: In some animal tests, levofloxacin has caused birth defects. Adequate studies in humans have not been done. The drug should be used during pregnancy only if potential benefits clearly justify the risks. Before you take levofloxacin, tell your doctor if you are pregnant or plan to become pregnant.

Breast Feeding: Levofloxacin passes into breast milk and may cause serious side effects in the nursing infant; use of the drug is discouraged when nursing.

Infants and Children: Levofloxacin is not recommended for use by persons under the age of 18 years, because it has been shown to interfere with bone development.

Special Concerns: If levofloxacin causes sensitivity to sunlight, stop taking the drug and try to avoid exposure to sunlight for the next 5 days; also, wear protective clothing and use a sunblock. Levofloxacin should not be taken by patients whose work makes it impossible to avoid exposure to sunlight. It is important to drink plenty of fluids while taking this drug.

OVERDOSE
Symptoms: No specific symptoms have been reported.

What to Do: If you have any reason to suspect an overdose, call your doctor, emergency medical services (EMS), or the nearest poison control center.

▼ INTERACTIONS

DRUG INTERACTIONS
Consult your doctor for specific advice if you are taking aminophylline, antacids, didanosine, iron supplements, sucralfate, or zinc salts. Also tell your doctor if you are taking any other prescription or over-the-counter drug.

FOOD INTERACTIONS
No known food interactions.

DISEASE INTERACTIONS
Caution is advised when taking levofloxacin. Consult your doctor if you have any other medical condition. Use of the drug can cause complications in patients with kidney disease, because this organ works to remove the medication from the body.

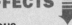

SIDE EFFECTS

SERIOUS
Serious reactions to levofloxacin are rare and include seizures, mental confusion, hallucinations, agitation, nightmares, depression, shortness of breath, unusual swelling in the face or extremities, and loss of consciousness. Also skin burning, redness, blisters, rash, or itching after exposure to sunlight and increased risk of tendinitis or tendon rupture. Call your doctor immediately.

COMMON
Increased sensitivity to sunlight (and increased risk of sunburn) for days following therapy.

LESS COMMON
Diarrhea, nausea and vomiting, stomach pain and upset, gas, headache, dizziness, restlessness, insomnia, changes in taste perception, drowsiness, itching, dry mouth, unusual body aches or pains.

LEVONORGESTREL IMPLANTS

BRAND NAME

Norplant

Available in: Implanted capsule
Available OTC? No   **As Generic?** No
Drug Class: Progestin (hormone)

▼ USAGE INFORMATION

WHY IT'S PRESCRIBED
As a birth control method.

HOW IT WORKS
The implant slowly releases levonorgestrel, a synthetic hormone, into the bloodstream. It prevents a woman's egg from developing fully and causes changes in the uterine lining that make it difficult for sperm to reach the egg. It may prevent ovulation in some patients.

▼ DOSAGE GUIDELINES

RANGE AND FREQUENCY
Six capsules are implanted under the skin of the upper arm. The capsules are placed in a fanlike position 15 degrees apart. They are removed after 5 years.

ONSET OF EFFECT
Within 24 hours if implanted within 7 days of the menstrual period.

DURATION OF ACTION
Up to 5 years.

DIETARY ADVICE
No special restrictions.

STORAGE
Not applicable.

MISSED DOSE
Not applicable; the drug is delivered continuously from the implant under the skin.

STOPPING THE DRUG
The decision to stop using the implant can be made whenever you choose, but the implants should be removed by your doctor.

PROLONGED USE
See your doctor at least once a year for periodic examinations and lab tests.

▼ PRECAUTIONS

Over 60: Not normally prescribed for postmenopausal women.

Driving and Hazardous Work: No special precautions are necessary.

Alcohol: No special precautions are necessary.

Pregnancy: Extensive studies have shown that no special risks to mother or child are associated with pregnancies occurring prior to or shortly after implantation of levonorgestrel capsules. Nevertheless, it is advisable to have the implants removed if pregnancy does occur.

Breast Feeding: Levonorgestrel passes into breast milk but has not been shown to cause problems. It can be used by nursing mothers who desire contraception.

Infants and Children: Levonorgestrel implants have not been shown to cause problems in teenagers. However, birth control methods that protect against sexually transmitted diseases (condoms, for example) are preferred for those in this age group.

Special Concerns: Do not have this implant inserted until you are sure you are not pregnant. Call your doctor immediately if one of the capsules falls out before the skin heals over the implant. No contraceptive method is perfect: If you suspect a pregnancy, you should call your doctor immediately. If you have any laboratory test, tell the health professional that you are using these contraceptives. Cigarette smoking or alcohol abuse can increase the risk of osteoporosis and blood clot formation. Implants should be removed if you

develop active thrombophlebitis (pain caused by a blot clot lodged in a blood vessel), thromboembolic disease, or jaundice (yellowish tinge to the eyes or skin), or if you will be immobilized for a significant period of time because of illness or some other factor. If you have a sudden unexplained vision problem, including changes in tolerance for contact lenses, you should be evaluated by an ophthalmologist.

OVERDOSE
Symptoms: Not applicable.

What to Do: Emergency instructions not applicable.

▼ INTERACTIONS

DRUG INTERACTIONS
Consult your doctor for specific advice if you are taking aminoglutethimide, carbamazepine, phenytoin, rifabutin, or rifampin.

FOOD INTERACTIONS
No known food interactions.

DISEASE INTERACTIONS
Caution is advised when using this contraceptive. Consult your doctor if you have any of the following: asthma, epilepsy, heart or circulation problems, kidney disease, liver disease, migraine headaches, breast disease, bleeding disorders, central nervous system disorders (including depression), diabetes, or high blood cholesterol.

⬇ SIDE EFFECTS ⬇

SERIOUS
Changes in or cessation of menstrual bleeding, unexpected or increased flow of breast milk, mental depression, skin rash, loss of or change in speech, impaired coordination or vision, severe and sudden shortness of breath. Call your doctor immediately.

COMMON
Stomach pain; swelling of face, ankles, or feet; mild headache; mood changes; unusual fatigue; weight gain; pain or irritation at site of implant.

LESS COMMON
Acne, breast pain or tenderness, hot flashes, insomnia, loss of sexual desire, loss or gain of scalp hair or body hair, brown spots on skin.

LEVOTHYROXINE SODIUM

Available in: Tablets, injection
Available OTC? No   **As Generic?** Yes
Drug Class: Hypothyroid agent

▼ USAGE INFORMATION

WHY IT'S PRESCRIBED
To treat patients with an underactive thyroid gland, goiter (enlarged thyroid gland), and benign (noncancerous) and malignant (cancerous) thyroid nodules.

HOW IT WORKS
Levothyroxine acts in the body as a substitute for natural thyroid hormone.

▼ DOSAGE GUIDELINES

RANGE AND FREQUENCY
Tablets—Adults and teenagers: 0.0016 mg per 2.2 lb (1 kg) a day. Children less than 6 months old: 0.025 to 0.05 mg once a day. Children 6 to 12 months old: 0.05 to 0.075 mg once a day. Children ages 1 to 5 years: 0.075 to 0.1 mg once a day. Children ages 6 to 12 years: 0.1 to 0.15 mg a day. Injection—Adults and teenagers: 0.05 to 0.1 mg into a vein or muscle once a day. Children less than 6 months old: 0.019 to 0.038 mg once a day. Children 6 to 12 months old: 0.038 to 0.056 mg once a day. Children ages 1 to 5 years: 0.056 to 0.075 mg once a day. Children ages 6 to 10 years: 0.075 to 0.113 mg once a day. Children ages 10 to 12: 0.113 to 0.15 mg once a day.

ONSET OF EFFECT
24 hours.

DURATION OF ACTION
1 to 3 weeks.

DIETARY ADVICE
Take it before breakfast on an empty stomach.

STORAGE
Store in a tightly sealed container away from moisture, heat, and direct light.

MISSED DOSE
If you miss your dose on one day, you may double the dose on the next day. If you miss two or more doses in a row, call your doctor.

STOPPING THE DRUG
The decision to stop taking the drug should be made in consultation with your doctor.

PROLONGED USE
If you must take this drug, it is very likely that lifelong therapy will be necessary. See your doctor regularly for routine tests and examinations to evaluate your condition.

▼ PRECAUTIONS

Over 60: Modification of the dosage may be required.

Driving and Hazardous Work: Avoid such activities until you determine how the medicine affects you.

Alcohol: Avoid alcohol.

Pregnancy: Using the recommended dose of levothyroxine has not been shown to cause birth defects. The dose may need to be changed during pregnancy. Consult your doctor for specific advice.

Breast Feeding: Using the recommended dose of levothyroxine has not been shown to cause problems while nursing. Consult your doctor for specific advice.

Infants and Children: No special problems are expected.

Special Concerns: You should wear a medical-alert bracelet or carry an identification card indicating that you are taking this medication.

OVERDOSE
Symptoms: Rapid heartbeat, chest pain, shortness of breath.

What to Do: Call your doctor, emergency medical services (EMS), or the nearest poison control center immediately.

▼ INTERACTIONS

DRUG INTERACTIONS
Consult your doctor for advice if you are taking anticoagulants, cholestyramine, colestipol, amphetamines, appetite suppressants, asthma medication, or cold, sinus, or allergy medications.

FOOD INTERACTIONS
No known food interactions.

DISEASE INTERACTIONS
Caution is advised when taking levothyroxine. Consult your doctor if you have any of the following: diabetes mellitus, diabetes insipidus, myxedema, an overactive thyroid gland, atherosclerosis (so-called hardening of the arteries), heart disease, high blood pressure, an underactive adrenal gland, or an underactive pituitary gland.

SIDE EFFECTS

SERIOUS
In rare instances, levothyroxine may cause severe headaches, skin rash, hives, rapid or irregular heartbeat, chest pain, or shortness of breath. These symptoms may signal an overdose or an allergic reaction. Seek emergency medical assistance immediately.

COMMON
No common side effects are associated with the use of levothyroxine.

LESS COMMON
Leg cramps, diarrhea, changes in menstrual cycle, changes in appetite, sweating, sensitivity to heat, shaking of the hands, fever, headache, insomnia, irritability, weight loss, vomiting, nervousness. These symptoms may indicate that your dose needs adjustment by your doctor.

LISINOPRIL

Available in: Tablets
Available OTC? No   **As Generic?** Yes
Drug Class: Angiotensin-converting enzyme (ACE) inhibitor

▼ USAGE INFORMATION

WHY IT'S PRESCRIBED
To control high blood pressure (hypertension). Also used to treat congestive heart failure (CHF) and left ventricular dysfunction (damage to the primary pumping chamber of the heart), and to minimize further kidney damage in diabetic patients with mild kidney disease.

HOW IT WORKS
Angiotensin-converting enzyme (ACE) inhibitors block an enzyme that produces angiotensin, a naturally occurring substance that causes blood vessels to constrict and also stimulates production of the adrenal hormone, aldosterone, which promotes sodium retention in the body. As a result, ACE inhibitor medications relax blood vessels (causing them to widen) and reduce sodium retention, which in turn lowers blood pressure and so decreases the workload of the heart.

▼ DOSAGE GUIDELINES

RANGE AND FREQUENCY
For high blood pressure: 5 to 40 mg once a day. For congestive heart failure: 2.5 to 20 mg once a day.

ONSET OF EFFECT
Within 1 hour.

DURATION OF ACTION
24 hours.

DIETARY ADVICE
Take lisinopril on an empty stomach about 1 hour before mealtime. Follow your doctor's dietary advice (including low-salt or low-cholesterol restrictions) to improve control over high blood pressure and heart disease. Avoid high-potassium foods such as bananas and citrus fruits and juices unless you are also taking medications that lower potassium levels, such as diuretics.

STORAGE
Store in a tightly sealed container away from heat and direct light.

MISSED DOSE
Take it as soon as you remember. If it is near the time for the next dose, skip the missed dose and resume your regular dosage schedule. Do not double the next dose.

STOPPING THE DRUG
Do not stop taking this drug abruptly; this may cause potentially serious health problems. Dosage should be reduced gradually according to your doctor's instructions.

PROLONGED USE
Lifelong therapy with lisinopril may be necessary. See your doctor regularly for examinations and tests if you must take this medicine for an extended period.

▼ PRECAUTIONS

Over 60: No unusual problems are expected in older patients.

Driving and Hazardous Work: Do not drive or engage in hazardous work until you determine how the medicine affects you.

Alcohol: Consume alcohol only in moderation, because it may increase the effect of the drug and cause an excessive drop in blood pressure. Consult your doctor for advice.

Pregnancy: Use of lisinopril during the last 6 months of pregnancy may cause severe defects in or death of the fetus. The drug should be discontinued if you are pregnant or plan to become pregnant.

Breast Feeding: Lisinopril may pass into breast milk;

caution is advised. Consult your doctor for advice.

Infants and Children: Children may be especially sensitive to the effects of lisinopril. Benefits must be weighed against potential risks; consult your pediatrician for advice.

OVERDOSE
Symptoms: Dizziness, confusion, faintness.

What to Do: Call your doctor, emergency medical services (EMS), or the nearest poison control center immediately.

▼ INTERACTIONS

DRUG INTERACTIONS
Consult your doctor if you are taking diuretics (especially potassium-sparing diuretics), potassium supplements or drugs containing potassium (check ingredient labels), lithium, anticoagulants (such as warfarin), indomethacin or other antiinflammatory drugs, or any over-the-counter medications (especially diet pills and cold remedies).

FOOD INTERACTIONS
Avoid low-salt milk and salt substitutes. Many of these products contain potassium.

DISEASE INTERACTIONS
Consult your doctor if you have systemic lupus erythematosus (SLE) or if you have had a prior allergic reaction to ACE inhibitor drugs. Lisinopril should be used with caution by patients with severe kidney disease or renal artery stenosis (narrowing of one or both of the arteries that supply blood to the kidneys).

▲ SIDE EFFECTS ▲

SERIOUS
Fever and chills; sore throat and hoarseness; sudden difficulty breathing or swallowing; swelling of the face, mouth, or extremities; impaired kidney function (ankle swelling, decreased urination); confusion; yellow discoloration of the eyes or skin (indicating liver disorder); intense itching; chest pain or palpitations; abdominal pain. Serious side effects are very rare; contact your doctor immediately.

COMMON
Dry, persistent cough.

LESS COMMON
Dizziness or fainting; skin rash; numbness or tingling in the hands, feet, or lips; unusual fatigue or muscle weakness; nausea; drowsiness; loss of taste; headache.

LISINOPRIL/HYDROCHLOROTHIAZIDE

Available in: Tablets
Available OTC? No   **As Generic?** Yes
Drug Class: Angiotensin-converting enzyme (ACE) inhibitor/diuretic

▼ USAGE INFORMATION

WHY IT'S PRESCRIBED
To treat high blood pressure (hypertension).

HOW IT WORKS
Angiotensin-converting enzyme (ACE) inhibitors such as lisinopril block an enzyme that produces angiotensin, a naturally occurring substance that causes blood vessels to constrict and stimulates production of the adrenal hormone aldosterone, which promotes sodium retention in the body. As a result, ACE inhibitors relax blood vessels (causing them to widen) and also reduce sodium retention, which lowers blood pressure and so decreases the workload of the heart. Hydrochlorothiazide (HCTZ), a diuretic, increases sodium and water in the urine output. By reducing the overall fluid volume in the body, diuretics reduce blood volume and so lower blood pressure.

▼ DOSAGE GUIDELINES

RANGE AND FREQUENCY
This combination medication comes in three strengths: lisinopril/hydrochlorothiazide 10/12.5, 20/12.5, and 20/25 mg. The dose ranges from 10 to 40 mg of lisinopril and 12.5 to 50 mg of hydrochlorothiazide a day. One or two tablets are taken once a day in the morning after breakfast.

ONSET OF EFFECT
Within 1 hour.

DURATION OF ACTION
Unknown.

DIETARY ADVICE
Follow your doctor's dietary advice (such as low-salt or low-fat restrictions) to improve control over high blood pressure and heart disease.

STORAGE
Store in a tightly sealed container away from moisture, heat, and direct light.

MISSED DOSE
Take it as soon as you remember. If it is near the time for the next dose, skip the missed dose and resume your regular dosage schedule. Do not double the next dose.

STOPPING THE DRUG
Discontinuing this drug abruptly may cause potentially serious problems. The dosage should be reduced gradually according to your doctor's instructions.

PROLONGED USE
Lifelong therapy may be required; see your doctor regularly for evaluation.

▼ PRECAUTIONS

Over 60: Adverse reactions may be more likely and more severe in older patients.

Driving and Hazardous Work: Do not drive or engage in hazardous work until you determine how the medicine affects you.

Alcohol: Consume alcohol only in moderation because it may increase the effect of the drug and cause an excessive drop in blood pressure. Consult your doctor for advice.

Pregnancy: Before taking this medication, tell your doctor if you are pregnant or plan to become pregnant. Use of this medicine during the last 6 months of pregnancy may cause severe defects in or death of the fetus.

Breast Feeding: Lisinopril may pass into breast milk; caution is advised. Consult your doctor for advice.

Infants and Children: Children may be especially sensitive to the effects of lisinopril. Consult your pedia-trician about the relative risks and benefits.

OVERDOSE
Symptoms: Overdose has not been reported; symptoms might include dizziness, faintness, or confusion.

What to Do: Although overdose is unlikely, call your doctor, emergency medical services (EMS), or the nearest poison control center immediately if you suspect that someone has taken a much larger dose than prescribed.

▼ INTERACTIONS

DRUG INTERACTIONS
Consult your doctor for specific advice if you are taking cholestyramine, colestipol, digitalis drugs, lithium, drugs or supplements containing potassium, or any over-the-counter drug (especially cold remedies and diet pills).

FOOD INTERACTIONS
Avoid low-salt milk and salt substitutes. Many of these products contain potassium.

DISEASE INTERACTIONS
Consult your doctor if you have systemic lupus erythematosus or if you have had a prior allergic reaction to ACE inhibitors. This medication should be used with caution by patients with severe kidney disease or renal artery stenosis (narrowing of one or both of the arteries that supply blood to the kidneys).

≡ SIDE EFFECTS ≡

SERIOUS
Fever and chills; sore throat and hoarseness; sudden difficulty breathing or swallowing; swelling of the face, mouth, or extremities; impaired kidney function (ankle swelling, decreased urination); confusion; yellow discoloration of the eyes or skin (indicating liver disorder); intense itching; chest pain or heartbeat irregularities; abdominal pain. Serious side effects are very rare; contact your doctor immediately.

COMMON
Dry, persistent cough.

LESS COMMON
Dizziness or fainting; skin rash; numbness or tingling in the hands, feet, or lips; change in color of the hands from white to blue to red (Raynaud's phenomenon) in cold weather; unusual fatigue or muscle weakness; loss of taste; nausea; drowsiness; headache; unusual dreams.

LORATADINE/PSEUDOEPHEDRINE

Available in: Extended-release tablets
Available OTC? No **As Generic?** No
Drug Class: Antihistamine/decongestant

▼ USAGE INFORMATION

WHY IT'S PRESCRIBED
To relieve the symptoms of seasonal allergic rhinitis (hay fever), which include runny nose, nasal congestion, and sneezing.

HOW IT WORKS
Loratadine blocks the effects of histamine, a naturally occurring substance that causes swelling, itching, sneezing, nasal discharge and congestion, and other symptoms of an allergic reaction. Pseudoephedrine narrows and constricts blood vessels to reduce blood flow to swollen nasal passages, which reduces nasal secretions, shrinks swollen nasal mucous membranes, and improves airflow through the nasal passages.

▼ DOSAGE GUIDELINES

RANGE AND FREQUENCY
The 12-hour formulation may be taken twice a day (every 12 hours). The 24-hour formulation should only be taken once a day. Tablets should be taken with a full glass of water.

ONSET OF EFFECT
Within 1 to 3 hours.

DURATION OF ACTION
12 to 24 hours or more.

DIETARY ADVICE
This drug can be taken without regard to meals. Take it with a full glass of water.

STORAGE
Store in a tightly sealed container away from moisture, heat, and direct light.

MISSED DOSE
Not applicable. This drug is taken as needed.

STOPPING THE DRUG
Not applicable. This drug is taken as needed.

PROLONGED USE
This drug is prescribed for short-term (seasonal) use only.

▼ PRECAUTIONS

Over 60: Adequate studies have not been done. However, older patients are more susceptible to the effects of the pseudoephedrine component.

Driving and Hazardous Work: The use of this drug should not impair your ability to perform such tasks safely. However, exercise caution if the drug makes you drowsy.

Alcohol: No special warnings.

Pregnancy: Adequate human studies have not been done. Discuss with your doctor the relative risks and benefits of using this drug while pregnant.

Breast Feeding: Both drugs pass into breast milk. Discuss with your doctor the relative risks and benefits of using this drug while nursing.

Infants and Children: Not recommended for use by children under age 12 years.

Special Concerns: Do not break or chew the tablet. Patients with a history of esophageal narrowing or difficulty swallowing should not take this drug.

OVERDOSE
Symptoms: Drowsiness, heartbeat irregularities, headache, giddiness, nausea, vomiting, sweating, increased thirst, chest pain, urination difficulties, muscle weakness and tenseness, anxiety, restlessness, insomnia, hallucinations, delusions, seizures, difficulty breathing.

What to Do: Call your doctor, emergency medical services (EMS), or the nearest poison control center immediately.

▼ INTERACTIONS

DRUG INTERACTIONS
This drug and MAO (monoamine oxidase) inhibitors should not be used within 14 days of each other. Consult your doctor for specific advice if you are taking beta-blockers, digitalis drugs, or over-the-counter antihistamines or decongestants.

FOOD INTERACTIONS
No known food interactions.

DISEASE INTERACTIONS
You should not take this drug if you have narrow-angle glaucoma, urinary retention, severe hypertension, or severe coronary artery disease. Caution is advised when taking this drug if you have any of the following: high blood pressure, heart disease, diabetes mellitus, increased eye pressure, hyperthyroidism, or enlarged prostate. Use of this drug may cause complications in patients with liver or kidney disease, because these organs work together to remove the medication from the body.

≡ SIDE EFFECTS ≡

SERIOUS
No serious side effects are associated with the use of loratadine/pseudoephedrine.

COMMON
Insomnia, dry mouth, drowsiness.

LESS COMMON
Nervousness, dizziness, indigestion.

LORAZEPAM

BRAND NAME

Ativan

Available in: Oral solution, tablets, injection
Available OTC? No   **As Generic?** Yes
Drug Class: Benzodiazepine tranquilizer; antianxiety agent

▼ USAGE INFORMATION

WHY IT'S PRESCRIBED
To treat anxiety and insomnia. Administered in a hospital setting, the injection form of lorazepam is used to treat a type of seizure disorder (status epilepticus) and is given as a sedative before surgery prior to the administration of anesthesia.

HOW IT WORKS
Lorazepam produces mild sedation by depressing activity in the central nervous system. In particular, the drug appears to enhance the effect of gamma-aminobutyric acid (GABA), a natural chemical that inhibits the firing of neurons and dampens the transmission of nerve signals, decreasing nervous excitation.

▼ DOSAGE GUIDELINES

RANGE AND FREQUENCY
For anxiety—Adults and teenagers: 1 to 2 mg every 8 or 12 hours, up to 6 mg a day. Older adults: 0.5 mg 2 times a day to start; the dose may be increased. For insomnia—Adults and teenagers: 1 to 2 mg taken at bedtime. Note: In all cases, use and dosage for children under 12 years of age must be determined by your doctor.

ONSET OF EFFECT
30 minutes to 2 hours for oral forms.

DURATION OF ACTION
12 to 24 hours.

DIETARY ADVICE
Can be taken with food to prevent gastrointestinal upset.

STORAGE
Store in a tightly sealed container away from moisture, heat, and direct light.

MISSED DOSE
Take it as soon as you remember. However, if it is near the time for the next dose, skip the missed dose and resume your regular dosage schedule. Do not double the next dose. For insomnia, do not take it unless your schedule allows a full night's sleep.

STOPPING THE DRUG
Never stop taking the drug abruptly; this can cause withdrawal symptoms. Dosage should be reduced gradually as directed by your doctor.

PROLONGED USE
Lorazepam may slowly lose its effectiveness with prolonged use. See your doctor for periodic evaluation if you must take this drug for an extended length of time.

▼ PRECAUTIONS

Over 60: Adverse reactions may be more likely and more severe in older patients. A lower dose may be necessary.

Driving and Hazardous Work: Lorazepam can impair mental alertness and physical coordination. Adjust your activities accordingly.

Alcohol: Avoid drinking alcoholic beverages.

Pregnancy: Use of lorazepam during pregnancy should be avoided if possible. Tell your doctor if you are pregnant or plan to become pregnant.

Breast Feeding: Lorazepam passes into breast milk; do not take this medication while you are nursing.

Infants and Children: Lorazepam should be used by children only under close medical supervision.

Special Concerns: Lorazepam use can lead to psychological or physical dependence. Short-term therapy (8 weeks or less) is typical; do not take the drug for a longer period unless so advised by your doctor. Never take more than the prescribed daily dose.

OVERDOSE
Symptoms: Extreme drowsiness, confusion, slurred speech, slow reflexes, poor coordination, staggering gait, tremor, slowed breathing, loss of consciousness.

What to Do: Call your doctor, emergency medical services (EMS), or the nearest poison control center immediately.

▼ INTERACTIONS

DRUG INTERACTIONS
Consult your doctor for specific advice if you are taking any drugs that depress the central nervous system, such as antihistamines, antidepressants or other psychiatric medications, barbiturates, sedatives, cough medicines, decongestants, and painkillers. Be sure your doctor knows about any over-the-counter drug you may take.

FOOD INTERACTIONS
None reported.

DISEASE INTERACTIONS
Consult your doctor if you have a history of alcohol or drug abuse, stroke or other brain disease, any chronic lung disease, hyperactivity, depression or other mental illness, myasthenia gravis, sleep apnea, epilepsy, porphyria, kidney disease, or liver disease.

⬇ SIDE EFFECTS ⬇

SERIOUS
Difficulty concentrating, outbursts of anger, other behavior problems, depression, hallucinations, low blood pressure (causing faintness or confusion), memory impairment, muscle weakness, skin rash or itching, sore throat, fever and chills, sores or ulcers in throat or mouth, unusual bruising or bleeding, extreme fatigue, yellowish tinge to eyes or skin. Call your doctor immediately.

COMMON
Drowsiness, loss of coordination, unsteady gait, dizziness, lightheadedness, slurred speech.

LESS COMMON
Change in sexual desire or ability, constipation, false sense of well-being (euphoria), nausea and vomiting, urinary problems, unusual fatigue.

LOSARTAN POTASSIUM

Available in: Tablets
Available OTC? No   **As Generic?** No
Drug Class: Antihypertensive/angiotensin II antagonist

▼ USAGE INFORMATION

WHY IT'S PRESCRIBED
To control high blood pressure (hypertension). This drug appears to have the same benefits as the class of antihypertensive drugs known as ACE (angiotensin-converting enzyme) inhibitors but without producing the common side effect (experienced by as many as 30% of patients) of a dry cough. Losartan may be used alone or in conjunction with other antihypertensive medications.

HOW IT WORKS
Losartan blocks the effects of angiotensin II, a naturally occurring substance that causes blood vessels to narrow. This medication causes the blood vessels to dilate, thereby lowering blood pressure and decreasing the workload of the heart.

▼ DOSAGE GUIDELINES

RANGE AND FREQUENCY
Adults: To start, 25 to 50 mg once a day. The usual maintenance dose is 25 to 100 mg taken once a day or divided into 2 doses. Chil-dren: Losartan is not recommended for children.

ONSET OF EFFECT
Within 1 hour.

DURATION OF ACTION
24 hours.

DIETARY ADVICE
Follow a healthy diet (low-salt, low-fat, low-cholesterol) as advised by your doctor to help control blood pressure and prevent heart disease.

STORAGE
Store losartan in a tightly sealed container away from moisture, heat, and direct light.

MISSED DOSE
Take it as soon as you remember. If it is near the time for the next dose, skip the missed dose and resume your regular dosage schedule. Do not double the next dose.

STOPPING THE DRUG
Take it as prescribed for the full treatment period. The decision to stop taking the drug should be made in consultation with your physician.

PROLONGED USE
Lifelong therapy may be necessary. However, if you do change certain health habits (for example, increasing exercise or losing weight), it may be possible to reduce the dose under your doctor's supervision.

▼ PRECAUTIONS

Over 60: Adverse reactions may be more likely and more severe in older patients.

Driving and Hazardous Work: Do not drive or engage in hazardous work until you determine how the medicine affects you.

Alcohol: Drink only in careful moderation. (See Special Concerns.)

Pregnancy: In certain ways, losartan is similar to a class of drugs that have caused damage to the unborn child when taken in the second or third trimester of pregnancy. Because safer, more effective medications can lower blood pressure during pregnancy and because adequate studies on the use of losartan during pregnancy have not been done, women who are pregnant or who are planning to become pregnant should not take this drug.

Breast Feeding: Losartan passes into breast milk; avoid use while nursing.

Infants and Children: The safety and effectiveness of this drug have not been established for children.

Special Concerns: Losartan may cause dizziness or light-headedness, which is most noticeable when you change position. This may lead to fainting, falls, and injury. Sit or lie down immediately if you feel dizzy or lightheaded. This side effect may be worsened by alcohol, hot weather, dehydration, fever, prolonged standing or sitting, or exercise.

OVERDOSE
Symptoms: Fainting, dizziness, weak pulse that might be very slow or very fast, nausea and vomiting, chest pain.

What to Do: Call your doctor, emergency medical services (EMS), or the nearest poison control center immediately.

▼ INTERACTIONS

DRUG INTERACTIONS
Consult your doctor for specific advice if you are taking diuretics; medicines or supplements containing potassium; salt substitutes; low-salt milk; NSAIDs; allopurinol; over-the-counter medications for colds, coughs, hay fever, asthma, sinus problems, or appetite control; or other prescription medications.

FOOD INTERACTIONS
No known food interactions.

DISEASE INTERACTIONS
Use of losartan may cause complications in patients with liver or kidney disease, because these organs work together to remove the medication from the body.

 SIDE EFFECTS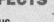

SERIOUS
Sudden difficulty breathing or swallowing; hoarseness; swelling of the face; mouth, hands, or throat; dizziness; cough; fever; and sore throat. Call your doctor immediately.

COMMON
Headache.

LESS COMMON
Back pain, fatigue, diarrhea, nasal congestion.

LOVASTATIN

BRAND NAME

Mevacor

Available in: Tablets
Available OTC? No   **As Generic?** Yes
Drug Class: Antilipidemic (cholesterol-lowering agent)

▼ USAGE INFORMATION

WHY IT'S PRESCRIBED
To treat high cholesterol. Usually prescribed after first lines of treatment—diet, weight loss, and exercise—fail to reduce total and low-density lipoprotein (LDL) cholesterol to acceptable levels. Lovastatin has also been approved for the primary prevention of coronary artery disease (CAD) in persons with no symptoms of CAD but who have average to modestly elevated levels of total and LDL cholesterol and below average high-density (HDL) cholesterol.

HOW IT WORKS
Lovastatin blocks the action of an enzyme required for the manufacture of cholesterol, thereby interfering with its formation. By lowering the amount of cholesterol in the liver cells, lovastatin increases the formation of receptors for LDL and thus reduces blood levels of total and LDL cholesterol. In addition to lowering LDL cholesterol levels, lovastatin modestly reduces triglyceride levels and raises HDL (the so-called "good") cholesterol.

▼ DOSAGE GUIDELINES

RANGE AND FREQUENCY
20 to 80 mg a day taken with meals. The 20-mg dose is taken with the evening meal; doses greater than 20 mg a day are taken in the morning and evening.

ONSET OF EFFECT
2 to 4 weeks.

DURATION OF ACTION
The effect persists for the duration of therapy.

DIETARY ADVICE
Cholesterol-lowering drugs are only one part of a total program that should include regular exercise and a healthy diet. The American Heart Association publishes a "Healthy Heart" diet, which is widely recommended.

STORAGE
Store lovastatin in a tightly sealed container away from moisture, heat, and direct light.

MISSED DOSE
Take your missed dose as soon as you remember. Take your next scheduled dose at the proper time and resume your regular dosage schedule. Do not take a double dose.

STOPPING THE DRUG
The decision to stop taking the drug should be made in consultation with your doctor. Once the medication is discontinued, blood cholesterol is likely to return to original elevated levels.

PROLONGED USE
Side effects are more likely with prolonged use. As you continue with lovastatin, your doctor will periodically order blood tests to evaluate liver function.

▼ PRECAUTIONS

Over 60: No special problems are expected in older patients.

Driving and Hazardous Work: The use of lovastatin should not impair your ability to perform such tasks safely.

Alcohol: No special precautions are necessary.

Pregnancy: Lovastatin should not be used during pregnancy or by women who are trying to become pregnant.

Breast Feeding: This drug is not recommended for women who are nursing.

Infants and Children: The drug can be effective, but safety is not known; it is rarely used in children. Consult your pediatrician.

Special Concerns: Important elements of treatment for high cholesterol include proper diet, weight loss, regular moderate exercise, and the avoidance of certain medications that may increase cholesterol levels. Because lovastatin has potential side effects, it is important that you maintain a recommended healthy diet and cooperate with other treatments your physician may suggest.

OVERDOSE
Symptoms: An overdose of lovastatin is unlikely.

What to Do: Emergency instructions not applicable.

▼ INTERACTIONS

DRUG INTERACTIONS
Consult your doctor if you are taking cyclosporine; gemfibrozil; niacin; antibiotics, especially erythromycin; or medications for fungal infections. All of these drugs may increase the risk of myositis (muscle inflammation) when taken with lovastatin and may lead to kidney failure.

FOOD INTERACTIONS
None reported.

DISEASE INTERACTIONS
Consult your doctor if you have any of the following problems: liver, kidney, or muscle disease or a medical history involving organ transplantation or recent surgery.

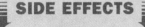

≣ SIDE EFFECTS ≣

SERIOUS
Fever, unusual or unexplained muscle aches and tenderness. Call your doctor right away.

COMMON
Side effects occur in only 1% to 2% of patients. These include constipation or diarrhea, dizziness or lightheadedness, bloating or gas, heartburn, nausea, skin rash, stomach pain, rise in liver enzymes.

LESS COMMON
Sleeping difficulty.

MEDROXYPROGESTERONE ACETATE

Available in: Tablets, injection
Available OTC? No **As Generic?** Yes
Drug Class: Progestin (hormone)

BRAND NAMES

Amen, Curretab, Cycrin, Depo-Provera, Provera

▼ USAGE INFORMATION

WHY IT'S PRESCRIBED
To treat amenorrhea (cessation of menstrual periods) and abnormal uterine bleeding. This drug also may be used as a contraceptive.

HOW IT WORKS
Medroxyprogesterone inhibits the secretion of pituitary hormones that regulate menstrual and reproductive cycles. The drug also alters activity of uterine cells, resulting in, among other changes, a thickening of the cervical mucus. Such changes make it less likely that a partner's sperm will reach and fertilize an egg.

▼ DOSAGE GUIDELINES

RANGE AND FREQUENCY
For amenorrhea—Tablets: 5 to 10 mg a day for 5 to 10 days. For abnormal uterine bleeding—Tablets: 5 to 10 mg a day for 5 to 10 days beginning on the 16th or 21st day of the menstrual cycle. For contraception: 1 depo (Depo-Provera) injection (150 mg) every 3 months. For use in treating menopause—Tablets: 10 mg a day for 10 to 14 days, together with estrogen in each 25-day cycle.

ONSET OF EFFECT
Varies with mode of delivery. Protection against pregnancy can begin immediately if injection is given within 5 days of the menstrual period.

DURATION OF ACTION
Tablets: 24 hours or more. Injection: More than 3 months.

DIETARY ADVICE
Take it with meals to prevent gastrointestinal upset.

STORAGE
Store it in a tightly sealed container away from heat and direct light.

MISSED DOSE
Take a missed dose of the tablet as soon as you remember. If it is near the time for the next dose, skip the missed dose and resume your regular dosage schedule. Do not double the next dose.

STOPPING THE DRUG
The decision to stop taking the drug should be made by your doctor.

PROLONGED USE
Consult your doctor about the need for periodic examinations and laboratory tests if you use this drug for an extended period.

▼ PRECAUTIONS

Over 60: No special problems are expected in older patients.

Driving and Hazardous Work: Do not drive or engage in hazardous work until you determine how the medicine affects you.

Alcohol: No special problems are expected.

Pregnancy: Before you use medroxyprogesterone, tell your doctor if you are pregnant or if you plan to become pregnant. This drug must not be used during pregnancy.

Breast Feeding: Medroxyprogesterone passes into breast milk; avoid or discontinue use while nursing.

Infants and Children: This medication is not recommended for young patients.

Special Concerns: Remember that no contraceptive method is foolproof; 1% of women using the medroxyprogesterone injections have become pregnant.

OVERDOSE
Symptoms: No specific symptoms have been reported.

What to Do: An overdose of medroxyprogesterone is unlikely to be life-threatening. However, if someone takes a much larger dose than prescribed, call your doctor, emergency medical services (EMS), or the nearest poison control center immediately.

▼ INTERACTIONS

DRUG INTERACTIONS
Consult your doctor for specific advice if you are taking aminoglutethimide, carbamazepine, phenytoin, rifabutin, or rifampin.

FOOD INTERACTIONS
No known food interactions.

DISEASE INTERACTIONS
Do not take medroxyprogesterone if you have known or suspected breast malignancies or tumors, acute liver disease or liver tumors, or active thrombophlebitis or thromboembolic disease. Consult your doctor if you have any of the following: asthma, epilepsy, migraine headaches, heart or circulation problems, bleeding problems, a history of thrombophlebitis or thromboembolic disease, diabetes mellitus, high blood cholesterol, kidney disease, risk factors for osteoporosis, or central nervous system disorders such as depression.

≡ SIDE EFFECTS ≡

SERIOUS
Abnormal menstrual bleeding; unexpected or increased flow of breast milk; mental depression; skin rash; loss of or change in speech, coordination, or vision; severe and sudden shortness of breath. Call your doctor immediately.

COMMON
Stomach pain; swelling of face, ankles, or feet; mild headache; mood changes; unusual fatigue; weight gain.

LESS COMMON
Acne, breast pain or tenderness, hot flashes, insomnia, loss of sexual desire, loss or gain of scalp hair or body hair, brown spots on skin.

MEFLOQUINE HYDROCHLORIDE

Available in: Tablets
Available OTC? No **As Generic?** No
Drug Class: Antiinfective/antimalarial

▼ USAGE INFORMATION

WHY IT'S PRESCRIBED
To treat mild to moderate acute malaria caused by strains of plasmodia (the parasite that causes malaria) that are susceptible to mefloquine—specifically, *Plasmodium falciparum* and *P. vivax*. Also used to prevent malaria caused by these strains.

HOW IT WORKS
Mefloquine is poisonous to the malarial parasite.

▼ DOSAGE GUIDELINES

RANGE AND FREQUENCY
Adults—To treat: 5 tablets (1,250 mg each) taken as a single dose. Patients with acute *P. vivax* malaria treated with mefloquine are at high risk of relapse. To avoid relapse after the initial treatment, patients should be treated with another antimalarial such as primaquine. To prevent: 250 mg once a week. Begin taking mefloquine 1 week prior to departure and continue taking the drug for 4 weeks on return. Children 6 months of age and older—To treat: 20 to 25 mg per 2.2 lb (1 kg) of body weight. Split the total dose into 2 doses 6 to 8 hours apart in order to reduce the risk and severity of side effects. To prevent: Your pediatrician will determine the appropriate dose.

ONSET OF EFFECT
Unknown.

DURATION OF ACTION
Up to 3 weeks.

DIETARY ADVICE
Do not take mefloquine on an empty stomach. Take with at least 8 oz of water.

STORAGE
Store it in a tightly sealed container away from moisture, heat, and direct light.

MISSED DOSE
If taking 1 or more doses a day, take it as soon as you remember. If it is near the time for the next dose, skip the missed dose and resume your regular dosage schedule. Do not double the next dose. If taking 1 weekly dose, take it as soon as possible, then resume regular schedule.

STOPPING THE DRUG
Take it as prescribed for the full treatment period.

PROLONGED USE
Periodic liver function tests and eye exams are recommended.

▼ PRECAUTIONS

Over 60: Adverse reactions may be more likely and more severe among this age group.

Driving and Hazardous Work: Avoid such activities until you determine how the medicine affects you. Dizziness and coordination difficulties may occur after the drug is discontinued.

Alcohol: No special warnings.

Pregnancy: The use of mefloquine during pregnancy is discouraged because of the risks it poses to the unborn child. Women of childbearing age should practice contraception during preventive therapy.

Breast Feeding: Mefloquine passes into breast milk; extreme caution is advised. Consult your physician for specific advice.

Infants and Children: Safety and effectiveness have not been established for children under the age of 6 months. Early vomiting has been associated with mefloquine use in children and with treatment failure. If a second dose is not tolerated, alternative antimalarial measures should be considered.

Special Concerns: If you take mefloquine once a week, take it on the same day every week. Malaria is spread by mosquitoes. Take appropriate precautions, such as using mosquito netting, to guard against being bitten by malaria-carrying mosquitoes.

OVERDOSE
Symptoms: Side effects may be more pronounced. (See Side Effects.)

What to Do: If you have reason to suspect overdose, call your doctor, emergency medical services (EMS), or the nearest poison control center immediately.

▼ INTERACTIONS

DRUG INTERACTIONS
Consult a doctor for advice if you are taking a beta-blocker, quinidine, quinine, chloroquine, antiarrhythmic drugs, calcium channel blockers, halofantrine, antihistamines, histamine (H1) blockers, tricyclic antidepressants, phenothiazines, or anticonvulsants. Also, tell your physician if you are taking any other prescription or over-the-counter drug.

FOOD INTERACTIONS
No known food interactions.

DISEASE INTERACTIONS
Consult your doctor for specific advice if you have a seizure or psychiatric disorder, impaired liver function, any eye condition, or heart disease.

 ## SIDE EFFECTS

SERIOUS
Slowed heartbeat, seizures. Severe anxiety, depression, restlessness, or confusion during preventive therapy may be signs of more serious psychiatric problems. Call your doctor immediately.

COMMON
Treatment-related: dizziness, muscle pain, nausea, fever, headache, vomiting, chills, diarrhea, skin rash, abdominal pain, fatigue, loss of appetite, ringing in the ears. Prevention-related: vomiting, nausea.

LESS COMMON
Treatment-related: hair loss, emotional problems, itching, fatigue. Prevention-related: dizziness, lightheadedness.

METFORMIN

Available in: Tablets, extended-release tablets
Available OTC? No   **As Generic?** Yes
Drug Class: Antidiabetic agent/biguanide

▼ USAGE INFORMATION

WHY IT'S PRESCRIBED
To lower abnormally high blood glucose (sugar) levels in patients with non-insulin-dependent (type 2) diabetes whose blood sugar levels cannot be adequately controlled by diet or exercise alone. The drug may be used alone or in conjunction with sulfonylurea drugs or insulin.

HOW IT WORKS
Metformin decreases the liver's production of glucose, inhibits the breakdown of fatty acids used to produce glucose, and increases the removal of glucose from muscle, the liver, and other body tissues where it is stored.

▼ DOSAGE GUIDELINES

RANGE AND FREQUENCY
Available in 500-mg, 850-mg, or 1,000-mg tablets; the extended-release tablets are available in 500-mg strength only and should not be used by patients under the age of 17 years. Initial dose: 500 mg a day taken with dinner. If tolerated, a second dose can be added to be taken with breakfast. The dose may be slowly increased (1 tablet every 1 or 2 weeks) to a maximum of 2,500 mg a day. Alternatively, 850 mg can be taken daily, increased by 850 mg every other week to a maximum of 2,550 mg per day.

ONSET OF EFFECT
Within 2 hours.

DURATION OF ACTION
From 12 to 15 hours.

DIETARY ADVICE
Take with meals to reduce risk of stomach upset.

STORAGE
Store it in a sealed container at room temperature away from heat and direct light.

MISSED DOSE
Take it with food as soon as you remember. However, if it is almost time for the next dose, skip the missed dose and resume your regular dosage schedule. Do not double the next dose.

STOPPING THE DRUG
Stop taking metformin only when your doctor advises.

PROLONGED USE
Because metformin helps manage diabetes but does not cure the disease, its use will continue as long as your blood glucose levels are being adequately controlled. If not, the metformin dosage may be adjusted or a different treatment prescribed.

▼ PRECAUTIONS

Over 60: Because metformin is metabolized in the kidneys, extra caution is necessary for thin, elderly patients with mild adrenal insufficiency (not often detected by the usual tests for kidney impairment).

Driving and Hazardous Work: No special precautions are necessary.

Alcohol: Excessive amounts of alcohol can increase the effect of metformin, possibly resulting in abnormally low blood glucose levels.

Pregnancy: Taking metformin during pregnancy is not advised. Consult your doctor if you become pregnant or plan to become pregnant; insulin is usually the treatment of choice for pregnant women who have diabetes.

Breast Feeding: Metformin passes into breast milk, although it has not been shown to cause harm to nursing infants.

Infants and Children: Glucophage may be used in children 10 years of age and older; Glucophage XR may be used in children 17 years of age and older.

OVERDOSE
Symptoms: Symptoms of lactic acidosis or hypoglycemia (see Serious Side Effects).

What to Do: Seek emergency medical assistance immediately.

▼ INTERACTIONS

DRUG INTERACTIONS
Consult your doctor if you are taking any of the following: amiloride, calcium channel blockers, cimetidine, digoxin, furosemide, morphine, procainamide, quinidine, quinine, ranitidine, trimethoprim, triamterene, or vancomycin.

FOOD INTERACTIONS
The amount and type of food you eat affect your blood glucose levels and must be taken into account while you receive metformin therapy.

DISEASE INTERACTIONS
Do not take metformin if you have a condition requiring careful control of blood glucose levels, such as severe infection; any condition contributing to abnormally low blood oxygen levels, such as congestive heart failure; metabolic acidosis (buildup of acid in the blood); a history of alcohol abuse; or kidney or liver disease.

≡ SIDE EFFECTS ≡

SERIOUS
In rare cases, metformin may lead to lactic acidosis, an abnormal and potentially life-threatening buildup of lactic acid in the blood. Symptoms include rapid, shallow breathing, unusual sleepiness or weakness, muscle pain, and abdominal distress. Metformin also occasionally causes abnormally low blood glucose levels (hypoglycemia); symptoms include blurred vision, cold sweats, confusion, anxiousness, rapid heartbeat, shakiness, and nausea. Seek medical assistance immediately.

COMMON
Diarrhea, nausea, vomiting, abdominal bloating, gas, diminished appetite. Usually, such symptoms are mild and transient. Consult your doctor if the symptoms persist or increase in severity.

LESS COMMON
Unpleasant or metallic taste in mouth.

METHOTREXATE

BRAND NAMES

Folex, Folex PFS, Mexate, Mexate-AQ, Rheumatrex

Available in: Tablets, injection
Available OTC? No   **As Generic?** Yes
Drug Class: Antineoplastic agent/antimetabolite; antipsoriatic; antirheumatic

▼ USAGE INFORMATION

WHY IT'S PRESCRIBED
To treat certain kinds of cancer, psoriasis, and rheumatoid arthritis.

HOW IT WORKS
Methotrexate interferes with the activity of an enzyme needed for the maintenance and replication of cells, especially those that divide and proliferate rapidly. Such cells include many types of cancer cells, as well as those that compose the bone marrow and the cells that line the mouth, intestine, and bladder. Consequently, in addition to its cancer-fighting effects, methotrexate may harm healthy tissues in the body, causing unpleasant or serious side effects. It is unknown how methotrexate works to ease rheumatoid arthritis, but this medication appears to modify the function of the immune system, whose activity is believed to play an important role in the progression of the disease.

▼ DOSAGE GUIDELINES

RANGE AND FREQUENCY
For psoriasis or rheumatoid arthritis—Tablets: 2.5 to 5 mg every 12 hours for 3 doses in 1 week or 7.5 to 10 mg once a week. Injection: 10 mg once a week. For cancer—Use and dose depend on type and stage of disease. Your doctor may alter dosage as needed. Consult your pediatrician for children's dose.

ONSET OF EFFECT
Unknown.

DURATION OF ACTION
Unknown.

DIETARY ADVICE
This drug is best taken 1 to 2 hours before meals.

STORAGE
Store in a tightly sealed container away from moisture, heat, and direct light.

MISSED DOSE
If you miss a dose, do not take the missed dose and do not double the next dose. Resume your regular schedule and check with your doctor.

STOPPING THE DRUG
The decision to stop taking the drug should be made by your doctor.

PROLONGED USE
See your doctor regularly for tests and examinations.

▼ PRECAUTIONS

Over 60: Adverse reactions may be more likely and more severe in older patients.

Driving and Hazardous Work: Avoid such activities until you determine how the medicine affects you.

Alcohol: Avoid alcohol.

Pregnancy: Methotrexate can cause birth defects and other problems; avoid use during pregnancy.

Breast Feeding: Methotrexate passes into breast milk and may cause serious side effects in the nursing infant; do not use it while breast feeding.

Infants and Children: Infants are more sensitive to the effects of methotrexate. No special problems are expected in older children.

Special Concerns: Methotrexate may lower your resistance to infection by reducing the number of white blood cells in the blood. Do not have any immunizations without your doctor's approval. Avoid contct with people with infections. Use care when shaving, trimming nails, or using sharp objects. Inform your doctor immediately if you have fever, chills, unusual bleeding or bruising, diarrhea, or a cough. Methotrexate may increase skin sensitivity to sunlight. Limit sun exposure until you see how the medicine affects you. After you stop taking methotrexate, you may experience back pain, blurred vision, confusion, seizures, dizziness, fever, or unusual fatigue; consult your doctor immediately.

OVERDOSE
Symptoms: Severe damage to the liver, kidneys, stomach, intestines, bone marrow, and lungs, causing a wide array of symptoms.

What to Do: If you suspect an overdose, seek medical assistance immediately.

▼ INTERACTIONS

DRUG INTERACTIONS
A number of drugs may interact with methotrexate. Ask your doctor for specific advice if you are taking any drugs that may affect the liver, such as azathioprine, retinoids, and sulfasalazine or any other prescription or over-the-counter medication.

FOOD INTERACTIONS
No known food interactions.

DISEASE INTERACTIONS
Consult your doctor if you have any of the following: a history of alcohol abuse, chicken pox, shingles, colitis, any disease of the immune system, kidney stones, any infection, intestinal blockage, kidney disease, liver disease, mouth sores or inflammation, or stomach ulcers.

 SIDE EFFECTS

SERIOUS
Black, tarry stools; bloody vomit; diarrhea; flushing or redness of skin; sores in mouth and on lips; stomach pain; blood in urine or stools; confusion; seizures; cough or hoarseness; fever or chills; pain in lower back or side; painful or difficult urination; red spots on skin; shortness of breath; swollen feet or lower legs; unusual bleeding or bruising; back pain; dark urine; drowsiness; dizziness; headache; joint pain; unusual fatigue; yellow-tinged eyes or skin. Call your doctor immediately.

COMMON
Loss of appetite, nausea and vomiting, minor mouth ulcers.

LESS COMMON
Acne, boils, pale skin, skin rash, or itching.

METHYLPHENIDATE HYDROCHLORIDE

Available in: Tablets, extended-release tablets
Available OTC? No   **As Generic?** Yes
Drug Class: Central nervous system stimulant

▼ USAGE INFORMATION

WHY IT'S PRESCRIBED
To treat attention-deficit hyperactivity disorder (ADHD). It is also used to treat narcolepsy.

HOW IT WORKS
Methylphenidate is thought to stimulate the release of norepinephrine, a natural hormone that promotes the transmission of nerve impulses in the brain. It works by decreasing restlessness and increasing attention in adults and children who cannot concentrate for very long, are easily distracted, or are unusually impulsive.

▼ DOSAGE GUIDELINES

RANGE AND FREQUENCY
For ADHD—Tablets: Adults and teenagers: 5 to 20 mg 2 to 3 times a day taken with or after meals. Children ages 6 to 12 years: To start, 5 mg 2 times a day. If needed, your doctor may increase the dose by 5 to 10 mg a week. Extended-release tablets: Adults, teenagers, and children ages 6 to 12 years: 20 mg 1 to 3 times a day every 8 hours. For narcolepsy—Tablets: Adults and teenagers: 5 to 20 mg 3 or 4 times a day taken with or after meals. Extended-release tablets: Adults and teenagers: 20 mg, 2 to 3 times a day.

ONSET OF EFFECT
Tablets: Usually within 30 minutes. Extended-release tablets: Usually between 30 and 60 minutes.

DURATION OF ACTION
Tablets: 4 to 6 hours. Extended-release tablets: 6 hours or longer.

DIETARY ADVICE
For attention-deficit hyperactivity disorder, this medicine should be taken with or after meals. For narcolepsy, it should be taken 30 to 45 minutes before meals.

STORAGE
Store methylphenidate in a tightly sealed container away from moisture, heat, and direct light.

MISSED DOSE
Take it as soon as you remember. If it is near the time for the next dose, skip the missed dose and resume your regular dosage schedule. Do not double the next dose.

STOPPING THE DRUG
The decision to stop taking the drug should be made by your doctor.

PROLONGED USE
See your doctor regularly for tests and examinations.

▼ PRECAUTIONS

Over 60: No special problems are expected.

Driving and Hazardous Work: Do not drive or engage in hazardous work until you determine how the medicine affects you.

Alcohol: Avoid alcohol.

Pregnancy: Adequate human studies have not been completed. Before taking methylphenidate, tell your doctor if you are pregnant or plan to become pregnant.

Breast Feeding: It is not known whether methylphenidate passes into breast milk; caution is advised. Consult your doctor for advice.

Infants and Children: This drug is not recommended for use by children under the age of 6 years. Older children may be especially likely to experience side effects such as loss of appetite, stomach pain, and weight loss.

Special Concerns: To prevent insomnia, do not take methylphenidate too close to bedtime. Your prescription cannot be refilled, so you must get a new one from your doctor to obtain more medication.

OVERDOSE
Symptoms: Agitation; confusion; delirium; seizures; dry mouth; false sense of wellbeing (euphoria); rapid, pounding, or irregular heartbeat; fever; sweating; severe headache; increased blood pressure; muscle twitching; trembling or tremors; vomiting.

What to Do: Call your doctor, emergency medical services (EMS), or the nearest poison control center immediately.

▼ INTERACTIONS

DRUG INTERACTIONS
Call your doctor for specific advice if you are taking caffeine; amantadine; appetite suppressants; tricyclic antidepressants; chlophedianol; pemoline; asthma medicine; amphetamines; medicine for colds, sinus problems, or allergies; nabilone; pimozide; or MAO (monoamine oxidase) inhibitors.

FOOD INTERACTIONS
Do not drink large amounts of caffeinated beverages, such as coffee, tea, soft drinks, cocoa, or chocolate milk.

DISEASE INTERACTIONS
Consult your doctor if you have Tourette's syndrome or other tics, glaucoma, epilepsy or another seizure disorder, high blood pressure, psychosis, severe anxiety, depression, or a history of alcohol or drug abuse.

SIDE EFFECTS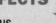

SERIOUS
Fast heartbeat, unusual bleeding or bruising, chest pain, fever, joint pain, increased heartbeat, skin rash or hives, uncontrolled body movements, blurred vision or other vision changes, seizures, sore throat and fever, unusual fatigue, weight loss, mood or mental changes. Call your doctor immediately.

COMMON
Loss of appetite, insomnia, nervousness.

LESS COMMON
Dizziness, stomach pain, drowsiness, nausea, headache.

METHYLPREDNISOLONE

Available in: Tablets, injection, enema
Available OTC? No **As Generic?** Yes
Drug Class: Corticosteroid

▼ USAGE INFORMATION

WHY IT'S PRESCRIBED
To treat numerous conditions that involve inflammation (a response by body tissues, producing redness, warmth, swelling, and pain). Such conditions include arthritis, allergic reactions, asthma, some skin diseases, multiple sclerosis flare-ups, and other autoimmune diseases. Also prescribed to treat deficiency of natural steroid hormones.

HOW IT WORKS
This hormone mimics the effects of the body's natural corticosteroids. It depresses the synthesis, release, and activity of inflammation-producing body chemicals. It also suppresses the activity of the immune system.

▼ DOSAGE GUIDELINES

RANGE AND FREQUENCY
Tablets: 4 to 160 mg a day, depending on condition, in 1 or more doses. Injection: 10 to 160 mg a day injected into a muscle or vein or 4 to 120 mg as needed injected into a muscle, joint, or lesion. Enema: 40 mg 3 to 7 times a week. Consult your pediatrician for children's dose.

ONSET OF EFFECT
Varies widely depending on form used.

DURATION OF ACTION
30 to 36 hours with tablets, 1 to 4 weeks after muscle injection, 1 to 5 weeks after other injections.

DIETARY ADVICE
Take it with food or milk to minimize stomach upset. Your doctor may recommend a low-salt, high-potassium, high-protein diet.

STORAGE
Store this medication in a tightly sealed container away from moisture, heat, and direct light. Do not freeze the liquid form.

MISSED DOSE
If you take several doses a day and it is close to the next dose, double the next dose. If you take 1 dose a day and you do not remember until the next day, skip the missed dose and do not double the next dose.

STOPPING THE DRUG
With long-term therapy, do not stop taking the drug abruptly; the dosage should be decreased gradually.

PROLONGED USE
Long-term use may lead to cataracts, diabetes, hypertension, or osteoporosis; see your doctor regularly.

▼ PRECAUTIONS

Over 60: Adverse reactions may be more likely and more severe in older patients.

Driving and Hazardous Work: Avoid such activities until you determine how the medicine affects you.

Alcohol: Alcohol may cause stomach problems; avoid it unless your physician approves occasional moderate drinking.

Pregnancy: Overuse during pregnancy can impair growth and development of the child.

Breast Feeding: Do not use this drug while nursing.

Infants and Children: Methylprednisolone may retard the development of bone and other tissues.

Special Concerns: This drug can lower your resistance to infection. Avoid immunizations with live vaccines. Patients undergoing long-term therapy should wear a medical-alert bracelet. Call a doctor if you develop a fever.

OVERDOSE
Symptoms: Fever, muscle or joint pain, nausea, dizziness, fainting, difficulty breathing. Prolonged overuse: Moon face, obesity, unusual hair growth, acne, loss of sexual function, muscle wasting.

What to Do: Seek medical assistance immediately.

▼ INTERACTIONS

DRUG INTERACTIONS
Consult your doctor for specific advice if you are taking aminoglutethimide, antacids, barbiturates, carbamazepine, griseofulvin, mitotane, phenylbutazone, phenytoin, primidone, rifampin, injectable amphotericin B, oral antidiabetes agents, insulin, digitalis drugs, diuretics, or medications containing potassium or sodium.

FOOD INTERACTIONS
Avoid excess sodium.

DISEASE INTERACTIONS
Consult your doctor if you have a history of bone disease, chicken pox, measles, gastrointestinal disorders, diabetes, recent serious infection, glaucoma, heart disease, hypertension, liver or kidney disorders, high blood cholesterol, thyroid problems, myasthenia gravis, or lupus.

≡ SIDE EFFECTS ≡

SERIOUS
Vision problems, frequent urination, increased thirst, rectal bleeding, blistering skin, confusion, hallucinations, paranoia, euphoria, depression, mood swings, redness and swelling at injection site. Call your doctor immediately.

COMMON
Increased appetite, indigestion, nervousness, insomnia, greater susceptibility to infections, increased blood pressure, slowed wound healing, weight gain, easy bruising, fluid retention.

LESS COMMON
Change in skin color, dizziness, headache, increased sweating, unusual growth of body or facial hair, increased blood sugar, peptic ulcers, adrenal insufficiency, muscle weakness, cataracts, glaucoma, osteoporosis.

METOPROLOL

Available in: Tablets, extended-release tablets (Injection is for hospital use only.)
Available OTC? No   **As Generic?** Yes
Drug Class: Beta-blocker

▼ USAGE INFORMATION

WHY IT'S PRESCRIBED
To treat mild to moderate high blood pressure or angina, to prevent or control heartbeat irregularities (cardiac arrhythmias), and to treat congestive heart failure. The injection is used in hospitals for emergency treatment of heart attack and is followed by maintenance with oral forms.

HOW IT WORKS
Metoprolol slows the rate and force of contraction of the heart by blocking certain nerve impulses, thus reducing blood pressure. By modifying nerve impulses to the heart, the drug also helps stabilize heart rhythm.

▼ DOSAGE GUIDELINES

RANGE AND FREQUENCY
For high blood pressure or angina—Adults: 100 to 400 mg a day in divided doses. Extended-release tablets: Up to 400 mg once a day. For treatment after a heart attack—Initial dose is 50 mg every 6 hours followed by a maintenance dose of 100 mg or more (up to 400 mg a day) 2 times a day for as long as the physician recommends. For congestive heart failure (Toprol-XL)—The exact dose will be determined by your doctor. Average dose is 25 mg once a day for 2 weeks in people with stable heart failure (NYHA class II) and 12.5 mg once a day in those with more severe heart failure. The dose may gradually be doubled every 2 weeks, up to 200 mg a day.

ONSET OF EFFECT
Within 15 minutes.

DURATION OF ACTION
6 to 12 hours; up to 24 hours with the extended-release tablet.

DIETARY ADVICE
Take it with food. Follow a low-salt or low-cholesterol diet to improve control over high blood pressure and heart disease.

STORAGE
Store metoprolol in a tightly sealed container away from heat and direct light.

MISSED DOSE
Take it as soon as you remember. However, if it is within 4 hours of your next dose (8 hours if using extended-release tablet), skip the missed dose and resume your regular dosage schedule. Do not double the next dose.

STOPPING THE DRUG
This drug should not be stopped suddenly; this may lead to angina and possibly a heart attack in patients with advanced heart disease. Slow reduction of the dose under doctor's close supervision for 2 to 3 weeks is advised.

PROLONGED USE
Lifelong therapy may be necessary. See your doctor for regular examinations.

▼ PRECAUTIONS

Over 60: Adverse reactions may be more likely and more severe in older patients.

Driving and Hazardous Work: Use caution until you determine how the medicine affects you.

Alcohol: Drink alcoholic beverages in careful moderation if at all. Alcohol may interact with the medication and cause a dangerous drop in blood pressure.

Pregnancy: Discuss with your doctor the relative risks and benefits of using this medication if you are pregnant.

Breast Feeding: Adverse effects in infants have not been documented.

Infants and Children: No special problems are expected.

OVERDOSE
Symptoms: Unusually slow or rapid heartbeat, severe dizziness or fainting, poor circulation in the hands (bluish skin), breathing difficulty, seizures.

What to Do: Call your doctor, emergency medical services (EMS), or the nearest poison control center immediately.

▼ INTERACTIONS

DRUG INTERACTIONS
Consult your doctor if you are taking amphetamines, oral antidiabetic agents, asthma medication, calcium channel blockers, clonidine, guanabenz, halothane, immunotherapy for allergies, insulin, MAO (monoamine oxidase) inhibitors, reserpine, other beta-blockers, or any over-the-counter medicine.

FOOD INTERACTIONS
None reported.

DISEASE INTERACTIONS
Metoprolol should be used with caution in people with diabetes, especially type 1, because the drug may mask symptoms of hypoglycemia. Consult your doctor if you have allergies or asthma, heart or blood vessel disease, hyperthyroidism, irregular (slow) heartbeat, myasthenia gravis, psoriasis, respiratory problems such as bronchitis or emphysema, kidney or liver disease, or a history of mental depression.

 SIDE EFFECTS

SERIOUS
Shortness of breath or wheezing; irregular or slow heartbeat (50 beats per minute or less); chest pain or tightness; swelling of the ankles, feet, and lower legs; mental depression. Call your doctor immediately.

COMMON
Dizziness or lightheadedness, especially when rising suddenly to a standing position; decreased sexual ability (erectile dysfunction) in men; unusual fatigue, weakness, or drowsiness; insomnia.

LESS COMMON
Anxiety, irritability, or nervousness; constipation; diarrhea; dry, sore eyes; itching; nausea or vomiting; nightmares or intensely vivid dreams; numbness or tingling.

METRONIDAZOLE

Available in: Cream, injection, topical and vaginal gel, tablets, extended-release tablets
Available OTC? No   **As Generic?** Yes
Drug Class: Antibacterial/antiprotozoal

▼ USAGE INFORMATION

WHY IT'S PRESCRIBED
To treat numerous bacterial infections, including certain sexually transmitted diseases, gynecological infections, amebiasis (amoeba infection in the intestine or liver), brain abscess or meningitis, pneumonia or other lung infections, blood poisoning, bone and joint infections, infections of the internal organs (including liver abscess and peritonitis), and skin infections.

HOW IT WORKS
Metronidazole kills bacteria and protozoa, probably by disrupting the organism's synthesis of DNA.

▼ DOSAGE GUIDELINES

RANGE AND FREQUENCY
The dose varies greatly depending on many factors, including the disorder being treated; the patient's age, weight, and general state of health; and the form of drug prescribed. Your doctor will determine the appropriate dosage regimen for you.

ONSET OF EFFECT
Unknown.

DURATION OF ACTION
Unknown.

DIETARY ADVICE
Oral forms of metronidazole can be taken with food to minimize stomach upset.

STORAGE
Store metronidazole in a tightly sealed container away from heat, moisture, and direct light. Do not refrigerate the liquid or topical forms.

MISSED DOSE
Take it as soon as you remember. If it is near the time for the next dose, skip the missed dose and resume your regular dosage schedule. Do not double the next dose.

STOPPING THE DRUG
Take it as prescribed for the full treatment period, even if you feel better before the scheduled end of therapy.

PROLONGED USE
If your symptoms do not improve or if they become worse after a few days, consult your doctor.

▼ PRECAUTIONS

Over 60: No special advice.

Driving and Hazardous Work: Avoid such activities until you determine how the medicine affects you.

Alcohol: A serious reaction, including possible flushing, rapid heartbeat, nausea, and vomiting, may occur if alcohol is consumed while taking this drug. Medications containing alcohol (cough syrups, for example) should also be carefully avoided, because they can cause the same reaction.

Pregnancy: Metronidazole has not caused birth defects in animals. Use of the oral forms during the first trimester is not recommended. Before you take metronidazole, tell your doctor if you are pregnant or plan to become pregnant.

Breast Feeding: Metronidazole passes into breast milk; avoid or discontinue use while nursing.

Infants and Children: The oral and injection forms are not expected to cause side effects different from or more severe than those in older persons. There is no information on the use of the topical forms by children.

Special Concerns: If you use the vaginal gel, wear cotton underwear, change it daily, and use a sanitary napkin to prevent leakage. Avoid using this medicine in or near the eyes. If it does get into your eyes, consult your doctor.

OVERDOSE
Symptoms: No cases of overdose have been reported.

What to Do: Emergency instructions not applicable.

▼ INTERACTIONS

DRUG INTERACTIONS
Consult your doctor for specific advice if you are taking cimetidine, lithium, anticoagulants, phenytoin, or phenobarbital. If you have taken disulfiram in the last 2 weeks, you should not take metronidazole. Also tell your doctor if you are taking any other prescription or over-the-counter medication.

FOOD INTERACTIONS
No known food interactions.

DISEASE INTERACTIONS
Consult your doctor if you have a history of blood disease, epilepsy or another central nervous system disorder, heart disease, or liver disease.

▼ SIDE EFFECTS

SERIOUS
Oral and injection forms: Pain, tingling, numbness, or weakness in hands or feet; seizures. Call your doctor immediately.

COMMON
Oral and injection forms: Diarrhea, dizziness, lightheadedness, headache, loss of appetite, nausea, vomiting, stomach pains or cramps. Vaginal gel: Vaginal itching; painful intercourse; thick, white vaginal discharge; irritation of sexual partner's penis; burning urination; more frequent urination; redness, stinging, or itching of genital area.

LESS COMMON
Oral and injection forms: Change in taste, dry mouth, sharp metallic taste in mouth. Cream and gel: Dry skin, skin irritation, watery eyes with burning or stinging. Vaginal gel: Dizziness, lightheadedness, diarrhea, furry tongue, loss of appetite, metallic taste in the mouth, nausea, vomiting.

MIRTAZAPINE

BRAND NAME

Remeron

Available in: Tablets
Available OTC? No   **As Generic?** No
Drug Class: Antidepressant

▼ USAGE INFORMATION

WHY IT'S PRESCRIBED
To treat symptoms of major depression.

HOW IT WORKS
The exact mechanism of action of mirtazapine is not known, but it affects levels of brain chemicals (norepinephrine and serotonin) that are thought to be linked to mood, emotions, and mental state.

▼ DOSAGE GUIDELINES

RANGE AND FREQUENCY
To start, 15 mg once a day at bedtime. The dose may be increased gradually by your doctor to no more than 45 mg a day.

ONSET OF EFFECT
Unknown.

DURATION OF ACTION
Unknown.

DIETARY ADVICE
No special restrictions.

STORAGE
Store it in a tightly sealed container away from heat, moisture, and direct light.

MISSED DOSE
Take it as soon as you remember. However, if it is near the time for the next day's dose, skip the missed dose and resume your regular dosage schedule. Do not double the next day's dose.

STOPPING THE DRUG
Take as prescribed for the full treatment period, even if you begin to feel better before the scheduled end of therapy. The decision to stop taking the drug should be made in consultation with your doctor.

PROLONGED USE
See your doctor regularly for tests and examinations if you take this medicine for a prolonged period. Prolonged use of mirtazapine can decrease the flow of saliva, which can increase the risk of cavities, periodontal disease, and other conditions.

▼ PRECAUTIONS

Over 60: No special problems have been reported.

Driving and Hazardous Work: Exercise caution until you determine how the medicine affects you. Drowsiness or lightheadedness can occur.

Alcohol: Avoid alcohol.

Pregnancy: In animal studies, mirtazapine did not cause birth defects but was shown to cause other problems. Human studies have not been done. Before you take mirtazapine, tell your doctor if you are pregnant or plan to become pregnant.

Breast Feeding: Mirtazapine may pass into breast milk; caution is advised. Consult your doctor for advice.

Infants and Children: The safety and effectiveness of mirtazapine use by infants and children have not been established.

Special Concerns: If dry mouth occurs, use sugar-free candy or gum for relief.

OVERDOSE
Symptoms: Severe drowsiness, disorientation, loss of memory, rapid heartbeat.

What to Do: Call your doctor, emergency medical services (EMS), or the nearest poison control center immediately.

▼ INTERACTIONS

DRUG INTERACTIONS
Mirtazapine and MAO inhibitors should not be used within 14 days of each other. Very serious side effects such as myoclonus (uncontrolled muscle jerking), hyperthermia (excessive rise in body temperature), nausea, vomiting, seizures, and extreme stiffness may result. Other drugs may interact with mirtazapine; consult your doctor for specific advice if you are taking central nervous system depressants, high blood pressure medication, diazepam, or kidney medication.

FOOD INTERACTIONS
No known food interactions.

DISEASE INTERACTIONS
Caution is advised when taking mirtazapine. Consult your doctor if you have heart or blood vessel disease or a history of seizures, drug abuse, or mental illness. Use of mirtazapine may cause complications in patients with liver or kidney disease, because these organs work together to remove the medication from the body.

☰ SIDE EFFECTS ☰

SERIOUS
Mood or mental changes, confusion, breathing difficulties, increased or decreased ability to move limbs, flulike symptoms, swelling of the lower extremities, skin rash, anxiety, agitation, extreme drowsiness, disorientation, loss of memory, rapid heartbeat. Call your doctor immediately.

COMMON
Dizziness, dry mouth, drowsiness, constipation, increased appetite, weight gain.

LESS COMMON
Muscle pains, unusual dreams, fatigue, back pain, vomiting, increased thirst, nausea, dizziness or fainting when getting up suddenly, sensitivity to touch, tremor, stomach pain, increased urination.

MOMETASONE FUROATE NASAL

Available in: Nasal spray
Available OTC? No   **As Generic?** No
Drug Class: Nasal corticosteroid

▼ USAGE INFORMATION

WHY IT'S PRESCRIBED
To prevent and treat the symptoms of allergic rhinitis (seasonal and perennial allergies such as hay fever).

HOW IT WORKS
Respiratory corticosteroids such as mometasone reduce or prevent inflammation of the lining of the airways, reduce the allergic response to inhaled allergens, and inhibit the secretion of mucus within the airways.

▼ DOSAGE GUIDELINES

RANGE AND FREQUENCY
Adults and teenagers: 2 sprays (50 micrograms [µg] in each spray) in each nostril once a day for a maximum daily dose of 200 µg. To prevent the symptoms of allergic rhinitis from developing, it is recommended that patients with known seasonal allergies begin taking mometasone 2 to 4 weeks before the anticipated start of the pollen season.

ONSET OF EFFECT
From 11 hours to 2 days.

DURATION OF ACTION
Mometasone is effective as long as you continue to take the medication.

DIETARY ADVICE
Mometasone can be used without regard to diet.

STORAGE
Store it in a tightly sealed container away from moisture, heat, and direct light.

MISSED DOSE
If you miss a dose on one day, resume your regular dosage schedule the next day. Do not double the next dose.

STOPPING THE DRUG
No special instructions.

PROLONGED USE
Consult your doctor about any need for periodic physical examinations and lab tests.

▼ PRECAUTIONS

Over 60: No special problems are expected.

Driving and Hazardous Work: Mometasone should not impair your ability to perform such tasks safely.

Alcohol: No special precautions are necessary.

Pregnancy: Nasal steroids have not been reported to cause birth defects if taken during pregnancy. Before using this drug, tell your doctor if you are pregnant or plan to become pregnant.

Breast Feeding: Mometasone may pass into breast milk; caution is advised. Consult your doctor for advice.

Infants and Children: Not recommended for use by children under age 12 years.

Special Concerns: Prior to your initial use of the inhaler, you must prime it by depressing the pump 10 times or until a fine mist appears. You may store the inhaler for up to 1 week without repriming. If it is unused for more than 1 week, reprime it by depressing the pump 2 times or until a fine mist appears. Avoid spraying the medication into your eyes.

OVERDOSE
Symptoms: No cases of overdose have been reported.

What to Do: An overdose with mometasone is unlikely. If someone takes a much larger dose than prescribed, call your doctor.

▼ INTERACTIONS

DRUG INTERACTIONS
Consult your doctor for advice if you are taking systemic corticosteroids, other inhaled corticosteroids, or any drugs that suppress the immune system.

FOOD INTERACTIONS
No known food interactions.

DISEASE INTERACTIONS
Consult your doctor if you have any other medical problem, particularly glaucoma, a herpes infection of the eye, a history of tuberculosis, liver disease, an underactive thyroid, or osteoporosis.

≡ SIDE EFFECTS ≡

SERIOUS
No serious side effects are associated with mometasone.

COMMON
Headache, increased susceptibility to viral infection, sore throat, nosebleeds or bloody nasal secretions.

LESS COMMON
Cough, increased susceptibility to upper respiratory infection, menstrual irregularities, bone pain, sinus pain.

MONTELUKAST

Available in: Tablets, chewable tablets
Available OTC? No   **As Generic?** No
Drug Class: Leukotriene receptor antagonist

▼ USAGE INFORMATION

WHY IT'S PRESCRIBED
To prevent and treat the symptoms of chronic asthma by preventing bronchospasm (contraction of the smooth muscle tissue surrounding the airways, which results in narrowing and obstruction of the air passages). Montelukast may be used in conjunction with other asthma treatments.

HOW IT WORKS
Montelukast blocks cell receptors for leukotrienes, naturally formed substances that cause inflammation and constriction of the airways. Unlike bronchodilators, which relieve the acute symptoms of an asthma attack, montelukast is prescribed to be taken regularly when no symptoms are present to reduce the chronic inflammation of the airways that causes asthma, thus preventing asthma attacks.

▼ DOSAGE GUIDELINES

RANGE AND FREQUENCY
Adults and children age 15 years and older: One 10-mg tablet a day taken in the evening. Children ages 6 to 14 years: One 5-mg chewable tablet a day taken in the evening. Children ages 2 to 5 years: One 4-mg chewable tablet a day taken in the evening.

ONSET OF EFFECT
Unknown.

DURATION OF ACTION
Unknown.

DIETARY ADVICE
Montelukast can be taken without regard to diet.

STORAGE
Store montelukast in a tightly sealed container away from moisture, heat, and direct light.

MISSED DOSE
If you miss a dose one day, do not double the dose the next day. Resume your regular dosage schedule.

STOPPING THE DRUG
The decision to stop taking the drug should be made in consultation with your doctor.

PROLONGED USE
No special problems are expected.

▼ PRECAUTIONS

Over 60: Adverse reactions may be more likely and more severe in this age group.

Driving and Hazardous Work: No special precautions are necessary.

Alcohol: No special precautions are necessary.

Pregnancy: Adequate human studies have not been done. Before taking montelukast, tell your doctor if you are pregnant or plan to become pregnant.

Breast Feeding: Montelukast may pass into breast milk; caution is advised. Consult your doctor for advice.

Infants and Children: Not recommended for use by children under age 2 years.

Special Concerns: Montelukast has no effect on an asthma attack that has already started. You should have a fast-acting inhaled bronchodilator on hand to treat an acute asthma attack in progress. Consult your doctor if you need to use inhaled bronchodilators more often than usual or if you are taking more than the maximum number of inhalations in a 24-hour period. Continue to take montelukast even when you are not experiencing any symptoms, as well as during periods of worsening asthma. In rare cases, if doses of systemic corticosteroids are reduced, montelukast may cause Churg-Strauss syndrome, a tissue disorder that sometimes strikes adult asthma patients and, if left untreated, can destroy organs. Early symptoms include fever, muscle aches, and weight loss. Montelukast should not be used as the sole treatment for exercise-induced bronchospasm.

OVERDOSE
Symptoms: No cases of overdose have been reported.

What to Do: An overdose of montelukast is unlikely. If someone takes a much larger dose than prescribed, call your doctor, emergency medical services (EMS), or the nearest poison control center immediately.

▼ INTERACTIONS

DRUG INTERACTIONS
Consult your doctor for specific advice if you are already taking phenobarbital or rifampin. Before you take montelukast, tell your doctor if you are allergic to any other prescription or over-the-counter medicine.

FOOD INTERACTIONS
No known food interactions.

DISEASE INTERACTIONS
If you have phenylketonuria, you should not use the chewable tablet form of montelukast, because it contains phenylalanine. Use of the drug may cause complications in those patients with severe liver disease, because this organ works to remove the medication from the body.

☰ SIDE EFFECTS ☰

SERIOUS
Skin rash (indicating potentially life-threatening allergic reaction), gastroenteritis (causing loss of appetite, nausea, vomiting, stomach upset, fever, and diarrhea). Call your doctor immediately.

COMMON
Headache.

LESS COMMON
Weakness, fatigue, fever, abdominal pain, indigestion, mouth ulcers, dizziness, nasal congestion, cough, flulike symptoms.

MUPIROCIN

BRAND NAME

Bactroban

Available in: Ointment, cream
Available OTC? No **As Generic?** Yes
Drug Class: Antibiotic

▼ USAGE INFORMATION

WHY IT'S PRESCRIBED
Mupirocin is prescribed for topical therapy of certain bacteria-related skin infections. Mupirocin may be used alone or is occasionally used in combination with a second antibiotic (which is usually taken in an oral form).

HOW IT WORKS
Mupirocin works by preventing bacterial cells from manufacturing vital cell proteins and forming protective cell walls. This action ultimately destroys the infecting bacterial organisms.

▼ DOSAGE GUIDELINES

RANGE AND FREQUENCY
Apply to affected skin 3 times a day. The site may be covered with a gauze dressing if desired.

ONSET OF EFFECT
Mupirocin begins antibacterial activity as soon as the ointment or cream is applied. Several days may be required, however, before its full effects become noticeable.

DURATION OF ACTION
Unknown.

DIETARY ADVICE
No special restrictions.

STORAGE
Store mupirocin in a tightly sealed container away from heat and direct light. Keep it away from moisture and extremes in temperature.

MISSED DOSE
Apply it as soon as you remember. If it is near the time for the next application, skip the missed one and resume your regular dosage schedule. Do not increase the quantity of medication with the next application.

STOPPING THE DRUG
Apply it as prescribed for the full treatment period, even if the affected area begins to feel better before the scheduled end of therapy.

PROLONGED USE
Therapy with this medication should not require more than 14 days in most cases. Extended use of mupirocin may increase the risk of undesirable side effects.

▼ PRECAUTIONS

Over 60: No special precautions for older patients.

Driving and Hazardous Work: The use of mupirocin should not impair your ability to perform such tasks safely.

Alcohol: No special precautions are necessary.

Pregnancy: Mupirocin has not been evaluated in pregnant women. It is likely that mupirocin is safe for use during pregnancy in certain situations. This should be determined by your doctor.

Breast Feeding: The drug is not thought to be significantly absorbed into the bloodstream. If excessive amounts of mupirocin were absorbed, however, it could pass into breast milk; consult your doctor for advice.

Infants and Children: Consult your pediatrician.

Special Concerns: Mupirocin should not be used by anyone with a history of allergic reaction to mupirocin or any of the ingredients in the ointment or cream (check the label carefully). As with any other antibiotic, mupirocin is useful only against types of bacteria that are susceptible to its effects. Therefore, it is important to tell your doctor if your condition has not improved or if it has worsened within 3 to 5 days of starting the drug. The particular bacteria causing your illness may be resistant to mupirocin, and a different antibiotic may be required. Avoid using this medicine near or around the eyes.

OVERDOSE
Symptoms: No cases of overdose have been reported.

What to Do: Overapplication of mupirocin is unlikely to be harmful. However, if someone swallows the medication, call your doctor, emergency medical services (EMS), or the nearest poison control center.

▼ INTERACTIONS

DRUG INTERACTIONS
No specific interactions have been reported. Consult your doctor or pharmacist if you are concerned about taking another prescription or non-prescription medication while you are using mupirocin.

FOOD INTERACTIONS
No known food interactions.

DISEASE INTERACTIONS
No disease interactions have been reported.

SIDE EFFECTS

SERIOUS
There are no serious side effects associated with the use of mupirocin.

COMMON
Mild stinging or burning sensation with initial application.

LESS COMMON
Persistent irritation or skin allergy with pain or discomfort (stinging or burning) at application site; itching, redness, rash, or dryness of the skin; nausea.

NABUMETONE

BRAND NAME

Relafen

Available in: Tablets
Available OTC? No   **As Generic?** Yes
Drug Class: Nonsteroidal antiinflammatory drug (NSAID)

▼ USAGE INFORMATION

WHY IT'S PRESCRIBED
To treat mild to moderate pain and inflammation caused by tendinitis, arthritis, bursitis, gout, soft tissue injuries, migraine and other vascular headaches, menstrual cramps, and other conditions. When patients fail to respond to one NSAID, another may be tried. The greatest effectiveness often requires trial and error of several different NSAIDs.

HOW IT WORKS
NSAIDs work by interfering with the formation of prosta-glandins, naturally occurring substances in the body that cause inflammation and make nerves more sensitive to pain impulses. NSAIDs also have other modes of action that are not as well understood.

▼ DOSAGE GUIDELINES

RANGE AND FREQUENCY
Adults: 1,000 mg once a day. It may be increased to a maximum of 2,000 mg a day. For children's dose, consult your pediatrician.

ONSET OF EFFECT
From 30 minutes to several hours or longer.

DURATION OF ACTION
Variable.

DIETARY ADVICE
Take with food; maintain your usual food and fluid intake.

STORAGE
Store in a tightly sealed container away from moisture, heat, and direct light.

MISSED DOSE
Take it as soon as you remember. However, if it is near the time for the next dose, skip the missed dose and resume your regular dosage schedule. Do not double the next dose.

STOPPING THE DRUG
The decision to stop taking the drug should be made in consultation with your doctor.

PROLONGED USE
Extended use can cause gastrointestinal problems, such as ulceration and bleeding, kidney dysfunction, and liver inflammation. Consult your doctor about the need for medical exams and lab tests.

▼ PRECAUTIONS

Over 60: Because of the potentially greater consequences of gastrointestinal side effects, the dose of NSAIDs for older patients, especially those over age 70, is often cut in half.

Driving and Hazardous Work: Avoid such activities until you determine how the medicine affects you.

Alcohol: Avoid alcohol when using this medication, because it increases the risk of stomach irritation.

Pregnancy: Avoid or discontinue this medication if you are pregnant or if you plan to become pregnant.

Breast Feeding: Nabumetone passes into breast milk; avoid use while breast feeding.

Infants and Children: May be used in exceptional circumstances; consult your doctor.

Special Concerns: Because NSAIDs can interfere with blood coagulation, this drug should be stopped at least 3 days prior to any surgery.

OVERDOSE
Symptoms: Severe nausea, vomiting, headache, confusion, seizures.

What to Do: Call your doctor, emergency medical services (EMS), or the nearest poison control center immediately.

▼ INTERACTIONS

DRUG INTERACTIONS
Do not take this drug with aspirin or any other NSAIDs without your doctor's approval. In addition, consult your doctor if you are taking antihypertensives, steroids, anticoagulants, antibiotics, itraconazole or ketoconazole, plicamycin, penicillamine, valproic acid, phenytoin, cyclosporine, digitalis drugs, lithium, methotrexate, probenecid, triamterene, or zidovudine.

FOOD INTERACTIONS
No known food interactions.

DISEASE INTERACTIONS
Consult your doctor if you have any of the following: bleeding problems, ulcers or inflammation of the stomach and intestines, diabetes mellitus, systemic lupus erythematosus (SLE, lupus), anemia, asthma, epilepsy, Parkinson's disease, kidney stones, or a history of heart disease or alcohol abuse. Use of nabumetone may cause complications in patients with liver or kidney disease, because these organs work together to remove the medication from the body.

 SIDE EFFECTS

SERIOUS
Shortness of breath or wheezing, with or without swelling of legs or other signs of heart failure; chest pain; peptic ulcer disease with vomiting of blood; black, tarry stools; decreasing kidney function. Call your doctor immediately.

COMMON
Nausea, vomiting, heartburn, diarrhea, constipation, headache, dizziness, sleepiness.

LESS COMMON
Ulcers or sores in mouth, depression, rashes or blistering of skin, ringing sound in the ears, unusual tingling or numbness of the hands or feet, seizures, blurred vision. Also, elevated potassium levels and decreased white/red blood cell counts; such problems can be detected by your doctor.

NAFARELIN ACETATE

BRAND NAME

Synarel

Available in: Nasal spray
Available OTC? Yes   **Available as Generic?** No
Drug Class: Gonadotropin-releasing hormone

▼ USAGE INFORMATION

WHY IT'S TAKEN
To relieve the pain and discomfort of endometriosis.

HOW IT WORKS
Nafarelin decreases the production of estrogen by the ovaries. Reduced blood estrogen levels lead to shrinking of endometrial tissue (uterine lining), which eases flare-ups of endometriosis.

▼ DOSAGE GUIDELINES

RANGE AND FREQUENCY
One spray of 200 micrograms (μg) into one nostril in the morning and 1 spray into the other nostril in the evening, beginning on day 2, 3, or 4 of the menstrual period.

ONSET OF EFFECT
After 4 weeks.

DURATION OF ACTION
3 to 6 months.

DIETARY ADVICE
No special restrictions.

STORAGE
Store container upright away from heat and direct light.

MISSED DOSE
Take it as soon as you remember. However, if it is near the time for the next dose, skip the missed dose and resume your regular dosage schedule. Do not double the next dose.

STOPPING THE DRUG
The decision to stop taking the drug should be made by your doctor.

PROLONGED USE
Your doctor should check your progress regularly during prolonged use.

▼ PRECAUTIONS

Over 60: This medicine is generally not used by older patients.

Driving and Hazardous Work: The use of nafarelin should not impair your ability to perform such tasks safely.

Alcohol: Avoid alcohol.

Pregnancy: Nafarelin is not recommended during pregnancy. When taking the drug, women should use nonhormonal contraception (methods other than birth control pills). If you think you are pregnant, stop taking the medicine and call your doctor immediately.

Breast Feeding: Nafarelin may pass into breast milk; caution is advised. Consult your doctor for advice.

Infants and Children: This drug is not recommended for use by prepubescent children.

Special Concerns: Tell your doctor if you smoke cigarettes or consume a lot of alcohol or caffeine. When using a new bottle of nafarelin spray, point the bottle away from you and pump about 7 times to prime it. Wipe the tip with a clean tissue or cloth each time you use the spray. Every 3 or 4 days, rinse the tip with warm water and wipe the tip for about 15 seconds; then dry it. To take a dose of nafarelin, first blow your nose gently. Hold your head forward a little, put the spray tip in the nostril, and aim for the back. Close the other nostril by pressing with a finger. After spraying, tilt your head back for a few seconds. Do not blow your nose.

OVERDOSE
Symptoms: No specific symptoms have been reported.

What to Do: An overdose of nafarelin is unlikely to be life-threatening. However, if someone takes a much larger dose than is recommended, call your doctor, emergency medical services (EMS), or the nearest poison control center immediately.

▼ INTERACTIONS

DRUG INTERACTIONS
Consult your doctor for specific advice if you are taking any nasal spray decongestant, adrenocorticoids, or anticonvulsant medication.

FOOD INTERACTIONS
No known food interactions.

DISEASE INTERACTIONS
Caution is advised when taking nafarelin. Consult your doctor if you have any menstrual disorder.

 SIDE EFFECTS

SERIOUS
Vaginal bleeding between menstrual periods; longer or heavier menstrual periods; shortness of breath, chest pain, joint pain, and hives caused by an allergic reaction; bloating or tenderness of the lower abdomen; unexpected or excess flow of milk. Call your doctor immediately.

COMMON
Acne, decreased sex drive, dryness of vagina, hot flashes, pain during intercourse, decreased breast size, palpitations, oily skin, cessation of menstrual periods.

LESS COMMON
Breast pain, headache, runny nose, mental depression, mood swings, rash, weight changes.

NARATRIPTAN HYDROCHLORIDE

Available in: Tablets
Available OTC? No   **As Generic?** No
Drug Class: Antimigraine/antiheadache drug

▼ USAGE INFORMATION

WHY IT'S PRESCRIBED
To treat severe, acute migraine headaches. Naratriptan is not intended as a migraine preventive or for use against any other kinds of pain or headache, including basilar and hemiplegic migraines. Your doctor will determine whether this medication is appropriate in your particular case.

HOW IT WORKS
The exact action mechanism of naratriptan is unknown.

▼ DOSAGE GUIDELINES

RANGE AND FREQUENCY
A single 1- or 2.5-mg tablet taken with water is generally effective. If the migraine returns or there is only partial symptomatic relief, the dose may be repeated once after 4 hours, but no more than 5 mg should be taken in any 24-hour period. Because individuals may vary in their response to naratriptan, your experience with the drug will determine the most appropriate initial dosage for you.

SIDE EFFECTS

SERIOUS
Chest pain or tightness; sudden or severe abdominal pain; shortness of breath; wheezing; heartbeat irregularities or palpitations; skin rash; hives; swelling of the eyelids, face, or lips. Seek emergency medical assistance immediately.

COMMON
Tingling, hot flashes, flushing, weakness, drowsiness or dizziness, fatigue, general feeling of illness.

LESS COMMON
There are no less common side effects associated with the use of naratriptan.

ONSET OF EFFECT
Within 1 to 3 hours.

DURATION OF ACTION
Up to 24 hours.

DIETARY ADVICE
The medication can be taken with or without food.

STORAGE
Store in a tightly sealed container away from moisture, heat, and direct light.

MISSED DOSE
Not applicable, because the drug is taken only when necessary.

STOPPING THE DRUG
Consult your doctor before discontinuing naratriptan.

PROLONGED USE
No special problems are expected. However, if you are at risk for coronary artery disease (see Special Concerns), you should undergo periodic medical tests and evaluation.

▼ PRECAUTIONS

Over 60: Naratriptan is not recommended for use in older patients.

Driving and Hazardous Work: Some people feel drowsy or dizzy during or after a migraine attack or after taking naratriptan. Avoid driving or other tasks requiring concentration if you have such symptoms.

Alcohol: No special warnings, although alcohol may trigger or exacerbate migraine headaches.

Pregnancy: Adequate human studies have not been done. Discuss with your doctor the relative risks and benefits of using the drug while pregnant.

Breast Feeding: Naratriptan may pass into breast milk; caution is advised. Consult your doctor for advice.

Infants and Children: The safety and effectiveness of naratriptan have not been established for patients under 18 years. Consult your pediatrician for advice.

Special Concerns: Serious but rare heart-related problems may occur after using naratriptan. Anyone at risk for unrecognized coronary artery disease, such as postmenopausal women, men over age 40, or those with risk factors for coronary artery disease (hypertension, high blood cholesterol levels, obesity, diabetes, strong family history of heart disease, or cigarette smoking), should have the first dose of naratriptan administered in a doctor's office. Naratriptan should not be used by any individual with any symptoms of heart disease (including chest pain or tightness or shortness of breath).

OVERDOSE

Symptoms: Increase in blood pressure resulting in light-headedness, tension in the neck, fatigue, and loss of coordination.

What to Do: An overdose of naratriptan is unlikely. If someone takes a much larger dose than prescribed, call your doctor, emergency medical services (EMS), or the nearest poison control center immediately.

▼ INTERACTIONS

DRUG INTERACTIONS
Do not take naratriptan within 24 hours of taking almotriptan, sumatriptan, rizatriptan, zolmitriptan, medication containing ergotamine, dihydroergotamine mesylate, or methysergide mesylate. Oral contraceptives may interact with naratriptan. Consult your doctor for advice.

FOOD INTERACTIONS
No known food interactions.

DISEASE INTERACTIONS
You should not take naratriptan if you have a history of angina, heart disease, stroke, uncontrolled hypertension, heartbeat irregularities, peripheral vascular disease, or severely impaired kidney or liver function.

NEFAZODONE HYDROCHLORIDE

BRAND NAME

Serzone

Available in: Tablets
Available OTC? No   **As Generic?** No
Drug Class: Antidepressant

▼ USAGE INFORMATION

WHY IT'S PRESCRIBED
To treat symptoms of major depression.

HOW IT WORKS
Nefazodone affects the levels of serotonin and norepinephrine, brain chemicals that are thought to be linked to mood, emotions, and mental state.

▼ DOSAGE GUIDELINES

RANGE AND FREQUENCY
Adults: To start, 100 mg once a day. The dose may then be gradually increased by your doctor to a maximum of 600 mg a day. Older adults: To start, 50 mg 1 or 2 times a day. The dose may then be gradually increased over time by your doctor.

ONSET OF EFFECT
The full effect may take several weeks.

DURATION OF ACTION
Unknown.

DIETARY ADVICE
Nefazodone can be taken without regard to diet.

STORAGE
Store in a tightly sealed container away from moisture, heat, and direct light.

MISSED DOSE
Take it as soon as you remember. However, if it is near the time for the next dose, skip the missed dose and resume your regular dosage schedule. Do not double the next dose.

STOPPING THE DRUG
Take it as prescribed for the full treatment period, even if you begin to feel better before the scheduled end of therapy. The decision to stop taking the drug should be made in consultation with your doctor.

PROLONGED USE
The usual course of therapy lasts 6 months to 1 year; some patients benefit from additional therapy.

▼ PRECAUTIONS

Over 60:
Adverse reactions may be more likely and more severe in older patients. A lower dose may be necessary.

Driving and Hazardous Work:
Proceed with caution until you determine how the medicine affects you. Drowsiness may occur.

Alcohol:
Avoid alcohol.

Pregnancy:
Nefazodone has not been shown to cause birth defects in animals. Adequate human studies have not been done. Before you take this medication, tell your doctor if you are pregnant or plan to become pregnant.

Breast Feeding:
Nefazodone may pass into breast milk; caution is advised.

Infants and Children:
Safety and effectiveness of the drug in children under 18 years have not been established.

Special Concerns:
Use sugar-free gum or candy for relief of dry mouth.

OVERDOSE

Symptoms: Lightheadedness, dizziness, confusion, fainting, nausea, vomiting, drowsiness.

What to Do: Call your doctor, emergency medical services (EMS), or the nearest poison control center immediately.

▼ INTERACTIONS

DRUG INTERACTIONS
Do not take nefazodone if you are taking terfenadine or astemizole. Nefazodone and monoamine oxidase (MAO) inhibitors should not be used within 14 days of each other. Very serious side effects such as myoclonus (uncontrolled muscle jerking), hyperthermia (excessive rise in body temperature), and extreme stiffness may result. For many patients, especially the elderly, the use of nefazodone in combination with triazolam is not recommended. Other drugs may also interact with nefazodone; consult your doctor if you are taking alprazolam, high blood pressure medication (antihypertensives), atorvastatin, simvastatin, central nervous system depressants (including cold medications, allergy drugs, narcotic pain relievers, and muscle relaxants), or tricyclic antidepressants.

FOOD INTERACTIONS
No known food interactions.

DISEASE INTERACTIONS
Consult your doctor if you have a history of drug or alcohol abuse, any heart condition, a history of seizures, any condition affecting blood vessels of the brain, symptoms of dehydration (such as confusion, irritability, flushed, dry skin, decreased urine output, and extreme thirst), or a history of mental disorders.

≡ SIDE EFFECTS ≡

SERIOUS
Blurred, partial loss of, or changes in vision; unsteadiness or clumsiness; skin rash; lightheadedness; ringing in the ears; prolonged or painful erection (lasting more than 4 hours). Call your doctor immediately.

COMMON
Drowsiness or dizziness, agitation, dry mouth, confusion, constipation or diarrhea, unusual dreams, heartburn, fever or chills, insomnia, loss of memory, headache, flushing, nausea or vomiting, increased appetite.

LESS COMMON
Joint pain, increased thirst, breast pain, cough, swelling of lower extremities, sore throat, trembling. Also unusual tingling, burning, or prickling sensations.

NEOMYCIN/POLYMYXIN B/HYDROCORTISONE OPHTHALMIC AND OTIC

Available in: Ophthalmic suspension, otic solution and suspension
Available OTC? No   **As Generic?** Yes
Drug Class: Antibiotic/corticosteroid combination

▼ USAGE INFORMATION

WHY IT'S PRESCRIBED
To treat or prevent bacterial infections of the eye or ear and to provide relief from eye or ear irritation and discomfort.

HOW IT WORKS
Ophthalmic and otic neomycin/polymyxin B/hydrocortisone kill bacteria by interfering with the genetic material of bacterial cells, preventing them from multiplying.

▼ DOSAGE GUIDELINES

RANGE AND FREQUENCY
Ophthalmic suspension: 1 drop every 3 to 4 hours. Otic solution and suspension for ear canal infection—Adults: 4 drops in the ear 3 to 4 times a day. Children: 3 drops in the ear 3 to 4 times a day.

ONSET OF EFFECT
Unknown.

DURATION OF ACTION
Unknown.

DIETARY ADVICE
No special restrictions.

STORAGE
Store it in a tightly sealed container away from moisture, heat, and direct light. Do not allow it to freeze.

MISSED DOSE
Apply it as soon as you remember. However, if it is near the time for the next dose, skip the missed dose and resume your regular dosage schedule. Do not double the next dose.

STOPPING THE DRUG
Use this drug as prescribed for the full treatment period, even if you begin to feel better before the scheduled end of therapy.

PROLONGED USE
Do not use the ear medication for more than 10 days unless your doctor directs otherwise. If you use the eye medication for a prolonged period, you should see your doctor regularly for tests and examinations.

▼ PRECAUTIONS

Over 60: No special problems are expected.

Driving and Hazardous Work: Do not drive or engage in hazardous work until you determine how the medicine affects your vision.

Alcohol: No special precautions are necessary.

Pregnancy: This medication is not likely to cause problems unless absorbed into the bloodstream; consult your doctor for advice.

Breast Feeding: This combination medication has not been shown to cause problems in nursing babies.

Infants and Children: No special precautions.

Special Concerns: To use the eye drops, first wash your hands. Tilt your head back. Gently apply pressure to the inside corner of the eyelid and with the index finger of the same hand, pull downward on the lower eyelid to make a space. Drop the medicine into this space and close your eye. Apply pressure for 1 or 2 minutes while keeping the eye closed without blinking. To use the ear drops, lie down or tilt your head so the infected ear faces up. Gently pull the earlobe up and back for adults (down and back for children) to straighten the ear canal. Drop the medicine into the ear. Keep the ear facing upward for 5 minutes (2 minutes for children) after inserting the drops to allow the medicine to reach the infection. If necessary, insert a cotton ball to prevent the medicine from leaking out. Make sure the applicator for eye or ear drops does not touch your eye, ear, finger, or any other surface. If your symptoms do not improve in a few days or if they become worse, contact your doctor.

OVERDOSE
Symptoms: No specific ones have been reported.

What to Do: An overdose of this medication is unlikely to be life-threatening. If a large volume enters the eye, flush fthe eye with water. If a large volume enters the ear or someone accidentally ingests the medicine, call your doctor, emergency medical services (EMS), or the nearest poison control center.

▼ INTERACTIONS

DRUG INTERACTIONS
Consult your doctor for specific advice if you are taking any other prescription or over-the-counter medication.

FOOD INTERACTIONS
No known food interactions.

DISEASE INTERACTIONS
Caution is advised when taking this combination antibiotic. Consult your doctor if you have any other eye or ear infection or medical problem.

⇊ SIDE EFFECTS ⇊

SERIOUS
Itching, rash, redness, swelling, or other eye or ear irritation that was not present before therapy. Call your doctor immediately.

COMMON
No common side effects have been reported with neomycin/polymyxin B/hydrocortisone.

LESS COMMON
Burning or stinging from the eye drops. There are no less common side effects associated with the ear preparation.

NIFEDIPINE

Available in: Extended-release tablets, capsules
Available OTC? No **As Generic?** Yes
Drug Class: Calcium channel blocker

▼ USAGE INFORMATION

WHY IT'S PRESCRIBED
To treat high blood pressure and to prevent attacks of angina pectoris (chest pain associated with coronary artery disease).

HOW IT WORKS
Nifedipine interferes with the movement of calcium into heart muscle cells and the smooth muscle cells in the walls of the arteries. This action relaxes blood vessels (causing them to widen), which lowers blood pressure, increases the blood supply to the heart, and decreases the heart's overall workload.

▼ DOSAGE GUIDELINES

RANGE AND FREQUENCY
Extended-release tablets: 30 or 60 mg once a day. The doses may be increased as determined by your doctor.

ONSET OF EFFECT
Within 20 minutes.

DURATION OF ACTION
Extended-release tablets: 12 to 24 hours.

DIETARY ADVICE
Nifedipine can be taken with or without food.

STORAGE
Store nifedipine in a tightly sealed container away from heat and direct light.

MISSED DOSE
Take it as soon as you remember. If it is near the time for the next dose, skip the missed dose and resume your regular dosage schedule. Do not double the next dose.

STOPPING THE DRUG
Do not stop taking this drug suddenly; this may cause potentially serious health problems. If therapy is to be discontinued, the dosage should be reduced gradually according to your doctor's instructions.

PROLONGED USE
You should see your doctor regularly for examinations and tests if you take this medicine for an extended period. Remember that this medicine controls high blood pressure but does not cure it. You may have to take nifedipine for the rest of your life.

▼ PRECAUTIONS

Over 60:
Adverse reactions may be more likely and more severe in older patients.

Driving and Hazardous Work:
Do not drive or engage in hazardous work until you determine how the medicine affects you.

Alcohol:
Avoid alcohol.

Pregnancy:
In animal studies, large doses of nifedipine have been shown to cause birth defects. Human studies have not been done. Before you take nifedipine, tell your doctor if you are pregnant or plan to become pregnant.

Breast Feeding:
Nifedipine passes into breast milk but has not been reported to cause problems; caution is advised. Consult your doctor for specific advice.

Infants and Children:
Although there is no specific information on the use of nifedipine in younger patients, the use of the capsule form is not recommended.

Special Concerns:
In addition to taking nifedipine, be sure to follow all special instructions about weight control and diet. Your doctor will advise you about which specific factors are most important for you. Check with your doctor before changing your diet.

OVERDOSE
Symptoms: Dizziness, slurred speech, confusion, weakness, drowsiness, nausea, abnormal heartbeat.

What to Do: Call your doctor, emergency medical services (EMS), or the nearest poison control center immediately.

▼ INTERACTIONS

DRUG INTERACTIONS
Consult your physician for specific advice if you are taking acetazolamide, amphotericin B, corticosteroids, dichlorphenamide, diuretics, methazolamide, beta-blockers, carbamazepine, cyclosporine, procainamide, quinidine, digitalis drugs, disopyramide, or the following eye medicines: betaxolol, levobunolol, metipranolol, or timolol.

FOOD INTERACTIONS
Avoid foods high in sodium.

DISEASE INTERACTIONS
Caution is advised when taking nifedipine. Consult your doctor if you have any of the following: abnormal heart rhythm, other disorders of the heart and blood vessels, mental depression, or Parkinson's disease. Use of the drug may cause complications in patients with liver or kidney disease, because these organs work together to remove the medication from the body.

≡ SIDE EFFECTS ≡

SERIOUS
Breathing difficulty, coughing, or wheezing; irregular or pounding heartbeat; chest pain; fainting. Call your doctor immediately.

COMMON
Headache; dizziness; skin flushing and feeling of warmth; swelling in the feet, ankles, or calves; palpitations.

LESS COMMON
Constipation or diarrhea, nausea, unusual fatigue and weakness, skin rash, increased urination, vision problems.

NITROFURANTOIN

BRAND NAMES

Furadantin, Furalan,
Furatoin, Macrobid,
Macrodantin,
Nitrofuracot

Available in: Capsules, oral suspension, tablets, extended-release capsules
Available OTC? No **As Generic?** Yes
Drug Class: Antiinfective

▼ USAGE INFORMATION

WHY IT'S PRESCRIBED
To treat urinary tract infections (UTIs).

HOW IT WORKS
Nitrofurantoin interferes with bacterial metabolism and cell wall formation. Eventually the bacteria die, bringing an end to the infection.

▼ DOSAGE GUIDELINES

RANGE AND FREQUENCY
Adults and teenagers–Capsules, oral suspension, tablets: 50 to 100 mg every 6 hours. Extended-release capsules: 100 mg every 12 hours. Children up to 12 years: Dosage must be determined by your doctor.

ONSET OF EFFECT
Within 1 hour.

DURATION OF ACTION
Capsules, oral suspension, tablets: 6 hours. Extended-release capsules: 24 hours.

DIETARY ADVICE
Nitrofurantoin should be taken with food or milk.

STORAGE
Store it in a tightly sealed container away from heat and direct light. Keep the oral suspension from freezing.

MISSED DOSE
Take it as soon as you remember. If it is near the time for the next dose, skip the missed dose and resume your regular dosage schedule. Do not double the next dose.

STOPPING THE DRUG
Take as prescribed for the full treatment period, even if you begin to feel better before the scheduled end of therapy.

PROLONGED USE
See your doctor regularly if you must take this drug for a prolonged period.

▼ PRECAUTIONS

Over 60: Adverse reactions may be more likely and more severe in older patients.

Driving and Hazardous Work: Do not drive or engage in hazardous work until you determine how the medicine affects you.

Alcohol: Avoid alcohol.

Pregnancy: Nitrofurantoin should not be taken within several weeks of the delivery date or during labor.

Breast Feeding: Nitrofurantoin passes into breast milk; avoid use while breast feeding.

Infants and Children: Nitrofurantoin is not recommended for use by infants younger than 1 month old.

Special Concerns: Nitrofurantoin may cause false results in some urine sugar tests for diabetes. If your symptoms do not improve or instead become worse within a few days, check with your doctor. When taking the oral suspension, be sure to shake the container forcefully before each dose. Use a specially marked measuring spoon or other device to dispense each dose, because a household teaspoon might not hold the correct amount. Tell your doctor if you have ever had an allergic reaction to nitrofurantoin or any related medicine, such as furazolidone, or if you are allergic to any other substance. When taking the extended-release capsule, swallow it whole without chewing.

OVERDOSE
Symptoms: Severe nausea, vomiting, diarrhea, loss of appetite.

What to Do: An overdose of nitrofurantoin is unlikely to be life-threatening. However, if someone takes a much larger dose than prescribed, call your doctor, emergency medical services (EMS), or the nearest poison control center.

▼ INTERACTIONS

DRUG INTERACTIONS
Consult your doctor for specific advice if you are taking acetohydroxamine; oral diabetes medicine; dapsone; furazolidone; methyldopa; procainamide; quinidine; sulfonamides; vitamin K; carbamazepine; chloroquine; cisplatin; cytarabine; vaccine for diphtheria, tetanus, and pertussis (DTP); disulfiram; ethotoin; hydroxychloroquine; lindane; lithium; mephenytoin; mexiletine; pemoline, phenytoin; pyridoxine; vincristine; probenecid; sulfinpyrazone; quinine; or any other antiinfective agent.

FOOD INTERACTIONS
No known food interactions.

DISEASE INTERACTIONS
Consult your doctor if you have any of the following: glucose-6-phosphate dehydrogenase (G6PD) deficiency, kidney disease, lung disease, or nerve damage.

SIDE EFFECTS

SERIOUS
Chest pain, chills, cough, fever, troubled breathing, dizziness, drowsiness, tingling or burning of face or mouth, sore throat, unusual weakness, unusual fatigue. Call your doctor immediately.

COMMON
Abdominal pain or stomach upset, diarrhea, nausea, vomiting, loss of appetite.

LESS COMMON
Dark yellow or brownish urine.

NITROGLYCERIN

Available in: Capsules, tablets, ointment, skin patch, aerosol
Available OTC? No   **As Generic?** Yes
Drug Class: Nitrate

▼ USAGE INFORMATION

WHY IT'S PRESCRIBED
To prevent or relieve attacks of angina (chest pain associated with heart disease).

HOW IT WORKS
Nitroglycerin relaxes the smooth muscle surrounding blood vessels and increases the supply of blood and oxygen to the heart. It also reduces the heart's workload and demand for oxygen.

▼ DOSAGE GUIDELINES

RANGE AND FREQUENCY
Ointment: 15 to 30 mg applied to skin every 6 to 8 hours. Skin patch: 1 patch applied every day, left on for 12 to 14 hours. Aerosol: 1 or 2 doses on or under the tongue at 5-minute intervals to relieve angina attack. Extended-release capsules: 2.5, 6.5, or 9 mg every 12 hours; can be taken every 8 hours. Extended-release tablets: 1.3, 2.6, or 6.5 mg every 12 hours; can be taken every 8 hours. Sublingual (under tongue) or buccal (inside the cheek) tablets: 0.15 to 0.6 mg repeated at 5-minute intervals to treat angina attack. If 3 tablets do not relieve pain, call your doctor.

ONSET OF EFFECT
Sublingual: 2 to 4 minutes. Buccal: 3 minutes. Oral: 20 to 45 minutes. Ointment and skin patch: 30 minutes.

DURATION OF ACTION
Sublingual: 30 to 60 minutes. Buccal: 5 hours. Oral: 8 to 12 hours. Ointment: 4 to 8 hours. Skin patch: Up to 24 hours.

DIETARY ADVICE
Oral forms used as a preventive should be taken 30 minutes before or 1 to 2 hours after meals.

STORAGE
Store it in a tightly sealed container away from moisture, heat, and direct light.

MISSED DOSE
Take it as soon as you remember you skipped a dose. If it is near the time for the next dose, skip the missed dose and resume your regular dosage schedule, as prescribed. Do not double the next dose.

STOPPING THE DRUG
The decision to stop taking nitroglycerin should be made by your doctor.

PROLONGED USE
See your doctor regularly for examinations and tests if you take this medicine for a prolonged period.

▼ PRECAUTIONS

Over 60: Adverse reactions may be more likely and more severe in older patients.

Driving and Hazardous Work: Do not drive or engage in hazardous work until you determine how the medicine affects you.

Alcohol: Avoid alcohol.

Pregnancy: Not recommended during pregnancy. Before taking nitroglycerin, be sure to tell your doctor if you are pregnant or plan to become pregnant.

Breast Feeding: Nitroglycerin may pass into breast milk; caution is advised. Consult your doctor for advice.

Infants and Children: No studies in infants and children have been done.

Special Concerns: The skin patch should be applied to different sites to prevent skin irritation.

OVERDOSE
Symptoms: Fast heartbeat, red and perspiring skin, headache, dizziness, palpitations, vision disturbances, nausea, vomiting, confusion, difficulty breathing.

What to Do: Call your doctor, emergency medical services (EMS), or the nearest poison control center immediately.

▼ INTERACTIONS

DRUG INTERACTIONS
Do not take nitroglycerin within 24 hours of taking sildenafil citrate. Sildenafil can enhance the action of nitrates (such as nitroglycerin), causing potentially dangerous decreases in blood pressure. Consult your doctor for specific advice if you are taking other heart medicines or drugs for hypertension.

FOOD INTERACTIONS
No known food interactions.

DISEASE INTERACTIONS
Consult your physician if you have any of the following: anemia, glaucoma, a recent head injury or stroke, a recent heart attack, or an overactive thyroid. Use of nitroglycerin may cause complications in patients with severe liver or kidney disease, because these organs work together to remove the medication from the body.

≣ SIDE EFFECTS ≣

SERIOUS
Blurred vision, severe or prolonged headache, skin rash, dry mouth. Call your doctor immediately.

COMMON
Flushing of face and neck, headache, nausea or vomiting, dizziness or lightheadedness when getting up, rapid heartbeat, restlessness.

LESS COMMON
Sore, reddened skin.

NORTRIPTYLINE HYDROCHLORIDE

BRAND NAMES

Aventyl, Pamelor

Available in: Capsules, oral solution
Available OTC? No   **As Generic?** Yes
Drug Class: Tricyclic antidepressant

▼ USAGE INFORMATION

WHY IT'S PRESCRIBED
To relieve symptoms of major depression, anxiety disorders, panic disorder, or chronic pain.

HOW IT WORKS
Nortriptyline affects levels of norepinephrine, a brain chemical that is thought to be linked to mood, emotions, and mental state.

▼ DOSAGE GUIDELINES

RANGE AND FREQUENCY
Adults: 25 mg 3 to 4 times a day; may be increased to a maximum dose of 150 mg a day. Teenagers: 25 to 50 mg a day. Children ages 6 to 12 years: 10 to 20 mg a day. Older adults: 25 to 100 mg a day; may be increased gradually by your doctor. Dosage is usually determined by blood level monitoring.

ONSET OF EFFECT
1 to 6 weeks.

DURATION OF ACTION
Unknown.

DIETARY ADVICE
To lessen stomach upset, take with food, unless your doctor instructs otherwise. Increase your intake of fiber and fluids.

STORAGE
Store it in a tightly sealed container away from heat, moisture, and direct light. Do not allow solution to freeze.

MISSED DOSE
If you take a one-time daily bedtime dose, do not take the missed dose in the morning because it may cause drowsiness. Call your doctor for specific advice. If you take more than 1 dose a day, take it as soon as you remember. If it is near the time for the next dose, skip the missed dose and resume your regular dosage schedule. Do not double the next dose.

STOPPING THE DRUG
Take it as prescribed for the full treatment period, even if you begin to feel better before the scheduled end of therapy. The decision to stop taking the drug should be made in consultation with your doctor.

PROLONGED USE
The usual course of therapy lasts 6 months to 1 year; some patients benefit from additional therapy.

▼ PRECAUTIONS

Over 60: Adverse reactions may be more likely and more severe in older patients. A lower dose may be necessary.

Driving and Hazardous Work: Use caution when driving or engaging in hazardous work until you determine how the medication affects you. Drowsiness or lightheadedness can occur.

Alcohol: Avoid alcohol.

Pregnancy: Adequate human studies have not been done. Consult your doctor for specific advice.

Breast Feeding: Nortriptyline passes into breast milk; do not use it while nursing.

Infants and Children: Not prescribed for children under the age of 6 years.

Special Concerns: This is a potentially dangerous drug, especially if taken in excess. Tricyclic antidepressants should not be within easy reach of suicidal patients. If dry mouth occurs, use candy or sugar-free gum for relief.

OVERDOSE
Symptoms: Difficulty breathing, severe fatigue, seizures, confusion, hallucinations, dilated pupils, irregular heartbeat, fever, impaired concentration.

What to Do: Call your doctor, emergency medical services (EMS), or the nearest poison control center immediately.

▼ INTERACTIONS

DRUG INTERACTIONS
Consult your doctor for specific advice if you are taking antithyroid agents, cimetidine, clonidine, guanadrel, guanethidine, metrizamide, appetite suppressants, isoproterenol, ephedrine, epinephrine, amphetamines, phenylephrine, antipsychotic drugs, pimozide, methyldopa, metyrosine, metoclopramide, pemoline, promethazine, trimeprazine, rauwolfia alkaloids, MAO inhibitors, or any drugs that depress the central nervous system.

FOOD INTERACTIONS
No known food interactions.

DISEASE INTERACTIONS
Consult your doctor if you have any of the following: a history of alcohol abuse, difficulty urinating, asthma, bipolar disorder, high blood pressure, stomach or intestinal problems, glaucoma, overactive thyroid, enlarged prostate, schizophrenia, seizures, a blood disorder, or kidney, heart, or liver disease.

 SIDE EFFECTS

SERIOUS
Confusion, heartbeat irregularities, hallucinations, seizures, extreme fatigue or drowsiness, blurred or altered vision, breathing difficulty, constipation, staring and absence of facial expression, impaired concentration, difficult urination, fever, extreme and persistent restlessness, loss of coordination and balance, difficulty swallowing or speaking, dilated pupils, eye pain, fainting. Also trembling, shaking, weakness, and stiffness in the extremities, and shuffling gait. Call your doctor immediately.

COMMON
Drowsiness or dizziness, headache, dry mouth or unpleasant taste, fatigue, heightened sensitivity to light, weight gain, nausea, increased appetite.

LESS COMMON
Heartburn, sleeping difficulty, diarrhea, increased or profuse sweating, vomiting.

OLANZAPINE

Available in: Tablets
Available OTC? No   **As Generic?** No
Drug Class: Neuroleptic; antipsychotic

▼ USAGE INFORMATION

WHY IT'S PRESCRIBED
To treat psychotic conditions (severe mental disorders characterized by distorted thoughts and perceptions), such as schizophrenia.

HOW IT WORKS
The exact mechanism of action of olanzapine is unknown. It appears to alter the activity of certain chemicals in the central nervous system to produce a tranquilizing and antipsychotic effect.

▼ DOSAGE GUIDELINES

RANGE AND FREQUENCY
Initial dose is 5 to 10 mg once daily. Dose may be increased by your doctor to a maximum of 20 mg a day.

ONSET OF EFFECT
Sedation may occur within minutes, but the onset of antipsychotic effect may take hours to occur or may not occur until days or weeks after the beginning of therapy.

DURATION OF ACTION
12 to 24 hours, but effects may persist for several days.

DIETARY ADVICE
No special restrictions.

STORAGE
Store in a tightly sealed container away from moisture, heat, and direct light.

MISSED DOSE
Take it as soon as you remember. However, if it is near the time for the next dose, skip the missed dose and resume your regular dosage schedule. Do not double the next dose.

STOPPING THE DRUG
The decision to stop taking the medication should be made in consultation with your physician.

PROLONGED USE
Consult your doctor about the need for follow-up evaluations and tests if you must take this drug for an extended period. Because olanzapine is a recently released drug, its risk

of inducing potentially irreversible tardive dyskinesia (involuntary movements of the jaw, lips, tongue, and body) is unknown.

▼ PRECAUTIONS

Over 60: No special problems are expected.

Driving and Hazardous Work: Do not drive or engage in hazardous work until you determine how the medicine affects you.

Alcohol: Avoid alcohol.

Pregnancy: Large doses of olanzapine reduced fetal survival in animal tests. Before you take olanzapine, tell your doctor if you are pregnant or plan to become pregnant.

Breast Feeding: Olanzapine may pass into breast milk; avoid use while nursing.

Infants and Children: The safety and effectiveness of olanzapine in children under 18 years have not been established.

Special Concerns: Avoid prolonged exposure to high temperatures or hot climates. Drink plenty of fluids and stay cool in the summertime. Avoid overexposure to sunlight until you determine if the drug heightens your skin's sensitivity to ultraviolet light.

OVERDOSE
Symptoms: Extreme drowsiness, slurred speech.

What to Do: Call your doctor, emergency medical services

(EMS), or the nearest poison control center immediately.

▼ INTERACTIONS

DRUG INTERACTIONS
The following drugs may interact with olanzapine. Consult your doctor for specific advice if you are taking carbamazepine, omeprazole, rifampin, high blood pressure medication, or any drugs that depress the central nervous system, including antihistamines, antidepressants or other psychiatric medications, barbiturates, sedatives, cough medicines, decongestants, and painkillers. Be sure your doctor knows about any over-the-counter medication you may be taking.

FOOD INTERACTIONS
No known food interactions.

DISEASE INTERACTIONS
Consult your doctor if you have Parkinson's disease or another movement disorder, glaucoma, epilepsy, liver disease, or kidney disease.

 SIDE EFFECTS

SERIOUS
Stiffness; shuffling gait; difficulty swallowing or speaking; persistent, uncontrolled chewing, lip smacking, or tongue movements; fever. Call your doctor immediately.

COMMON
Drowsiness, headache, dizziness, constipation, dry mouth, blurred vision, runny nose.

LESS COMMON
Stomach pain, unclear speech or stuttering, muscle tightness, faintness, increased appetite, increased cough, watering of mouth, insomnia, joint pain, nausea, vomiting, sore throat, rapid heartbeat, increased thirst, urinary incontinence, weight loss.

ORLISTAT

Available in: Capsules
Available OTC? No   **As Generic?** No
Drug Class: Lipase inhibitor

▼ USAGE INFORMATION

WHY IT'S PRESCRIBED
To achieve weight loss and weight maintenance in obesity when used in conjunction with a reduced-calorie diet and appropriate physical activity. Orlistat is indicated for patients with an initial body mass index (BMI) of 30 or greater (see Special Concerns for information on BMI calculation) and for those with a BMI greater than 27 who also have other risk factors such as high blood pressure, high blood cholesterol, and diabetes.

HOW IT WORKS
Orlistat inhibits the activity of lipases, intestinal enzymes required for the digestion of dietary fats. Orlistat prevents the breakdown of a portion of ingested fat. The undigested fat cannot be absorbed and is excreted in the feces. At full dosage, orlistat can reduce the absorption of fat by about 30%.

▼ DOSAGE GUIDELINES

RANGE AND FREQUENCY
120 mg (1 capsule) 3 times a day at mealtime.

ONSET OF EFFECT
Within 24 to 48 hours.

DURATION OF ACTION
48 to 72 hours.

DIETARY ADVICE
Take with liquid during or up to 1 hour after each main meal containing fat. Follow a balanced, reduced-calorie diet. The daily intake of fat (approximately ⅓ of the calories), carbohydrate, and protein should be spread out over the three meals. If a meal is missed or contains no fat, the dose of orlistat can be skipped. Because orlistat can also reduce the absorption of fat-soluble vitamins, a multivitamin supplement (containing vitamins A, D, and E and beta-carotene) should also be taken once a day at least 2 hours before or after ingesting orlistat.

STORAGE
Store it in a tightly sealed container away from moisture, heat, and direct light.

MISSED DOSE
If you miss a dose, take it if you remember within 1 hour of eating. However, if more than 1 hour has passed, skip the missed dose and return to your regular schedule. Do not double the next dose.

STOPPING THE DRUG
The decision to stop taking the drug should be made in consultation with your doctor.

PROLONGED USE
The safety and effectiveness of this medication have not been determined beyond 2 years of use.

▼ PRECAUTIONS

Over 60: No specific studies of orlistat have been done on older patients.

Driving and Hazardous Work: The use of orlistat should not impair your ability to perform such tasks safely.

Alcohol: No special precautions are necessary.

Pregnancy: Adequate human studies have not been done. Before taking orlistat, tell your doctor if you are pregnant or plan to become pregnant.

Breast Feeding: It is unknown whether orlistat passes into breast milk. However, do not take the drug while nursing. Consult your doctor for advice.

Infants and Children: Safety and effectiveness have not been established for children under 18 years.

Special Concerns: A medical cause for obesity (such as hypothyroidism) should be ruled out before taking orlistat. Consult your doctor or a nutritionist for information about a nutritionally balanced, reduced-calorie diet and an exercise program. The BMI can be calculated by dividing your weight in pounds by your height in inches squared and then multiplying by 705.

OVERDOSE
Symptoms: No cases of overdose have been reported.

What to Do: An overdose of orlistat is unlikely. If someone takes a much larger dose than prescribed, call your doctor.

▼ INTERACTIONS

DRUG INTERACTIONS
The following drugs may interact with orlistat. Consult your doctor for specific advice if you are taking: statin (cholesterol-lowering) drugs, cyclosporine, warfarin, another weight loss medication (such as sibutramine or phentermine), or any other prescription or over-the-counter medicines.

FOOD INTERACTIONS
Orlistat reduces the absorption of fat-soluble vitamins A, D, E, and K and beta-carotene. Gastrointestinal side effects may increase after the consumption of high-fat foods or with a diet high in fat (more than 30% of the day's total calories from fat).

DISEASE INTERACTIONS
This medication should not be used if you have chronic malabsorption or gallbladder problems. Consult your doctor if you have an eating disorder (anorexia or bulimia).

⬇ SIDE EFFECTS ⬇

SERIOUS
No serious side effects have yet been reported.

COMMON
Oily spotting, gas with discharge, fecal urgency, oily stool, anal leakage, increased defecation, fecal incontinence.

LESS COMMON
Abdominal pain or discomfort.

OSELTAMIVIR PHOSPHATE

Available in: Capsules, oral suspension
Available OTC? No   **As Generic?** No
Drug Class: Antiviral

▼ USAGE INFORMATION

WHY IT'S PRESCRIBED
To treat and prevent infection from influenza type A or B. Oseltamivir can reduce the severity of symptoms and shorten the duration of flu episodes.

HOW IT WORKS
Oseltamivir is believed to interfere with the synthesis of the viral enzyme neuraminidase, which is needed in order for the virus to infect cells in the respiratory tract and elsewhere in the body. The drug affects only certain susceptible strains of the influenza type A or B viruses.

▼ DOSAGE GUIDELINES

RANGE AND FREQUENCY
For treatment—Adults and teenagers: 75 mg twice a day for 5 days. Treatment should be initiated as soon as possible and no more than 2 days after the onset of signs or symptoms of the flu. Children 12 years and under: Consult your pediatrician. For prevention—Adults and teenagers: 75 mg once a day for 7 days. Therapy should be initiated within 2 days of exposure. For prevention during a community outbreak: 75 mg once a day for up to 6 weeks.

ONSET OF EFFECT
Unknown.

DURATION OF ACTION
Unknown.

DIETARY ADVICE
No special restrictions.

STORAGE
Store this medication in a tightly sealed container away from moisture, heat, and direct light. Do not allow oral suspensions to freeze.

MISSED DOSE
Take it as soon as you remember. If it is near (within 2 hours) the time for the next dose, skip the missed dose and resume your regular dosage schedule. Do not double the next dose.

STOPPING THE DRUG
It is important to take oseltamivir for the full treatment period as prescribed. Do not stop taking the drug before the scheduled end of therapy even if you begin to feel better; this may lead to a relapse.

PROLONGED USE
If your symptoms do not improve or if they become worse in a few days, consult your doctor.

▼ PRECAUTIONS

Over 60: No special problems are expected.

Driving and Hazardous Work: Do not drive or engage in hazardous work until you determine how the medicine affects you.

Alcohol: No special precautions are necessary.

Pregnancy: Adequate studies have not been completed. Discuss the relative risks and benefits of using this medication while you are pregnant with your doctor.

Breast Feeding: Oseltamivir may pass into breast milk, but it is unknown if this poses any risks to the nursing infant. Consult your doctor for specific advice.

Infants and Children: The safety and effectiveness of this drug for treatment have not been established for children under the age of 1 year. The safety and effectiveness of this drug for prevention have not been established for children under the age of 13 years.

Special Concerns: This medication is not a substitute for a flu shot. Continue to receive your annual flu shot. Shake the oral suspension well before use.

OVERDOSE
Symptoms: No cases have been reported. However, nausea and vomiting are probable symptoms.

What to Do: If you have any reason to suspect an overdose, call your doctor, emergency medical services (EMS), or the nearest poison control center.

▼ INTERACTIONS

DRUG INTERACTIONS
No known drug interactions.

FOOD INTERACTIONS
No known food interactions.

DISEASE INTERACTIONS
The dose of oseltamivir should be lowered in patients with severe kidney disease. Safety has not been determined in people with liver disease.

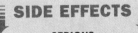

⬇ SIDE EFFECTS ⬇

SERIOUS
No serious side effects are associated with oseltamivir.

COMMON
Nausea and vomiting.

LESS COMMON
Bronchitis, insomnia, dizziness.

OXAPROZIN

Available in: Caplets
Available OTC? No   **As Generic?** Yes
Drug Class: Nonsteroidal antiinflammatory drug (NSAID)

▼ USAGE INFORMATION

WHY IT'S PRESCRIBED
To treat mild to moderate pain and inflammation caused by tendinitis, arthritis, bursitis, gout, soft tissue injuries, migraine and other vascular headaches, menstrual cramps, and other conditions. When patients fail to respond to one NSAID, another may be tried. The greatest effectiveness often requires trial and error of several different NSAIDs.

HOW IT WORKS
NSAIDs work by interfering with the formation of prostaglandins, naturally occurring substances in the body that cause inflammation and make nerves more sensitive to pain impulses. NSAIDs also have other modes of action that are not as well understood.

▼ DOSAGE GUIDELINES

RANGE AND FREQUENCY
Adults: 1,200 mg once a day. The maximum daily dose is 1,800 mg divided into smaller amounts taken 2 or 3 times a day. Children: Consult your pediatrician.

ONSET OF EFFECT
From 30 minutes to several hours or longer.

DURATION OF ACTION
Varies.

DIETARY ADVICE
Take it with food; maintain your usual food and fluid intake.

STORAGE
Store it in a tightly sealed container away from moisture, heat, and direct light.

MISSED DOSE
Take it as soon as you remember. If it is near the time for the next dose, skip the missed dose and resume your regular dosage schedule. Do not double the next dose.

STOPPING THE DRUG
The decision to stop taking the drug should be made in consultation with your doctor.

PROLONGED USE
Prolonged use can cause gastrointestinal problems such as ulceration and bleeding, kidney dysfunction, and liver inflammation. Consult your doctor about the need for medical examinations and laboratory tests.

▼ PRECAUTIONS

Over 60: Because of the potentially greater consequences of gastrointestinal side effects, the dose of NSAIDs for older patients, especially those over age 70, is often cut in half.

Driving and Hazardous Work: Avoid such activities until you determine how the medicine affects you.

Alcohol: Avoid alcohol when using this medication because it increases the risk of stomach irritation.

Pregnancy: Avoid or discontinue using this drug if you are pregnant or if you plan to become pregnant.

Breast Feeding: Oxaprozin passes into breast milk; avoid use while nursing.

Infants and Children: May be used in exceptional circumstances; consult your doctor.

Special Concerns: Because NSAIDs can interfere with blood coagulation, this drug should be stopped at least 3 days prior to any surgery.

OVERDOSE
Symptoms: Severe nausea, vomiting, headache, seizures, confusion.

What to Do: Call your doctor, emergency medical services (EMS), or the nearest poison control center immediately.

▼ INTERACTIONS

DRUG INTERACTIONS
Do not take this drug with aspirin or any other NSAIDs without your doctor's approval. In addition, consult your doctor if you are taking antihypertensives, steroids, anticoagulants, antibiotics, itraconazole or ketoconazole, plicamycin, penicillamine, valproic acid, phenytoin, cyclosporine, digitalis drugs, lithium, methotrexate, probenecid, triamterene, or zidovudine.

FOOD INTERACTIONS
No known food interactions.

DISEASE INTERACTIONS
Consult your doctor if you have any of the following: bleeding problems, ulcers or inflammation of the stomach and intestines, diabetes, systemic lupus erythematosus (SLE, lupus), anemia, asthma, epilepsy, Parkinson's disease, kidney stones, or a history of heart disease or alcohol abuse. Use of oxaprozin may cause complications in patients with liver or kidney disease, because these organs work together to remove the medication from the body.

☰ SIDE EFFECTS ☰

SERIOUS
Shortness of breath or wheezing, with or without swelling of legs or other signs of heart failure; chest pain; peptic ulcer disease with vomiting of blood; black, tarry stools; decreasing kidney function. Call your doctor immediately.

COMMON
Nausea, vomiting, heartburn, diarrhea, constipation, headache, dizziness, sleepiness.

LESS COMMON
Ulcers or sores in mouth, depression, rashes or blistering of skin, ringing sound in the ears, unusual tingling or numbness of the hands or feet, seizures, blurred vision. Also elevated potassium levels, decreased blood counts; such problems can be detected by your doctor.

OXYCODONE HYDROCHLORIDE

Available in: Oral solution, tablets, controlled-release tablets
Available OTC? No   **As Generic?** No
Drug Class: Opioid (narcotic) analgesic

▼ USAGE INFORMATION

WHY IT'S PRESCRIBED
To relieve moderate to severe pain.

HOW IT WORKS
Opioid analgesics such as oxycodone relieve pain by acting on specific areas of the central nervous system (the brain and spinal cord) that process pain signals from nerves throughout the body.

▼ DOSAGE GUIDELINES

RANGE AND FREQUENCY
Adults: 5 mg every 3 to 6 hours or 10 mg 3 to 4 times a day as needed. Children: Dosages must be determined by your pediatrician. Controlled-release tablets: Your doctor will determine the proper dosage for you.

ONSET OF EFFECT
10 to 15 minutes.

DURATION OF ACTION
3 to 6 hours.

DIETARY ADVICE
This medication can be taken with food or milk to lessen stomach upset.

STORAGE
Store it in a tightly sealed container away from moisture, heat, and direct light. Do not freeze the liquid form.

MISSED DOSE
If you are taking oxycodone on a fixed schedule, take it as soon as you remember. If it is near the time for the next dose, skip the missed dose and resume your regular dosage schedule. Do not double the next dose.

STOPPING THE DRUG
The decision to stop taking the drug should be made by your doctor.

PROLONGED USE
You should see your doctor regularly for tests and physical examinations if you must take this medication for an extended period. Prolonged use of oxycodone can cause physical dependence.

▼ PRECAUTIONS

Over 60: Adverse reactions may be more likely and more severe in older patients.

Driving and Hazardous Work: Avoid such activities until you determine how the medicine affects you.

Alcohol: Avoid alcohol.

Pregnancy: Human studies have not been done. Before using this drug, tell your doctor if you are pregnant or plan to become pregnant. Overuse during pregnancy can cause drug dependence in the fetus.

Breast Feeding: Oxycodone may pass into breast milk; caution is advised. Consult your doctor for advice.

Infants and Children: Adverse reactions to oxycodone may be more likely and more severe in children. Consult your doctor.

Special Concerns: If you feel that the medication is not working properly after a few weeks, do not increase the dose on your own. Consult your doctor. Before having surgery, tell the doctor or dentist in charge that you are taking this drug. The controlled-release tablets are prescribed for use only in opioid-tolerant patients requiring daily doses of 160 mg or more.

OVERDOSE
Symptoms: Confusion; severe drowsiness, weakness, or dizziness; slurred speech; small, pinpoint pupils; cold, clammy skin; slow breathing; seizures; loss of consciousness.

What to Do: Call your doctor, emergency medical services (EMS), or the nearest poison control center immediately.

▼ INTERACTIONS

DRUG INTERACTIONS
Consult your doctor for specific advice if you are taking carbamazepine or other medicine for seizures, barbiturates, sedatives, cough medicines, decongestants, antidepressants, other prescription pain medications, monoamine oxidase (MAO) inhibitors, naltrexone, rifampin, or zidovudine.

FOOD INTERACTIONS
No known food interactions.

DISEASE INTERACTIONS
Consult your doctor if you have any of the following: a history of alcohol or drug abuse; emotional illness; brain disorders or head injury; seizures; lung disease; prostate problems or other problems with urination; gallstones; colitis; heart, or kidney, liver, or thyroid disease.

SIDE EFFECTS

SERIOUS
Serious side effects of oxycodone are indistinguishable from those of overdose: Confusion; severe drowsiness, weakness, or dizziness; slurred speech; small, pinpoint pupils; cold, clammy skin; slow breathing; seizures; loss of consciousness.

COMMON
Dizziness or lightheadedness, nausea or vomiting, drowsiness, constipation, itching.

LESS COMMON
Swelling in the feet, sweating, false sense of well-being (euphoria), urinary retention.

OXYCODONE/ACETAMINOPHEN

Available in: Capsules, oral solution, tablets
Available OTC? No   **As Generic?** Yes
Drug Class: Opioid (narcotic) analgesic

▼ USAGE INFORMATION

WHY IT'S PRESCRIBED
To relieve moderate to severe pain when nonprescription pain relievers prove inadequate. A narcotic analgesic such as oxycodone, in combination with acetaminophen, may provide better pain relief than either medicine taken alone. Used together, relief may be achieved at lower doses of the two drugs.

HOW IT WORKS
Opioid medications such as oxycodone relieve pain by acting on specific areas of the central nervous system (the brain and the spinal cord) that process pain signals from nerves throughout the body. Acetaminophen appears to interfere with the action of prostaglandins, naturally occurring hormone-like substances in the body that cause inflammation and make nerves more sensitive to pain impulses.

▼ DOSAGE GUIDELINES

RANGE AND FREQUENCY
Adults: 1 capsule or tablet every 4 to 6 hours or 1 tsp of the oral solution every 4 to 6 hours.

ONSET OF EFFECT
Unknown.

DURATION OF ACTION
Unknown.

DIETARY ADVICE
This medication can be taken with food or milk to lessen stomach irritation.

STORAGE
Store in a tightly sealed container away from moisture, heat, and direct light.

MISSED DOSE
If you are taking the drug on a fixed schedule, take it as soon as you remember. However, if it is near the time for the next dose, skip the missed dose and resume your regular dosage schedule. Do not double the next dose.

STOPPING THE DRUG
The decision to stop taking the drug should be made by your doctor.

PROLONGED USE
See your doctor regularly for examinations and laboratory tests if long-term therapy is required. Prolonged use of narcotic drugs such as oxycodone can cause physical dependence; prolonged use of acetaminophen at high doses can cause liver damage.

▼ PRECAUTIONS

Over 60: Adverse reactions may be more likely and more severe in older patients.

Driving and Hazardous Work: Do not drive or engage in hazardous work until you determine how the medicine affects you.

Alcohol: Avoid alcohol.

Pregnancy: Human studies have not been done. Before you use this drug, tell your doctor if you are pregnant or plan to become pregnant. Overuse of the medication while you are pregnant can cause drug dependence in the fetus.

Breast Feeding: It is not known whether this medication passes into breast milk; caution is advised. Consult your doctor for advice.

Infants and Children: Adverse reactions may be more likely and more severe in children.

Special Concerns: If you feel that the medication is not working properly after a few weeks, do not increase the dose. Consult your doctor.

OVERDOSE
Symptoms: Severe dizziness or drowsiness; cold, clammy skin; difficult or slow breathing or shortness of breath; severe confusion; seizures; stomach cramps or pain; diarrhea; low blood pressure; constricted pupils of eyes; increased sweating; nausea or vomiting; irregular heartbeat; severe weakness.

What to Do: Call your doctor, emergency medical services (EMS), or the nearest poison control center immediately.

▼ INTERACTIONS

DRUG INTERACTIONS
Consult your doctor for specific advice if you are taking any prescription or over-the-counter drugs, especially drugs with acetaminophen; central nervous system depressants such as antihistamines or medicine for hay fever, allergies, or colds; barbiturates; seizure medications; muscle relaxants; anesthetics; tranquilizers, sedatives, or sleep aids.

FOOD INTERACTIONS
No known food interactions.

DISEASE INTERACTIONS
Consult your physician if you have a head injury or brain disease, an underactive thyroid, an enlarged prostate, seizures, kidney or liver disease, gallbladder problems, a blood disorder, or a history of alcohol or drug abuse.

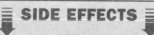
SIDE EFFECTS

SERIOUS
Bloody, dark, or cloudy urine; severe pain in lower back or side; pale or black, tarry stools; yellowish tinge to the eyes or skin; hallucinations; frequent urge to urinate; painful or difficult urination; sudden decrease in amount of urine; unusual bleeding or bruising; irregular heartbeat; skin rash, hives, or itching; unusual excitement; swelling of face; confusion; trembling or uncontrolled muscle movements; redness or flushing of face. Call your doctor immediately.

COMMON
Dizziness, lightheadedness, nausea or vomiting, drowsiness, constipation.

LESS COMMON
Allergic reaction, false sense of well-being (euphoria), depression, loss of appetite, blurring or change in vision, headache, sweating.

PAROXETINE HYDROCHLORIDE

Available in: Tablets, oral suspension
Available OTC? No   **As Generic?** No
Drug Class: Selective serotonin reuptake inhibitor (SSRI) antidepressant

▼ USAGE INFORMATION

WHY IT'S PRESCRIBED
To treat symptoms of major (classic) depression, obsessive-compulsive disorder, panic disorder, and social anxiety disorder.

HOW IT WORKS
Paroxetine affects levels of serotonin, an important brain chemical called a neurotransmitter, that is thought to be linked to mood, emotions, and mental state.

▼ DOSAGE GUIDELINES

RANGE AND FREQUENCY
Adults: To start, 20 mg once a day, usually taken in the morning; dose may be gradually increased by your doctor to 50 mg a day. Older adults: To start, 10 mg once a day; the dosage may be gradually increased by your doctor to 40 mg a day.

ONSET OF EFFECT
From 1 to 4 weeks.

DURATION OF ACTION
Unknown.

DIETARY ADVICE
This drug can be taken without regard to diet.

STORAGE
Store it in a tightly sealed container away from moisture, heat, and direct light.

MISSED DOSE
Take it as soon as you remember. If it is near the time for the next dose, skip the missed dose and resume your regular dosage schedule. Do not double the next dose.

STOPPING THE DRUG
Take as prescribed for the full treatment period, even if you begin to feel better. The decision to stop taking the drug should be made in consultation with your doctor. The dosage should be gradually tapered over 1 to 2 weeks.

PROLONGED USE
The usual course of therapy for depression lasts 6 months to 1 year; some patients may benefit from additional therapy.

▼ PRECAUTIONS

Over 60: Adverse reactions may be more likely and more severe in older patients. A lower dose may be necessary for people in this age group.

Driving and Hazardous Work: Use caution when driving or engaging in hazardous work until you determine how the medicine affects you.

Alcohol: Avoid alcohol.

Pregnancy: Adequate studies of paroxetine use during pregnancy have not been done. Before you take this medication, tell your doctor if you are pregnant or plan to become pregnant.

Breast Feeding: Paroxetine passes into breast milk; caution is advised. Consult your doctor for advice.

Infants and Children: The safety and effectiveness of paroxetine use in children have not been established.

Special Concerns: Take paroxetine at least 6 hours before bedtime to prevent insomnia, unless it causes drowsiness.

OVERDOSE
Symptoms: Agitation or irritability, severe drowsiness, dizziness, coma, dilated pupils, severe dry mouth, rapid heartbeat, trembling, severe nausea and vomiting.

What to Do: Call your doctor, emergency medical services (EMS), or the nearest poison control center immediately.

▼ INTERACTIONS

DRUG INTERACTIONS
Paroxetine and monoamine oxidase (MAO) inhibitors should not be used within 14 days of each other. Very serious side effects such as myoclonus (uncontrolled muscle spasms), hyperthermia (excessive rise in body temperature), and extreme stiffness may result. Do not take paroxetine with thioridazine; dangerous heart rhythm irregularities may result. Tryptophan, warfarin, sumatriptan, naratriptan, rizatriptan, and zolmitriptan may also interact with paroxetine; consult your doctor for advice.

FOOD INTERACTIONS
No known food interactions.

DISEASE INTERACTIONS
Caution is advised when taking paroxetine. Consult your doctor if you have a history of alcohol or drug abuse or a seizure disorder. Use of paroxetine may cause complications in patients with liver or kidney disease, because these organs work together to remove the medication from the body.

 SIDE EFFECTS

SERIOUS
Muscle pain or fatigue, lightheadedness or fainting, rash, agitation or irritability, severe drowsiness, dilated pupils, severe dry mouth, rapid heartbeat, trembling, severe nausea or vomiting. Call your doctor immediately.

COMMON
Insomnia, dizziness, sexual dysfunction, unusual fatigue, loss of initiative, nausea or vomiting, constipation, difficulty urinating, headache, trembling.

LESS COMMON
Decreased sexual desire, blurred vision, increased or decreased appetite, weight gain or loss, heartbeat irregularities, change in sense of taste. Also tingling, prickling, or burning feeling.

PENICILLIN V

Available in: Tablets, delayed-release tablets, liquid
Available OTC? No   **As Generic?** Yes
Drug Class: Penicillin antibiotic

USAGE INFORMATION

WHY IT'S PRESCRIBED
To treat a variety of bacterial infections, including those of the ear, nose, and throat; skin and soft tissues; genitourinary tract; and respiratory tract. It is also prescribed before surgery or dental work in patients at risk for endocarditis (infection of the lining of the heart, which may damage the heart's valves).

HOW IT WORKS
Penicillin V destroys susceptible bacteria by interfering with their ability to produce cell walls as they multiply.

DOSAGE GUIDELINES

RANGE AND FREQUENCY
Adults: 500 to 2,000 mg a day for infections, 2,000 mg to prevent bacterial endocarditis, or as ordered by physician. Children: 15 to 50 mg per 2.2 lb (1 kg) of body weight per day in divided doses to treat infections. To prevent infection after dental surgery: 2 g (1 g for children) 30 to 60 minutes before procedure, then 1 g (500 mg for children) 6 hours afterward.

ONSET OF EFFECT
Unknown.

DURATION OF ACTION
Up to 6 hours.

DIETARY ADVICE
Take it on an empty stomach 1 to 2 hours before or 3 to 4 hours after a meal.

STORAGE
Store in a tightly sealed container away from heat and direct light.

MISSED DOSE
Take it as soon as you remember. If it is near the time for the next dose, skip the missed dose and resume your regular dosage schedule. Do not double the next dose.

STOPPING THE DRUG
It is very important to take this drug as prescribed for the full treatment period. Stopping the medicine prematurely may lead to serious complications.

PROLONGED USE
Prolonged use of any antibiotic increases the risk of superinfection (a more severe and drug-resistant infection); caution is advised.

PRECAUTIONS

Over 60: No special problems are expected.

Driving and Hazardous Work: The use of penicillin should not impair your ability to perform such tasks safely.

Alcohol: No special precautions are necessary.

Pregnancy: Adequate studies of penicillin antibiotic use during pregnancy have not been done; however, no problems have been reported.

Breast Feeding: Penicillin V may pass into breast milk and cause problems in the nursing infant; avoid use while nursing.

Infants and Children: No special problems are expected.

Special Concerns: Penicillin V can cause false results on some urine sugar tests for patients with diabetes. If severe diarrhea occurs as a side effect of penicillin V, do not take antidiarrheal drugs; call your doctor. Oral contraceptives may not be effective while you are taking penicillin; consider other methods of birth control. Those who are prone to asthma, hay fever, hives, or allergies may be more likely to have an allergic reaction to a penicillin antibiotic medication.

OVERDOSE
Symptoms: Severe nausea, vomiting, diarrhea, seizures.

What to Do: An overdose of penicillin is unlikely to be life-threatening. However, if someone takes a much larger dose than prescribed, call your doctor or local emergency medical services (EMS) right away.

INTERACTIONS

DRUG INTERACTIONS
Consult your physician for specific advice if you are taking aminoglycosides, angiotensin-converting enzyme (ACE) inhibitors, diuretics, potassium supplements or drugs containing potassium, anticoagulants or other anticlotting drugs, nonsteroidal antiinflammatory drugs, oral contraceptives, sulfinpyrazone, cholestyramine, colestipol, methotrexate, probenecid, or rifampin.

FOOD INTERACTIONS
Acidic foods or juices can reduce the antibiotic effect.

DISEASE INTERACTIONS
Consult your doctor if you have a history of allergies, asthma, congestive heart failure, gastrointestinal disorders (especially colitis associated with the use of antibiotics), or impaired kidney function.

 SIDE EFFECTS

SERIOUS
Irregular, rapid, or labored breathing; lightheadedness or sudden fainting; joint pain; fever; severe abdominal pain and cramping with watery or bloody stools; severe allergic reaction (marked by sudden swelling of the lips, tongue, face, or throat; breathing difficulty; skin rash, itching, or hives); unusual bleeding or bruising; yellowish tinge to eyes or skin. Call your doctor immediately.

COMMON
Mild rash, mild diarrhea, nausea, vomiting, headache, vaginal discharge and itching, pain or white patches in the mouth or on the tongue.

LESS COMMON
Diminished urine output, chills, weakness, fatigue.

PHENAZOPYRIDINE HYDROCHLORIDE

Available in: Tablets
Available OTC? Yes   **As Generic?** Yes
Drug Class: Urinary analgesic

BRAND NAMES

Azo-Standard, Baridium, Eridium, Geridium, Phenazodine, Pyridiate, Pyridium, Urodine, Urogesic, Viridium

▼ USAGE INFORMATION

WHY IT'S PRESCRIBED
For short-term relief of symptoms caused by irritation of the urinary tract. Such symptoms include burning, pain, and discomfort during urination, as well as an increased urge to urinate with only small amounts of urine passed on each occasion. Irritation of the urinary tract commonly occurs as a result of bladder infection; phenazopyridine can ease symptoms but will not cure such an infection.

HOW IT WORKS
Phenazopyridine passes through—and has a local anesthetic effect on the lining of—the urinary tract, thus relieving the discomfort associated with infection or inflammation.

▼ DOSAGE GUIDELINES

RANGE AND FREQUENCY
Adults: 200 mg 3 times a day. Children: 1.8 mg per lb of body weight 3 times a day.

ONSET OF EFFECT
Unknown.

DURATION OF ACTION
Unknown.

DIETARY ADVICE
This medication is best taken with or after meals to minimize stomach upset.

STORAGE
Store it in a tightly sealed container away from heat, moisture, and direct light.

MISSED DOSE
Take it as soon as you remember. If it is near the time for the next dose, skip the missed dose and resume your regular dosage schedule. Do not double the next dose.

STOPPING THE DRUG
The decision to stop taking the drug should be made by your doctor. If it is being taken with an antibiotic, it should be taken for only 2 days (6 doses).

PROLONGED USE
Phenazopyridine is intended only for short-term use.

▼ PRECAUTIONS

Over 60: No special problems are expected.

Driving and Hazardous Work: Do not drive or engage in hazardous work until you determine how the medicine affects you.

Alcohol: No special precautions are necessary.

Pregnancy: Adequate human studies have not been done. Before taking phenazopyridine, tell your doctor if you are pregnant or plan to become pregnant.

Breast Feeding: Phenazopyridine may pass into breast milk; caution is advised. Consult your doctor for advice.

Infants and Children: No special problems are expected.

Special Concerns:
Phenazopyridine causes the urine to turn reddish orange. This is harmless, but it may stain clothing. The drug may also cause permanent staining or discoloration of soft contact lenses; it is best to wear glasses while taking this drug. For diabetic patients, phenazopyridine may cause false test results with sugar and urine ketone tests. Do not chew the tablets; chewing may cause permanent discoloration of teeth. Do not use any leftover medicine for future urinary tract infections without consulting your doctor.

OVERDOSE
Symptoms: Fatigue, paleness, shortness of breath, heart palpitations, bloody or cloudy urine, decreased urine output, swelling of the ankles and calves, lower back or flank pain, nausea or vomiting.

What to Do: An overdose is unlikely, but call your doctor, emergency medical services (EMS), or the nearest poison control center immediately if symptoms of overdose occur.

▼ INTERACTIONS

DRUG INTERACTIONS
Some drugs may interact with phenazopyridine. Consult your doctor for specific advice if you are taking any prescription or over-the-counter medication.

FOOD INTERACTIONS
No known food interactions.

DISEASE INTERACTIONS
Caution is advised when taking phenazopyridine. Consult your doctor if you have any of the following: glucose-6-phosphate dehydrogenase (G6PD) deficiency, hepatitis, uremia, pyelonephritis (kidney infection) during pregnancy, or other kidney disease.

≡ SIDE EFFECTS ≡

SERIOUS
Serious side effects are rare. Call your doctor immediately if you experience any of the following: difficulty breathing; swelling of the face, fingers, feet, or lower legs; blue or purple-blue skin color; unusual fatigue; fever; confusion; sudden decrease in urine output; shortness of breath; tightness in the chest; skin rash; yellow discoloration of the eyes or skin; unusual weight gain.

COMMON
Reddish-orange urine.

LESS COMMON
Indigestion, dizziness, stomach cramps or pain, headache.

PHENOBARBITAL

Available in: Capsules, elixir, tablets, injection
Available OTC? No **As Generic?** Yes
Drug Class: Barbiturate

▼ USAGE INFORMATION

WHY IT'S PRESCRIBED
Primarily used for sedation before surgery and to control certain types of seizures. With the availability of newer sleep-inducing drugs, it is now rarely used for short-term treatment of insomnia.

HOW IT WORKS
Barbiturates such as phenobarbital act as powerful sedatives by reducing activity in the central nervous system (the brain and spinal cord).

▼ DOSAGE GUIDELINES

RANGE AND FREQUENCY
For sedation— Adult oral dose: 30 to 120 mg 2 or 3 times a day, not to exceed 400 mg a day. Children's oral dose: 2 mg per 2.2 lb (1 kg) of body weight 3 times a day. For seizures— Adult oral dose: 60 to 250 mg a day. Children's oral dose: 1 to 6 mg per 2.2 lb of body weight per day. For insomnia— Adult oral dose: 100 to 320 mg at bedtime. Dosages for injectable forms of the drug will be determined by your doctor.

ONSET OF EFFECT
About 1 hour.

DURATION OF ACTION
10 to 12 hours.

DIETARY ADVICE
Tablets may be crushed and taken with fluid or food.

STORAGE
Store it in a tightly sealed container away from heat, moisture, and direct light.

MISSED DOSE
If you are taking phenobarbital regularly, take the missed dose as soon as you remember. If it is near the time for the next dose, skip the missed dose and resume your regular dosage schedule. Do not double the next dose.

STOPPING THE DRUG
The decision to stop taking the drug should be made by your doctor. There is a risk of withdrawal side effects when the drug is stopped suddenly.

⬇ SIDE EFFECTS ⬇

SERIOUS
Excitability, confusion, or excessive sedation to the point you cannot be awakened. Also yellow discoloration of eyes or skin; swollen eyelids, face, or lips; wheezing; rash (may be signs of drug allergy); sores on the lips or mouth. Call your doctor immediately.

COMMON
Clumsiness, unsteadiness, persistent drowsiness, dizziness or lightheadedness.

LESS COMMON
Anxiety or nervousness, nightmares, insomnia, constipation, feeling faint, irritability, headache, nausea or vomiting.

PROLONGED USE
Barbiturates may be habit-forming, and prolonged use may increase the risk of dependency. Phenobarbital, as well as other barbiturates, is used only for short-term treatment of insomnia. It usually is not effective when used for longer than 14 days.

▼ PRECAUTIONS

Over 60: Adverse reactions may be more likely and more severe in older patients and may require that smaller doses be used.

Driving and Hazardous Work: Because of sedative effects, do not drive or engage in hazardous work until you determine how the medicine affects you.

Alcohol: Avoid alcohol; its sedative effects are additive to those of the drug.

Pregnancy: Phenobarbital can cause birth defects and problems during pregnancy. Before you take phenobarbital, be sure to tell your doctor if you are pregnant or plan to become pregnant.

Breast Feeding: Phenobarbital passes into breast milk in small amounts and can cause side effects in breast-feeding infants. Consult your doctor for advice.

Infants and Children: As with older patients, infants and children are sensitive to the effects of phenobarbital.

Special Concerns: Phenobarbital may cause physical or mental dependence. Check with your doctor if you feel overly sedated or if you suffer withdrawal side effects when you stop taking the drug.

OVERDOSE
Symptoms: Severe sedation or excessive drowsiness, confusion, severe weakness, slurred speech, staggering walk, shortness of breath or troubled breathing.

What to Do: Call your doctor, emergency medical services (EMS), or the nearest poison control center immediately.

▼ INTERACTIONS

DRUG INTERACTIONS
Consult your doctor for specific advice if you are taking other seizure medications, central nervous system depressants, warfarin (blood thinner), or oral contraceptives. Phenobarbital may make oral contraceptives less effective.

FOOD INTERACTIONS
No known food interactions.

DISEASE INTERACTIONS
Caution is advised when taking phenobarbital. Consult your doctor if you have any of the following: kidney disease, liver disease, porphyria, anemia, hyperactivity, mental depression, or a history of alcohol or drug abuse.

PHENYTOIN

DiPhen, Dilantin, Diphenylan, Phenytex

Available in: Prompt and extended capsules, chewable tablets, oral suspension
Available OTC? No   **As Generic?** Yes
Drug Class: Anticonvulsant

▼ USAGE INFORMATION

WHY IT'S PRESCRIBED
To prevent or control seizures in the treatment of certain types of epilepsy and other conditions.

HOW IT WORKS
Phenytoin is thought to depress the activity of certain parts of the brain and to suppress the irregular and uncontrolled firing of neurons that causes seizures.

▼ DOSAGE GUIDELINES

RANGE AND FREQUENCY
Adults: 200 to 500 mg a day in 1 to 3 doses a day. Children: 5 to 300 mg a day as a single dose or in 2 divided doses. Some patients require higher doses. A low dose is used to start and then is gradually increased by your doctor.

ONSET OF EFFECT
Several hours.

DURATION OF ACTION
Maximum effect lasts for 24 hours or longer; effectiveness then gradually decreases.

DIETARY ADVICE
Take it with food to minimize stomach upset. Tablets may be crushed, chewed, or swallowed whole.

STORAGE
Store it in a tightly sealed container away from moisture, heat, and direct light.

MISSED DOSE
Take it as soon as you remember. Be especially careful about not missing a dose if you are taking this drug only once daily.

STOPPING THE DRUG
This medication should never be stopped abruptly; this may cause seizures. The dose is typically tapered over a period of weeks under the supervision of your doctor.

PROLONGED USE
This drug is often taken for prolonged periods. See your doctor for periodic checkups.

▼ PRECAUTIONS

Over 60: Older patients may require lower doses to minimize side effects.

Driving and Hazardous Work: Do not drive or engage in hazardous work until you determine how the medicine affects you.

Alcohol: May contribute to excessive drowsiness.

Pregnancy: Anticonvulsant drugs are associated with an increased risk of birth defects. However, seizures during pregnancy can also increase the risks to the unborn child. Discuss with your doctor the potential risks and benefits of using this drug during pregnancy. Folate supplementation is recommended beginning 1 to 2 months before conception and throughout pregnancy.

Breast Feeding: Phenytoin passes into breast milk, although at low levels. Consult your doctor for advice.

Infants and Children: No special problems are expected.

Special Concerns: The generic version of this drug is not recommended. Do not change the brand of phenytoin you are taking without consulting your doctor. The suspension form of phenytoin should be shaken well before you take it. Your doctor may advise you to wear a medical-alert bracelet or carry an identification card saying that you are taking this medication.

OVERDOSE
Symptoms: Blurred or double vision, difficulty walking, severe clumsiness or unsteadiness, severe confusion, dizziness or drowsiness.

What to Do: Call your doctor, emergency medical services (EMS), or the nearest poison control center immediately.

▼ INTERACTIONS

DRUG INTERACTIONS
Many other drugs may interact with phenytoin, including other anticonvulsants (carbamazepine, phenobarbital, primidone, valproic acid), allopurinol, amiodarone, anticancer drugs, chloramphenicol, chlorpheniramine, cimetidine, diazoxide, dicumarol, disulfiram, isoniazid, loxapine, phenylbutazone, rifampin, sulfonamides, trazodone, trimethoprim.

FOOD INTERACTIONS
No known food interactions.

DISEASE INTERACTIONS
Caution is advised in those with liver or kidney disease, because these organs work together to remove the medication from the body.

▼ SIDE EFFECTS

SERIOUS
Fever, sore throat, swollen glands, pointlike rash on the skin or mucous membranes, blistering or peeling, mouth sores or bleeding gums, easy bruising, pallor, weakness, confusion, or seizures may be a sign of a potentially fatal blood disorder or other complication. Call your doctor immediately.

COMMON
Sedation, lethargy, nervousness, dizziness, thickened gums, excessive growth of body and facial hair. High doses may cause abnormal movements of the eyes, mouth, tongue, or limbs. Prolonged use may cause mild nerve impairment in the arms or legs.

LESS COMMON
Constipation, acne, mild skin rash, incoordination. There are numerous additional possible side effects; consult your doctor if you are concerned about any adverse or unusual reactions.

PIOGLITAZONE HYDROCHLORIDE

Available in: Tablets
Available OTC? No   **As Generic?** No
Drug Class: Thiazolidinedione/antidiabetic agent

▼ USAGE INFORMATION

WHY IT'S PRESCRIBED
As a single therapeutic agent or as an adjunct (supplemental) therapy to a sulfonylurea, metformin, or insulin to control blood glucose levels in patients with non-insulin-dependent (type 2) diabetes.

HOW IT WORKS
Pioglitazone increases the body's sensitivity and response to insulin.

▼ DOSAGE GUIDELINES

RANGE AND FREQUENCY
To start, 15 to 30 mg once a day. For people taking only pioglitazone and who do not respond adequately, the dose may be increased by a doctor to no more than 45 mg once a day. If monotherapy does not control blood glucose, combination therapy should be considered. If hypoglycemia occurs when taking pioglitazone in combination with a sulfonylurea or insulin, it may be necessary to decrease the dose of the sulfonylurea or insulin.

ONSET OF EFFECT
Within 1 week.

DURATION OF ACTION
Unknown.

DIETARY ADVICE
Pioglitazone may be taken with or without food.

STORAGE
Store it in a tightly sealed container away from heat, moisture, and direct light.

MISSED DOSE
If it is the same day, take the missed dose as soon as you remember. If you miss an entire day's dose, resume your regular dosage schedule the next day and do not double the next dose.

STOPPING THE DRUG
The decision to stop taking pioglitazone should be made in consultation with your physician.

PROLONGED USE
See your doctor regularly for liver function tests if you must take pioglitazone for an extended period of time.

▼ PRECAUTIONS

Over 60: No special problems are expected.

Driving and Hazardous Work: Pioglitazone should not impair your ability to perform such tasks safely.

Alcohol: Drink only in moderation, if at all.

Pregnancy: Adequate studies of pioglitazone use during pregnancy have not been done. In general, insulin is the treatment of choice for controlling blood glucose levels during pregnancy. Pioglitazone should not be used during pregnancy unless your doctor believes the potential benefit justifies the potential risk to the fetus. Pioglitazone may stimulate ovulation in premenopausal women who have stopped ovulating. Contraception may be advised.

Breast Feeding: Pioglitazone may pass into breast milk; do not use it while nursing.

Infants and Children: Safety and effectiveness of pioglitazone have not been established in children.

Special Concerns: Another thiazolidinedione drug, troglitazone, has been associated with rare, serious, and sometimes fatal, liver-related side effects. Although no similar side effects have been reported for pioglitazone, liver function tests are recommended just prior to treatment, every 2 months for the first year, and periodically thereafter. If you develop unexplained symptoms of liver dysfunction, such as nausea, vomiting, abdominal pain, fatigue, loss of appetite, or dark urine, call your doctor immediately. It is important to follow your doctor's advice on diet, exercise, and other measures to help control diabetes.

OVERDOSE
Symptoms: No specific ones have been reported.

What to Do: No cases of overdose have been reported, but if someone takes a much larger dose than prescribed, call your doctor, emergency medical services (EMS), or the nearest poison control center immediately.

▼ INTERACTIONS

DRUG INTERACTIONS
No known drug interactions.

FOOD INTERACTIONS
No known food interactions.

DISEASE INTERACTIONS
Pioglitazone should not be taken by those with type 1 diabetes or for the treatment of diabetic ketoacidosis. Caution is advised if you have edema or heart failure. Consult your doctor prior to using pioglitazone if you have any type of liver abnormality.

 SIDE EFFECTS

SERIOUS
No serious side effects have been associated with the use of pioglitazone.

COMMON
Upper respiratory tract infection, sore throat.

LESS COMMON
Headache, sinusitis, muscle pain, tooth disorder, edema (swelling).

POTASSIUM CHLORIDE

Available in: Liquid, soluble granules, powder, tablets, sustained-release capsules
Available OTC? No **As Generic?** Yes
Drug Class: Electrolyte

▼ USAGE INFORMATION

WHY IT'S PRESCRIBED
To restore or maintain proper potassium levels in the body. Potassium is an electrolyte, a mineral that helps maintain proper fluid balance. It is also vital in the transmission of nerve impulses.

HOW IT WORKS
Potassium chloride is absorbed into body fluids and taken into the cells, where it is part of a number of metabolic actions, especially those that involve the release of energy. It also aids in the conduction of nerve impulses responsible for muscle movement and heart contraction.

▼ DOSAGE GUIDELINES

RANGE AND FREQUENCY
20 milliequivalents (mEq) to 100 mEq daily in divided doses. A single dose should not exceed 20 mEq.

ONSET OF EFFECT
Unknown.

DURATION OF ACTION
Unknown.

DIETARY ADVICE
It must be taken after meals or with food and a glass of water or other liquid. Follow all special dietary guidelines as outlined by your doctor.

STORAGE
Store it in a tightly sealed container away from heat and direct light. Keep liquid forms of potassium refrigerated, but do not allow them to freeze.

MISSED DOSE
If you remember within 2 hours, take the missed dose with food or liquids and resume your regular dosage schedule. If you remember after 2 hours, skip the missed dose and return to your regular dosage schedule. Do not double the next dose.

STOPPING THE DRUG
Do not stop taking potassium without first consulting your physician. Be very careful not to stop taking potassium abruptly if you are also taking digitalis drugs (digoxin).

PROLONGED USE
Extended use requires periodic testing of blood potassium levels by your doctor.

▼ PRECAUTIONS

Over 60: Older people may be at greater risk of retaining too much potassium because of age-related changes in the kidneys' ability to excrete it. Older patients should have their potassium levels checked regularly.

Driving and Hazardous Work: No special problems are expected.

Alcohol: No special problems are expected.

Pregnancy: Potassium supplements are considered safe during pregnancy if used exactly as prescribed.

Breast Feeding: Potassium may pass into breast milk. Consult your doctor for specific advice.

Infants and Children: Although the safety and effectiveness of potassium use by children have not been established, no specific problems have been documented.

Special Concerns: Remember that the foods in your diet must also be considered when calculating your total intake of potassium. Be certain to read all labels carefully, especially on all products labeled "low-sodium," such as canned foods and some breads, many of which contain potassium. Do not crush sustained-release forms. Swallow tablets without chewing, sucking, or crushing. Be sure the powder form is completely dissolved before ingesting it.

OVERDOSE
Symptoms: Irregular heartbeat; muscle weakness, which may progress to paralysis of the diaphragm and interfere with breathing.

What to Do: Call your doctor, emergency medical services (EMS), or the nearest poison control center immediately.

▼ INTERACTIONS

DRUG INTERACTIONS
The following drugs may interact adversely with potassium chloride. Consult your doctor for advice if you are taking digitalis drugs, potassium-sparing diuretics, thiazide diuretics, NSAIDs, beta-blockers, heparin, triamterene, anticholinergics, or ACE inhibitors.

FOOD INTERACTIONS
To prevent ingestion of too much potassium, discuss your diet with your doctor. Foods high in potassium include avocados, bananas, broccoli, dried fruits, grapefruit, beans, meats, nuts, spinach, low-salt milk, squash, melon, brussels sprouts, zucchini, frozen orange juice, and tomatoes.

DISEASE INTERACTIONS
Consult your doctor if you have any of the following medical conditions: intestinal obstruction, dehydration, severe diarrhea, compression of the esophagus, delayed gastric emptying, peptic ulcer, heart blockage, or a predisposition to retaining the mineral potassium.

⬇ SIDE EFFECTS ⬇

SERIOUS
Numbness or tingling in the hands, feet, or lips; slowed or irregular heartbeat; breathing difficulty; unusual fatigue or weakness; confusion. Stop taking the drug and consult your doctor at once.

COMMON
Diarrhea, abdominal discomfort, gas, nausea and vomiting.

LESS COMMON
Black or bloody stools, pain when swallowing. Consult your doctor if such symptoms persist.

PRAVASTATIN

Available in: Tablets
Available OTC? No   **As Generic?** No
Drug Class: Antilipidemic (cholesterol-lowering agent)

▼ USAGE INFORMATION

WHY IT'S PRESCRIBED
To treat high cholesterol. Usually prescribed after first lines of treatment—diet, weight loss, and exercise—fail to reduce total and low-density lipoprotein (LDL) cholesterol to acceptable levels.

HOW IT WORKS
Pravastatin blocks the action of an enzyme required for the manufacture of cholesterol, thereby interfering with its formation. By lowering the amount of cholesterol in the liver cells, pravastatin increases the formation of receptors for LDL and thus reduces blood levels of total and LDL cholesterol. In addition to lowering LDL cholesterol, pravastatin modestly reduces triglyceride levels and raises high-density lipoprotein (HDL; the so-called "good") cholesterol.

▼ DOSAGE GUIDELINES

RANGE AND FREQUENCY
The initial dose is 10 to 20 mg once a day. The dose may be increased to a maximum of 40 mg per day. The drug is most effective when taken in the evening.

ONSET OF EFFECT
2 to 4 weeks.

DURATION OF ACTION
The effect persists for the duration of therapy.

DIETARY ADVICE
Cholesterol-lowering drugs are only one part of a total program that should include regular exercise and a healthy diet. The American Heart Association publishes a "Healthy Heart" diet, which is recommended.

STORAGE
Store it in a tightly sealed container away from heat and direct light.

MISSED DOSE
Take it as soon as you remember. Take the next scheduled dose at the proper time and resume your regular dosage schedule as prescribed. Do not double the next dose.

STOPPING THE DRUG
The decision to stop taking the drug should be made in consultation with your doctor. Once the medication is discontinued, blood cholesterol will probably return to its original elevated level.

PROLONGED USE
Side effects are more likely with prolonged use. As you continue with pravastatin, your doctor will periodically order blood tests to evaluate liver function.

▼ PRECAUTIONS

Over 60: No special problems are expected.

Driving and Hazardous Work: The use of pravastatin should not impair your ability to perform such tasks safely.

Alcohol: No special precautions are necessary.

Pregnancy: Pravastatin should not be used during pregnancy or by women who plan to become pregnant in the near future.

Breast Feeding: This drug is not recommended for women who are nursing.

Infants and Children: Long-term effects of pravastatin in children have not been determined. It is rarely used in young patients; consult your doctor.

Special Concerns: Important elements of treatment for high cholesterol include proper diet, weight loss, regular moderate exercise, and the avoidance of certain medications that may increase cholesterol levels. Because pravastatin has potential side effects, it is important that you maintain a recommended healthy diet and cooperate with other treatments your physician may suggest.

OVERDOSE
Symptoms: Overdose is unlikely to occur.

What to Do: Emergency instructions not applicable.

▼ INTERACTIONS

DRUG INTERACTIONS
Consult your doctor if you are taking cyclosporine; gemfibrozil; niacin; antibiotics, especially erythromycin; or medications for fungus infections. All of these drugs may increase the risk of myositis (muscle inflammation) when taken with pravastatin and may lead to kidney failure.

FOOD INTERACTIONS
No known food interactions.

DISEASE INTERACTIONS
Consult your doctor if you have any of the following problems: liver, kidney, or muscle disease or a medical history involving organ transplantation or recent surgery.

≡ SIDE EFFECTS ≡

SERIOUS
Fever, unusual or unexplained muscle aches and tenderness. Call your doctor right away.

COMMON
Side effects occur in only 1% to 2% of patients. These include constipation or diarrhea, dizziness, gas, headache, heartburn, nausea, skin rash, stomach pain, and an increase in liver enzymes (detectable by your doctor).

LESS COMMON
Insomnia.

PREDNISONE

Available in: Oral suspension, syrup, tablets
Available OTC? No   **As Generic?** Yes
Drug Class: Corticosteroid

▼ USAGE INFORMATION

WHY IT'S PRESCRIBED
To treat numerous conditions that involve inflammation (a response by body tissues, producing redness, warmth, swelling, and pain). Such conditions include arthritis, allergic reactions, asthma, some skin diseases, multiple sclerosis flare-ups, and other autoimmune diseases. Also prescribed to treat deficiency of natural steroid hormones.

HOW IT WORKS
Prednisone mimics the effects of the body's natural corticosteroid hormones. It depresses the synthesis, release, and activity of inflammation-producing body chemicals. It also suppresses the activity of the immune system.

▼ DOSAGE GUIDELINES

RANGE AND FREQUENCY
Adults and teenagers—For severe inflammation or to suppress the immune system: 5 to 100 mg a day in divided doses. For multiple sclerosis: 200 mg daily for 1 week, then 80 mg every other day for 1 month. Children: Consult your pediatrician.

ONSET OF EFFECT
Variable.

DURATION OF ACTION
Variable.

DIETARY ADVICE
It can be taken with food or milk to minimize stomach upset. Your doctor may suggest a low-salt, high-potassium, high-protein diet.

STORAGE
Store it in a tightly sealed container away from moisture, heat, and direct light. Do not allow liquid forms to freeze.

MISSED DOSE
Take it as soon as you remember. If you take several doses a day and it is close to the next dose, double the next dose. If you take 1 dose a day and you do not remember until the next day, skip the missed dose and do not double the next dose.

STOPPING THE DRUG
With long-term therapy, do not stop taking the drug abruptly; the dosage should be decreased gradually.

PROLONGED USE
Long-term use may lead to cataracts, diabetes, hypertension, or osteoporosis; see your doctor for regular examinations.

▼ PRECAUTIONS

Over 60: Adverse reactions may be more likely and more severe in older adults.

Driving and Hazardous Work: Avoid such activities until you determine how the medicine affects you.

Alcohol: Alcohol may cause stomach problems; avoid it unless your physician approves occasional moderate drinking.

Pregnancy: Overuse during pregnancy can retard the child's growth and cause other developmental problems. Consult your doctor.

Breast Feeding: Do not use this drug while nursing.

Infants and Children: Prednisone may retard the growth and development of bone and other tissues.

Special Concerns: This drug can lower resistance to infection. Avoid immunizations with live vaccines. Patients undergoing long-term therapy should wear a medical-alert bracelet. Call your doctor if you develop a fever.

OVERDOSE
Symptoms: Fever, muscle or joint pain, nausea, dizziness, fainting, difficulty breathing. Prolonged overuse: Moon face, obesity, unusual hair growth, acne, loss of sexual function, muscle wasting.

What to Do: Call your doctor, emergency medical services (EMS), or the nearest poison control center immediately.

▼ INTERACTIONS

DRUG INTERACTIONS
Consult your doctor for specific advice if you are taking aminoglutethimide, antacids, barbiturates, carbamazepine, griseofulvin, mitotane, phenylbutazone, phenytoin, primidone, rifampin, injectable amphotericin B, oral antidiabetes agents, insulin, digitalis drugs, diuretics, or medications containing potassium or sodium.

FOOD INTERACTIONS
Avoid excess sodium.

DISEASE INTERACTIONS
Consult your doctor if you have a history of bone disease, chicken pox, measles, gastrointestinal disorders, diabetes, glaucoma, heart disease, hypertension, liver or kidney disorders, high blood cholesterol, thyroid problems, myasthenia gravis, or lupus or have recently had a serious problem.

☰ SIDE EFFECTS ☰

SERIOUS
Vision problems, frequent urination, increased thirst, rectal bleeding, blistering skin, confusion, hallucinations, paranoia, euphoria, depression, mood swings, redness and swelling at injection site. Call your doctor immediately.

COMMON
Increased appetite, indigestion, nervousness, insomnia, greater susceptibility to infections, increased blood pressure, slowed wound healing, weight gain, easy bruising, fluid retention.

LESS COMMON
Change in skin color, dizziness, headache, increased sweating, unusual growth of body or facial hair, increased blood sugar, peptic ulcers, adrenal insufficiency, muscle weakness, cataracts, glaucoma, osteoporosis.

PROMETHAZINE HYDROCHLORIDE

Available in: Tablets, syrup, injection, suppositories
Available OTC? No **As Generic?** Yes
Drug Class: Antihistamine

▼ USAGE INFORMATION

WHY IT'S PRESCRIBED
To relieve the symptoms of hay fever and other allergies, to prevent motion sickness, and to treat nausea and vomiting. Promethazine may also be used in some patients for its sedative effect.

HOW IT WORKS
Promethazine interferes with but does not block the release and action of histamine, a naturally occurring substance in the body that causes swelling, itching, sneezing, watery eyes, hives, and other symptoms of allergic reaction. Promethazine also has an anticholinergic effect, meaning that this medication blocks the transmission of certain nerve impulses, which in turn relaxes the smooth muscle tissue that controls activity in the bladder, stomach, intestine, lungs, and other organ systems. This effect thereby helps to ease the symptoms of motion sickness, nausea, gastrointestinal upset, and anxiety.

▼ DOSAGE GUIDELINES

RANGE AND FREQUENCY
Tablets or syrup—For allergies: Adults and teenagers: 10 to 12.5 mg 4 times a day, before meals and at bedtime, or 25 mg at bedtime. Children 2 years and older: 5 to 12.5 mg 3 times a day or 25 mg at bedtime. For nausea and vomiting: Adults and teenagers: 25 mg for first dose, then 10 to 25 mg every 4 to 6 hours as needed. Children 2 years and older: 10 to 25 mg every 4 to 6 hours. To prevent motion sickness: Adults and teenagers: 25 mg taken 30 to 60 minutes before traveling. Children 2 years and older: 10 to 25 mg 30 to 60 minutes before traveling. For dizziness: Adults and teenagers: 25 mg 2 times a day. Children 2 years and older: 10 to 25 mg 2 times a day. As a sedative: Adults and teenagers: 25 to 50 mg. Children 2 years and older: 10 to 25 mg. Injection—For allergies: Adults and teenagers: 25 mg into a vein or muscle. Children 2 years and older: 6.25 to 12.5 mg 3 times a day into a muscle or 25 mg at bedtime. For nausea and vomiting: Adults and teenagers: 12.5 to 25 mg every 4 hours into a vein or muscle. Children 2 years and older: 12.5 to 25 mg every 4 to 6 hours into a muscle. As a sedative: Adults and teens: 25 to 50 mg injected into a vein or muscle. Children 2 years and older: 12.5 to 25 mg into a muscle. Suppositories—For allergies: Adults and teens: 25 mg at first; 25 mg 2 hours later if needed. Children 2 years and older: 6.25 to 12.5 mg 3 times a day or 25 mg at bedtime. For nausea and vomiting: Adults and teenagers: 25 mg at first, then 12.5 to 25 mg every 4 to 6 hours if needed. Children 2 years and older: 12.5 to 25 mg every 4 to 6 hours. For dizziness: Adults and teenagers: 25 mg 2 times a day. Children 2 years and older: 12.5 to 25 mg 2 times a day. As a sedative: Adults and teenagers: 25 to 50 mg. Children 2 years and older: 12.25 to 25 mg.

ONSET OF EFFECT
15 to 60 minutes orally or by suppository; 20 minutes after injection.

DURATION OF ACTION
Up to 12 hours.

DIETARY ADVICE
Take it with food or milk to lessen stomach irritation.

STORAGE
Store in a tightly sealed container away from heat and direct light at room temperature. Do not store the tablets in a place with excessive moisture, such as the bathroom medicine cabinet. Do not allow the syrup or injection to freeze.

MISSED DOSE
Take it as soon as you remember. If it is near the time for the next dose, skip the missed dose and resume your regular dosage schedule. Do not double the next dose.

STOPPING THE DRUG
You should take it as prescribed for the full treatment period, but you may stop taking the drug if you are feeling better before the scheduled end of therapy.

PROLONGED USE
See your doctor regularly if you take this medicine for a prolonged period. Prolonged use of this antihistamine may decrease salivary flow, which may lead to thrush (white, furry patches in the mouth caused by fungal infection), periodontal disease (disease and decay of the teeth, gums, jaw, and other supportive structures in the mouth), dental caries (cavities), and gingivitis (gum disease). Practice good oral hygiene to prevent these disorders.

▼ PRECAUTIONS

Over 60: Adverse reactions may be more likely and more severe in older patients.

≣ SIDE EFFECTS ≣

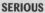

SERIOUS
Sore throat and fever, unusual fatigue, unusual bleeding or bruising. Call your doctor immediately.

COMMON
Drowsiness, thickening of mucus.

LESS COMMON
Blurred vision; confusion; difficult or painful urination; dizziness; dry mouth, nose, or throat; increased sensitivity of skin to sunlight; faintness; increased sweating; stinging or burning of rectum (suppository form); loss of appetite; ringing or buzzing in ears; skin rash; fast heartbeat; unusual excitement or irritability.

Driving and Hazardous Work: Do not drive or engage in hazardous work until you determine how the medicine affects you.

Alcohol: Avoid alcohol.

Pregnancy: Promethazine has not been shown to cause birth defects in animals. Thorough human studies have not been done. However, if the mother takes the drug during the 2 weeks before delivery, the baby may have jaundice or problems with blood clotting. Before you take it, tell your doctor if you are pregnant or plan to become pregnant.

Breast Feeding: Promethazine passes into breast milk; avoid or discontinue use while nursing. The flow of breast milk may be decreased as a result of the medication.

Infants and Children: Adverse reactions, such as seizures, may be more common and more severe in infants and children. It is not recommended for children with a history of breathing difficulty while sleeping or with a family history of sudden infant death syndrome (SIDS). Children and adolescents with signs of Reye's syndrome should not take this drug, especially by injection. Its side effects may be mistaken for symptoms of Reye's syndrome.

Special Concerns: If you have an allergy test, stop taking promethazine 4 days before the test and tell the doctor that you were taking promethazine.

OVERDOSE

Symptoms: Clumsiness; insomnia; seizures; severe dryness of mouth, nose, or throat; redness of face; hallucinations; muscle spasms; trouble breathing; jerky movements of head and face; dizziness; trembling and shaking of the hands.

What to Do: Call your doctor, emergency medical services (EMS), or the nearest poison control center immediately.

▼ INTERACTIONS

DRUG INTERACTIONS
Consult your doctor for specific advice if you are taking amoxapine, antipsychotics, medications containing alcohol, barbiturates, methyldopa, metoclopramide, metyrosine, epinephrine, metrizamide, pemoline, pimozide, rauwolfia alkaloids, anticholinergics, central nervous system depressants, maprotiline, other antihistamines, tricyclic antidepressants, levodopa, or monoamine oxidase (MAO) inhibitors.

FOOD INTERACTIONS
No known food interactions.

DISEASE INTERACTIONS
Consult your doctor if you have any of the following: blood disease, heart or blood vessel disease, enlarged prostate, urinary tract blockage, epilepsy, glaucoma, Reye's syndrome, jaundice, or liver disease.

PROPOXYPHENE/ACETAMINOPHEN

Available in: Tablets
Available OTC? No   **As Generic?** Yes
Drug Class: Opioid (narcotic) analgesic

BRAND NAMES

Darvocet-N 100, Darvocet-N 50, E-Lor, Propacet 100, Wygesic

▼ USAGE INFORMATION

WHY IT'S PRESCRIBED
To relieve mild to moderate pain.

HOW IT WORKS
Opioids such as propoxyphene relieve pain by acting on specific areas of the spinal cord and the brain that process pain signals from nerves throughout the body. Acetaminophen appears to interfere with the action of prostaglandins, naturally occurring substances in the body that cause inflammation and make nerves more sensitive to pain impulses.

▼ DOSAGE GUIDELINES

RANGE AND FREQUENCY
Adults: 1 or 2 tablets, depending on strength, every 4 to 6 hours. Children: Dose must be determined individually by your pediatrician.

ONSET OF EFFECT
Within 2 hours.

DURATION OF ACTION
Unknown.

DIETARY ADVICE
It can be taken with food to lessen stomach irritation.

STORAGE
Store it in a tightly sealed container away from moisture, heat, and direct light.

MISSED DOSE
If you are taking the drug on a fixed schedule, take it as soon as you remember. If it is near the time for the next dose, skip the missed dose and resume your regular dosage schedule. Do not double the next dose.

STOPPING THE DRUG
The decision to stop taking this medication should be made only in consultation with your doctor.

PROLONGED USE
You should see your doctor regularly for tests and examinations if you take this medication for a prolonged period. Prolonged use can cause nerve damage as well as physical dependence.

▼ PRECAUTIONS

Over 60: Adverse reactions may be more likely and more severe in older patients.

Driving and Hazardous Work: Do not drive or engage in hazardous work until you determine how the medicine affects you.

Alcohol: Avoid alcohol.

Pregnancy: Propoxyphene has not caused birth defects in animals. Human studies have not been done. Before you use this medication, tell your doctor if you are pregnant or plan to become pregnant. Overuse of the medication during pregnancy can cause physical dependence in the newborn.

Breast Feeding: Propoxyphene and acetaminophen pass into breast milk and may cause sedation in the nursing infant. Consult your doctor for advice.

Infants and Children: Adverse reactions may be more likely and more severe in children. Consult your pediatrician for advice.

Special Concerns: If you feel that the medication is not working properly after a few weeks, do not increase the dose on your own. Consult your doctor.

OVERDOSE
Symptoms: Severe dizziness or drowsiness; cold, clammy skin; difficult or slow breathing or shortness of breath; severe confusion; seizures; stomach cramps or pain; diarrhea; low blood pressure; increased sweating; constricted pupils; nausea or vomiting; irregular heartbeat; severe weakness.

What to Do: Call your doctor, emergency medical services (EMS), or the nearest poison control center immediately.

▼ INTERACTIONS

DRUG INTERACTIONS
Consult your doctor for specific advice if you are taking any prescription or over-the-counter drugs, especially other drugs containing acetaminophen, or central nervous system depressants, which include antihistamines or decongestants for hay fever, allergies, or colds; barbiturates; seizure medication; muscle relaxants; anesthetics; and tranquilizers, sedatives, or sleep-inducing medications.

FOOD INTERACTIONS
No known food interactions.

DISEASE INTERACTIONS
Consult your doctor if you have a head injury or brain disease, an underactive thyroid, an enlarged prostate, seizures, kidney or liver disease, gall bladder problems, a blood disorder, or a history of alcohol or drug abuse.

≡ SIDE EFFECTS ≡

SERIOUS
Bloody, dark, or cloudy urine; severe pain in the lower back or side; pale or black, tarry stools; yellow discoloration of eyes or skin (jaundice); hallucinations; frequent urge to urinate; painful or difficult urination; sudden decrease in urine output; increased sweating; unusual bleeding or bruising; irregular heartbeat; skin rash, hives, or itching; excitability; ringing or buzzing in the ears; pinpoint red spots on skin; sore throat and fever; confusion; trembling or uncontrolled muscle movements; redness, flushing, or swelling of the face. Call your doctor immediately.

COMMON
Dizziness, lightheadedness, constipation, nausea, vomiting, drowsiness, unusual fatigue.

LESS COMMON
Stomach pain, false sense of well-being (euphoria), depression, loss of appetite, blurred vision, nightmares or unusual dreams, dry mouth, headache, nervousness, insomnia.

PROPRANOLOL HYDROCHLORIDE

Available in: Extended-release capsules, oral solution, tablets, injection
Available OTC? No   **As Generic?** Yes
Drug Class: Beta-blocker

▼ USAGE INFORMATION

WHY IT'S PRESCRIBED
To treat angina, mild to moderate high blood pressure, irregular heartbeat (cardiac arrhythmias), hypertrophic cardiomyopathy (weakness of the heart muscle), heart attack, pheochromocytoma, tremors, and migraine headaches.

HOW IT WORKS
Propranolol blocks nerve impulses to various parts of the body, which accounts for its many effects. For example, propranolol slows the heart rate and force of the contraction (which helps lower blood pressure), decreases the heart's oxygen requirement (which helps prevent angina), and helps stabilize heart rhythm.

▼ DOSAGE GUIDELINES

RANGE AND FREQUENCY
Adults—For angina: 80 to 320 mg a day in 2, 3, or 4 doses.
For high blood pressure: 40 mg 2 times a day; may be increased up to 640 mg a day. For irregular heartbeat: 10 to 30 mg 3 or 4 times a day. For cardiomyopathy: 20 to 40 mg 3 or 4 times a day. For pheochromocytoma: 30 to 160 mg a day in divided doses. For preventing migraine headache: 20 mg 4 times a day; may be increased to 240 mg a day. For trembling: 40 mg 2 times a day; may be increased to 320 mg a day. Children—For high blood pressure: 0.5 mg to 4 mg per 2.2 lb (1 kg) of body weight a day. For irregular heartbeat: 0.5 to 4 mg per 2.2 lb of body weight a day in divided doses.

ONSET OF EFFECT
Within 30 minutes.

DURATION OF ACTION
Up to 12 hours.

DIETARY ADVICE
Mix the concentrated oral solution with water, juice, or a carbonated drink.

STORAGE
Store it in a tightly sealed container away from heat and direct light.

MISSED DOSE
Take it as soon as you remember. If it is near the time for the next dose, skip the missed dose and resume your regular dosage schedule. Do not double the next dose.

STOPPING THE DRUG
Do not stop taking this drug suddenly; the dosage must be slowly tapered under your physician's close supervision.

PROLONGED USE
Lifelong therapy with propranolol may be necessary; prolonged use may be associated with a greater incidence of side effects. Regular monitoring and evaluation by your doctor are advised.

▼ PRECAUTIONS

Over 60: Adverse reactions may be more likely and more severe in older patients.

Driving and Hazardous Work: Avoid such activities until you determine how the drug affects you.

Alcohol: Avoid alcohol.

Pregnancy: Consult your doctor to weigh the risks and benefits of using propranolol during pregnancy.

Breast Feeding: Propranolol passes into breast milk; caution is advised.

Infants and Children: The correct dosage will be determined by your pediatrician.

Special Concerns: Take extra care during exercise or hot weather to avoid dizziness and fainting. Check your pulse often; if it is slower than usual or less than 50 beats a minute, call your doctor.

OVERDOSE
Symptoms: Unusually slow or rapid heartbeat, severe dizziness or fainting, poor circulation in the hands (bluish skin), breathing difficulty, seizures.

What to Do: Call your doctor, emergency medical services (EMS), or the nearest poison control center immediately.

▼ INTERACTIONS

DRUG INTERACTIONS
Consult your doctor for specific advice if you are taking allergy shots, aminophylline, caffeine, oxtriphylline, theophylline, oral antidiabetics, insulin, calcium channel blockers, clonidine, guanabenz, or monoamine oxidase (MAO) inhibitors.

FOOD INTERACTIONS
No known food interactions.

DISEASE INTERACTIONS
It must be used with caution in people with diabetes, especially for insulin-dependent diabetes, because the drug may mask symptoms of hypoglycemia. Consult a doctor if you have allergies, bronchitis, emphysema, heart or blood vessel disease (including congestive heart failure and peripheral vascular disease), mental depression, myasthenia gravis, psoriasis, hyperthyroidism, kidney disease, or liver disease.

 ≡ SIDE EFFECTS ≡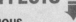

SERIOUS
Shortness of breath or wheezing; irregular or slow heartbeat (50 beats per minute or less); pain or feelings of tightness or pressure in the chest; swelling of the ankles, feet, and lower legs; depression. Call your doctor immediately.

COMMON
Dizziness or lightheadedness, especially when rising suddenly to a standing position; decreased sexual ability (erectile dysfunction) in men; unusual fatigue, weakness, or drowsiness; insomnia.

LESS COMMON
Anxiety, irritability; constipation; diarrhea; dry eyes; itching; nausea or vomiting; nightmares or intensely vivid dreams; numbness, tingling, or prickling in the fingers, toes, or scalp.

QUINAPRIL HYDROCHLORIDE

Available in: Tablets
Available OTC? No **As Generic?** No
Drug Class: Angiotensin-converting enzyme (ACE) inhibitor

▼ USAGE INFORMATION

WHY IT'S PRESCRIBED
To control high blood pressure (hypertension), to treat congestive heart failure (CHF), to treat patients with left ventricular dysfunction (damage to the pumping chamber of the heart), and to minimize further kidney damage in diabetics with mild kidney disease.

HOW IT WORKS
Angiotensin-converting enzyme (ACE) inhibitors block an enzyme that produces angiotensin, a naturally occurring substance that causes blood vessels to constrict and stimulates production of the adrenal hormone, aldosterone, which promotes sodium retention in the body. As a result, ACE inhibitors relax blood vessels (causing them to widen) and reduces sodium retention, which lowers blood pressure and so decreases the workload of the heart.

▼ DOSAGE GUIDELINES

RANGE AND FREQUENCY
10 mg once a day. Dosage may be increased to 20 to 80 mg a day taken in 1 or 2 doses.

ONSET OF EFFECT
Within 1 hour.

DURATION OF ACTION
24 hours.

DIETARY ADVICE
Take quinapril on an empty stomach about 1 hour before mealtime. Follow your doctor's dietary advice (such as low-salt or low-cholesterol restrictions) to improve control over high blood pressure and heart disease. Avoid high-potassium foods, such as bananas and citrus fruits and juices, unless you are also taking drugs that lower potassium levels, such as diuretics.

STORAGE
Store it in a tightly sealed container away from heat and direct light.

MISSED DOSE
Take it as soon as you remember. If it is near the time for the next dose, skip the missed dose and resume your regular dosage schedule. Do not double the next dose.

STOPPING THE DRUG
Do not stop taking this drug abruptly; this may cause potentially serious health problems. Dosage should be reduced gradually according to your doctor's instructions.

PROLONGED USE
Lifelong therapy may be necessary. See your doctor for regular evaluation.

▼ PRECAUTIONS

Over 60: No special advice.

Driving and Hazardous Work: Avoid such activities until you determine how the medicine affects you.

Alcohol: Consume alcohol only in moderation because it may increase the effect of the drug and cause an excessive drop in blood pressure.

Pregnancy: Use of quinapril during the last 6 months of pregnancy may cause severe defects in or even death of the fetus. The drug should be discontinued if you are pregnant or plan to become pregnant.

Breast Feeding: Quinapril may pass into breast milk; caution is advised. Consult your doctor for advice.

Infants and Children: The safety and efficacy of quinapril use by infants and children have not been established. Benefits must be weighed against potential risks; consult your pediatrician for specific advice.

OVERDOSE
Symptoms: None reported.

What to Do: Overdose is unlikely, but call your doctor, emergency medical services (EMS), or the nearest poison control center immediately if you suspect that someone has taken a much larger dose than prescribed.

▼ INTERACTIONS

DRUG INTERACTIONS
Consult your doctor if you are taking diuretics (especially potassium-sparing diuretics), potassium supplements or drugs containing potassium (check ingredient labels), lithium, anticoagulants (such as warfarin), indomethacin or other antiinflammatory drugs, or any over-the-counter medicines (especially cold remedies and diet pills).

FOOD INTERACTIONS
Avoid low-salt milk and salt substitutes. Many of these products contain potassium. Avoid large servings of high-potassium foods such as bananas and citrus fruits or juices.

DISEASE INTERACTIONS
Consult your doctor if you have systemic lupus erythematosus (SLE) or if you have had a prior allergic reaction to ACE inhibitors. Quinapril should be used with caution by patients with severe kidney disease or renal artery stenosis (narrowing of one or both of the arteries that supply blood to the kidneys).

SIDE EFFECTS

SERIOUS
Fever and chills; sore throat and hoarseness; sudden difficulty breathing or swallowing; swelling of the face, mouth, or extremities; impaired kidney function (ankle swelling, decreased urination); confusion; yellow discoloration of the eyes or skin (indicating liver disorder); intense itching; chest pain or palpitations; abdominal pain. Serious side effects are very rare; contact your doctor immediately.

COMMON
Dry, persistent cough.

LESS COMMON
Dizziness or fainting; skin rash; numbness or tingling in the hands, feet, or lips; unusual fatigue or muscle weakness; nausea; drowsiness; loss of taste; headache.

RALOXIFENE HYDROCHLORIDE

Available in: Tablets
Available OTC? No   **As Generic?** No
Drug Class: Selective estrogen receptor modulator (SERM)

▼ USAGE INFORMATION

WHY IT'S PRESCRIBED
For the treatment and prevention of osteoporosis in postmenopausal women. Unlike estrogen, raloxifene does not stimulate overgrowth of the endometrium (the tissue lining the uterus) and thus does not increase the risk of uterine cancer.

HOW IT WORKS
Healthy bone tissue is continuously remodeled (broken down and then reformed); the minerals and other components of bone are reabsorbed by certain cells and then replaced by new bone formation. Raloxifene suppresses the activity of the cells that resorb bone; consequently, the breakdown of bone tissue occurs more slowly than the laying down of new bone. This action preserves bone density and strength.

▼ DOSAGE GUIDELINES

RANGE AND FREQUENCY
One 60-mg tablet a day.

ONSET OF EFFECT
Unknown.

DURATION OF ACTION
Unknown.

DIETARY ADVICE
Raloxifene may be taken at any time of day without regard to a meal schedule. Patients are generally advised to take calcium and vitamin D supplements to aid bone formation.

STORAGE
Store it in a tightly sealed container away from moisture, heat, and direct light.

MISSED DOSE
If you miss a dose one day, do not double the dose the next day.

STOPPING THE DRUG
The decision to stop taking this medication should be made in consultation with your doctor.

PROLONGED USE
Clinical research studies have not yet determined the drug's safety and effectiveness beyond 3 years of use.

≡ SIDE EFFECTS ≡

▼ SERIOUS ▼
No serious side effects have been reported.

COMMON
Increased incidence of infections, flulike symptoms, hot flashes, joint pain, sinusitis, unexpected weight gain.

LESS COMMON
Leg cramps, mild chest pain, fever, migraine, indigestion, vomiting, flatulence, stomach upset, swelling of the legs and feet, muscle pain, insomnia, sore throat, increased cough, pneumonia, laryngitis, rash, sweating, yeast infection, urinary tract infection, white vaginal discharge.

▼ PRECAUTIONS

Over 60: No special advice.

Driving and Hazardous Work: No special warnings.

Alcohol: Alcohol should be restricted in high-risk women because it is a risk factor for osteoporosis.

Pregnancy: Raloxifene is normally not prescribed to premenopausal women. Raloxifene should not be given to pregnant women.

Breast Feeding: Raloxifene should not be used by nursing mothers.

Infants and Children: Not for use by children.

Special Concerns: Patients taking raloxifene are encouraged to engage in regular weight-bearing exercise and should avoid cigarettes and limit alcohol, which inhibit healthy bone production. Unlike estrogen replacement therapy, raloxifene does not reduce hot flashes in postmenopausal women.

OVERDOSE
Symptoms: No cases of overdose have been reported.

What to Do: An overdose with raloxifene is unlikely. If someone takes a much larger dose than prescribed, call your doctor.

▼ INTERACTIONS

DRUG INTERACTIONS
Estrogen should not be taken concurrently with raloxifene. Because cholestyramine reduces absorption of raloxifene, the two drugs should not be taken at the same time of day. Consult your doctor if you are taking any of the following medications that may interact with raloxifene: warfarin, indomethacin, clofibrate, naproxen, ibuprofen, diazepam, or diazoxide.

FOOD INTERACTIONS
No known food interactions.

DISEASE INTERACTIONS
You should not take raloxifene if you have any history of thromboembolic disease, including deep vein thrombosis, pulmonary embolism, and retinal vein thrombosis. Raloxifene must be used with caution by patients with impaired liver function; consult your doctor for specific advice about your own case.

RAMIPRIL

Available in: Tablets
Available OTC? No **As Generic?** No
Drug Class: Angiotensin-converting enzyme (ACE) inhibitor

▼ USAGE INFORMATION

WHY IT'S PRESCRIBED
To control high blood pressure (hypertension); to treat congestive heart failure; to treat patients with left ventricular dysfunction (damage to the pumping chamber of the heart); to reduce risk of heart attack, stroke, and death from cardiovascular causes; and to minimize further kidney damage in diabetics with mild kidney disease.

HOW IT WORKS
Angiotensin-converting enzyme (ACE) inhibitors block an enzyme that produces angiotensin, a naturally occurring substance that causes blood vessels to constrict and stimulates production of the adrenal hormone, aldosterone, which promotes sodium retention in the body. As a result, ACE inhibitors relax blood vessels (causing them to widen) and reduces sodium retention, which lowers blood pressure and so decreases the workload of the heart.

▼ DOSAGE GUIDELINES

RANGE AND FREQUENCY
2.5 mg to 20 mg per day taken in 1 or 2 doses.

ONSET OF EFFECT
Within 1 to 2 hours.

DURATION OF ACTION
24 hours.

DIETARY ADVICE
Take it on an empty stomach about 1 hour before mealtime. Follow your doctor's dietary advice (such as low-salt or low-cholesterol restrictions) to improve control over high blood pressure and heart disease. Avoid high-potassium foods such as bananas and citrus fruits and juices unless you are also taking medications that lower potassium levels, such as diuretics.

STORAGE
Store it in a tightly sealed container away from heat and direct light. Avoid extremes in temperature.

MISSED DOSE
Take it as soon as you remember. If it is near the time for the next dose, skip the missed dose and resume your regular dosage schedule. Do not double the next dose.

STOPPING THE DRUG
Do not stop taking this drug abruptly; this may cause potentially serious health problems. Dosage should be reduced gradually according to your doctor's instructions.

PROLONGED USE
Lifelong therapy may be necessary. See your doctor for regular examinations and tests if you must take this medication for a prolonged period of time.

▼ PRECAUTIONS

Over 60: No special advice.

Driving and Hazardous Work: Do not drive or engage in hazardous work until you determine how the medicine affects you.

Alcohol: Consume alcohol only in moderation because it may increase the effect of the drug and cause an excessive drop in blood pressure. Consult your doctor for advice.

Pregnancy: Use of ramipril during the last 6 months of pregnancy may cause severe defects in or even death of the fetus. The drug should be discontinued if you are pregnant or plan to become pregnant.

Breast Feeding: Ramipril may pass into breast milk; caution is advised. Consult your doctor for advice.

Infants and Children: Children may be especially sensitive to the effects of ramipril. Benefits must be weighed against potential risks; consult your pediatrician for advice.

OVERDOSE
Symptoms: Dizziness or fainting caused by extremely low blood pressure.

What to Do: Call your doctor, emergency medical services (EMS), or local hospital.

▼ INTERACTIONS

DRUG INTERACTIONS
Consult your doctor if you are taking diuretics (especially potassium-sparing diuretics), potassium supplements or drugs containing potassium (check ingredient labels), lithium, anticoagulants (such as warfarin), indomethacin or other antiinflammatory drugs, or any over-the-counter medications (especially cold remedies and diet pills).

FOOD INTERACTIONS
Avoid low-salt milk and salt substitutes. Many of these products contain potassium. Avoid consuming large servings of high-potassium foods such as bananas and citrus fruits or juices.

DISEASE INTERACTIONS
Consult your doctor if you have systemic lupus erythematosus (SLE) or if you have had a prior allergic reaction to ACE inhibitors. Ramipril should be used with caution by patients with severe kidney disease or renal artery stenosis (narrowing of one or both of the arteries that supply blood to the kidneys).

≡ SIDE EFFECTS ≡

SERIOUS
Fever and chills; sore throat and hoarseness; sudden difficulty breathing or swallowing; swelling of the face, mouth, or extremities; impaired kidney function (ankle swelling, decreased urination); confusion; yellow discoloration of the eyes or skin (indicating liver disorder); intense itching; chest pain or palpitations; abdominal pain. Serious side effects are very rare; contact your doctor immediately.

COMMON
Dry, persistent cough.

LESS COMMON
Dizziness or fainting; skin rash; numbness or tingling in the hands, feet, or lips; unusual fatigue or muscle weakness; nausea; drowsiness; loss of taste; headache.

RANITIDINE

Available in: Capsules, tablets, injection, syrup, granules
Available OTC? Yes   **As Generic?** Yes
Drug Class: Histamine (H2) blocker

▼ USAGE INFORMATION

WHY IT'S PRESCRIBED
To treat ulcers of the stomach and duodenum, conditions that cause increased stomach acid production (such as Zollinger-Ellison syndrome), erosive esophagitis (severe, chronic inflammation of the esophagus), and gastroesophageal reflux (backwash of stomach acid into the esophagus, resulting in heartburn).

HOW IT WORKS
Ranitidine blocks the action of histamine (a compound produced in the body's cells), which in turn decreases the stomach's secretion of hydrochloric acid. Once stomach acid production is decreased, the body is better able to heal itself.

▼ DOSAGE GUIDELINES

RANGE AND FREQUENCY
Adults—Oral dose: 150 mg, 2 times a day, in the morning and at bedtime, or 300 mg once daily before bedtime.

Injection: 50 mg every 6 to 8 hours. Patients with Zollinger-Ellison syndrome may require up to 6 g per day taken orally. For treatment of heartburn with the over-the-counter form: 75 mg as needed, not to exceed 150 mg a day. Children—Consult your pediatrician for appropriate individual dosage.

ONSET OF EFFECT
30 to 60 minutes.

DURATION OF ACTION
Up to 13 hours.

DIETARY ADVICE
Avoid foods that cause stomach irritation.

STORAGE
Store away from heat and direct light. Keep liquid form from freezing.

MISSED DOSE
Take it as soon as you remember. If it is near the time for the next dose, skip the missed dose and resume your regular dosage schedule. Do not double the next dose.

STOPPING THE DRUG
Take the prescription-strength medicine for the full treatment period, even if you begin to feel better before the scheduled end of therapy.

PROLONGED USE
Do not take nonprescription-strength ranitidine for more than 2 weeks unless you have been otherwise instructed by your doctor.

▼ PRECAUTIONS

Over 60: Adverse reactions may be more likely and more severe in older patients.

Driving and Hazardous Work: Do not drive or engage in hazardous work until you determine how the medicine affects you.

Alcohol: Avoid drinking alcohol. Ranitidine may increase blood alcohol levels.

Pregnancy: Risks vary, depending on the patient and dosage. Consult your doctor.

Breast Feeding: Ranitidine passes into breast milk and may pose harm to the child; avoid or discontinue use while nursing.

Infants and Children: Ranitidine is not recommended for young patients, although it has not been shown to cause any side effects or problems different from those in adults when used for short periods of time.

Special Concerns: Avoid cigarette smoking because it may increase stomach acid secretion and thus worsen the disease. Do not take ranitidine if you have ever had an allergic reaction to a histamine (H2) blocker. If stomach pain becomes worse while using the drug, be sure to tell your doctor right away.

OVERDOSE
Symptoms: Vomiting, diarrhea, breathing problems, slurred speech, rapid heartbeat, delirium.

What to Do: Call your doctor, emergency medical services (EMS), or the nearest poison control center immediately.

▼ INTERACTIONS

DRUG INTERACTIONS
Consult your doctor for specific advice if you are taking antacids, antidepressants, aspirin, beta-blockers, caffeine, diazepam, glipizide, ketoconazole, lidocaine, phenytoin, procainamide, theophylline, or warfarin.

FOOD INTERACTIONS
Carbonated drinks, caffeine-containing beverages, citrus fruits and juices, and other acidic foods or liquids may irritate the stomach or interfere with the therapeutic action of ranitidine.

DISEASE INTERACTIONS
Patients with kidney disease should not use ranitidine or should use it in smaller, limited doses under careful supervision by a physician.

 ## ≣ SIDE EFFECTS ≣

SERIOUS
Irregular heart rhythm (palpitations), slowed heartbeat, severe blood problems resulting in unusual bleeding, bruising, fever, chills, and increased susceptibility to infection. Call your doctor immediately.

COMMON
Headache, fatigue, drowsiness, dizziness, nausea, vomiting, abdominal pain, diarrhea, constipation.

LESS COMMON
Blurred vision, decreased sexual desire or function, swelling of breasts in males or females, temporary hair loss, hallucinations, depression, insomnia, skin rash, hives, or redness.

REPAGLINIDE

Available in: Tablets
Available OTC? No   **As Generic?** No
Drug Class: Antidiabetic agent

▼ USAGE INFORMATION

WHY IT'S PRESCRIBED
As an adjunct therapy to dietary measures and exercise to help control blood sugar levels in patients with type 2 diabetes mellitus. Repaglinide is the first in a new class of oral antidiabetic medications designed to control blood glucose levels following meals.

HOW IT WORKS
Repaglinide stimulates the pancreas to produce more insulin. Increased insulin levels reduce blood glucose by promoting the transport of glucose into muscle cells and other tissues, where it is used as a source of energy. The rapid onset and short duration of repaglinide's action make it effective in controlling glucose levels after a meal.

▼ DOSAGE GUIDELINES

RANGE AND FREQUENCY
Dosage must be determined for each patient individually, based on blood glucose levels and response to the drug. The recommended dosage range is 0.5 to 4 mg taken 15 to 30 minutes before meals. Repaglinide may be taken before meals 2, 3, or 4 times a day depending on the patient's meal pattern. The maximum recommended daily dose is 16 mg.

ONSET OF EFFECT
30 to 60 minutes.

DURATION OF ACTION
1 to 2 hours.

DIETARY ADVICE
Doses should be taken 15 to 30 minutes before meals.

STORAGE
Store in a tightly sealed container away from moisture, heat, and direct light.

MISSED DOSE
If you miss a dose, take it with the next meal. Do not double the next dose.

STOPPING THE DRUG
Do not stop taking the drug without your doctor's approval.

PROLONGED USE
Prolonged use increases the risk of adverse effects. Periodic physical examinations and blood tests to monitor glucose levels are needed.

▼ PRECAUTIONS

Over 60: Older patients may be more susceptible to adverse effects, especially hypoglycemia.

Driving and Hazardous Work: Caution is advised until you have reached a stable dosing regimen that does not produce episodes of hypoglycemia.

Alcohol: Limit alcohol intake; hypoglycemia is more likely to occur after the consumption of alcohol.

Pregnancy: Repaglinide is not usually given during pregnancy. Insulin is the treatment of choice for pregnant women with diabetes.

Breast Feeding: Repaglinide may pass into breast milk; consult your doctor for advice.

Infants and Children: Safety and effectiveness of repaglinide have not been established.

Special Concerns: Follow your doctor's advice about diet, exercise, and weight control carefully. These aspects of treatment are just as essential to the proper control of diabetes as taking the medication. Always be sure to carry some form of medical identification that indicates you have diabetes and that lists all of the drugs you are taking.

OVERDOSE
Symptoms: Excessive hunger, nausea, anxiety, cold sweats, drowsiness, rapid heartbeat, weakness, changes in mental state, loss of consciousness (indications of hypoglycemia). Overdose is most likely to occur when caloric intake is deficient, after or during more exercise than usual, or after consumption of more than a small amount of alcohol.

What to Do: Call your doctor, emergency medical services (EMS), or local hospital immediately.

▼ INTERACTIONS

DRUG INTERACTIONS
Consult your doctor if you are taking antifungal agents such as ketoconazole or miconazole, as well as antibiotics, rifampin, barbiturates, carbamazepine, aspirin or other nonsteroidal antiinflammatory drugs (NSAIDs), sulfonamides, chloramphenicol, probenecid, monoamine oxidase (MAO) inhibitors, beta-blockers, diuretics, corticosteroids, phenothiazines, estrogens, oral contraceptives, phenytoin, calcium channel blockers, sympathomimetics, or isoniazid.

FOOD INTERACTIONS
A special diet is essential for proper control of blood glucose levels.

DISEASE INTERACTIONS
Do not use repaglinide if you have type 1 diabetes mellitus. Use of repaglinide may cause complications in patients with impaired liver or kidney function, because these organs are both involved in removing the medication from the body.

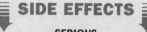

▤ SIDE EFFECTS ▤

SERIOUS
Hypoglycemia (blood sugar levels that are too low), resulting in shakiness, headache, cold sweats, anxiety, and changes in mental state. Immediately ingest food or drink containing sugar. Inform your doctor about the frequency and timing of hypoglycemic events.

COMMON
Increased incidence of upper respiratory or sinus infection, headache, back pain, joint pain, diarrhea.

LESS COMMON
Constipation, indigestion, urinary tract infection, mild allergic reaction.

RIMANTADINE HYDROCHLORIDE

BRAND NAME

Flumadine

Available in: Syrup, tablets
Available OTC? No   **As Generic?** No
Drug Class: Antiviral

▼ USAGE INFORMATION

WHY IT'S PRESCRIBED
To prevent or treat type A influenza.

HOW IT WORKS
Rimantadine interferes with the activity of the virus's genetic material, blocking an essential step in the the process of viral replication. The drug affects only certain susceptible strains of the influenza type A virus.

▼ DOSAGE GUIDELINES

RANGE AND FREQUENCY
Adults and children age 10 years and older: 100 mg 2 times a day or 200 mg once a day. Children up to age 10: 2.3 mg per lb of body weight once a day; the dose should not exceed a total of 150 mg daily. Frail, older adults or those with impaired liver or kidney function: 100 mg once a day. The drug should be continued for about 7 days.

ONSET OF EFFECT
Unknown. For prevention of the flu, take rimantadine prior to or immediately after exposure to someone who has influenza.

DURATION OF ACTION
Unknown.

DIETARY ADVICE
Take it on an empty stomach at least 1 hour before or 2 hours after a meal.

STORAGE
Store it in a tightly sealed container away from heat and direct light. Do not allow the syrup to freeze.

MISSED DOSE
Take it as soon as you remember. If it is near the time for the next dose, skip the missed dose and resume your regular dosage schedule. Do not double the next dose.

STOPPING THE DRUG
It is important to take rimantadine for the full treatment period as prescribed, whether for treatment or prevention of influenza. If you have the flu, do not stop taking the drug before the scheduled end of therapy even if you begin to feel better; this may lead to a relapse.

PROLONGED USE
If your symptoms do not improve or if they become worse in a few days, you should consult your doctor. You should see your doctor regularly for tests and examinations if you take this medicine for a prolonged period.

▼ PRECAUTIONS

Over 60: Adverse reactions may be more likely and more severe; a smaller dose is commonly prescribed.

Driving and Hazardous Work: Do not drive or engage in hazardous work until you determine how the medicine affects you.

Alcohol: Avoid alcohol.

Pregnancy: Rimantadine has been shown to cause birth defects in animals. Human studies have not been done. Before you take rimantadine, tell your physician if you are pregnant or if you plan to become pregnant.

Breast Feeding: Rimantadine may pass into breast milk, but it is unknown if this poses any risks to the nursing infant. Consult your doctor for specific advice.

Infants and Children: In tests, rimantadine did not cause unusual side effects or problems in children over 1 year of age. Tests in children under 1 year of age have not been done. Consult your pediatrician for advice.

Special Concerns: Ask your doctor about receiving an influenza vaccine (flu shot) if you have not yet had one. If you are taking the syrup form of rimantadine, use a special measuring spoon to dispense the dose accurately. If the medicine causes insomnia, take it several hours before going to bed.

OVERDOSE
Symptoms: Agitation, heart rhythm abnormalities.

What to Do: An overdose of rimantadine is unlikely to be life-threatening. However, if someone takes a much larger dose than prescribed, call your doctor, emergency medical services (EMS), or the nearest poison control center.

▼ INTERACTIONS

DRUG INTERACTIONS
Other drugs may interact with rimantadine; consult your doctor for specific advice if you are taking any other prescription or over-the-counter medication.

FOOD INTERACTIONS
No known food interactions.

DISEASE INTERACTIONS
Consult your doctor if you have a history of epilepsy or other seizures. Use of the drug may cause complications in patients with liver or kidney disease, because these organs work together to remove the medication from the body.

 SIDE EFFECTS

SERIOUS
No serious side effects are associated with rimantadine.

COMMON
Nausea and vomiting, mild diarrhea.

LESS COMMON
Dizziness, trouble concentrating, nervousness, dry mouth, loss of appetite, stomach pain, unusual fatigue, insomnia.

RISEDRONATE SODIUM

Available in: Tablets
Available OTC? No   **As Generic?** No
Drug Class: Bisphosphonate inhibitor of bone resorption

▼ USAGE INFORMATION

WHY IT'S PRESCRIBED
To treat and prevent osteoporosis in postmenopausal
women. Also used to prevent
and treat steroid-induced
osteoporosis in men and
women who are either beginning or continuing treatment
with steroids (such as prednisone) for chronic diseases
and to treat Paget's disease,
a disorder characterized by
rapid breakdown and reformation of bone, which can
lead to fragility and malformation of bones.

HOW IT WORKS
Healthy bones are continuously remodeled (broken
down and then reformed);
the minerals and other bone
components are reabsorbed
by one set of cells (osteoclasts) and replaced by
another set of cells to form
new bone. Risedronate
suppresses the activity of
osteoclasts; consequently,
the breakdown of bone tissue
occurs more slowly than the
laying down of new bone. As
a result, bone density and
strength are preserved.

▼ DOSAGE GUIDELINES

RANGE AND FREQUENCY
For treatment and prevention
of osteoporosis (both postmenopausal and steroid-
induced): 5 mg a day.
For Paget's disease: 30 mg
once a day for 2 months.

ONSET OF EFFECT
Unknown.

DURATION OF ACTION
Unknown.

DIETARY ADVICE
Take risedronate with a full
glass of plain water. Taking
the drug with any food or
beverage (including mineral
water) other than plain water
is likely to reduce the absorption of the drug from the
intestine. Take the tablets
at least 30 minutes before
the first food or drink of the
day (other than plain water).
The drug must be taken in
an upright position. Maintain
adequate vitamin D and
calcium intake; however,
vitamin or mineral supplements should be taken no
less than 2 hours after
taking risedronate.

STORAGE
Store it in a tightly sealed
container away from mois-
ture, heat, and direct light.

MISSED DOSE
If you miss a dose on one
day, do not double the dose
the next day. Resume your
regular dosage schedule.

STOPPING THE DRUG
Take it as prescribed for the
full treatment period. The
decision to stop taking the
drug should be made in consultation with your physician.

PROLONGED USE
For Paget's disease: Risedronate is usually prescribed
for a 2-month course of
therapy. A second round of
treatment may be considered
after this 2-month period.
Consult your doctor.

▼ PRECAUTIONS

Over 60: No special problems are expected.

**Driving and Hazardous
Work:** Do not drive or
engage in hazardous work
until you determine how the
medicine affects you.

Alcohol: No special precautions are necessary.

Pregnancy: Consult your
doctor about whether the
benefits of taking the medicine outweigh the potential
risks to the unborn child.

Breast Feeding: Risedronate
may pass into breast milk;
caution is advised. Consult
your doctor for specific
advice about your particular
situation.

Infants and Children: Safety
and effectiveness have not
been established for children
under age 18 years.

Special Concerns: Remain
upright for at least 30 minutes
after taking this medication.
If you develop symptoms of
esophageal disease (such as
difficulty or pain when swallowing; chest pain, specifically
behind the sternum; or
severe or persistent heartburn), contact your doctor
before continuing risedronate.

OVERDOSE
Symptoms: No cases of overdose have been reported.

What to Do: If someone
takes a much larger dose
than prescribed, call your
doctor, emergency medical
services (EMS), or a poison
control center.

▼ INTERACTIONS

DRUG INTERACTIONS
If needed, antacids that contain calcium, aluminum, or
magnesium should be taken
no sooner than 2 hours after
taking risedronate.

FOOD INTERACTIONS
No known food interactions,
although risedronate works
best when taken on an empty
stomach.

DISEASE INTERACTIONS
Kidney impairment or a
gastrointestinal disease may
increase the risk of side
effects. Low blood calcium
levels and vitamin D deficiency must be treated before
using risedronate.

 SIDE EFFECTS

SERIOUS
Serious side effects are rare and may include chest pain
and swelling of the arms, legs, face, lips, tongue, or throat.

COMMON
Flulike symptoms, diarrhea, abdominal pain, nausea,
constipation, joint pain, headache, dizziness, skin rash.

LESS COMMON
Weakness, growth of tumors, belching, bone pain, leg
cramps, muscle weakness, bronchitis, sinus infection,
ringing in the ears, dry eye.

RISPERIDONE

Available in: Tablets, oral solution
Available OTC? No   **As Generic?** No
Drug Class: Antipsychotic

▼ USAGE INFORMATION

WHY IT'S PRESCRIBED
To treat psychotic conditions (severe mental disorders characterized by distorted thoughts, perceptions, and emotions), such as schizophrenia.

HOW IT WORKS
The exact mechanism of action of risperidone is unknown. It appears to alter the activity of certain chemicals in the central nervous system to produce a tranquilizing and antipsychotic effect.

▼ DOSAGE GUIDELINES

RANGE AND FREQUENCY
Adults and teenagers: 2 to 6 mg a day in 1 or 2 divided doses. Dosage may be adjusted by your doctor, if needed, at intervals of not less than 1 week. Older adults: To start, 0.5 mg 2 times a day; may be increased to 3 mg a day.

ONSET OF EFFECT
Sedation may occur within minutes, but the onset of antipsychotic effect may take hours to occur or may not occur until days or weeks after the beginning of therapy.

DURATION OF ACTION
At least 12 to 24 hours, although effects may persist for several days.

DIETARY ADVICE
No special restrictions.

STORAGE
Store it in a tightly sealed container away from moisture, heat, and direct light.

MISSED DOSE
Take it as soon as you remember. However, if it is near the time for the next dose, skip the missed dose and resume your regular dosage schedule. Do not double the next dose.

STOPPING THE DRUG
The decision to stop taking the drug should be made in consultation with your doctor.

PROLONGED USE
Prolonged use may lead to tardive dyskinesia (involuntary movements of the jaw, lips, tongue, and, in rare cases, the arms, legs, hands, or body). Consult your doctor about the need for follow-up evaluations and tests if you must take this drug for an extended period.

▼ PRECAUTIONS

Over 60: Adverse reactions may be more likely and more severe in older patients.

Driving and Hazardous Work: Do not drive or engage in hazardous work until you determine how the medicine affects you.

Alcohol: Avoid alcohol.

Pregnancy: Adequate studies have not been done. Before you take risperidone, tell your doctor if you are pregnant or plan to become pregnant.

Breast Feeding: It is not known if risperidone passes into breast milk; caution is advised. Consult your doctor for specific advice.

Infants and Children: Risperidone is not commonly prescribed for patients under 18 years of age.

Special Concerns: Avoid prolonged exposure to high temperatures or hot climates. Drink plenty of fluids and stay cool in the summertime. Avoid overexposure to sunlight until you determine if the drug heightens your skin's sensitivity to ultraviolet light.

OVERDOSE
Symptoms: Drowsiness, rapid heartbeat, low blood pressure, seizures.

What to Do: Call your doctor, emergency medical services (EMS), or the nearest poison control center immediately.

▼ INTERACTIONS

DRUG INTERACTIONS
Other drugs may interact with risperidone. Consult your doctor for advice if you are taking an antidepressant, bromocriptine, carbamazepine, clozapine, high blood pressure medication, levodopa, pergolide, or any medications that depress the central nervous system, including antihistamines, cold remedies, decongestants, and tranquilizers.

FOOD INTERACTIONS
No known food interactions.

DISEASE INTERACTIONS
Consult your doctor if you have Parkinson's disease or any movement disorder, glaucoma, epilepsy, liver disease, kidney disease, heart disease.

≡ SIDE EFFECTS ≡

SERIOUS
Rapid heartbeat, profuse sweating, seizures, difficulty breathing, neck stiffness, swelling of the tongue, difficulty swallowing. Also a rare condition can develop called neuroleptic malignant syndrome, characterized by stiffness or spasms of the muscles, high fever, and confusion or disorientation. Call your doctor immediately.

COMMON
Nausea, reduced perspiration, dry mouth, blurred vision, drowsiness, shaking of the hands, muscle stiffness, stooped posture.

LESS COMMON
Difficult urination, menstrual irregularities, breast pain or swelling, unexpected weight gain, uncontrolled movements of the tongue, fever, chills, sore throat, unusual bruising or bleeding, heart palpitations, skin rash, itching, increased sensitivity of the skin to sunlight.

RIVASTIGMINE TARTRATE

Available in: Capsules, oral solution
Available OTC? No   **As Generic?** No
Drug Class: Reversible cholinesterase inhibitor

BRAND NAME
Exelon

▼ USAGE INFORMATION

WHY IT'S PRESCRIBED
To treat mild to moderate Alzheimer's disease.

HOW IT WORKS
The exact mechanism of action is unknown. However, rivastigmine is believed to work by inhibiting acetyl-cholinesterase enzymes, which reduces the breakdown of acetylcholine, a brain chemical crucial to memory. An acetylcholine deficiency is thought to result in the severe memory loss associated with Alzheimer's disease.

▼ DOSAGE GUIDELINES

RANGE AND FREQUENCY
To start, 1.5 mg twice a day. After 2 weeks of treatment, your doctor may increase the dose to 3 mg twice a day. The dose may be further increased at no less than 2-week intervals to 4.5 mg twice a day and then to the maximum dose of 6 mg twice a day, if tolerated.

ONSET OF EFFECT
Unknown.

DURATION OF ACTION
Unknown.

DIETARY ADVICE
Rivastigmine should be taken with meals in the morning and evening. The oral solution may be swallowed directly from the syringe or mixed with a small glass of water, cold fruit juice, or soda.

STORAGE
Store it in a tightly sealed container away from moisture, heat, and direct light. Do not freeze the oral solution.

MISSED DOSE
Take it as soon as you remember, unless the time for your next scheduled dose is within the next 2 hours. If so, do not take the missed dose. Take your next scheduled dose at the proper time and resume your regular dosage schedule. Do not double the next dose. If therapy has been interrupted for several days or longer, consult your doctor.

STOPPING THE DRUG
The decision to stop taking the drug should be made in consultation with your doctor.

PROLONGED USE
No problems are expected with long-term use.

▼ PRECAUTIONS

Over 60: No special advice.

Driving and Hazardous Work: Do not drive or engage in hazardous work until you determine how the medicine affects you.

Alcohol: Avoid alcohol while using this medication.

Pregnancy: In some animal studies, large doses of rivastigmine were shown to cause problems. Before you take rivastigmine, tell your doctor if you are pregnant or plan to become pregnant.

Breast Feeding: It is not known whether rivastigmine passes into breast milk; caution is advised. Consult your doctor for specific advice.

Infants and Children: Rivastigmine is not intended for use in children.

Special Concerns: Before you have any surgery or dental or emergency treatment, tell the doctor or dentist in charge that you are taking rivastigmine. Rivastigmine will not cure Alzheimer's disease and will not stop the disease from getting worse, but it will improve cognitive ability of some patients. Caretakers should be instructed in the correct way to administer the oral solution of rivastigmine.

OVERDOSE
Symptoms: Severe nausea, vomiting, increased salivation, sweating, slow heartbeat, low blood pressure, irregular breathing, unconsciousness, increased muscle weakness, and even death.

What to Do: Call your doctor, emergency medical services (EMS), or the nearest poison control center immediately.

▼ INTERACTIONS

DRUG INTERACTIONS
NSAIDs (nonsteroidal anti-inflammatory drugs) may increase the risk of peptic ulcer or gastrointestinal bleeding when taken with rivastigmine.

FOOD INTERACTIONS
No known food interactions.

DISEASE INTERACTIONS
Caution is advised when taking rivastigmine. Consult your doctor if you have asthma, epilepsy or a history of seizures, heart problems, intestinal blockage, stomach or duodenal ulcer, liver disease, or urinary problems.

SIDE EFFECTS

SERIOUS
Possible gastrointestinal bleeding. No other serious side effects are associated with the use of rivastigmine.

COMMON
Significant nausea, vomiting, loss of appetite, and weight loss. Other common side effects include heartburn, weakness, dizziness, diarrhea, abdominal pain.

LESS COMMON
Increased sweating, fatigue, malaise, headache, drowsiness, tremor, flatulence, insomnia, depression, anxiety.

ROFECOXIB

BRAND NAME

Vioxx

Available in: Tablets, oral suspension
Available OTC? No   **As Generic?** No
Drug Class: Nonsteroidal antiinflammatory drug (NSAID)/COX-2 inhibitor

▼ USAGE INFORMATION

WHY IT'S PRESCRIBED
For the management of chronic osteoarthritis pain. Rofecoxib is also used in the short-term relief of acute general and menstrual pain.

HOW IT WORKS
By inhibiting the activity of the enzyme cyclooxygenase-2 (COX-2), rofecoxib reduces the synthesis of prostaglandins that play a role in causing arthritis pain and inflammation. It does not inhibit the activity of COX-1, the enzyme involved in the synthesis of prostaglandins that help protect against stomach ulcers and other health problems.

▼ DOSAGE GUIDELINES

RANGE AND FREQUENCY
For osteoarthritis: To start, 12.5 mg once a day. Your doctor may increase the dose to 25 mg once a day if adequate relief is not achieved with the lower dose. For acute or menstrual pain: 50 mg once a day. To minimize potential gastrointestinal side effects, the lowest effective dose should be used for the shortest possible time. Use of rofecoxib for more than 5 days for relief of acute pain has not been studied.

ONSET OF EFFECT
For acute pain: Within 45 minutes. For osteoarthritis: Unknown.

DURATION OF ACTION
Unknown.

DIETARY ADVICE
Rofecoxib may be taken with or without food.

STORAGE
Store it in a tightly sealed container away from moisture, heat, and direct light. Do not refrigerate the oral suspension.

MISSED DOSE
If you do not remember until the next day, skip the missed dose and resume your regular dosage schedule. Do not double the next dose.

STOPPING THE DRUG
The decision to stop taking the drug should be made in consultation with your doctor.

PROLONGED USE
The risk of gastrointestinal side effects may be increased with extended use.

▼ PRECAUTIONS

Over 60: No special problems are expected. Therapy should be started with the lowest recommended dose.

Driving and Hazardous Work: No special problems are expected.

Alcohol: Avoid alcohol when using this medication because it increases the risk of stomach irritation.

Pregnancy: Discuss with your doctor the relative risks and benefits of using this drug while you are pregnant. Do not use rofecoxib during the last trimester.

Breast Feeding: Rofecoxib may pass into breast milk; caution is advised. Consult your doctor for advice on whether to discontinue nursing or discontinue the drug.

Infants and Children: The safety and effectiveness of this drug have not been established for children under the age of 18 years.

OVERDOSE
Symptoms: No cases of overdose have been reported. Symptoms may include lethargy; drowsiness; nausea; vomiting; abdominal pain; black, tarry stools; breathing difficulty; and coma.

What to Do: If you suspect an overdose or if someone takes a much larger dose than prescribed, call your doctor, emergency medical services (EMS), or the nearest poison control immediately.

▼ INTERACTIONS

DRUG INTERACTIONS
Do not take this drug with aspirin or any other NSAIDs without your doctor's approval. In addition, consult your doctor if you are taking furosemide, angiotensin-converting enzyme (ACE) inhibitors, methotrexate, lithium, rifampin, or warfarin.

FOOD INTERACTIONS
No known food interactions.

DISEASE INTERACTIONS
Rofecoxib should not be taken by people who have experienced asthma, hives, or allergic-type reactions after taking aspirin or other nonsteroidal antiinflammatory drugs (NSAIDs). Consult your doctor if you have any of the following: bleeding problems, inflammation or ulcers of the stomach and intestines, asthma, high blood pressure, or heart failure. Use of the drug may cause complications in patients with liver or kidney disease, because these organs both work to remove the medication from the body.

 SIDE EFFECTS

SERIOUS
Stomach ulcers. Black, tarry stools may signal stomach bleeding. Symptoms of liver disease (nausea, fatigue, lethargy, itching, yellowish discoloration of the eyes or skin, fluid retention). Call your doctor immediately.

COMMON
Indigestion, mild swelling, heartburn, nausea, increased blood pressure.

LESS COMMON
Flatulence, sore throat, upper respiratory tract infection, back pain, and mild abdominal pain.

ROSIGLITAZONE MALEATE

BRAND NAME

Avandia

Available in: Tablets
Available OTC? No   **As Generic?** No
Drug Class: Thiazolidinedione/antidiabetic agent

▼ USAGE INFORMATION

WHY IT'S PRESCRIBED
As a single therapeutic agent or as an adjunct (supplemental) therapy to metformin to control blood glucose (sugar) levels in patients with type 2 (non-insulin-dependent) diabetes.

HOW IT WORKS
Rosiglitazone increases the body's sensitivity and response to its own insulin.

▼ DOSAGE GUIDELINES

RANGE AND FREQUENCY
To start, 4 mg once a day (in the morning) or in 2 divided doses (in the morning and evening). Patients not responding adequately to 4 mg a day after 12 weeks may have their dose increased by their doctor to 8 mg once a day or in 2 divided doses.

ONSET OF EFFECT
Within 2 to 4 weeks.

DURATION OF ACTION
Unknown.

DIETARY ADVICE
Rosiglitazone may be taken with or without food.

STORAGE
Store it in a tightly sealed container away from moisture, heat, and direct light.

MISSED DOSE
Take it as soon as you remember. If it is near the time for the next dose, skip the missed dose and resume your regular dosage schedule. Do not double the next dose.

STOPPING THE DRUG
The decision to stop taking the drug should be made in consultation with your doctor.

PROLONGED USE
See your doctor regularly for liver function tests if you take rosiglitazone for an extended period.

▼ PRECAUTIONS

Over 60: No special problems are expected.

Driving and Hazardous Work: The use of rosiglitazone should not impair your ability to perform such tasks safely.

Alcohol: Drink alcohol only in moderation.

Pregnancy: Adequate studies of rosiglitazone use during pregnancy have not been done. In general, insulin is the treatment of choice for controlling blood glucose levels during pregnancy. Rosiglitazone should not be used during pregnancy unless your doctor believes the potential benefit justifies the potential risk to the fetus. Rosiglitazone may stimulate ovulation in premenopausal women who have stopped ovulating. Contraception may be advised.

Breast Feeding: Rosiglitazone may pass into breast milk; do not use it while nursing.

Infants and Children: The safety and effectiveness of rosiglitazone have not been established in children.

Special Concerns: Another thiazolidinedione drug, troglitazone, has been associated with rare, serious, and sometimes fatal liver-related side effects. Although no similar side effects have been reported for rosiglitazone, liver function tests are often recommended just prior to treatment, every 2 months for the first year, and periodically thereafter. If you develop unexplained symptoms of liver dysfunction, such as nausea, vomiting, abdominal pain, fatigue, loss of appetite, or dark urine, call your doctor immediately. It is important to follow your doctor's advice about diet, exercise, and other measures to help control your diabetes.

OVERDOSE
Symptoms: No specific symptoms have been reported.

What to Do: No cases of overdose have been reported, but if someone takes a much larger dose than prescribed, call your doctor, emergency medical services (EMS), or the nearest poison control center immediately.

▼ INTERACTIONS

DRUG INTERACTIONS
No known drug interactions.

FOOD INTERACTIONS
No known food interactions.

DISEASE INTERACTIONS
Rosiglitazone should not be taken by those with type 1 diabetes or for the treatment of diabetic ketoacidosis. Caution is advised if you have edema or heart failure. Consult your doctor prior to using rosiglitazone if you have any type of liver abnormality.

 **SIDE EFFECTS**

SERIOUS
No serious side effects have been associated with rosiglitazone.

COMMON
Weight gain.

LESS COMMON
Upper respiratory tract infection, headache, edema (swelling).

SALMETEROL XINAFOATE

Available in: Inhalation aerosol, inhalation powder
Available OTC? No   **As Generic?** No
Drug Class: Bronchodilator/sympathomimetic

▼ USAGE INFORMATION

WHY IT'S PRESCRIBED
Salmeterol is used to dilate air passages in the lungs that have become narrowed as a result of disease or inflammation. This drug is used to treat asthma and chronic obstructive pulmonary disease.

HOW IT WORKS
Salmeterol widens constricted airways in the lungs by relaxing the smooth muscles that surround the bronchial passages.

▼ DOSAGE GUIDELINES

RANGE AND FREQUENCY
This drug may be used when needed to relieve breathing difficulty. Adults and teenagers—Inhalation aerosol: 2 inhalations twice daily approximately 12 hours apart. Inhalation powder: 1 inhalation twice a day approximately 12 hours apart.

ONSET OF EFFECT
Within 15 minutes.

DURATION OF ACTION
Up to 12 hours.

DIETARY ADVICE
Maintain your usual food and fluid intake. Increase fluids if you have a fever or diarrhea, in hot weather, or during exercise.

STORAGE
Store it in a tightly sealed container away from moisture, heat, and direct light.

MISSED DOSE
Take it as soon as you remember. If it is near the time for the next dose, skip the missed dose and resume your regular dosage schedule. Do not double the next dose.

STOPPING THE DRUG
The decision to stop taking the drug should be made by your doctor.

PROLONGED USE
It may not be necessary to finish the recommended course of therapy. Consult your doctor.

▼ PRECAUTIONS

Over 60: Adverse reactions may be more likely and more severe in older patients.

Driving and Hazardous Work: Do not drive or engage in hazardous work until you determine how the medicine affects you.

Alcohol: No special warnings.

Pregnancy: Safety of use during pregnancy has not been established. Consult your doctor.

Breast Feeding: It is not known if salmeterol passes into breast milk. Mothers who wish to breast-feed while taking this drug should discuss the matter with their doctor.

Infants and Children: Use of salmeterol inhalation aerosol is not recommended for children younger than 12 years.

Special Concerns: This medication takes 15 minutes to work. Do not use salmeterol for acute or sudden attacks or for worsening asthma. Pay heed to any asthma attack or other breathing difficulty that does not improve after your usual rescue treatment. Seek help immediately if you feel as if your lungs are persistently constricted, if you are using more than the recommended number of treatments or puffs per day, or if you feel that a recent attack is somehow different from others. Do not wash the device for the inhalation powder; keep it dry.

OVERDOSE
Symptoms: Chest pain or heaviness; irregular, fluttering, racing, or pounding heartbeat; dizziness; lightheadedness; severe weakness; fainting; severe headache; muscle tremors or shaking.

What to Do: Call your doctor, emergency medical services (EMS), or the nearest poison control center immediately.

▼ INTERACTIONS

DRUG INTERACTIONS
Consult your doctor for specific advice if you are taking beta-blockers.

FOOD INTERACTIONS
No known food interactions.

DISEASE INTERACTIONS
Consult your doctor if you have a history of any of the following: heart disease or heartbeat irregularities, high blood pressure, anxiety disorders, or a thyroid condition.

 SIDE EFFECTS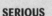

SERIOUS
Salmeterol may become ineffective if used too often, resulting in more severe breathing difficulty that does not improve. Signs include persistent wheezing, coughing, or shortness of breath; confusion; bluish color of lips or fingernails; and the inability to speak. Other side effects include chest pain or heaviness; irregular, racing, fluttering, or pounding heartbeat; lightheadedness; fainting; severe weakness; and severe headache.

COMMON
Headache, sore throat, runny or stuffy nose.

LESS COMMON
Abdominal pain, diarrhea, nausea, cough, muscle aches.

SAQUINAVIR

BRAND NAMES

Fortovase, Invirase

Available in: Capsules
Available OTC? No   **As Generic?** No
Drug Class: Antiviral/protease inhibitor

▼ USAGE INFORMATION

WHY IT'S PRESCRIBED
To treat HIV (human immuno-deficiency virus) infection in combination with other drugs. Although not a cure for HIV, saquinavir may suppress replication of the virus and delay progression of the disease.

HOW IT WORKS
Saquinavir blocks the activity of a viral protease, an enzyme that HIV needs to reproduce. Blocking the protease causes HIV to make copies that cannot infect new cells.

▼ DOSAGE GUIDELINES

RANGE AND FREQUENCY
Adults and teenagers 16 years and older: 600 mg 3 times a day in combination with other antiretroviral drugs. Higher doses (up to 1,200 mg 3 times a day) are sometimes used. Lower doses (400 mg 2 times a day) are used when saquinavir is combined with ritonavir, a similar drug.

ONSET OF EFFECT
Unknown. With most anti-retroviral drugs, an early response can be seen within the first few days of therapy, but the maximum effect may take 12 to 16 weeks.

DURATION OF ACTION
Unknown.

DIETARY ADVICE
It should be taken within 2 hours after a full meal.

STORAGE
Capsules should be refrigerated. If it is brought to room temperature, store it in a tightly sealed container away from heat and direct light and use within 3 months.

MISSED DOSE
Take it as soon as you remember. However, if it is near the time for the next dose, skip the missed dose and resume your regular dosage schedule. Do not double the next dose.

STOPPING THE DRUG
The decision to stop taking the drug should be made in consultation with your doctor.

PROLONGED USE
See your doctor regularly for tests and examinations.

▼ PRECAUTIONS

Over 60: No special studies have been done.

Driving and Hazardous Work: Avoid such activities until you determine how the medicine affects you.

Alcohol: Avoid alcohol if liver function is impaired.

Pregnancy: Human studies have not been done. Nevertheless, the drug is being used increasingly in combination with other antiretroviral drugs to treat pregnant HIV-infected women.

Breast Feeding: It is unknown whether saquinavir passes into breast milk; however, women with HIV should not breast-feed to avoid transmitting the virus to an uninfected child.

Infants and Children: The safety and effectiveness in children under the age of 16 years have not been established.

Special Concerns: Use of saquinavir does not eliminate the risk of passing the AIDS virus to other persons. You should take appropriate pre-ventive measures. If saquinavir increases skin sensitivity to sunlight, wear tightly woven clothing and use sunscreen. Do not substitute one brand of saquinavir for another without consulting your doctor. They may not be equal in strength.

OVERDOSE
Symptoms: No cases of overdose have been reported.

What to Do: If you have reason to suspect an overdose, call your doctor, emergency medical services (EMS), or the nearest poison control.

▼ INTERACTIONS

DRUG INTERACTIONS
Saquinavir should not be used at the same time as triazolam, midazolam, statins (cholesterol-lowering drugs), or ergotamine/belladonna alkaloids. Consult your doctor if you are taking any other medication, especially rifampin, rifabutin, nevirapine, or sildenafil. Some drugs, such as ketoconazole, delavirdine, ritonavir, and nelfinavir, are used in combination with saquinavir because they increase its blood levels and, possibly, its effectiveness.

FOOD INTERACTIONS
Fatty foods and grapefruit juice enhance the body's absorption of saquinavir. Food may reduce side effects.

DISEASE INTERACTIONS
Consult your doctor if you have any other medical condition. Use of saquinavir may cause complications in patients with liver disease, because this organ works to remove the medication from the body.

 ## SIDE EFFECTS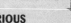

SERIOUS
High blood sugar (diabetes) has occurred in patients taking drugs of this class, although a cause-and-effect relationship has not been established. Contact your doctor if you develop increased thirst or excessive urination. Other side effects include psychosis, thoughts of suicide, and lung disease.

COMMON
Burning, prickling, numbness, or tingling sensations in various parts of the body; confusion; seizures; headache; loss of muscle coordination; diarrhea; abdominal discomfort; nausea; skin rash; increased skin sensitivity to light; general weakness.

LESS COMMON
Loss of appetite, kidney stones, urinary tract bleeding, hair loss, swelling of the eyelid, nail problems, night sweats, small bumplike growths on the skin, impotence, anxiety attack, leg cramps.

SERTRALINE HYDROCHLORIDE

BRAND NAME

Zoloft

Available in: Capsules, tablets
Available OTC? No   **As Generic?** No
Drug Class: Selective serotonin reuptake inhibitor (SSRI) antidepressant

▼ USAGE INFORMATION

WHY IT'S PRESCRIBED
To treat symptoms of major depression, obsessive-compulsive disorder, and panic disorder.

HOW IT WORKS
Sertraline affects levels of serotonin, a hormonelike brain chemical that is thought to be linked to changes in a person's mood, emotions, and mental state.

▼ DOSAGE GUIDELINES

RANGE AND FREQUENCY
Adults: To start, 50 mg once a day in the morning or in the evening. Dose may be gradually increased by your doctor to 200 mg a day. Older adults: To start, 12.5 to 25 mg once a day. Dose may be gradually increased by your doctor to 200 mg a day. Children ages 6 to 12 years: To start, 25 mg once a day. Children ages 13 to 17 years: To start, 50 mg once a day. Dose may be gradually in-creased by your pediatrician.

ONSET OF EFFECT
1 to 4 weeks.

DURATION OF ACTION
Unknown.

DIETARY ADVICE
No special restrictions.

STORAGE
Store it in a tightly sealed container away from moisture, heat, and direct light.

MISSED DOSE
Take it as soon as you remember. If it is near the time for the next dose, skip the missed dose and resume your regular dosage schedule. Do not double the next dose.

STOPPING THE DRUG
Take it as prescribed for the full treatment period. When it is time to stop therapy, your dosage will be tapered gradually by your doctor.

PROLONGED USE
The usual course of therapy lasts 6 months to 1 year; some patients benefit from additional therapy.

▼ PRECAUTIONS

Over 60: No special problems have been reported.

Driving and Hazardous Work: Use caution when driving or engaging in hazardous work until you determine how the medicine affects you.

Alcohol: Avoid alcohol.

Pregnancy: Adequate studies of sertraline use during pregnancy have not been done. Before you take sertraline, tell your doctor if you are currently pregnant or if you plan to become pregnant.

Breast Feeding: It is not known whether sertraline passes into breast milk; caution is advised. Consult your doctor for specific advice.

Infants and Children: The safety and effectiveness of the use of sertraline in children under age 6 years have not been established.

Special Concerns: Take sertraline at least 6 hours before bedtime to prevent insomnia, unless it causes drowsiness.

OVERDOSE
Symptoms: Sleepiness, nausea, vomiting, rapid heartbeat, anxiety, dilated pupils.

What to Do: Call your doctor, emergency medical services (EMS), or the nearest poison control center immediately.

▼ INTERACTIONS

DRUG INTERACTIONS
Sertraline and monoamine oxidase (MAO) inhibitors should not be used within 14 days of each other. Very serious side effects such as myoclonus (uncontrolled muscle spasms), hyperthermia (excessive rise in body temperature), and extreme stiffness may result. The following drugs may also interact with sertraline; consult your doctor for advice if you are taking cimetidine, digitoxin, warfarin, sumatriptan, naratriptan, zolmitriptan, oral antidiabetic agents (such as tolbutamide), tricyclic antidepressants, or any prescription or over-the-counter drugs that depress the central nervous system, including antihistamines, barbiturates, sedatives, cough medicines, and decongestants.

FOOD INTERACTIONS
No known food interactions.

DISEASE INTERACTIONS
Consult your doctor if you have a history of alcohol or drug abuse. Use of sertraline may cause complications in patients with liver or kidney disease, because these organs work together to remove the medication from the body.

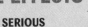

SIDE EFFECTS

SERIOUS
Skin rash, hives, or itching; unusually fast speech; fever; extreme agitation. Call your doctor immediately.

COMMON
Insomnia, diarrhea, sexual dysfunction, decrease in appetite, weight loss, drowsiness, headache, dry mouth, stomach cramps, abdominal pain, gas, trembling, fatigue, loss of initiative.

LESS COMMON
Anxiety, agitation, increased appetite, blurred or altered vision, constipation, heartbeat irregularities, flushing, unusual feeling of warmth, vomiting.

SIBUTRAMINE HYDROCHLORIDE MONOHYDRATE

BRAND NAME

Meridia

Available in: Capsules
Available OTC? No   **As Generic?** No
Drug Class: Inhibitor of neurotransmitter reuptake

▼ USAGE INFORMATION

WHY IT'S PRESCRIBED
To aid in the medical management of obesity in conjunction with a carefully supervised diet and exercise program. Sibutramine is only recommended for overweight people with a body mass index (BMI) greater than 30 or greater than 27 in people with other medical risk factors such as diabetes or high blood pressure.

HOW IT WORKS
Sibutramine affects the appetite control center in the brain by inhibiting the reuptake of neurotransmitters like serotonin. The resulting increase in their availability suppresses appetite.

▼ DOSAGE GUIDELINES

RANGE AND FREQUENCY
To start, 10 mg once a day. Dose may be increased up to 15 mg once a day.

ONSET OF EFFECT
Significant weight changes may take several weeks or months to develop.

DURATION OF ACTION
When taking sibutramine regularly, most people lose weight within the first 6 months. Weight loss is maintained for duration of therapy.

DIETARY ADVICE
It can be taken with a meal or on an empty stomach.

STORAGE
Store it in a tightly sealed container away from moisture, heat, and direct light.

MISSED DOSE
If you miss a dose one day, do not double the dose the next day. Resume your regular dosage schedule.

STOPPING THE DRUG
The decision to stop taking the drug should be made in consultation with your doctor.

PROLONGED USE
The safety and effectiveness have not been determined beyond 2 years of use.

▼ PRECAUTIONS

Over 60: No specific studies have been done.

Driving and Hazardous Work: Do not drive or engage in hazardous work until you determine how the medicine affects you.

Alcohol: Sibutramine may increase the sedative effects of alcohol. Consult your doctor for specific advice.

Pregnancy: Sibutramine should not be used by pregnant women. Before taking sibutramine, tell your doctor if you are pregnant or plan to become pregnant.

Breast Feeding: Sibutramine should not be used by nursing mothers.

Infants and Children: Children under the age of 16 years should not use sibutramine.

Special Concerns: Meridia and other diet drugs have been associated with an increased risk of potentially grave cardiovascular and cardiopulmonary problems. If you experience any unusual or disturbing adverse effects, stop taking sibutramine and call your doctor immediately.

OVERDOSE
Symptoms: No cases of overdose have been reported.

What to Do: If someone takes a much larger dose than prescribed or a child swallows the drug, call your doctor, emergency medical services (EMS), or the nearest poison control immediately.

▼ INTERACTIONS

DRUG INTERACTIONS
You should not take sibutramine if you take monoamine oxidase (MAO) inhibitors, other weight loss medications, medications for depression, migraine medications, dihydroergotamine, meperidine, fentanyl, pentazocine, dextromethorphan (found in many cough medicines), lithium, or tryptophan. Sibutramine may interact with ketoconazole, erythromycin, over-the-counter cough and cold medications, allergy medicines, and decongestants. Consult your doctor for specific advice.

FOOD INTERACTIONS
No known food interactions.

DISEASE INTERACTIONS
You should not take sibutramine if you have coronary artery disease, angina, cardiac arrhythmia, history of heart attack, congestive heart failure, history of stroke, anorexia nervosa, history of seizures, or narrow-angle glaucoma. Sibutramine can substantially raise blood pressure in some patients. Use of sibutramine may cause complications in patients with liver or kidney disease, because these organs work together to remove the medication from the body. Consult your doctor if you have a history of migraines, mental depression, Parkinson's disease, thyroid disorders, osteoporosis, gallbladder disease, a major eating disorder (such as bulimia nervosa), or any other medical problem.

▒ SIDE EFFECTS ▒

SERIOUS
No serious side effects have yet been reported. However, if you experience symptoms that were not present before taking the medication, such as shortness of breath or chest pain, call your doctor.

COMMON
Dry mouth, constipation, insomnia.

LESS COMMON
Headache, increased sweating, increased blood pressure and heart rate.

SILDENAFIL CITRATE

Available in: Tablets
Available OTC? No   **As Generic?** No
Drug Class: Phosphodiesterase type 5 inhibitor

▼ USAGE INFORMATION

WHY IT'S PRESCRIBED
To treat erectile dysfunction (impotence), which may occur in association with atherosclerosis, vascular disease or other circulatory problems, diabetes, kidney disease, hormonal abnormalities, neurological disease or injury, severe depression, or other psychological difficulties.

HOW IT WORKS
Sildenafil selectively inhibits the action of an enzyme (phosphodiesterase type 5) that breaks down a substance that relaxes smooth muscles and permits blood flow that engorges the columns of erectile tissue in the penis. Unlike other treatments for erectile dysfunction, which produce erections with or without sexual arousal, sildenafil allows the patient to respond naturally to sexual stimulation.

▼ DOSAGE GUIDELINES

RANGE AND FREQUENCY
The recommended dose for most patients is 50 mg taken approximately 1 hour before sexual activity. The dose may be increased to no more than 100 mg or decreased to 25 mg. Your doctor will help determine the correct dose. Do not take the drug more than once in a 24-hour period.

ONSET OF EFFECT
Within 30 minutes to 4 hours.

DURATION OF ACTION
Unknown.

DIETARY ADVICE
No special recommendations.

STORAGE
Store it in a tightly sealed container away from moisture, heat, and direct light.

MISSED DOSE
Not applicable.

STOPPING THE DRUG
Not applicable.

PROLONGED USE
Sildenafil treats but does not cure erectile dysfunction. Patients must continue using sildenafil to maintain its benefit; lifelong therapy may be needed.

▼ PRECAUTIONS

Over 60: No special problems are expected.

Driving and Hazardous Work: This drug should not impair your ability to perform such tasks safely.

Alcohol: No special precautions are necessary. However, alcohol is known to decrease sexual function.

Pregnancy: Not applicable; sildenafil is not approved for use by women.

Breast Feeding: Not applicable; sildenafil is not approved for use by women.

Infants and Children: Not applicable; sildenafil is not to be used by children.

Special Concerns: Sildenafil does not offer any protection against sexually transmitted diseases. Appropriate measures (for example, using condoms) should be taken to ensure adequate protection against sexually transmitted diseases, including infection with the human immunodeficiency virus (HIV). Sildenafil should be taken only by men who have been clinically evaluated for and diagnosed with erectile dysfunction by a doctor.

OVERDOSE
Symptoms: No cases of overdose have been reported.

What to Do: An overdose of sildenafil is unlikely. If someone takes a much larger dose than prescribed, call your doctor.

▼ INTERACTIONS

DRUG INTERACTIONS
Sildenafil can enhance the action of nitrates (such as nitroglycerin, which is used to treat episodes of angina), causing potentially dangerous decreases in blood pressure. Therefore, sildenafil should not be used by patients taking nitrates of any kind. Use of sildenafil in conjunction with other erectile dysfunction medications is not recommended. Consult your doctor if you are taking protease inhibitors such as ritonavir and saquinavir, which may affect levels of sildenafil in the blood.

FOOD INTERACTIONS
No known food interactions.

DISEASE INTERACTIONS
Caution is advised when taking sildenafil. Consult your doctor if you have a history of any of the following: high or very low blood pressure; structural deformity of the penis; a bleeding disorder; heart attack, stroke, or life-threatening arrhythmia within the past 6 months; heart failure; coronary heart disease; retinitis pigmentosa; peptic ulcer; sickle cell anemia; multiple myeloma; or leukemia.

≣ SIDE EFFECTS ≣

SERIOUS
Rarely, a painful or prolonged erection (lasting more than 4 hours) may occur. If an erection does not resolve on its own in a reasonable amount of time, seek medical help promptly. If the erection does resolve on its own, consult your doctor for specific guidelines. Serious cardiovascular events such as heart attack, cardiac arrhythmias, cerebral hemorrhage, and transient ischemic attack have been reported following the use of sildenafil. However, it is unclear whether these events are caused by sildenafil, the presence of preexisting cardiovascular risk factors sexual activity, or a combination of these factors.

COMMON
Headache, flushing, indigestion. Such side effects are generally mild to moderate and usually short-lived.

LESS COMMON
Nasal congestion, vision abnormalities, bloodshot or burning eyes, diarrhea, blood in the urine.

SIMVASTATIN

Available in: Tablets
Available OTC? No   **As Generic?** No
Drug Class: Antilipidemic (cholesterol-lowering agent)

▼ USAGE INFORMATION

WHY IT'S PRESCRIBED
To treat high cholesterol. Also used to reduce the risk of stroke or transient ischemic attack ("mini-stroke") in patients with high cholesterol and coronary artery disease. Usually prescribed after the first lines of treatment—diet, weight loss, and exercise—fail to reduce total cholesterol and low-density lipoprotein (LDL) cholesterol to acceptable levels.

HOW IT WORKS
Simvastatin blocks the action of an enzyme required for the manufacture of cholesterol, thereby interfering with its formation. By lowering the amount of cholesterol in the liver cells, simvastatin increases the formation of receptors for low-density lipoprotein (LDL) cholesterol and thus reduces blood levels of total and LDL cholesterol. In addition to lowering LDL cholesterol, simvastatin modestly reduces triglyceride levels and raises high-density lipoprotein (HDL; the so-called "good") cholesterol levels in the blood.

▼ DOSAGE GUIDELINES

RANGE AND FREQUENCY
The initial dose is 10 to 40 mg once a day. It may be increased to a maximum of 80 mg per day. Simvastatin is most effective when taken in the evening.

ONSET OF EFFECT
2 to 4 weeks.

DURATION OF ACTION
The effect persists for the duration of therapy.

DIETARY ADVICE
Cholesterol-lowering drugs are only one part of a total program that should include regular exercise and a healthy diet. The American Heart Association publishes a "Healthy Heart" diet, which is recommended.

STORAGE
Store it in a tightly sealed container away from heat and direct light.

MISSED DOSE
Take it as soon as you remember. Take your next dose at the proper time and resume your regular dosage schedule. Do not double the next dose.

STOPPING THE DRUG
The decision to stop taking the drug should be made in consultation with your doctor. Once the medication is discontinued, blood cholesterol is likely to return to original elevated levels.

PROLONGED USE
Side effects are more likely with prolonged use. As you continue with simvastatin, your doctor will periodically order blood tests to evaluate liver function.

▼ PRECAUTIONS

Over 60: No special problems are expected in older patients.

Driving and Hazardous Work: The use of simvastatin should not impair your ability to perform such tasks safely.

Alcohol: No special precautions are necessary.

Pregnancy: It should not be used during pregnancy or by women who plan to become pregnant in the near future.

Breast Feeding: This drug is not recommended for women who are nursing.

Infants and Children: The long-term effects of simvastatin in children have not been determined. It is rarely used for children; consult your pediatrician.

Special Concerns: Important elements of treatment for high cholesterol include proper diet, weight loss, regular moderate exercise, and the avoidance of certain medications that may increase cholesterol levels. Because simvastatin has potential side effects, it is important that you maintain a recommended healthy diet and cooperate with other treatments your physician may suggest.

OVERDOSE
Symptoms: No specific symptoms have been reported; overdose is unlikely.

What to Do: Emergency instructions not applicable.

▼ INTERACTIONS

DRUG INTERACTIONS
Consult your doctor if you are taking cyclosporine; gemfibrozil; niacin; antibiotics, especially erythromycin; HIV protease inhibitors; or medications for fungus infections. All of these drugs may increase the risk of myositis (muscle inflammation) when taken with simvastatin and may lead to kidney failure.

FOOD INTERACTIONS
No known food interactions.

DISEASE INTERACTIONS
Consult your doctor if you have liver, kidney, or muscle disease or a medical history involving organ transplantation or recent surgery.

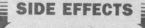

≣ SIDE EFFECTS ≣

SERIOUS
Fever, unusual or unexplained muscle aches and tenderness. Call your doctor right immediately.

COMMON
Side effects occur in only 1% to 2% of patients. They may include constipation or diarrhea, dizziness or lightheadedness, bloating or gas, heartburn, nausea, skin rash, stomach pain, rise in liver enzymes.

LESS COMMON
Insomnia.

SPIRONOLACTONE

Available in: Tablets
Available OTC? No   **As Generic?** Yes
Drug Class: Potassium-sparing diuretic

▼ USAGE INFORMATION

WHY IT'S PRESCRIBED
As adjunctive (supplementary) treatment with other diuretics to increase excretion of sodium and water in the urine while conserving potassium. Spironolactone may be used on its own in patients with liver disease or primary hyperaldosteronism, a life-threatening disorder that occurs when the adrenal glands secrete too much of the hormone aldosterone.

HOW IT WORKS
Spironolactone blocks the effect of aldosterone in the kidneys to increase excretion of sodium and water in the urine while conserving potassium. In conjunction with thiazide or loop diuretics, it reduces the overall fluid volume in the body, which helps control symptoms of liver disease, heart disease, and kidney disease.

▼ DOSAGE GUIDELINES

RANGE AND FREQUENCY
Adults: 100 to 400 mg a day in 2 to 4 doses. Children: 1 to 3 mg per 2.2 lb (1 kg) of body weight in 1 to 4 doses a day.

ONSET OF EFFECT
1 to 2 days.

DURATION OF ACTION
2 to 3 days.

DIETARY ADVICE
Take it with meals to enhance absorption.

STORAGE
Store it in a tightly sealed container away from heat and direct light.

MISSED DOSE
Take it as soon as you remember. If it is near the time for the next dose, skip the missed dose and resume your regular dosage schedule. Do not double the next dose.

STOPPING THE DRUG
The decision to stop taking the drug should be made by your doctor.

PROLONGED USE
You should see your doctor periodically for tests if you take this medicine for a prolonged period.

 SIDE EFFECTS

SERIOUS
Skin rash or itching, shortness of breath, cough or hoarseness, fever or chills, pain in lower back or side, painful or difficult urination. Call your doctor immediately.

COMMON
Nausea, vomiting, diarrhea.

LESS COMMON
Dizziness, headache, sweating, decreased sexual ability, breast tenderness, breast enlargement in men, increased hair growth in females, irregular menstrual periods.

▼ PRECAUTIONS

Over 60: No special precautions are necessary.

Driving and Hazardous Work: The use of spironolactone should not impair your ability to perform such tasks safely.

Alcohol: No special warnings.

Pregnancy: This drug has not been shown to cause birth defects in animals; human tests have not been done. In any case, spironolactone is not usually prescribed during pregnancy.

Breast Feeding: Spironolactone passes into breast milk but has not been reported to cause problems. Consult your doctor for advice about its use while nursing.

Infants and Children: No special problems are expected.

OVERDOSE
Symptoms: Acute electrolyte imbalance causing central nervous system disturbances.

What to Do: An overdose of spironolactone is unlikely to be life-threatening. However, if someone takes a much larger dose than prescribed, call your doctor, emergency medical services (EMS), or the nearest poison control.

▼ INTERACTIONS

DRUG INTERACTIONS
Consult your doctor for specific advice if you are taking cyclosporine, digoxin, lithium, or medicines or supplements containing potassium. Also, because angiotensin-converting enzyme (ACE) inhibitors block aldosterone production, spironolactone is not useful in patients taking this type of medication.

FOOD INTERACTIONS
Avoid consuming large servings of high-potassium foods, which include bananas, melons, prunes, citrus fruits and juices (and most fruits in general), avocados, potatoes, nuts, baked beans, brussels sprouts, and skim milk.

DISEASE INTERACTIONS
Caution is advised when taking spironolactone. Consult your doctor if you have any of the following: kidney stones, menstrual problems, breast enlargement, liver disease, or kidney disease.

SUMATRIPTAN SUCCINATE

BRAND NAME

Imitrex

Available in: Tablets, injection, nasal spray
Available OTC? No   **As Generic?** No
Drug Class: Antimigraine/antiheadache drug

▼ USAGE INFORMATION

WHY IT'S PRESCRIBED
To treat severe, acute migraine headaches (sumatriptan is not effective against any other kinds of pain or headache). Because of the risk of side effects, sumatriptan is generally used only when other treatments prove ineffective.

HOW IT WORKS
Sumatriptan appears to activate chemical messengers that cause blood vessels in the brain to constrict, thus lessening the effects of a migraine. It relieves not only the pain, but also nausea, vomiting, sensitivity to sound and light, and other symptoms associated with migraines.

▼ DOSAGE GUIDELINES

RANGE AND FREQUENCY
Tablets: A single dose of 25 to 100 mg taken with fluid is generally effective. If the headache returns or there is only partial relief, additional single doses of up to 50 mg may be given at intervals of at least 2 hours, but no more than 200 mg should be taken in a 24-hour period. Injection—Initial dose: 6 mg injection. Additional doses: Another 6-mg injection separated by at least 1 hour. Nasal spray: A single dose of 5, 10, or 20 mg into one nostril. A 10-mg dose may be achieved by administering a 5-mg dose in each nostril. If the headache returns or there is only partial relief, an additional single dose of up to 20 mg may be given at an interval of at least 2 hours, but no more than 40 mg should be taken in a 24-hour period.

ONSET OF EFFECT
Tablets: Within 30 minutes. Injection: Within 10 to 20 minutes. Nasal spray: Within 15 to 30 minutes.

DURATION OF ACTION
Unknown, but the peak effect occurs within 1 to 4 hours.

DIETARY ADVICE
No special recommendations.

STORAGE
Keep it away from heat and direct light; do not allow solution to freeze.

MISSED DOSE
Not applicable.

STOPPING THE DRUG
Consult your doctor before discontinuing sumatriptan.

PROLONGED USE
Consult your doctor if you have used sumatriptan for three migraine episodes and have not had relief, if there is no improvement in symptoms after several weeks of use, or if migraines increase in severity or frequency.

▼ PRECAUTIONS

Over 60: Sumatriptan is not recommended for use in older patients.

Driving and Hazardous Work: Sumatriptan may cause drowsiness or dizziness. Avoid such activities until you determine how it affects you.

Alcohol: No special warnings; alcohol may trigger or exacerbate migraine headaches.

Pregnancy: Do not use this drug while pregnant.

Breast Feeding: Do not use this drug while nursing.

Infants and Children: Not recommended for children.

Special Concerns:
Rare but serious heart-related problems may occur after sumatriptan use. Anyone at risk for unrecognized coronary artery disease—such as postmenopausal women, men over age 40, or those with heart disease risk factors—should have the first dose of sumatriptan administered in a doctor's office. It should not be used by those with any symptoms of active heart disease (chest pain or tightness, shortness of breath).

OVERDOSE
Symptoms: No overdoses have been reported.

What to Do: Although overdose is unlikely, if you take a much larger dose than prescribed, call your doctor, emergency medical services (EMS), or the nearest poison control center immediately.

▼ INTERACTIONS

DRUG INTERACTIONS
Do not take sumatriptan within 24 hours of taking any other migraine drug. Consult your doctor for advice if you are taking antidepressants, selective serotonin reuptake inhibitors (SSRIs), or lithium.

FOOD INTERACTIONS
See Dietary Advice.

DISEASE INTERACTIONS
You should not take sumatriptan if you have a history of coronary artery disease, especially angina, heart attack, Prinzmetal's angina, or uncontrolled hypertension. It should be used with caution in patients with liver disease or severe kidney dysfunction.

 SIDE EFFECTS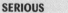

SERIOUS
Chest pain (mild to severe) or feeling of heaviness or pressure in the chest; wheezing or shortness of breath and rapid, shallow, or irregular breathing; puffiness or swelling of the eyelids, face or, lips; hives; intense itching. Seek emergency medical assistance immediately.

COMMON
Pain, burning, or redness at injection site; a general feeling of warmth or heat; a feeling of numbness, tightness, or tingling; mild pain of the jaw, mouth, tongue, throat, nose, or sinuses; dizziness; drowsiness; feeling cold or weak; feeling flushed or lightheaded; muscle aches, cramps, or stiffness; nausea or vomiting.

LESS COMMON
Mild chest pain; heaviness or pressure in the chest or neck; anxiety; feeling tired or ill; vision changes.

TAMOXIFEN CITRATE

Available in: Tablets
Available OTC? No   **As Generic?** Yes
Drug Class: Antiestrogen; antineoplastic (anticancer) agent

▼ USAGE INFORMATION

WHY IT'S PRESCRIBED
To treat breast cancer in women and men and to help reduce the incidence of breast cancer in women at high risk.

HOW IT WORKS
Tamoxifen blocks the effects of the hormone estrogen on certain organs in the body. Because the growth of some types of breast cancer is stimulated by estrogen, tamoxifen interferes with the growth of such tumors.

▼ DOSAGE GUIDELINES

RANGE AND FREQUENCY
For treatment and prevention: 20 mg a day in 2 10-mg doses.

ONSET OF EFFECT
Several weeks.

DURATION OF ACTION
Several weeks.

DIETARY ADVICE
It is recommended that tamoxifen be taken after breakfast and after dinner. Swallow the tablet whole with a glass of water.

STORAGE
Store it in a tightly sealed container away from moisture, heat, and direct light.

MISSED DOSE
Take it as soon as you remember and resume your regular dosage schedule.

STOPPING THE DRUG
The decision to stop taking the drug should be made by your doctor.

PROLONGED USE
See your doctor regularly for tests and examinations if you take this drug for a prolonged period. Tamoxifen does not prevent all breast cancers, so women taking the drug for prevention should continue to have regular breast exams and mammograms.

▼ PRECAUTIONS

Over 60: No different side effects or problems are expected in older patients.

Driving and Hazardous Work: No special precautions.

Alcohol: No special problems are expected, but you should consult your doctor.

Pregnancy: Tamoxifen may cause miscarriage, birth defects, fetal death, and unexpected vaginal bleeding and so should not be taken during pregnancy. Avoid becoming pregnant for at least 2 months after stopping tamoxifen. Notify your doctor and stop taking tamoxifen immediately if pregnancy occurs.

Breast Feeding: Tamoxifen may pass into breast milk; do not nurse while taking it.

Infants and Children: Tamoxifen is not prescribed for infants and children.

Special Concerns: Women should have regular gynecological examinations while taking tamoxifen and for months or years after discontinuing it, because the medication may increase the long-term risk of uterine cancer. Tamoxifen may change or stop a woman's normal menstrual cycle, but she may still be fertile. A reliable birth control method other than oral contraceptives (barrier method) should therefore be used while taking this drug. Tamoxifen for breast cancer risk reduction has not been studied in women under the age of 35. Risk factors for breast cancer include early age at first menstruation, late age at first pregnancy, no pregnancies, breast cancer in a first-degree relative, history of previous breast biopsies, or high-risk changes seen on a biopsy.

OVERDOSE
Symptoms: Nausea, vomiting, irregular heartbeat, tremor, dizziness, seizures, exaggerated reflexes.

What to Do: Call your doctor, emergency medical services (EMS), or the nearest poison control center immediately.

▼ INTERACTIONS

DRUG INTERACTIONS
You should not take tamoxifen to prevent breast cancer if you are taking anticoagulants (such as warfarin). Consult your doctor for advice if you are taking antacids, cimetidine, famotidine, ranitidine, or birth control pills.

FOOD INTERACTIONS
No known food interactions.

DISEASE INTERACTIONS
Consult your doctor if you have a medical history that includes any of the following: cataracts or other vision disturbances, high blood levels of cholesterol or triglycerides, blood clots, low white blood cell or platelet count. Tamoxifen should not be taken to prevent breast cancer by women with a history of deep vein thrombosis or pulmonary embolism.

⯈ SIDE EFFECTS ⯇

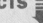

SERIOUS
Endometrial cancer (menstrual irregularities, abnormal nonmenstrual vaginal bleeding, changes in vaginal discharge, pelvic pain or pressure); deep vein thrombosis and pulmonary embolism (pain or swelling in legs, shortness of breath, sudden chest pain, coughing up blood); cataracts; new breast lumps; confusion, weakness, or drowsiness; yellowish tinge to eyes or skin. Call your doctor promptly.

COMMON
Hot flashes, weight gain.

LESS COMMON
Bone pain, headache, nausea or vomiting, skin dryness or rash, changes in menstrual period, vaginal discharge, itching in genital area of women, depression, erectile dysfunction (impotence) or decreased sexual interest in men. Other side effects include high blood calcium levels and liver dysfunction; such problems can be detected by your doctor.

TAMSULOSIN HYDROCHLORIDE

Available in: Capsules
Available OTC? No   **As Generic?** No
Drug Class: Benign prostatic hyperplasia (BPH) therapy agent

▼ USAGE INFORMATION

WHY IT'S PRESCRIBED
To treat symptoms of urinary difficulty that occur with benign prostatic hyperplasia (BPH)—a noncancerous enlargement of the prostate gland. BPH is extremely common among men over the age of 50.

HOW IT WORKS
By blocking a specific (alpha) receptor, tamsulosin relaxes muscle tissue in the prostate and the opening of the bladder. Note that tamsulosin will not shrink the prostate; symptoms may worsen and surgery may eventually be required. Unlike other alpha-receptor blockers used to treat BPH, tamsulosin is not used to treat hypertension.

▼ DOSAGE GUIDELINES

RANGE AND FREQUENCY
0.4 mg once a day. It should be taken 30 minutes after the same meal every day. If patients fail to respond to the 0.4-mg dose after 2 to 4 weeks of therapy, they may increase the dose to 0.8 mg once a day.

ONSET OF EFFECT
Unknown.

DURATION OF ACTION
Unknown.

DIETARY ADVICE
There are no dietary restrictions. However, tamsulosin should be taken 30 minutes after the same meal every day. Do not chew, crush, or open the capsules.

STORAGE
Store it in a tightly sealed container away from moisture, heat, and direct light.

MISSED DOSE
If therapy is discontinued or interrupted for several days at either the 0.4-mg dose or the 0.8-mg dose, therapy should be started again with the 0.4-mg once-daily dose.

STOPPING THE DRUG
Take tamsulosin as prescribed for the full treatment period.

PROLONGED USE
If you take this drug for an extended period, see your doctor regularly so that changes in prostate size can be monitored.

▼ PRECAUTIONS

Over 60: No special problems are expected.

Driving and Hazardous Work: Tamsulosin may impair mental functioning, causing drowsiness, lightheadedness, or dizziness, especially when you take the medication for the first time. Caution is advised; for 24 hours after the initial dose, avoid driving or other activities requiring mental alertness. Effects should diminish after taking several doses.

Alcohol: Alcohol may increase effects of dizziness or fainting; drink in moderation.

Pregnancy: Tamsulosin is not indicated for use by women.

Breast Feeding: Tamsulosin is not indicated for use by women.

Infants and Children: Tamsulosin is not indicated for use by children.

Special Concerns: The first dose is likely to cause dizziness or lightheadedness. Take the drug at night and get out of bed slowly the next day. Be cautious when exercising and during hot weather. Tell your primary care physician if you are planning to have surgery requiring general anesthesia, including dental surgery. Do not chew, crush, or open the capsules.

OVERDOSE
Symptoms: An overdose is unlikely to occur. Possible symptoms after an excessive dose may include severe headache or orthostatic hypotension (see Less Common Side Effects).

What to Do: If someone takes a much larger dose than prescribed, keep the patient lying down and call your doctor, emergency medical services (EMS), or the nearest poison control center immediately.

▼ INTERACTIONS

DRUG INTERACTIONS
Tamsulosin should not be used in conjunction with other BPH therapy agents. Consult your doctor if you are taking either cimetidine or warfarin, which may interact with tamsulosin.

FOOD INTERACTIONS
None reported.

DISEASE INTERACTIONS
None reported.

 SIDE EFFECTS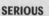

SERIOUS
No serious side effects have been reported.

COMMON
Headache, increased susceptibility to infection, joint pain, back pain, muscle pain, dizziness, runny nose, diarrhea, abnormal ejaculation.

LESS COMMON
Mild chest pain, drowsiness, insomnia, decreased libido, sore throat, cough, sinus infection, nausea, mouth pain, vision problems. The drug may also promote orthostatic hypotension (episodes of low blood pressure are most likely to occur when rising quickly from a seated or lying position), which produces symptoms of lightheadedness, dizziness, confusion, or fainting.

TEMAZEPAM

BRAND NAME

Restoril

Available in: Capsules, tablets
Available OTC? No   **As Generic?** Yes
Drug Class: Benzodiazepine tranquilizer

▼ USAGE INFORMATION

WHY IT'S PRESCRIBED
To treat insomnia.

HOW IT WORKS
Temazepam generally produces mild sedation by depressing activity in the central nervous system. In particular, temazepam appears to enhance the effect of gamma-aminobutyric acid (GABA), a natural chemical that inhibits the firing of neurons and dampens nerve-signal transmission, thus decreasing nervous excitation.

▼ DOSAGE GUIDELINES

RANGE AND FREQUENCY
Adults: 15 mg taken at bedtime. Older adults: To start, 7.5 mg taken at bedtime. The dose may be increased. Use and dose for children under 18 years must be determined by your doctor.

ONSET OF EFFECT
Unknown.

DURATION OF ACTION
Unknown. It may take more than 2 hours.

DIETARY ADVICE
Take it 30 minutes before bedtime with a full glass of water. Temazepam can be taken with food to prevent gastrointestinal upset.

STORAGE
Store in a tightly sealed container away from heat and direct light.

MISSED DOSE
Take it as soon as you remember, unless it is late at night. Do not take the medicine unless your schedule allows a full night's sleep.

STOPPING THE DRUG
Discontinuing the drug abruptly may produce withdrawal symptoms (sleep disruption, nervousness, irritability, diarrhea, abdominal cramps, muscle aches, memory impairment). The dosage should be reduced gradually according to your doctor's instructions.

PROLONGED USE
This medication may slowly lose its effectiveness, and adverse reactions are more likely to occur with prolonged use. You should see your doctor for periodic evaluation if you must take it for an extended time.

▼ PRECAUTIONS

Over 60: Adverse reactions may be more likely and more severe. A lower dose may be warranted.

Driving and Hazardous Work: Do not drive or engage in hazardous work until you determine how the medicine affects you.

Alcohol: Avoid alcohol.

Pregnancy: Use during pregnancy should be avoided if possible. Be sure to tell your doctor if you are pregnant or plan to become pregnant.

Breast Feeding: Temazepam passes into breast milk; do not take it while nursing.

Infants and Children: Safety and effectiveness have not been established for children under age 18 years.

Special Concerns: Temazepam use can lead to psychological or physical dependence if the drug is not taken in strict accordance with your doctor's instructions. Never take more than the prescribed daily dose.

OVERDOSE
Symptoms: Extreme drowsiness, confusion, slurred speech, slow reflexes, poor coordination, staggering gait, tremor, slowed breathing, loss of consciousness.

What to Do: Call your doctor, emergency medical services (EMS), or the nearest poison control center immediately.

▼ INTERACTIONS

DRUG INTERACTIONS
Consult your physician for advice if you are taking drugs that depress the central nervous system; these include antihistamines, antidepressants or other psychiatric medications, barbiturates, sedatives, cough medicines, decongestants, and painkillers. Be sure your doctor knows about any over-the-counter drug you may take.

FOOD INTERACTIONS
None reported.

DISEASE INTERACTIONS
Consult your doctor if you have a history of alcohol or drug abuse, stroke or other brain disease, any chronic lung disease, glaucoma, hyperactivity, depression or other mental illness, sleep apnea, myasthenia gravis, epilepsy, porphyria, kidney disease, or liver disease.

≡ SIDE EFFECTS ≡

SERIOUS
Difficulty concentrating, outbursts of anger, other behavior problems, depression, convulsions, hallucinations, low blood pressure (causing faintness or confusion), memory impairment, muscle weakness, skin rash or itching, sore throat, fever and chills, sores or ulcers in throat or mouth, unusual bruising or bleeding, extreme fatigue, yellowish tinge to eyes or skin. Call your doctor immediately.

COMMON
Loss of coordination, unsteady gait, lightheadedness, dizziness, drowsiness, slurred speech.

LESS COMMON
Stomach cramps or pain, vision disturbances, change in sexual desire or ability, constipation or diarrhea, dry mouth or watering mouth, false sense of well-being (euphoria), rapid or pounding heartbeat, headache, muscle spasms, nausea and vomiting, urinary problems, trembling.

TERAZOSIN

BRAND NAME

Hytrin

Available in: Tablets, capsules
Available OTC? No   **As Generic?** Yes
Drug Class: Antihypertensive; benign prostatic hyperplasia (BPH) therapy agent

▼ USAGE INFORMATION

WHY IT'S PRESCRIBED
To lower and control high blood pressure (hypertension) and to treat symptoms of urinary difficulty that occur with benign prostatic hyperplasia (BPH). Findings from a major clinical trial indicate that terazosin is associated with a high incidence of cardiovascular complications. The American Academy of Cardiology has recommended that physicians reconsider use of terazosin in the treatment of hypertensive patients on a case-by-case basis.

HOW IT WORKS
Terazosin helps control hypertension by relaxing blood vessels and permitting them to expand, which decreases blood pressure. For BPH, it helps relax the muscles in the prostate gland and the opening of the bladder, improving the passage of urine.

▼ DOSAGE GUIDELINES

RANGE AND FREQUENCY
For high blood pressure: Initially, 1 mg taken at bedtime, then 1 to 5 mg once daily. For children, the dose and frequency must be determined by the pediatrician. For BPH: Initially, 1 mg taken at bedtime, then 5 to 10 mg once daily.

ONSET OF EFFECT
Within 15 minutes, with peak blood pressure effect within 2 to 3 hours. When used to treat urinary difficulty associated with BPH, within 4 to 6 weeks.

DURATION OF ACTION
24 hours.

DIETARY ADVICE
Terazosin can be taken before, with, or after meals.

STORAGE
Store it in a tightly sealed container away from moisture, heat, and direct light.

MISSED DOSE
Take it as soon as possible the same day. If it is the next day, skip the missed dose. Do not double the dose. Resume your regular dosage schedule.

STOPPING THE DRUG
Do not discontinue taking the medication suddenly, even if you start to experience side effects. Consult your physician. If terazosin is discontinued for several days, you may need to start therapy over, using the initial dosing regimen.

PROLONGED USE
When taking the medication for hypertension, blood pressure measurement is recommended at regular intervals.

▼ PRECAUTIONS

Over 60: Older persons are generally more sensitive to terazosin and more likely to experience adverse side effects, especially when rising from a lying or seated position. Rise slowly to minimize symptoms.

Driving and Hazardous Work: Terazosin may impair mental ability, causing drowsiness, lightheadedness, or dizziness, especially when you take the medication for the first time. Caution is advised; avoid driving or other activities requiring mental alertness for 24 hours after the initial dose. Effects should diminish after several doses.

Alcohol: Alcohol may increase effects of dizziness or fainting; drink in strict moderation if at all.

Pregnancy: Well-controlled studies have not been done. Consult your physician if you are pregnant or if you plan to become pregnant.

Breast Feeding: It is not known whether terazosin passes into breast milk. Consult your physician for specific advice.

Infants and Children: Adequate studies of terazosin use in this age group have not been performed. Discuss the risks and benefits with your pediatrician.

Special Concerns: Be sure to notify your doctor if you are taking nonprescription medications for asthma, colds, cough, allergy, or appetite suppression. These drugs can increase blood pressure and cause other complications if they are taken with terazosin.

OVERDOSE
Symptoms: Extremely low blood pressure (hypotension), with accompanying fatigue, weakness, headache, palpitations, fainting, or dizziness.

What to Do: Call your doctor, emergency medical services (EMS), or the nearest poison control center immediately.

▼ INTERACTIONS

DRUG INTERACTIONS
Several drugs may interact with terazosin, including anti-inflammatory medications, especially indomethacin, which can cause fluid and sodium retention, and estrogen, which can reduce the antihypertensive effects of the drug. Consult your doctor.

FOOD INTERACTIONS
None are expected.

DISEASE INTERACTIONS
Consult your physician if you have kidney disease, severe heart disease, or chest pain caused by angina pectoris. Terazosin may aggravate these conditions.

⇊ SIDE EFFECTS ⇊

SERIOUS
No serious side effects have been reported.

COMMON
Dizziness.

LESS COMMON
Chest pain; lightheadedness or fainting, especially when rising quickly from a seated or lying position. Such symptoms are more common when you first take the medication, and generally diminish over time. These symptoms tend to recur when the dosage is increased. Take it at bedtime to minimize such problems.

TERBINAFINE HYDROCHLORIDE

Available in: Tablets, topical cream
Available OTC? Yes **As Generic?** No
Drug Class: Antifungal

▼ USAGE INFORMATION

WHY IT'S PRESCRIBED
The tablets are used only to treat fungal infections of the fingernails and toenails (tinea unguium). The cream is used to treat fungal infections of the skin, such as tinea corporis (ringworm), tinea cruris (jock itch), and tinea pedis (athlete's foot).

HOW IT WORKS
Terbinafine inhibits an enzyme essential for the production of substances vital for the reproduction and survival of some types of fungal organisms.

▼ DOSAGE GUIDELINES

RANGE AND FREQUENCY
Tablets: 250 mg once a day for 6 weeks for fingernail fungus; 250 mg once a day for 12 weeks for toenail fungus. Cream: Apply a thin film of medicine to the affected area 1 to 2 times a day for ring-worm or jock itch, 2 times a day for athlete's foot. Apply the cream for at least 1 week but no longer than 4 weeks.

ONSET OF EFFECT
Tablets: The optimal effect is seen several months after the completion of treatment. Cream: Unknown.

DURATION OF ACTION
Unknown.

DIETARY ADVICE
Terbinafine can be taken or applied without regard to meals.

STORAGE
Store it in a tightly sealed container away from moisture, heat, and direct light. Do not allow the cream to freeze.

MISSED DOSE
It is important to not miss any doses. Take or apply as soon as you remember. If you do not remember until the next day, skip the missed dose and resume your regular dosage schedule. Do not double the next dose and do not use excessive amounts of the cream.

STOPPING THE DRUG
Take terbinafine tablets as prescribed for the full treatment period.

PROLONGED USE
Side effects are more likely to occur with prolonged use. Tests of liver function are recommended if the tablets are used for longer than 6 weeks.

▼ PRECAUTIONS

Over 60: No special advice.

Driving and Hazardous Work: No special precautions.

Alcohol: No special warnings.

Pregnancy: Terbinafine tablets are not recommended for pregnant women.

Breast Feeding: Avoid use of the tablets while nursing.

Infants and Children: Terbinafine is not recommended for children under the age of 18 years.

Special Concerns: Wash your hands before and after applying the cream. Do not allow topical terbinafine to come into contact with your eyes, nose, and mouth. If using terbinafine for ringworm, wear loose-fitting, well-ventilated clothing and avoid excess heat and humidity. Use of a bland, absorbent powder such as talcum once or twice a day after the cream has been applied and absorbed by the skin is recommended. If using the medication for jock itch, do not wear underwear that is tight or made from synthetic materials; wear loose-fitting cotton underwear. If using terbinafine for athlete's foot, dry your feet carefully after bathing and wear clean cotton socks with sandals or well-ventilated shoes. Before applying the medication, wash the affected area with soap and warm water and dry thoroughly.

OVERDOSE
Symptoms: Tablets: nausea, vomiting, abdominal pain, dizziness, rash, frequent urination, and headache.

What to Do: Call your doctor as soon as possible.

▼ INTERACTIONS

DRUG INTERACTIONS
Consult your doctor if you are taking rifampin, cimetidine, or any other preparation that is to be applied to the same area of skin as terbinafine cream.

FOOD INTERACTIONS
No known food interactions.

DISEASE INTERACTIONS
Use of terbinafine tablets may cause complications in patients with liver or kidney disease, because these organs work together to remove the medication from the body. Consult your doctor if you have a history of alcohol abuse (a potential cause of liver disease).

 SIDE EFFECTS

SERIOUS
Serious side effects with terbinafine are rare. However, terbinafine tablets may cause liver dysfunction; severe skin reactions such as Stevens-Johnson syndrome; severe blood disorders, potentially resulting in increased susceptibility to infection, uncontrolled bleeding or other problems; or severe allergic reactions. Seek emergency medical assistance immediately.

COMMON
Headache, diarrhea, rash, stomach pain, indigestion, nausea.

LESS COMMON
Tablets may cause flatulence, itching, skin eruptions, loss of taste, weakness, fatigue, vomiting, joint and muscle pain, or hair loss. Terbinafine cream may cause redness, itching, burning, blistering, swelling, oozing, or other signs of skin irritation not present before using the drug.

TETRACYCLINE HYDROCHLORIDE

Available in: Capsules, tablets, liquid, topical forms, ophthalmic forms, injection
Available OTC? No   **As Generic?** Yes
Drug Class: Tetracycline antibiotic

▼ USAGE INFORMATION

WHY IT'S PRESCRIBED
To treat infections caused by bacteria or protozoa (tiny single-celled organisms); also to treat acne.

HOW IT WORKS
Tetracycline kills bacteria and protozoa by inhibiting the manufacture of specific proteins needed by the organisms to survive.

▼ DOSAGE GUIDELINES

RANGE AND FREQUENCY
Oral forms (capsules, tablets, liquid) for bacterial and protozoal infections: 500 to 2,000 mg 1 to 4 times a day as determined by your doctor. Topical forms (cream, topical ointment, topical solution) for acne or skin infections: Apply 1 or 2 times a day to affected areas. Ophthalmic forms (opthalmic ointment, ophthalmic solution) for eye infections: Apply once every 2 to 12 hours as determined by your doctor.

ONSET OF EFFECT
Unknown.

DURATION OF ACTION
Unknown.

DIETARY ADVICE
Oral forms are best taken on an empty stomach with a full glass of water.

STORAGE
Store it in a tightly sealed container away from heat and direct light. Refrigerate liquid forms but do not freeze them.

MISSED DOSE
Take it as soon as you remember. If it is near the time for the next dose, skip the missed dose and resume your regular dosage schedule. Do not double the next dose.

STOPPING THE DRUG
Take it as prescribed for the full treatment period, even if you begin to feel better before the scheduled end of therapy.

PROLONGED USE
It may increase susceptibility to infections by microorganisms resistant to antibiotics.

▼ PRECAUTIONS

Over 60: It is not known whether tetracycline causes different or more severe adverse reactions in older patients than it does in younger persons.

Driving and Hazardous Work: Do not drive or engage in hazardous work until you determine how the medicine affects you.

Alcohol: It is advisable to abstain from alcohol when fighting an infection.

Pregnancy: Tetracycline should not be used during pregnancy.

Breast Feeding: Tetracycline passes into breast milk and may be harmful to the nursing infant. The patient must choose between using the drug or breast feeding.

Infants and Children: Tetracycline should be used by children younger than 8 years of age only if other antibiotics are unlikely to be effective, because it can cause permanent tooth staining.

Special Concerns: If tetracycline causes increased sensitivity of your skin to sunlight, wear protective clothing, use a sunscreen with an SPF (sun protection factor) of 15 or higher, and try to avoid direct exposure to sunlight, especially between 10 A.M. and 3 P.M. Before having surgery, tell the doctor or dentist in charge that you are taking tetracycline. If you use makeup, it is best to apply only water-based cosmetics and to keep the amount to a minimum during tetracycline therapy for the skin. The drug can reduce the effectiveness of oral contraceptives. You should use a different method of birth control while taking this antibiotic. Absorption of tetracycline may be altered if you take antacids.

OVERDOSE
Symptoms: Severe nausea, vomiting, diarrhea, difficulty swallowing.

What to Do: An overdose is unlikely to be life-threatening. However, if someone takes a much larger dose than prescribed, call your doctor, emergency medical services (EMS), or the nearest poison control center immediately.

▼ INTERACTIONS

DRUG INTERACTIONS
Consult your physician for advice if you are taking antacids, calcium supplements, cholestyramine, choline and magnesium salicylates, medicines containing iron, laxatives containing magnesium, or oral contraceptives.

FOOD INTERACTIONS
Avoid dairy products while taking tetracycline.

DISEASE INTERACTIONS
Consult your doctor if you have a history of kidney disease or liver disease.

SIDE EFFECTS

SERIOUS
Increased frequency of urination, increased thirst, unusual fatigue, discoloration of skin and mucous membranes. Call your doctor immediately.

COMMON
Stomach cramps and discomfort, diarrhea, nausea, vomiting, increased sensitivity of skin to sunlight, itching in genital or rectal area, sore mouth or tongue, dizziness, lightheadedness, or unsteadiness.

LESS COMMON
No less common side effects have been reported.

THEOPHYLLINE

Available in: Tablets, capsules, extended release forms, elixir, syrup, oral solution
Available OTC? No   **As Generic?** Yes
Drug Class: Bronchodilator/xanthine

▼ USAGE INFORMATION

WHY IT'S PRESCRIBED
Theophylline is used to reduce the frequency and severity of breathing problems in people with asthma, emphysema, bronchitis, and other lung disorders.

HOW IT WORKS
An asthma attack occurs when the smooth muscles in the bronchial passages of the lungs go into a spasm (bronchospasm). Theophylline relaxes these muscles, helping widen the constricted airways and restore normal breathing.

▼ DOSAGE GUIDELINES

RANGE AND FREQUENCY
Adults not currently taking any theophylline medications: Your physician will prescribe a "loading dose," which is based on your weight and taken only once. This is followed by a daily maintenance dose, usually 300 to 600 mg a day taken in 1 or 2 doses. Patients given extended-release capsules: After the loading dose, take one-half of the total daily dose at 12-hour intervals, unless otherwise directed by your doctor. Adults currently taking theophylline: Dose is determined by blood level of theophylline. Children: Consult a pediatrician.

ONSET OF EFFECT
Variable.

DURATION OF ACTION
Variable.

DIETARY ADVICE
Avoid large amounts of foods or beverages containing caffeine, including colas. Otherwise, maintain your usual food and fluid intake.

STORAGE
Store in a tightly sealed container away from heat and direct light. Keep it away from moisture and extremes in temperature.

MISSED DOSE
Take it as soon as you remember. If it is near the time for the next dose, skip the missed dose and resume your regular dosage schedule. Do not double the next dose.

STOPPING THE DRUG
The decision to stop taking the drug should be made by your doctor.

PROLONGED USE
Therapy with this medication may require months or years.

▼ PRECAUTIONS

Over 60: Adverse reactions may be more likely and more severe in older patients.

Driving and Hazardous Work: Do not drive or engage in hazardous work until you determine how the medicine affects you.

Alcohol: Avoid alcohol.

Pregnancy: Discuss the relative risks with your doctor. Generally, this drug should be used only if necessary and if a substitute cannot be prescribed.

Breast Feeding: Theophylline passes into breast milk and may be toxic to nursing infants; avoid or discontinue use while breast feeding.

Infants and Children: Theophylline has been used in children of all ages. Consult your pediatrician for specific dosages. Theophylline elixir contains alcohol and should not be used by children.

Special Concerns: You will need periodic blood tests to determine theophylline levels. Do not switch brands of theophylline, and especially do not switch between extended-release forms and other forms without notifying your doctor. Inform your doctor if you have stopped smoking; tobacco affects the level of theophylline in the blood.

OVERDOSE
Symptoms: Abdominal pain; bloody vomiting; disorientation, extreme anxiety, or unusual behavior; seizures; twitching, trembling, or shaking; rapid, pounding, or irregular heartbeat; dizziness, lightheadedness, or fainting.

What to Do: Call your doctor, emergency medical services (EMS), or the nearest poison control center immediately.

▼ INTERACTIONS

DRUG INTERACTIONS
Consult your doctor for specific advice if you are taking beta-blockers, cimetidine, ciprofloxacin, clarithromycin, enoxacin, erythromycin, fluvoxamine, mexiletine, pentoxifylline, propranolol, tacrine, thiabendazole, ticlopidine, troleandomycin, moricizine, phenytoin, or rifampin.

FOOD INTERACTIONS
Your doctor may suggest that you restrict caffeine intake.

DISEASE INTERACTIONS
Consult your doctor if you have a history of convulsions, heart failure, liver disease, or underactive thyroid.

≡ SIDE EFFECTS ≡

SERIOUS
Vomiting; trembling; confusion; rapid, irregular, or pounding pulse; chest pain; dizziness; convulsions; skin rashes.

COMMON
Restlessness, insomnia, loss of appetite, nervousness, irritability, nausea.

LESS COMMON
Heartburn, diarrhea.

TOLTERODINE TARTRATE

BRAND NAME

Detrol

Available in: Tablets
Available OTC? No   **As Generic?** No
Drug Class: Anticholinergic

▼ USAGE INFORMATION

WHY IT'S PRESCRIBED
To treat overactive bladder with symptoms of urinary frequency, urgency, or urge incontinence.

HOW IT WORKS
Tolterodine decreases the urge to urinate by blocking nerve receptors that trigger contractions of the bladder.

▼ DOSAGE GUIDELINES

RANGE AND FREQUENCY
Adults: 2 mg twice a day. Dose may be lowered by your doctor to 1 mg twice a day, depending on response to the medication. Adults with impaired liver function: No more than 1 mg twice a day.

ONSET OF EFFECT
Unknown.

DURATION OF ACTION
Unknown.

DIETARY ADVICE
Tolterodine can be taken with or without food. It's best to maintain your usual food and fluid intake.

STORAGE
Store it in a tightly sealed container away from moisture, heat, and direct light.

MISSED DOSE
Take it as soon as you remember. If it is near the time for the next dose, skip the missed dose and resume your regular dosage schedule. Do not double the next dose.

STOPPING THE DRUG
The decision to stop taking the drug should be made in consultation with your physician.

PROLONGED USE
See your doctor periodically if you must take this drug for a prolonged period.

▼ PRECAUTIONS

Over 60: No special problems are expected in older patients.

Driving and Hazardous Work: The use of tolterodine should not impair your ability to perform such tasks safely.

Alcohol: No special problems are expected.

Pregnancy: No human studies have been done with tolterodine. Before taking this medication, tell your doctor if you are pregnant or plan to become pregnant.

Breast Feeding: Tolterodine may pass into breast milk; avoid use while nursing. Consult your doctor for specific advice.

Infants and Children: Not recommended for use by children under the age of 18 years.

OVERDOSE
Symptoms: Drowsiness, mental confusion, dizziness, loss of coordination, dry mouth.

What to Do: Few cases of overdose have been reported. However, if someone takes a much larger dose than prescribed, call your doctor, emergency medical services (EMS), or the nearest poison control center immediately.

▼ INTERACTIONS

DRUG INTERACTIONS
The following drugs may interact with tolterodine. Consult your doctor for specific advice if you are taking fluoxetine, macrolide antibiotics, or antifungal drugs.

FOOD INTERACTIONS
There are no known food interactions.

DISEASE INTERACTIONS
You should not take tolterodine if you have urinary retention, gastric retention, or uncontrolled narrow-angle glaucoma. Tolterodine should be used with caution in patients with liver or kidney disease, because these organs work together to remove the medication from the body.

≣ SIDE EFFECTS ≣

SERIOUS
Chest pain. Consult your doctor immediately.

COMMON
Headache, constipation, indigestion, dry eye, dry mouth.

LESS COMMON
Numbness, tingling or prickling sensation, abdominal pain, flatulence, nausea or vomiting, bronchitis, cough, dry skin, nervousness, drowsiness, blurred vision.

TRAMADOL HYDROCHLORIDE

Available in: Tablets
Available OTC? No   **As Generic?** Yes
Drug Class: Analgesic

▼ USAGE INFORMATION

WHY IT'S PRESCRIBED
To help manage moderate to somewhat severe pain, such as that occurring after joint surgery and certain gynecological procedures (cesarean section, for example).

HOW IT WORKS
Tramadol acts on the central nervous system to block pain transmission signals. The drug works like narcotic analgesics, and although it is not a narcotic, it can be habit-forming, leading to mental and physical drug dependence.

▼ DOSAGE GUIDELINES

RANGE AND FREQUENCY
1 or 2 tablets (50 mg each) every 6 hours as needed. For severe pain, your doctor may prescribe 2 tablets for the first dose.

ONSET OF EFFECT
Usually within 1 hour, with a peak effect at 2 hours.

DURATION OF ACTION
6 to 7 hours.

DIETARY ADVICE
Tramadol can be taken with or without food.

STORAGE
Store it in a tightly sealed container away from heat and direct light.

MISSED DOSE
Take it as soon as you remember. However, if it is near the time for the next dose, skip the missed dose and resume your regular dosage schedule. Do not double the next dose.

STOPPING THE DRUG
The decision to stop taking the drug should be made by your doctor.

PROLONGED USE
You should see your doctor regularly for tests and examinations if you take this drug for a prolonged period.

▼ PRECAUTIONS

Over 60: Tramadol stays longer in the bodies of older patients than younger ones; your doctor may adjust the dose accordingly.

Driving and Hazardous Work: Do not drive or engage in hazardous work until you determine how the medicine affects you.

Alcohol: Do not consume alcohol while taking tramadol because this medication may compound the drug's sedative effect on the central nervous system.

Pregnancy: Tramadol has caused birth defects and other problems in animals. Human studies have not been done. Before you take the drug, tell your doctor if you are pregnant or are planning to become pregnant.

Breast Feeding: Tramadol passes into breast milk; avoid or discontinue use while breast feeding.

Infants and Children: Safety and effectiveness have not been established for the use of tramadol in children under 16 years old.

Special Concerns: Before undergoing any kind of surgery, including dental surgery, be sure your doctor or dentist knows that you are taking tramadol.

OVERDOSE

Symptoms: Breathing difficulty, seizures, vomiting.

What to Do: Call your doctor, emergency medical services (EMS), or the nearest poison control center immediately.

▼ INTERACTIONS

DRUG INTERACTIONS
Consult your doctor for specific advice if you are taking carbamazepine, anesthetics, monoamine oxidase (MAO) inhibitors, or any drugs known to depress the central nervous system, including sedatives, tranquilizers, sleeping pills, antihistamines, other prescription pain medicines, barbiturates, medications for seizures, or muscle relaxants.

FOOD INTERACTIONS
No known food interactions.

DISEASE INTERACTIONS
Caution is advised when taking tramadol. Consult your doctor if you have severe abdominal or stomach conditions or a history of alcohol abuse, drug abuse, head injury, or seizure disorders. Use of tramadol may cause complications in patients with liver or kidney disease, because these organs work together to remove the medication from the body.

≡ SIDE EFFECTS ≡

SERIOUS
Blurred vision, difficulty urinating, frequent urge to urinate, blisters under the skin, change in walking balance, dizziness or lightheadedness when getting up, fainting, fast heartbeat, memory loss, hallucinations, shortness of breath. Also numbness, tingling, pain, or weakness in hands or feet; redness, swelling, and itching of skin; trembling and shaking of hands or feet; trouble performing routine tasks. Call your doctor immediately.

COMMON
Dizziness, vertigo, headache, drowsiness, nausea, vomiting, constipation.

LESS COMMON
Weakness, lack of energy, anxiety, confusion, euphoria, nervousness, insomnia, visual disturbances, stomach upset, dry mouth, diarrhea, abdominal pain, loss of appetite, gas, menopausal symptoms, sweating, muscle spasm, rash.

TRAZODONE

Available in: Tablets
Available OTC? No **As Generic?** Yes
Drug Class: Antidepressant

▼ USAGE INFORMATION

WHY IT'S PRESCRIBED
To treat symptoms of major depression. It may be taken with selective serotonin reuptake inhibitor (SSRI) antidepressants such as fluoxetine, sertraline, and paroxetine when these drugs cause insomnia.

HOW IT WORKS
Trazodone helps balance levels of serotonin, a brain chemical that is profoundly linked to mood, emotions, and mental state.

▼ DOSAGE GUIDELINES

RANGE AND FREQUENCY
Adults: To start, 50 mg 3 times a day, or 75 mg 2 times a day, or 100 mg at bedtime. The dose may be gradually increased by your doctor to 400 mg a day. Older adults: To start, 25 mg 3 times a day or 50 mg at bedtime. The dose may be increased by your doctor.

ONSET OF EFFECT
1 to 4 weeks.

DURATION OF ACTION
Unknown.

DIETARY ADVICE
It can be taken with a meal or light snack to reduce the chance of dizziness and to increase the absorption of the drug by the body.

STORAGE
Store it in a tightly sealed container away from moisture, heat, and direct light.

MISSED DOSE
Take it as soon as you remember, unless the time for your next scheduled dose is within the next 4 hours. If so, do not take the missed dose. Take your next scheduled dose at the proper time and resume your regular dosage schedule. Do not double the next dose.

STOPPING THE DRUG
Take as prescribed for the full treatment period, even if you begin to feel better before the scheduled end of therapy. The decision to stop taking the drug should be made in consultation with your doctor.

PROLONGED USE
The usual course of therapy lasts for 6 months to 1 year; some patients benefit from additional therapy beyond that period.

≡ SIDE EFFECTS ≡

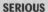

SERIOUS
Muscle twitching, confusion. Call your doctor immediately.

COMMON
Drowsiness, dry mouth, dizziness, lightheadedness, unpleasant taste in mouth, nausea and vomiting, headache.

LESS COMMON
Blurred vision, muscle pains, diarrhea, constipation, unusual fatigue.

▼ PRECAUTIONS

Over 60: Adverse reactions may be more likely and more severe in older patients. Lower doses may be needed.

Driving and Hazardous Work: Use caution when driving or engaging in hazardous work until you determine how the medicine affects you. Drowsiness may occur.

Alcohol: Avoid alcohol.

Pregnancy: Adequate studies of trazodone use during pregnancy have not been done. Before you take trazodone, tell your doctor if you are pregnant or plan to become pregnant.

Breast Feeding: Trazodone passes into breast milk; caution is advised. Consult your doctor for specific advice.

Infants and Children: The safety and effectiveness have not been established for infants and children.

OVERDOSE
Symptoms: Severe nausea and vomiting, loss of coordination, drowsiness.

What to Do: Call your doctor, emergency medical services (EMS), or the nearest poison control center immediately.

▼ INTERACTIONS

DRUG INTERACTIONS
The following drugs may interact with trazodone. Consult your doctor for specific advice if you are taking high blood pressure medication, central nervous system depressants (including cold and allergy drugs, narcotic pain relievers, and muscle relaxants), fluoxetine, or tricyclic antidepressants.

FOOD INTERACTIONS
No known food interactions.

DISEASE INTERACTIONS
Caution is advised when taking trazodone. Consult your doctor if you have a history of alcohol abuse or any heart condition. Use of trazodone may cause complications in patients with liver or kidney disease, because these organs work together to remove the medication from the body.

TRETINOIN

BRAND NAMES

Avita, Renova, Retin-A, Retinoic Acid

Available in: Cream, gel, liquid
Available OTC? No   **As Generic?** Yes
Drug Class: Acne drug

▼ USAGE INFORMATION

WHY IT'S PRESCRIBED
Tretinoin is used to treat mild to moderate acne.

HOW IT WORKS
Although the exact mechanism of action of tretinoin is unknown, the drug appears to affect skin cells so that they are shed in a more normal fashion, therefore "unplugging" blackheads and whiteheads (comedones), the initial changes in acne formation.

▼ DOSAGE GUIDELINES

RANGE AND FREQUENCY
Adults: Apply once daily at bedtime.

ONSET OF EFFECT
Variable, usually within 2 to 6 weeks after starting therapy.

DURATION OF ACTION
The effect of tretinoin typically persists for as long as the medication continues to be applied.

DIETARY ADVICE
No special restrictions.

STORAGE
Store it in a tightly sealed container away from heat and direct light. Keep it away from moisture and extremes in temperature. The gel form of this medication is flammable; keep it away from heat and open flame.

MISSED DOSE
This drug is applied once every 24 hours at night. If you miss a day, resume your regular dosage schedule the next day. There is no need to apply extra medication with the next dose to compensate for the missed dose.

STOPPING THE DRUG
Use it as prescribed for the full treatment period, even if you show signs of improvement before the scheduled end of therapy.

PROLONGED USE
Therapy with this medication is frequently long term.

≡ SIDE EFFECTS ≡

SERIOUS
No serious side effects are associated with regular applications of of tretinoin when used as directed.

COMMON
Mild redness and peeling or excessive dryness at the site of application.

LESS COMMON
Irritation or allergy with severe redness, swelling, blistering, pain, rash, or crusting at sites of application; changes in pigment (either lightening or darkening of skin color). These problems generally improve when the medication is stopped or reduced in dosage or frequency of application. Consult your doctor.

▼ PRECAUTIONS

Over 60: No special problems are expected.

Driving and Hazardous Work: No special precautions are necessary.

Alcohol: No special precautions are necessary.

Pregnancy: Avoid or discontinue tretinoin if you are pregnant or if you are trying to become pregnant.

Breast Feeding: Tretinoin may pass into breast milk; caution is advised. Consult your doctor for advice.

Infants and Children: The drug is not recommended for children.

Special Concerns: People with a history of allergy to tretinoin or any other ingredients in the medication should not use the product. Do not apply large amounts of tretinoin to your skin with the expectation of better or faster results. This will lead to unnecessary irritation of affected skin and surrounding areas. Sunburned skin is more susceptible to irritation from tretinoin, and application should be avoided. Avoid excessive exposure to sunlight or use of sunlamps. Keep this medication away from your eyes, mouth, and nostrils or severe irritation and redness may result. Do not apply tretinoin to inflamed skin. If your skin becomes reddened and painful while using tretinoin, discontinue use of the medication and call your doctor. If you are using cosmetics, gently cleanse the skin to be treated before applying the medication.

OVERDOSE
Symptoms: Excessive application of tretinoin may lead to severe irritation of the skin.

What to Do: If tretinoin is ingested, call your doctor, emergency medical services (EMS), or the nearest poison control center.

▼ INTERACTIONS

DRUG INTERACTIONS
Consult your doctor for specific advice if you are taking other acne medications that are applied to the same area of skin, including prescription and nonprescription treatments containing sulfur, resorcinol, alpha-hydroxy acids, or salicylic acid; medicated soaps, abrasives, cleansers, or cosmetics; topical preparations with a high concentration of alcohol, astringents, extract of lime, or spices; and medications used for a drying effect.

FOOD INTERACTIONS
No known food interactions.

DISEASE INTERACTIONS
Caution is advised when using tretinoin. Consult your doctor if you have eczema.

TRIAMCINOLONE INHALANT AND NASAL

Available in: Nasal spray, oral inhalation
Available OTC? No   **As Generic?** No
Drug Class: Respiratory corticosteroid

▼ USAGE INFORMATION

WHY IT'S PRESCRIBED
Oral inhalation: To treat bronchial asthma. Nasal spray: To treat allergic rhinitis (seasonal or perennial allergies such as hay fever) and to prevent recurrence of nasal polyps after surgical removal.

HOW IT WORKS
Respiratory corticosteroids such as triamcinolone primarily reduce or prevent inflammation of the lining of the airways (the underlying cause of asthma), reduce the allergic response to inhaled allergens, and inhibit the secretion of mucus within the airways.

▼ DOSAGE GUIDELINES

RANGE AND FREQUENCY
Adults and children ages 12 years and older—Oral inhalation: 2 inhalations of 100 micrograms (µg) each 3 or 4 times a day. Maximum dose is 16 inhalations a day. In some patients, maintenance can be achieved when the total daily dose is given 2 times a day. Nasal spray: 2 sprays (55 µg each) in each nostril once a day. It can be increased to 440 µg per day in 1 or up to 4 doses. After relief is achieved, it can be decreased to as little as 1 spray (55 µg) in each nostril once a day.

ONSET OF EFFECT
Usually within 1 week; it may take 3 weeks for the full effect to occur.

DURATION OF ACTION
Several days.

DIETARY ADVICE
No special restrictions.

STORAGE
Store it in a tightly sealed container away from heat and direct light.

MISSED DOSE
Take it as soon as you remember. However, if it is near the time for the next dose, skip the missed dose and resume your regular dosage schedule. Do not double the next dose.

STOPPING THE DRUG
The decision to stop taking the drug should be made only after consultation with your doctor.

PROLONGED USE
Consult your doctor about the need for regular periodic medical tests and examinations if you must take this drug for a prolonged period.

▼ PRECAUTIONS

Over 60: No special problems are expected with older patients.

Driving and Hazardous Work: The use of triamcinolone should not impair your ability to perform such tasks safely.

Alcohol: No special precautions are necessary.

Pregnancy: Inhaled or nasal steroids have not been reported to cause birth defects if taken during pregnancy. Before using such drugs, tell your doctor if you are or if you are planning to become pregnant.

Breast Feeding: Triamcinolone may pass into breast milk; caution is advised. Consult your doctor for advice.

Infants and Children: No special problems are expected in children, but the lowest possible dose should be used.

Special Concerns: Inhaled steroids will not help an asthma attack in progress. Inhaled steroids can lower resistance to yeast infections of the mouth, throat, or voice box. To prevent yeast infections, gargle or rinse your mouth with water after each use; do not swallow the water. Know how to use the spray properly; read and follow the directions that come with the device. Before you have surgery, tell the doctor or dentist that you are using a steroid.

OVERDOSE
Symptoms: No specific ones have been reported.

What to Do: Call your doctor, emergency medical services (EMS), or the nearest poison control center if you have any reason to suspect an overdose.

▼ INTERACTIONS

DRUG INTERACTIONS
Consult your physician for advice if you are taking systemic corticosteroids, other inhaled corticosteroids, or any drugs that suppress the immune system.

FOOD INTERACTIONS
No known food interactions.

DISEASE INTERACTIONS
Consult your physician if you have any of the following: nasal septal ulcers, ocular herpes simplex, or any fungal, bacterial, or systemic viral infection. If you are exposed to chicken pox or measles, tell your doctor at once.

≡ SIDE EFFECTS ≡

SERIOUS
No serious side effects have been reported.

COMMON
Oral inhalation: Sore throat, white patches in mouth or throat, hoarseness. Nasal spray: Nosebleeds or bloody nasal secretions, nasal burning or irritation, sore throat.

LESS COMMON
Eye pain, watering eyes, gradual decrease of vision, stomach pain and digestive disturbances.

TRIMETHOPRIM/SULFAMETHOXAZOLE

BRAND NAMES
Bactrim, Cotrim, Septra, Sulfamethoprim, Uro-D/S, Uroplus

Available in: Tablets, injection
Available OTC? No **As Generic?** Yes
Drug Class: Antiinfective

▼ USAGE INFORMATION

WHY IT'S PRESCRIBED
To treat urinary tract infections, ear infections, chronic bronchitis, *Pneumocystis carinii* pneumonia (a lung infection commonly seen in patients with compromised immune systems), traveler's diarrhea, and other types of diarrheal disease.

HOW IT WORKS
This drug is a combination of two active ingredients. Both trimethoprim and sulfamethoxazole kill or inhibit growth of bacteria by disrupting their ability to make necessary proteins.

▼ DOSAGE GUIDELINES

RANGE AND FREQUENCY
For common bacterial infections—Adults: The usual dose is 1 double-strength (DS) tablet 2 times a day. Duration of therapy depends on the type of infection and will be determined by your doctor. For alternative dosages and for treatment of children, consult your pediatrician; dosages can vary considerably depending on age, weight, and kidney function.

ONSET OF EFFECT
Unknown.

DURATION OF ACTION
Unknown.

DIETARY ADVICE
Tablets should be taken with a full glass of water and can be taken with food to lessen stomach upset.

STORAGE
Store it in a tightly sealed container away from heat and direct light.

MISSED DOSE
Take it as soon as you remember. However, if it is near the time for the next dose, skip the missed dose and resume your regular dosage schedule. Do not double the next dose.

STOPPING THE DRUG
Take the drug as prescribed for the full treatment period, even if you begin to feel better before the scheduled end of therapy.

PROLONGED USE
See your doctor regularly for tests and examinations if you must take this medicine for an extended period.

▼ PRECAUTIONS

Over 60: Adverse reactions may be more likely and more severe in older patients.

Driving and Hazardous Work: Do not drive or engage in hazardous work until you determine how the medicine affects you.

Alcohol: No special problems are expected, although it is generally advisable to abstain from alcohol when fighting an infection.

Pregnancy: Trimethoprim with sulfamethoxazole has caused birth defects in animals. Human studies have not been done. It should be used during pregnancy only if the benefits clearly outweigh the possible risks. Before you take this medication, tell your doctor if you are pregnant or plan to become pregnant.

Breast Feeding: Trimethoprim with sulfamethoxazole passes into breast milk; avoid or discontinue use while nursing.

Infants and Children: This medication is not recommended for use by children under the age of 2 months.

Special Concerns: Some patients experience increased sensitivity to sunlight, so take preventive measures. Use sunscreen, wear protective clothing, and avoid exposure to the sun. Patients with acquired immunodeficiency syndrome (AIDS) may have a higher incidence of side effects, especially rash. Nonetheless, trimethoprim with sulfamethoxazole remains valuable for treating a number of problems associated with this disease.

OVERDOSE
Symptoms: Loss of appetite, nausea, vomiting, dizziness, headache, drowsiness, depression, confusion, altered mental status, fever, blood in urine, yellow skin or eyes.

What to Do: Call your doctor, emergency medical services (EMS), or the nearest poison control center immediately.

▼ INTERACTIONS

DRUG INTERACTIONS
The following drugs may interact with trimethoprim with sulfamethoxazole. Consult your doctor for specific advice if you are taking cyclosporine, methotrexate, phenytoin, procainamide, sulfonylureas, or warfarin.

FOOD INTERACTIONS
No known food interactions.

DISEASE INTERACTIONS
Use of sulfamethoxazole may cause complications in patients with liver or kidney disease, because these organs work together to remove the medication from the body. This drug can also cause complications in patients with certain types of anemia. Consult your doctor for specific advice if you have any other medical condition.

SIDE EFFECTS

SERIOUS
Skin rash, sore throat, fever, joint pain, shortness of breath, pale skin, reddish spots on skin, unusual bleeding or bruising. Call your doctor immediately.

COMMON
Nausea, vomiting, loss of appetite, allergic skin reactions, itching, hives.

LESS COMMON
Abdominal pain, diarrhea, seizures, dizziness, ringing in ears, headache, hallucinations, depression, unusual sensitivity to sunlight.

VALACYCLOVIR HYDROCHLORIDE

Available in: Tablets
Available OTC? No   **As Generic?** No
Drug Class: Antiviral

▼ USAGE INFORMATION

WHY IT'S PRESCRIBED
To treat the symptoms of shingles (herpes zoster). Also used for the treatment and suppression of genital herpes.

HOW IT WORKS
Valacyclovir is converted in the body to acyclovir, which interferes with the activity of enzymes needed for the replication of viral DNA in cells, thus preventing the virus from multiplying. Although it cannot cure herpes infections, it can relieve symptoms and speed the healing of herpes lesions. It may also reduce the duration of any lingering pain (postherpetic neuralgia).

▼ DOSAGE GUIDELINES

RANGE AND FREQUENCY
For shingles: Adults: 1 g 3 times a day for 7 days. To treat initial episodes of genital herpes: 1 g 2 times a day for 10 days. To treat recurrent genital herpes: 500 mg 2 times a day for 5 days. For suppression of chronic recurrent genital herpes: 1 g once a day. In patients with a history of 9 or fewer recurrences per year: 500 mg once a day.

ONSET OF EFFECT
Within 30 minutes.

DURATION OF ACTION
Unknown.

DIETARY ADVICE
No special restrictions.

STORAGE
Store in a tightly sealed container away from heat, moisture, and direct light.

MISSED DOSE
Take it as soon as you remember. If it is near the time for the next dose, skip the missed dose and resume your regular dosage schedule. Do not double the next dose.

STOPPING THE DRUG
The decision to stop taking the drug should be made with your doctor.

PROLONGED USE
The usual course of therapy lasts 7 to 10 days. If for any reason you must take it for a longer period, see your doctor for regular tests and exams.

▼ PRECAUTIONS

Over 60: No special problems are expected, although a smaller dose may be necessary for those with a history of impaired renal (kidney) function.

Driving and Hazardous Work: Exercise caution until you determine how the medication affects you.

Alcohol: No special warnings.

Pregnancy: Human studies of valacyclovir use during pregnancy have not been done, but birth defects or other problems have not been reported. Before you take valacyclovir, tell your doctor if you are pregnant or plan to become pregnant.

Breast Feeding: Valacyclovir may pass into breast milk. It is unknown if this poses any risks to the nursing infant; no problems have been reported. Consult your doctor for advice.

Infants and Children: The safety and effectiveness of this drug for children have not been established.

Special Concerns: Keep the body areas affected by shingles or herpes clean and dry, and wear comfortable, loose-fitting clothes to avoid irritation. Start taking valacyclovir as soon as possible after the symptoms appear, ideally within 72 hours. Do not take valacyclovir if you have ever had an allergic reaction to antiviral drugs.

OVERDOSE
Symptoms: No cases of overdose of valacyclovir have been reported. If an overdose were to occur, symptoms likely would be those of acute kidney failure, which include blood in the urine; passing only small amounts of urine; swelling of the ankles, hands, face, or other areas; shortness of breath; itching; fever; and flank pain.

What to Do: Seek medical assistance immediately.

▼ INTERACTIONS

DRUG INTERACTIONS
Consult your doctor if you are taking any other prescription or over-the-counter medication, especially cimetidine or probenecid. These drugs slow the kidney's removal of valacyclovir, increasing the possibility of adverse side effects.

FOOD INTERACTIONS
No known food interactions.

DISEASE INTERACTIONS
Caution is advised when taking valacyclovir. Use of valacyclovir may cause complications in patients with kidney disease, because these organs work to remove the drug from the body. Consult your doctor if you have a weakened immune system; for example, if you are infected with the human immunodeficiency virus (HIV) or are taking immunosuppressant drugs to prevent organ rejection after a kidney or bone marrow transplant. Use of valacyclovir by patients with weakened immune systems can cause extreme side effects that may be fatal.

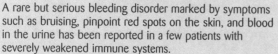

≣ SIDE EFFECTS ≣

SERIOUS
A rare but serious bleeding disorder marked by symptoms such as bruising, pinpoint red spots on the skin, and blood in the urine has been reported in a few patients with severely weakened immune systems.

COMMON
Headache, nausea.

LESS COMMON
Constipation or diarrhea, loss of appetite, dizziness, stomach pain, vomiting, unusual fatigue.

VALPROIC ACID (VALPROATE; DIVALPROEX SODIUM)

Available in: Capsules, syrup
Available OTC? No **As Generic?** Yes
Drug Class: Anticonvulsant

▼ USAGE INFORMATION

WHY IT'S PRESCRIBED
To control certain types of seizures in the treatment of epilepsy and other disorders. Also used to treat acute mania in the treatment of bipolar disorder.

HOW IT WORKS
Valproic acid is thought to depress the activity of certain parts of the brain and suppress the abnormal firing of neurons that causes seizures.

▼ DOSAGE GUIDELINES

RANGE AND FREQUENCY
Adults and children: 7 to 27 mg per lb of body weight in 3 or 4 divided doses. Higher doses may be required. A low dose is used to start; it may be gradually increased by your doctor to achieve maximum therapeutic benefit with a minimum of side effects.

ONSET OF EFFECT
Within several hours.

DURATION OF ACTION
Maximum effect lasts for 12 hours or longer. Effectiveness then gradually decreases.

DIETARY ADVICE
Take it with food to minimize stomach upset. The syrup can be taken with liquids, but avoid carbonated beverages because the combination can irritate the mouth and throat.

STORAGE
Store it in a tightly sealed container away from moisture, heat, and direct light. Do not allow the syrup to freeze.

MISSED DOSE
Take it as soon as you remember. If it is almost time for the next dose, skip the missed dose and resume your regular dosage schedule. Do not double the next dose without your doctor's approval.

STOPPING THE DRUG
Abruptly stopping this drug may cause seizures. Your doctor will taper the dose over a period of weeks.

PROLONGED USE
See your doctor regularly for tests if you must take this drug for a prolonged period.

▼ PRECAUTIONS

Over 60: Older patients may require lower doses to minimize side effects.

Driving and Hazardous Work: This drug may cause drowsiness or dizziness. Do not drive or engage in hazardous work until you determine how it affects you.

Alcohol: May contribute to excessive drowsiness.

Pregnancy: Valproic acid is associated with an increased risk of birth defects when taken during pregnancy. However, seizures during pregnancy can also increase the risks to the fetus. Discuss with your doctor the potential risks and benefits of using this drug during pregnancy. Folate supplementation is recommended starting 1 to 2 months before conception and throughout pregnancy.

Breast Feeding: Valproic acid passes into breast milk, although at low levels. Consult your doctor for specific advice before nursing.

Infants and Children: Adverse reactions may be more likely and more severe in children.

Special Concerns: The generic version of this drug is not recommended. Your doctor may advise you to wear a medical-alert bracelet or carry an identification card saying that you are taking this drug.

OVERDOSE
Symptoms: Restlessness, sleepiness, hallucinations, trembling arms and hands, loss of consciousness.

What to Do: Call your doctor, emergency medical services (EMS), or the nearest poison control center immediately.

▼ INTERACTIONS

DRUG INTERACTIONS
Valproic acid can interact with many drugs, including other anticonvulsants (carbamazepine, clonazepam, ethosuximide, felbamate, lamotrigine, phenobarbital, phenytoin, primidone), antacids, aspirin and other nonsteroidal antiinflammatory drugs (NSAIDs), barbiturates, cholestyramine, haloperidol, heparin, isoniazid, loxapine, monoamine oxidase (MAO) inhibitors, maprotiline, phenobarbital, tricyclic antidepressants, and warfarin.

FOOD INTERACTIONS
No known food interactions.

DISEASE INTERACTIONS
Special caution is advised if you have a history of blood disease, brain disease, or kidney or liver disease.

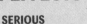

SIDE EFFECTS

SERIOUS
Severe abdominal pain and vomiting, muscle weakness and lethargy, yellow discoloration of the skin or eyes, facial swelling, abnormal bleeding or bruising, or seizures may be a sign of liver failure or other potentially fatal complications. Call your doctor immediately.

COMMON
Nausea and vomiting, heartburn, diarrhea, cramps, loss of appetite and weight loss, increased appetite and weight gain, hair loss, tremor, dizziness, confusion, clumsiness or unsteadiness, sedation.

LESS COMMON
Drowsiness, restlessness, constipation, unusual excitability, skin rash, headache, blurred or double vision, irritability or other changes in mental state. There are numerous additional side effects; consult your doctor if you are concerned about any adverse or unusual reactions.

VALSARTAN

Available in: Capsules
Available OTC? No   **As Generic?** No
Drug Class: Antihypertensive/angiotensin II antagonist

▼ USAGE INFORMATION

WHY IT'S PRESCRIBED
To control high blood pressure. This drug appears to have the same benefits as the class of antihypertensive drugs known as angiotensin-converting enzyme (ACE) inhibitors, without producing the common side effect (experienced by as many as 30% of patients) of a dry cough. Your doctor may prescribe valsartan to be used by itself or in conjunction with other antihypertensive medications.

HOW IT WORKS
Valsartan blocks the effects of angiotensin II, a naturally occurring substance that causes blood vessels to narrow. Valsartan causes the blood vessels to dilate, thereby lowering blood pressure and decreasing the workload of the heart.

▼ DOSAGE GUIDELINES

RANGE AND FREQUENCY
To start, 80 mg once a day. The dose may be increased by your doctor to a maximum dose of 320 mg a day.

ONSET OF EFFECT
Within 2 to 4 weeks.

DURATION OF ACTION
Unknown.

DIETARY ADVICE
Follow a healthy diet (low-salt, low-fat, low-cholesterol) as advised by your doctor to help control blood pressure and prevent heart disease.

STORAGE
Store it in a tightly sealed container away from moisture, heat, and direct light.

MISSED DOSE
Take it as soon as you remember. If it is near the time for the next dose, skip the missed dose and resume your regular dosage schedule. Do not double the next dose.

STOPPING THE DRUG
Take it as prescribed for the full treatment period. The decision to stop taking the drug should be made in consultation with your physician.

PROLONGED USE
Lifelong therapy may be necessary. If you change certain health habits (increasing exercise or losing weight, for example), a reduced dose may be possible under a doctor's supervision.

▼ PRECAUTIONS

Over 60: No special problems are expected.

Driving and Hazardous Work: Do not drive or engage in hazardous work until you determine how the medicine affects you.

Alcohol: No special precautions are necessary.

Pregnancy: In certain ways, valsartan is similar to a class of drugs that have caused damage to the unborn child when taken in the second or third trimester of pregnancy. Because safer, more effective medications can lower blood pressure during pregnancy and because adequate studies on the use of valsartan during pregnancy have not been done, women who are pregnant or planning to become pregnant should not take it.

Breast Feeding: Valsartan may pass into breast milk; caution is advised. Consult your doctor for advice.

Infants and Children: The safety and effectiveness of use by children have not been established.

Special Concerns: Valsartan may cause dizziness or light-headedness, which is most noticeable when you change position. This may lead to fainting, falls, and injury. Sit or lie down immediately if you feel dizzy or lightheaded.

This side effect may be worsened by alcohol, hot weather, dehydration, fever, prolonged standing, prolonged sitting, or exercise.

OVERDOSE
Symptoms: Fainting, dizziness, weak pulse that might be very slow or very fast, nausea, vomiting, confusion, chest pain.

What to Do: An overdose of valsartan is unlikely to be life-threatening. However, if someone takes a much larger dose than prescribed, call your doctor, emergency medical services (EMS), or the nearest poison control center immediately.

▼ INTERACTIONS

DRUG INTERACTIONS
No drug interactions have yet been observed with valsartan. Consult your doctor for specific advice if you are taking any other medication, including other high blood pressure drugs. Valsartan can be taken together with diuretics or other medications for high blood pressure if your doctor approves.

FOOD INTERACTIONS
No known food interactions.

DISEASE INTERACTIONS
Caution is advised when taking valsartan. Use of valsartan may cause complications in patients with liver or kidney disease, because these organs work together to remove the medication from the body.

SIDE EFFECTS

SERIOUS
No serious side effects have been reported.

COMMON
No common side effects have been reported.

LESS COMMON
Headache, dizziness, upper respiratory infection, cough, diarrhea, rhinitis, sinusitis, nausea, viral infection, abdominal pain, fatigue, edema, joint pains, heart palpitations, skin rash, constipation, dry mouth, gas, anxiety, insomnia, erectile dysfunction (impotence) in men.

VENLAFAXINE

BRAND NAMES

Effexor, Effexor XR

Available in: Tablets, extended-release capsules
Available OTC? No   **As Generic?** No
Drug Class: Antidepressant

▼ USAGE INFORMATION

WHY IT'S PRESCRIBED
To treat symptoms of major depression and generalized anxiety disorder (GAD).

HOW IT WORKS
Venlafaxine helps balance levels of serotonin and norepinephrine, which are brain chemicals that are profoundly linked to mood, emotions, and mental state.

▼ DOSAGE GUIDELINES

RANGE AND FREQUENCY
Tablets—Adults: 75 mg a day in 2 or 3 divided doses. The dose may be gradually increased by your doctor to 375 mg a day. Extended-release capsules: 75 mg once a day. The dose may be increased by up to 75 mg at a time at intervals of not less than 4 days up to a maximum dose of 225 mg a day.

ONSET OF EFFECT
2 weeks or more.

DURATION OF ACTION
Unknown.

DIETARY ADVICE
Venlafaxine should be taken with meals.

STORAGE
Store it in a tightly sealed container away from moisture, heat, and direct light.

MISSED DOSE
Tablets: Take it as soon as you remember, unless the time for your next scheduled dose is within the next 2 hours. If so, skip the missed dose, take the next scheduled dose, and resume your regular schedule. Do not double the next dose. Extended-release capsules: If you miss a dose on one day, do not double the dose the next day.

STOPPING THE DRUG
Take as prescribed for the full treatment period.

PROLONGED USE
See your doctor regularly for tests and examinations if you must take this medicine for an extended period.

▼ PRECAUTIONS

Over 60: No special problems are expected.

Driving and Hazardous Work: Do not drive or engage in hazardous work until you determine how the medicine affects you.

Alcohol: Avoid alcohol.

Pregnancy: Adequate studies of venlafaxine use during pregnancy have not been done. Before you take venlafaxine, tell your doctor if you are pregnant or plan to become pregnant.

Breast Feeding: It is not known whether venlafaxine passes into breast milk; caution is advised. Consult your doctor for specific advice.

Infants and Children: The safety and effectiveness of venlafaxine use by children have not been established.

Special Concerns: Venlafaxine can cause an elevation in blood pressure. Therefore, blood pressure should be monitored regularly, especially in the first several months of drug therapy.

OVERDOSE
Symptoms: Extreme drowsiness or fatigue.

What to Do: Call your doctor, emergency medical services (EMS), or the nearest poison control center immediately.

▼ INTERACTIONS

DRUG INTERACTIONS
Venlafaxine and monoamine oxidase (MAO) inhibitors should not be used within 14 days of each other. Serious side effects such as myoclonus (uncontrolled muscle spasms), hyperthermia (excessive rise in body temperature), and extreme stiffness may result. Consult your doctor for specific advice if you are taking any other prescription or over-the-counter medication.

FOOD INTERACTIONS
No known food interactions.

DISEASE INTERACTIONS
Consult your physician if you have a history of any of the following: high or low blood pressure, alcohol or drug abuse, heart disease, or seizures. Use of venlafaxine may cause complications in patients with liver or kidney disease, because these organs work together to remove the medication from the body.

 ## SIDE EFFECTS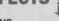

SERIOUS
Headache, changes in or blurred vision, decreased sexual ability or desire, difficulty urinating, itching, skin rash, chest pain, heartbeat irregularities, changes in moods or mental state, extreme drowsiness or fatigue. Call your physician immediately.

COMMON
Fatigue, dizziness or drowsiness, anxiety, dry mouth, changes in taste, loss of appetite, nausea, vomiting, chills, diarrhea, constipation, prickly sensation of skin, heartburn, increased sweating, runny nose, stomach gas or pain, insomnia, unusual dreams, weight loss.

LESS COMMON
Frequent yawning, twitching.

VERAPAMIL HYDROCHLORIDE

Available in: Extended-release capsules, tablets, injection
Available OTC? No   **As Generic?** Yes
Drug Class: Calcium channel blocker

▼ USAGE INFORMATION

WHY IT'S PRESCRIBED
To treat high blood pressure (hypertension), angina pectoris (chest pain associated with heart disease), and heartbeat irregularities (cardiac arrhythmias).

HOW IT WORKS
Verapamil interferes with the movement of calcium into heart muscle cells and the smooth muscle cells in the walls of the arteries. This action relaxes blood vessels (causing them to widen), which lowers blood pressure, increases the blood supply to the heart, and decreases the heart's overall workload.

▼ DOSAGE GUIDELINES

RANGE AND FREQUENCY
Adults: 40 to 160 mg 3 times a day. Your doctor may increase the dose as necessary, up to a maximum of 480 mg a day. Extended-release capsules: 200 to 480 mg once a day. Extended-release tablets: 120 mg once a day to 240 mg every 12 hours. Children: The dose will be determined by a pediatrician.

ONSET OF EFFECT
Oral forms: 1 to 2 hours. Injection: 1 to 5 minutes.

DURATION OF ACTION
Extended-release capsules: 24 hours. Tablets: 8 to 10 hours. Injection: 1 to 6 hours.

DIETARY ADVICE
Take oral forms with food.

STORAGE
Store it in a tightly sealed container away from heat and direct light.

MISSED DOSE
Take it as soon as you remember. If it is near the time for the next dose, skip the missed dose and resume your regular dosage schedule. Do not double the next dose.

STOPPING THE DRUG
Do not stop taking this drug suddenly; this may cause potentially serious health problems. If therapy is to be discontinued, dosage should be reduced gradually according to doctor's instructions.

PROLONGED USE
Lifetime therapy with verapamil may be necessary; regular medical exams and tests are important in such cases.

▼ PRECAUTIONS

Over 60: Adverse reactions may be more likely and more severe in older patients.

Driving and Hazardous Work: Do not drive or engage in hazardous work until you determine how the medicine affects you.

Alcohol: Avoid alcohol.

Pregnancy: Large doses of verapamil have been shown to cause birth defects in animals; human studies have not been done. Before you take verapamil, tell your doctor if you are pregnant or plan to become pregnant.

Breast Feeding: Verapamil passes into breast milk but has not been reported to cause problems; caution is advised. Consult your doctor for advice.

Infants and Children: Oral doses for children 1 to 15 years old must be determined by your pediatrician.

Special Concerns: In addition to taking verapamil, be sure to follow all special instructions on weight control and diet. Your doctor will advise you about which specific factors are most important for you. Check with your doctor before making changes in your diet. Extended-release forms should not be crushed or chewed.

OVERDOSE

Symptoms: Extremely slow heartbeat and heart palpitations; dizziness or fainting (caused by excessively low blood pressure).

What to Do: Call your doctor, emergency medical services (EMS), or the nearest poison control center immediately.

▼ INTERACTIONS

DRUG INTERACTIONS
Consult your physician for specific advice if you are taking acetazolamide, amphotericin B, corticosteroids, dichlorphenamide, diuretics, methazolamide, beta-blockers, carbamazepine, cyclosporine, lithium, procainamide, quinidine, digitalis, disopyramide or the following eye medicines: betaxolol, levobunolol, metipranolol, or timolol.

FOOD INTERACTIONS
Avoid foods high in sodium.

DISEASE INTERACTIONS
Caution is advised when taking verapamil. Consult your doctor if you have any of the following: abnormal heart rhythm or other disorders of the heart and blood vessels, mental depression, or Parkinson's disease. Verapamil may cause complications in patients with liver or kidney disease, because these organs work together to remove the medication from the body.

SIDE EFFECTS

SERIOUS
Breathing difficulty, coughing, or wheezing; irregular or pounding heartbeat; chest pain; extreme dizziness; fainting. Call your doctor immediately.

COMMON
Headache; dizziness; constipation; flushing and a feeling of warmth; swelling in the feet, ankles, or calves; heart palpitations.

LESS COMMON
Diarrhea, nausea, unusual fatigue and weakness, skin rash, increased urination, ringing in the ears.

WARFARIN

BRAND NAMES
Coumadin, Panwarfin

Available in: Tablets, injection
Available OTC? No   **As Generic?** Yes
Drug Class: Anticoagulant

▼ USAGE INFORMATION

WHY IT'S PRESCRIBED
To prevent blood clot formation in patients who are suffering from heart, lung, and blood vessel disorders that could lead to heart attack, stroke, or other problems.

HOW IT WORKS
Warfarin blocks the action of vitamin K, a compound necessary for blood clotting.

▼ DOSAGE GUIDELINES

RANGE AND FREQUENCY
Adults: To start, 5 to 10 mg daily taken once a day. Long-term, usually 2 to 10 mg a day taken once a day. Children: The dose must be determined by a pediatrician. It should be taken at the same time every day.

ONSET OF EFFECT
36 to 48 hours.

DURATION OF ACTION
24 to 96 hours.

DIETARY ADVICE
Warfarin can be taken with liquid or food.

STORAGE
Store it in a tightly sealed container away from heat and direct light.

MISSED DOSE
If you miss a dose, take it as soon as you remember, unless it is almost time for the next dose. In that case, skip the missed dose and go back to your regular schedule. Do not double the next dose.

STOPPING THE DRUG
Take it as prescribed for the full treatment period, even if you begin to feel better before the scheduled end of therapy. The decision to stop taking the drug should be made by your doctor.

PROLONGED USE
Regular tests of prothrombin time (a simple test that measures the time it takes for one stage of blood coagulation to occur) are needed when taking this drug. Your doctor may also take stool and urine samples periodically to check for the presence of blood.

▼ PRECAUTIONS

Over 60: Adverse reactions may be more likely and more severe in older patients.

Driving and Hazardous Work: Avoid this if you have blurred vision or feel dizzy. Avoid activities that could cause injury.

Alcohol: Use it with caution. Alcohol can increase or decrease the effect of warfarin. Generally, consume no more than one drink a day.

Pregnancy: Warfarin may cause birth defects. Do not use during pregnancy.

Breast Feeding: Warfarin passes into breast milk. Do not use while nursing.

Infants and Children: Not recommended for children under 18 years.

OVERDOSE
Symptoms: Bleeding gums, uncontrolled nosebleeds, blood in the urine or stools.

What to Do: Discontinue use and call your doctor, emergency medical services (EMS), or the nearest poison control center right away.

▼ INTERACTIONS

DRUG INTERACTIONS
Consult your doctor for specific advice if you are taking steroid drugs, acetaminophen, allopurinol, aminogluthemide, antibiotics, antiarrhythmic heart drugs, androgens, antacids, antifungal drugs, antihistamines, aspirin, antidiabetic drugs, disulfiram, barbiturates, benzodiazepine tranquilizers, calcium supplements, chloramphenicol, any cholesterol-lowering drugs, or a nonsteroidal antiinflammatory drug (NSAID).

FOOD INTERACTIONS
Avoid green, leafy vegetables and other foods that are rich in vitamin K (liver, broccoli, cauliflower, kale, spinach, and cabbage). Intake of too much vitamin K can override the anticlotting effect of warfarin and render the drug useless. On the other hand, certain substances can interfere with the absorption of vitamin K so much that normal, healthy clotting (necessary for wounds to heal) is impaired. Megadoses of vitamin E can do this, as can fish oil supplements and foods high in omega-3 fatty acids. These substances can enhance the effect of anticlotting drugs so much that a tendency to hemorrhage may result.

DISEASE INTERACTIONS
Consult your doctor about taking warfarin if you have high blood pressure, diabetes, serious liver or kidney disease, or a severe allergy.

≡ SIDE EFFECTS ≡

SERIOUS
Allergic reaction (marked by wheezing, breathing difficulty, hives, or swelling of lips, tongue, and throat); bleeding into skin and soft tissue; abnormal bleeding from nose, gastrointestinal tract, urinary tract, or uterus; severe infection; excessive or unexpected menstrual bleeding; black vomit; bruises or purple marks on skin. Consult your doctor immediately.

COMMON
No common side effects have been reported.

LESS COMMON
Loss of appetite, unusual weight loss, nausea, vomiting, skin rash, diarrhea, cramping.

ZAFIRLUKAST

Available in: Tablets
Available OTC? No   **As Generic?** No
Drug Class: Leukotriene receptor antagonist

▼ USAGE INFORMATION

WHY IT'S PRESCRIBED
To prevent the symptoms of asthma on a maintenance basis and also to prevent bronchospasm (contraction of the smooth muscle tissue surrounding the airways, which results in narrowing and obstruction of the air passages). Zafirlukast may be used in conjunction with other asthma treatments.

HOW IT WORKS
Zafirlukast blocks receptors for leukotrienes, chemicals that cause inflammation and constriction of the bronchial airways. Unlike bronchodilators, which relieve an acute asthma attack, zafirlukast is taken regularly when no symptoms are present to reduce the chronic airway inflammation that underlies asthma. This prevents symptomatic asthma attacks.

▼ DOSAGE GUIDELINES

RANGE AND FREQUENCY
Adults and teenagers: 20 mg twice a day. Children ages 7 to 11 years: 10 mg twice a day. Doses are usually taken in the morning and evening on an empty stomach (at least 1 hour before or 2 hours after eating).

ONSET OF EFFECT
Within 1 week.

DURATION OF ACTION
Unknown.

DIETARY ADVICE
Zafirlukast should be taken 1 hour before or 2 hours after meals. Taking it with a high-fat or high-protein meal reduces its availability in the body by 40%.

STORAGE
Store it in a tightly sealed container away from heat and direct light.

MISSED DOSE
Take it as soon as you remember. If it is near the time for the next dose, skip the missed dose and resume your regular dosage schedule. Do not double the next dose.

STOPPING THE DRUG
The decision to stop the drug should be made by a doctor.

PROLONGED USE
No problems are expected. It is important to take zafirlukast every day, even during symptom-free periods.

▼ PRECAUTIONS

Over 60: In clinical trials, mild or moderate infections, primarily of the respiratory tract, occurred more often than expected in older patients. The rate of infection was proportional to the dose of zafirlukast taken. Other adverse reactions were no more likely or more severe in older patients than in younger persons.

Driving and Hazardous Work: Do not drive or engage in hazardous work until you determine how the medication affects you.

Alcohol: No special warnings.

Pregnancy: In some animal studies, zafirlukast caused birth defects and other problems. Human studies have not been done. Before you take zafirlukast, tell your doctor if you are pregnant or plan to become pregnant.

Breast Feeding: Zafirlukast passes into breast milk; do not use it while nursing.

Infants and Children: The safety and effectiveness of zafirlukast in children under the age of 7 years have not been established.

Special Concerns: Zafirlukast has no effect on an asthma attack already in progress. In very rare cases, the drug may cause Churg-Strauss syndrome, a tissue disorder that strikes adult asthma patients and, if untreated, can destroy organs. Early symptoms include fever, muscle aches, and weight loss.

OVERDOSE
Symptoms: None.

What to Do: Call your doctor if you suspect an overdose.

▼ INTERACTIONS

DRUG INTERACTIONS
Consult your doctor for specific advice if you are taking aspirin, carbamazepine, cyclosporine, felodipine, isradipine, nicardipine, nifedipine, nimodipine, phenytoin, tolbutamide, erythromycin, terfenadine, theophylline, or warfarin. Patients who are taking warfarin or any other anticoagulant should have their prothrombin time monitored closely and appropriate changes made in the anticoagulant dosage when they start taking zafirlukast. Before you take zafirlukast, tell your doctor if you are allergic to any over-the-counter or prescription medicine.

FOOD INTERACTIONS
No known food interactions.

DISEASE INTERACTIONS
Consult your doctor if you have any other medical condition. Use of zafirlukast can cause complications in patients with liver disease, because this organ works to remove the medication from the body.

⟱ SIDE EFFECTS ⟱

SERIOUS
Burning or prickling sensation, skin rash. A rare side effect with high doses is liver dysfunction (symptoms include abdominal pain, nausea, fatigue, lethargy, itching, yellow discoloration of the eyes or skin, and flulike symptoms). Call your doctor immediately.

COMMON
Headache.

LESS COMMON
Weakness, abdominal pain, back pain, diarrhea, dizziness, mouth ulcers, nausea, vomiting.

ZALEPLON

Available in: Capsules
Available OTC? No   **As Generic?** No
Drug Class: Sedative/hypnotic

▼ USAGE INFORMATION

WHY IT'S PRESCRIBED
For the short-term treatment of insomnia and other sleep-related problems.

HOW IT WORKS
By depressing activity in the central nervous system (the brain and spinal cord), zaleplon causes drowsiness and mild sedation. Because the drug is metabolized more quickly than similar medications, zaleplon is associated with a lower incidence of such common side effects as daytime drowsiness.

▼ DOSAGE GUIDELINES

RANGE AND FREQUENCY
The appropriate dosage will be determined by your doctor. The recommended dosage for adults: 10 mg. Debilitated patients and people over 60: 5 mg. Zaleplon should only be taken at bedtime or after the patient has gone to bed and has difficulty falling asleep.

ONSET OF EFFECT
Within 1 hour.

DURATION OF ACTION
About 4 hours.

DIETARY ADVICE
Do not take it after a heavy, high-fat meal. The absorption of zaleplon may be slowed, thereby reducing the drug's effectiveness.

STORAGE
Store it in a tightly sealed container away from moisture, heat, and direct light.

MISSED DOSE
If you forget to take the medication at bedtime and you are unable to fall asleep, you can still take the drug unless it is within 4 hours of when you need to be awake.

STOPPING THE DRUG
The decision to stop taking the drug should be made in consultation with your doctor.

PROLONGED USE
Zaleplon is usually prescribed only for short-term therapy (lasting several days or up to 4 weeks). See your doctor for periodic evaluations if you must take this drug for a longer time. Persistent insomnia may be a sign of an underlying medical problem.

▼ PRECAUTIONS

Over 60: Adverse reactions may be more likely in older patients. Smaller doses are usually prescribed.

Driving and Hazardous Work: Avoid such activities until you determine how this medication affects you.

Alcohol: Avoid alcohol.

Pregnancy: In large doses, zaleplon has been shown to slow the progress of fetal development in animals. Human studies have not been done. Zaleplon is not recommended for use by pregnant women. Before you take zaleplon, be sure to tell your doctor if you are pregnant or plan to become pregnant.

Breast Feeding: Zaleplon passes into breast milk, but its effect on the nursing infant is unknown. Women who are nursing should not take this medication.

Infants and Children: Safety and effectiveness have not been established for patients under age 18 years.

Special Concerns: When you stop taking zaleplon, you may have trouble falling asleep for the first few nights.

OVERDOSE
Symptoms: Severe drowsiness, breathing difficulty, severe clumsiness or unsteadiness, severe dizziness, severe nausea and vomiting, slow heartbeat, vision problems.

What to Do: Call your doctor, emergency medical services (EMS), or the nearest poison control center immediately.

▼ INTERACTIONS

DRUG INTERACTIONS
Other drugs may interact with zaleplon. Consult your doctor for specific advice if you are taking rifampin, phenytoin, carbamazepine, phenobarbital, or other drugs that depress the central nervous system; these include antihistamines, other psychiatric medications, barbiturates, sedatives, cough medicines, decongestants, and painkillers. Be sure your doctor knows about any over-the-counter medication you may be taking.

FOOD INTERACTIONS
No known food interactions.

DISEASE INTERACTIONS
Caution is advised when taking zaleplon. Consult your doctor if you have a history of drug dependence or alcohol abuse, chronic respiratory disease (including asthma, bronchitis, or emphysema), mental depression, or sleep apnea. Using zaleplon may cause complications in patients with liver disease, because this organ works to remove the medication from the body.

 SIDE EFFECTS

SERIOUS
Hallucinations, abnormal thoughts or behavior, confusion or disorientation, unsteadiness, dizziness, lightheadedness, unusual nervousness, agitation, difficulty breathing. Call your doctor immediately.

COMMON
Daytime drowsiness, general pain or discomfort, memory problems, headache.

LESS COMMON
Abdominal pain, weakness, fever.

ZANAMIVIR

Available in: Inhalant
Available OTC? No   **As Generic?** No
Drug Class: Antiviral

▼ USAGE INFORMATION

WHY IT'S PRESCRIBED
To treat type A or type B influenza. Zanamivir can reduce the severity of symptoms and shorten the duration of flu episodes.

HOW IT WORKS
Zanamivir is believed to interfere with the synthesis of the viral enzyme neuraminidase, which a virus needs in order to infect cells in the respiratory tract and elsewhere in the body. The drug affects only certain susceptible strains of the influenza type A or type B viruses.

▼ DOSAGE GUIDELINES

RANGE AND FREQUENCY
Adults and teenagers: 2 inhalations (one 5-mg blister per inhalation) every 12 hours for 5 days. On the first day of treatment, 2 doses should be taken if possible, provided there is at least 2 hours between doses. On subsequent days, follow the dosage schedule outlined above. Treatment should be initiated within 2 days after the onset of symptoms of the flu.

ONSET OF EFFECT
Unknown.

DURATION OF ACTION
Unknown.

DIETARY ADVICE
No special restrictions.

STORAGE
Store in a tightly sealed container away from heat and direct light.

MISSED DOSE
Take it as soon as you remember that you have missed your dose. If it is near the time for the next dose, skip the missed dose and resume your regular dosage schedule. Do not double the next dose.

STOPPING THE DRUG
It is important to take zanamivir for the full treatment period as prescribed. Do not stop taking the drug before the scheduled end of therapy, even if you begin to feel better; this may lead to a relapse.

PROLONGED USE
If your symptoms do not improve or if they become worse in a few days, you should consult your doctor.

▼ PRECAUTIONS

Over 60: No special problems are expected.

Driving and Hazardous Work: Avoid such activities until you determine how the medicine affects you.

Alcohol: No special warnings.

Pregnancy: Adequate studies have not been completed. Discuss with your doctor the relative risks and benefits of using this drug while pregnant.

Breast Feeding: Zanamivir may pass into breast milk, but it is unknown if this poses any risks to the nursing infant. Consult your doctor for specific advice.

Infants and Children: Zanamivir is not recommended for children under the age of 12 years.

Special Concerns: Zanamivir should be administered using the Diskhaler device. See your doctor for instructions and a demonstration of the proper use of this device.

OVERDOSE
Symptoms: No specific ones have been reported.

What to Do: If you have any reason to suspect an overdose, call your doctor, emergency medical services (EMS), or the nearest poison control center.

▼ INTERACTIONS

DRUG INTERACTIONS
No known drug interactions.

FOOD INTERACTIONS
No known food interactions.

DISEASE INTERACTIONS
Consult your doctor if you have any respiratory illness, such as chronic obstructive pulmonary disease (COPD) or asthma.

⩵ SIDE EFFECTS ⩵

SERIOUS
There are no serious side effects associated with the use of zanamivir.

COMMON
There are no common side effects associated with the use of zanamivir.

LESS COMMON
Dizziness.

ZIDOVUDINE (AZT)

BRAND NAME

Retrovir

Available in: Capsules, syrup, injection
Available OTC? No   **As Generic?** No
Drug Class: Antiviral

▼ USAGE INFORMATION

WHY IT'S PRESCRIBED
To treat human immuno-deficiency virus (HIV) infection in combination with other drugs and to prevent passage of the virus from pregnant women to their babies. Although not a cure for HIV, this drug may suppress the replication of the virus and delay the progression of the disease. Also used to treat HIV-related dementia and HIV-related thrombocytopenia (low platelet count).

HOW IT WORKS
Zidovudine (AZT) interferes with the activity of enzymes needed for the replication of DNA in viral cells, thus preventing HIV from reproducing.

▼ DOSAGE GUIDELINES

RANGE AND FREQUENCY
For HIV infection—Adults and teenagers: Capsules: 200 mg 3 times a day or 300 mg 2 times a day. Injection (given until oral dose can be taken): 0.9 mg per lb of body weight injected slowly into a vein every 4 hours (6 times a day). To prevent the transmission of HIV to newborns— For pregnant women: Capsules: 100 mg 5 times a day from 14th week of pregnancy to delivery. Injection: 0.9 mg per lb of body weight for first hour of delivery, followed by 0.45 mg per lb until the baby is delivered. For newborns: Syrup: 0.9 mg per lb of body weight starting within 12 hours of birth and continuing for 6 weeks. Higher doses (up to 1,200 mg per day) are sometimes used to treat HIV-related dementia or thrombocytopenia.

ONSET OF EFFECT
Unknown. With most anti-retroviral drugs, an early response can be seen within the first few days of therapy, but the maximum effect may take 12 to 16 weeks.

DURATION OF ACTION
Unknown. The effects of zidovudine may be prolonged if the medication is used in combination with other effective drugs and the virus is maximally suppressed.

≣ SIDE EFFECTS ≣

SERIOUS
Anemia (low red blood cell count) causing paleness, fatigue, or shortness of breath; fever. If such symptoms occur, call your doctor right away.

COMMON
Headaches, nausea, muscle aches, insomnia, mood swings, stomach upset, loss of appetite.

LESS COMMON
Bands of discoloration on the fingernails; hepatitis (liver inflammation, which may cause yellowish discoloration of skin and eyes).

DIETARY ADVICE
Take it with food to minimize side effects.

STORAGE
Store it in a tightly sealed container away from heat and direct light.

MISSED DOSE
Take the drug as soon as you remember. If it is near the time for the next dose, skip the missed dose and resume your regular dosage schedule. Do not double the next dose.

STOPPING THE DRUG
The decision to stop taking the drug should be made in consultation with your doctor.

PROLONGED USE
See your doctor regularly for tests and examinations as long as you take this drug.

▼ PRECAUTIONS

Over 60: No special studies have been done on older patients. A lower dose may be necessary, especially if kidney function is impaired.

Driving and Hazardous Work: Do not drive or engage in hazardous work until you determine how the medicine affects you.

Alcohol: Avoid alcohol if liver function is impaired.

Pregnancy: Zidovudine can decrease the risk of passing HIV to the unborn child; in animal studies, it has not caused birth defects.

Breast Feeding: Women who are infected with HIV should not breast-feed to avoid transmitting the virus to an uninfected child.

Infants and Children: The usage and dosage of zidovudine for infants and children must be determined by your doctor.

Special Concerns: Use of zidovudine does not eliminate the risk of passing HIV to other persons. You should take appropriate preventive measures.

OVERDOSE
Symptoms: Sudden nausea and vomiting; headache, dizziness, or drowsiness.

What to Do: Seek medical assistance right away.

▼ INTERACTIONS

DRUG INTERACTIONS
Consult your doctor for specific advice if you are taking amphotericin B (by injection), anticancer agents, thyroid drugs, azathioprine, chloramphenicol, colchicine, cyclophosphamide, flucytosine, ganciclovir, interferon, mercaptopurine, methotrexate, plicamycin, clarithromycin, or probenecid. Also consult your doctor for specific advice if you are taking any other prescription or over-the-counter medication.

FOOD INTERACTIONS
Zidovudine may be better tolerated if taken with food.

DISEASE INTERACTIONS
Caution is advised when taking zidovudine. Consult your doctor if you have anemia or another blood problem or liver disease.

ZOLMITRIPTAN

Available in: Tablets
Available OTC? No   **As Generic?** No
Drug Class: Antimigraine/antiheadache drug

▼ USAGE INFORMATION

WHY IT'S PRESCRIBED
To treat severe, acute migraine headaches. This medication is not intended as a migraine preventive or for use against any other kinds of pain or headache, including basilar and hemiplegic migraines. Your doctor will determine whether zolmitriptan is appropriate in your particular case.

HOW IT WORKS
The exact mechanism of zolmitriptan's action is unknown.

▼ DOSAGE GUIDELINES

RANGE AND FREQUENCY
A single dose ranging from half of a 2.5-mg tablet to one 5-mg tablet is generally effective. If the migraine returns or there is only partial relief, the dose may be repeated once after 2 hours, but no more than 10 mg should be taken in a 24-hour period. Because the individual response to zolmitriptan may vary, your doctor will determine the appropriate dosage. A general recommendation is to take one 2.5-mg tablet as the initial dose.

ONSET OF EFFECT
Within 2 hours.

DURATION OF ACTION
Up to 24 hours.

DIETARY ADVICE
The medication can be taken with or without food.

STORAGE
Store it in a tightly sealed container away from moisture, heat, and direct light.

MISSED DOSE
Not applicable; the drug is taken only when necessary.

STOPPING THE DRUG
Consult your doctor before discontinuing zolmitriptan.

PROLONGED USE
No special problems are expected. Patients at risk for heart disease should undergo periodic medical tests and evaluation.

≣ SIDE EFFECTS ≣

SERIOUS
Serious side effects with zolmitriptan are rare. However, zolmitriptan may cause a heart attack; chest pain or tightness; sudden or severe abdominal pain; shortness of breath; wheezing; heartbeat irregularities; swelling of face, eyelids, or lips; skin rash; or hives. Seek emergency medical assistance immediately.

COMMON
Hot flashes or chills, numbness, prickling or tingling sensations, dry mouth, dizziness, drowsiness, weakness.

LESS COMMON
Indigestion, nausea, muscle ache.

▼ PRECAUTIONS

Over 60: Zolmitriptan is not recommended for use in older patients.

Driving and Hazardous Work: Do not drive or engage in dangerous work until you determine how the medication affects you.

Alcohol: No special warnings, although alcohol may trigger or exacerbate migraines.

Pregnancy: Do not use zolmitriptan without first consulting your doctor if you are pregnant or if you suspect you might be pregnant.

Breast Feeding: Zolmitriptan may pass into breast milk; consult your doctor.

Infants and Children: The safety and effectiveness for patients under age 18 years have not been established.

Special Concerns: Serious but rare heart-related problems may occur after using zolmitriptan. Anyone at risk for unrecognized coronary artery disease—such as postmenopausal women, men over the age of 40, or people with known risk factors for heart disease (hypertension, high blood cholesterol levels, obesity, diabetes, a strong family history of heart disease, or cigarette smoking)—should have the first dose of the medication administered in a doctor's office. Zolmitriptan should not be used by those with any symptoms of active heart disease (chest pain or tightness, shortness of breath).

OVERDOSE

Symptoms: Increase in blood pressure resulting in lightheadedness, tension in the neck, fatigue, and loss of coordination.

What to Do: An overdose with zolmitriptan is unlikely. If someone takes a much larger dose than prescribed, call your doctor, emergency medical services (EMS), or the nearest poison control center immediately.

▼ INTERACTIONS

DRUG INTERACTIONS
Do not take zolmitriptan within 24 hours of taking almotriptan, naratriptan, sumatriptan, rizatriptan, medication containing ergotamine, dihydroergotamine mesylate, or methysergide mesylate. Zolmitriptan and monoamine oxidase (MAO) inhibitors such as phenelzine, tranylcypromine, procarbazine, and selegiline should not be used within 14 days of each other. Zolmitriptan should be used with caution in patients taking SSRIs (selective serotonin reuptake inhibitors), which include fluoxetine, fluvoxamine, paroxetine, and sertraline.

FOOD INTERACTIONS
See Dietary Advice.

DISEASE INTERACTIONS
You should not take zolmitriptan if you have a history of angina, heart disease, stroke, uncontrolled hypertension, heartbeat irregularities, or peripheral vascular disease. Zolmitriptan should be used with caution in patients with liver disease or severely impaired kidney function.

ZOLPIDEM TARTRATE

Available in: Tablets
Available OTC? No   **As Generic?** No
Drug Class: Sedative/hypnotic

▼ USAGE INFORMATION

WHY IT'S PRESCRIBED
For the short-term treatment of insomnia.

HOW IT WORKS
Zolpidem depresses activity in the central nervous system (the brain and spinal cord), which causes drowsiness and mild sedation.

▼ DOSAGE GUIDELINES

RANGE AND FREQUENCY
Adults: 10 mg at bedtime. Patients over 60: 5 mg at bedtime.

ONSET OF EFFECT
Within minutes.

DURATION OF ACTION
2 to 4 hours.

DIETARY ADVICE
Zolpidem may be taken without regard to diet, although it generally works faster on an empty stomach.

STORAGE
Store it in a tightly sealed container away from heat and direct light.

MISSED DOSE
Take the drug as soon as you remember, unless it is late at night. Do not take the drug unless your schedule permits 7 or 8 hours of sleep.

STOPPING THE DRUG
The decision to stop taking the drug should be made in consultation with your doctor. Discontinuing the drug abruptly may produce withdrawal symptoms (including sleep disruption, nervousness, irritability, diarrhea, abdominal cramps, muscle aches, memory impairment). The dosage should be reduced gradually according to your doctor's instructions.

PROLONGED USE
Zolpidem is usually prescribed only for short-term therapy (lasting several days or up to 2 weeks). See your doctor for periodic evaluations if you must take this medicine for a longer time. Persistent insomnia may be a sign of an underlying medical problem.

▼ PRECAUTIONS

Over 60: Adverse reactions may be more likely and more severe in older patients. Smaller doses usually are prescribed.

Driving and Hazardous Work: Zolpidem may impair mental alertness and physical coordination. Adjust your activities accordingly.

Alcohol: Avoid alcohol.

Pregnancy: In large doses, zolpidem has been shown to slow the progress of fetal development in animals. Human studies have not been done. Before you take the drug, be sure to tell your doctor if you are pregnant or plan to become pregnant.

Breast Feeding: Zolpidem passes into breast milk, but its effect on the nursing infant is unknown. Consult your doctor for advice.

Infants and Children: Safety and effectiveness have not been established for patients under age 18 years.

Special Concerns: When you stop taking zolpidem, you may have trouble falling asleep for the first few nights.

OVERDOSE
Symptoms: Severe drowsiness, breathing difficulty, severe clumsiness or unsteadiness, severe dizziness, severe nausea and vomiting, slow heartbeat, vision problems.

What to Do: Call your doctor, emergency medical services (EMS), or the nearest poison control center immediately.

▼ INTERACTIONS

DRUG INTERACTIONS
Other drugs may interact with zolpidem. Consult your doctor for specific advice if you are taking tricyclic antidepressants (such as amitriptyline, clomipramine, doxepin, or nortriptyline) or other drugs that depress the central nervous system; these include antihistamines, barbiturates, other psychiatric medications, sedatives, cough medicines, decongestants, and painkillers. Be sure your doctor knows about any over-the-counter medication you may take.

FOOD INTERACTIONS
No known food interactions.

DISEASE INTERACTIONS
Caution is advised when taking zolpidem. Consult your doctor if you have a history of alcohol abuse or drug dependence, sleep apnea, chronic respiratory disease (including asthma, bronchitis, or emphysema), or mental depression. Use of zolpidem may cause complications in patients with liver or kidney disease, because these organs work together to remove the medication from the body.

 ≡ SIDE EFFECTS ≡

SERIOUS
Hallucinations, abnormal thoughts or behavior, confusion or disorientation, unsteadiness, dizziness, lightheadedness, unusual nervousness, agitation, difficulty breathing. Call your doctor immediately.

COMMON
Daytime drowsiness, diarrhea, general pain or discomfort, memory problems, nausea, bizarre or unusually vivid dreams, vomiting.

LESS COMMON
Stomach discomfort, agitation, feelings of panic, convulsions, muscle cramps, nausea, vomiting, unusual fatigue, uncontrolled weeping, worsening of emotional problems, vision problems, dry mouth.

A-to-Z
Over-the-Counter
Drug Profiles

ACETAMINOPHEN

Available in: Capsules, caplets, tablets, powder, liquid, suppositories
Available as Generic? Yes
Drug Class: Analgesic; antipyretic (fever reducer)

BRAND NAMES

Aceta, Actamin, Anacin-3, Apacet, Aspirin Free Anacin, Atasol, Banesin, Dapa, Datril Extra-Strength, Feverall, Genapap, Genebs, Liquiprin, Neopap, Oraphen-PD, Panadol, Phenaphen, Redutemp, Snaplets-FR, Suppap, Tapanol, Tylenol, Valorin

▼ USAGE INFORMATION

WHY IT'S TAKEN
To treat mild to moderate pain and fever, including simple headaches, muscle aches, and mild forms of arthritis. Acetaminophen is useful for patients who cannot take aspirin, such as those taking anticoagulants or suffering from gastrointestinal ulcers or bleeding disorders.

HOW IT WORKS
Acetaminophen appears to interfere with the action of prostaglandins, substances in the body that cause inflammation and make nerves more sensitive to pain impulses. It also relieves fever, probably by acting on the heat-regulating center of the brain.

▼ DOSAGE GUIDELINES

RANGE AND FREQUENCY
Adults and teenagers: 325 to 650 mg every 4 to 6 hours or 1 g 3 to 4 times a day as needed. Extended-release caplets: 2 every 8 hours. Maximum dosage with short-term therapy should not exceed 4 g a day; with long-term therapy, it should not exceed 2.6 g a day unless otherwise prescribed by your doctor. Children 12 years and under: Consult a pediatrician for the proper dose. The liquid form may be recommended for young children.

ONSET OF EFFECT
Within 15 to 30 minutes.

DURATION OF ACTION
3 to 4 hours; 8 hours for extended-release form.

DIETARY ADVICE
Take it with water 30 minutes before or 2 hours after meals. It may be taken with milk to minimize stomach upset. If you are on a salt-restricted diet, be sure to take into account the sodium present in the powder form of acetaminophen.

STORAGE
Store it in a tightly sealed container away from heat and direct light. Refrigerate liquid forms (to make them more palatable) and rectal suppositories. Do not allow the medication to freeze.

MISSED DOSE
Take it as soon as you remember. If it is near the time for the next dose, skip the missed dose and resume your regular dosage schedule. Do not double the next dose.

STOPPING THE DRUG
Unless directed otherwise by your doctor, limit use to 5 days for children under 12 years and 10 days for adults.

PROLONGED USE
Prolonged use may lead to liver problems, kidney problems, or anemia in some patients. Talk to your doctor about the need for periodic physical examinations and laboratory tests.

▼ PRECAUTIONS

Over 60: Adverse reactions may be more likely and more severe in older patients; lower doses may be necessary.

Driving and Hazardous Work: No problems are expected.

Alcohol: Avoid alcohol; combining the two can cause serious liver problems. Patients with a history of alcohol abuse should not use acetaminophen except under close supervision by a doctor.

Pregnancy: No problems have been reported. Consult your doctor if you are or plan to become pregnant.

Breast Feeding: No problems have been reported.

Infants and Children: No problems are expected; however, some formulations are sweetened with aspartame, which should not be consumed by children with phenylketonuria.

OVERDOSE
Symptoms: Nausea, vomiting, appetite loss, abdominal pain, excessive sweating, confusion, drowsiness or exhaustion, stomach tenderness, heartbeat irregularities, yellowing of the skin and eyes.

What to Do: If you suspect an overdose, seek medical aid immediately, even if no symptoms are present. Steps must be taken promptly to avoid potentially fatal liver damage.

▼ INTERACTIONS

DRUG INTERACTIONS
Consult your doctor for specific advice if you are taking anticoagulants (such as warfarin), aspirin, an nonsteroidal antiinflammatory drug (NSAID), barbiturates, carbamazepine, hydantoins, rifampin, sulfinpyrazone, isoniazid, nicotine, or zidovudine.

FOOD INTERACTIONS
No known food interactions.

DISEASE INTERACTIONS
Consult your doctor before taking this drug if you have liver or kidney disease, diabetes mellitus, phenylketonuria, or a history of alcohol abuse.

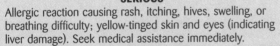

≣ SIDE EFFECTS ≣

SERIOUS
Allergic reaction causing rash, itching, hives, swelling, or breathing difficulty; yellow-tinged skin and eyes (indicating liver damage). Seek medical assistance immediately.

COMMON
No common side effects have been reported.

LESS COMMON
Sore throat and fever (not present before treatment and not caused by the condition being treated); extreme fatigue or weakness; unexplained bleeding or bruising; blood in urine; painful, decreased, or frequent urination.

ACETAMINOPHEN/ASPIRIN/CAFFEINE

BRAND NAMES

Buffets II, Duradyne, Excedrin Extra Strength, Excedrin Migraine, Gelpirin, Goody's Extra Strength Tablets, Goody's Headache Powders, Supac, Vanquish Caplets

Available in: Tablets, caplets, oral powder
Available as Generic? No
Drug Class: Analgesic

▼ USAGE INFORMATION

WHY IT'S TAKEN
For the temporary relief of mild to moderate pain associated with arthritis or migraines.

HOW IT WORKS
Acetaminophen and aspirin both appear to interfere with the production of prostaglandins, naturally occurring substances in the body that cause inflammation and make nerves more sensitive to pain impulses. Caffeine is believed to enhance the effectiveness of pain relievers.

▼ DOSAGE GUIDELINES

RANGE AND FREQUENCY
Because the amount of each of the components varies with different brands, consult your doctor for the appropriate dose. The following are general guidelines. Adults and teenagers—Tablets and caplets: 1 to 2 pills every 3 to 6 hours as needed and depending on the strength of the product. Do not take more than 8 pills in a 24-hour period. Oral powder: 1 packet followed immediately by a full glass of water every 6 hours. Children: Generally not recommended for children.

ONSET OF EFFECT
Unknown.

DURATION OF ACTION
Unknown.

DIETARY ADVICE
It should be taken with food or a full glass of water to minimize stomach upset.

STORAGE
Store it in a tightly sealed container protected from heat, moisture, and direct light.

MISSED DOSE
Skip the missed dose and then resume your regular dosage schedule. Do not double the next dose.

STOPPING THE DRUG
You may stop taking the drug whenever you choose.

PROLONGED USE
This combination is indicated for short-term use only. Side effects are more likely with prolonged use.

▼ PRECAUTIONS

Over 60: Adverse reactions may be more common and more severe.

Driving and Hazardous Work: This drug may cause drowsiness or vision difficulties.

Alcohol: Do not consume more than 2 alcoholic beverages a day.

Pregnancy: Discuss with your doctor the relative risks and benefits of using this drug while pregnant. This drug should not be used during the last 3 months of pregnancy.

Breast Feeding: This drug may pass into breast milk; consult your doctor for specific advice.

Infants and Children: Consult your pediatrician. This drug is not recommended for children under 16 years, because the aspirin component may cause a rare but life-threatening liver condition known as Reye's syndrome.

Special Concerns: Be sure your doctor knows you are taking this medication; it can interfere with the results of some blood and urine tests. Patients allergic to aspirin should not take this drug.

OVERDOSE
Symptoms: Nausea and vomiting, disorientation, seizures, rapid breathing, ringing or buzzing in the ears, fever, appetite loss, abdominal pain, excessive sweating, drowsiness or exhaustion, stomach tenderness, heartbeat irregularities, yellow discoloration of the skin and eyes, agitation, anxiety, restlessness, delirium.

What to Do: Call your doctor, emergency medical services (EMS), or the nearest poison control center immediately.

▼ INTERACTIONS

DRUG INTERACTIONS
Consult your doctor before taking this drug if you are currently taking any of the following: blood pressure medication, gout or arthritis drugs, anticoagulants such as warfarin, antidiabetic agents, steroids, seizure medication, NSAIDs, barbiturates, nicotine, zidovudine (AZT), isoniazid, a central nervous system stimulant, a monoamine oxidase (MAO) inhibitor, amantadine, OTC cold and allergy medications, or asthma medicine.

FOOD INTERACTIONS
Do not drink large amounts of beverages containing caffeine, such as coffee, tea, cola, cocoa, or chocolate milk.

DISEASE INTERACTIONS
Consult your doctor if you have liver or kidney disease, diabetes mellitus, phenylketonuria, asthma, a bleeding disorder, congestive heart failure, gout, high blood pressure, thyroid disease, a peptic ulcer, anxiety, panic attacks, agoraphobia, insomnia, or a history of alcohol abuse.

≣ SIDE EFFECTS ≣

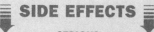

SERIOUS
Difficulty swallowing; dizziness, lightheadedness, or fainting; flushing, redness, or change in color of skin; difficulty breathing, shortness of breath, tightness in the chest, or wheezing; sudden decrease in urine output; swelling of face, eyelids, or lips; black or tarry stools; unusual bleeding or bruising; yellow discoloration of the skin and eyes (indicating liver damage). Call your doctor immediately.

COMMON
Indigestion, nausea and vomiting, stomach pain.

LESS COMMON
Sleeping difficulty, nervousness, irritability.

ALUMINUM SALTS

Available in: Tablets, capsules, oral suspension, gel
Available as Generic? Yes
Drug Class: Antacid

▼ USAGE INFORMATION

WHY IT'S TAKEN
To treat heartburn, acid indigestion, sour stomach, peptic ulcers, gastritis, esophagitis, and gastroesophageal reflux. May also be used to treat or prevent excess phosphate in the blood or to prevent urinary phosphate stones.

HOW IT WORKS
Aluminum salts neutralize stomach acid and reduce the action of pepsin, a digestive enzyme. This provides symptomatic relief from excess stomach acid.

▼ DOSAGE GUIDELINES

RANGE AND FREQUENCY
1 to 2 tablets or capsules or 1 tsp to 2 tbsp suspension or gel as often as every 2 hours, up to 12 times per day. Take the dose between meals unless your doctor directs otherwise. When using it as sole treatment of peptic ulcer or esophagitis, take it 1 and 3 hours after meals and at bedtime. Tablets should be chewed.

ONSET OF EFFECT
Within minutes.

DURATION OF ACTION
20 minutes to 3 hours.

DIETARY ADVICE
Avoid a low-phosphate diet during prolonged use unless your doctor directs otherwise. Some recommended high-phosphate foods include red meat, poultry, fish, eggs, dark green leafy vegetables, dairy products, and nuts.

STORAGE
Store in a tightly sealed container and protect from heat, moisture, and direct light. Refrigerate liquid forms.

MISSED DOSE
Take it as soon as you remember. Do not double the next dose.

STOPPING THE DRUG
Take it as directed.

PROLONGED USE
Do not take it for more than 2 weeks unless your doctor recommends otherwise.

▼ PRECAUTIONS

Over 60: Constipation or intestinal trouble is more common in older persons. Older patients who have or who are at high risk for osteoporosis or other bone disorders should avoid frequent use of this medicine.

Driving and Hazardous Work: No special precautions are necessary.

Alcohol: Alcohol decreases the effect of antacids.

Pregnancy: Consult your doctor before taking aluminum salts while pregnant.

Breast Feeding: Antacids containing aluminum pass into breast milk. It is unknown whether this poses any risk to nursing infants. Consult your doctor for advice.

Infants and Children: Antacids should not be given to children under age 6 years unless otherwise instructed by a physician.

Special Concerns: Use over-the-counter antacids only occasionally unless otherwise directed by your doctor. Persistent heartburn that is not readily relieved by antacids may be a signal of a heart attack or another serious disorder. In such cases, seek medical help promptly.

OVERDOSE
Symptoms: Shallow breathing, dry mouth, constipation or diarrhea, confusion, headache, weakness or fatigue, bone pain, stupor.

What to Do: Seek medical assistance immediately.

▼ INTERACTIONS

DRUG INTERACTIONS
Other medications may lose their effectiveness when taken within 1 hour of antacids. Consult your doctor for specific advice if you are taking amphetamines, bisacodyl, citrates, chenodiol, digoxin, enteric-coated medications, iron salts, isoniazid, ketoconazole, mecamylamine, methenamine, penicillamine, phosphates, nitrofurantoin, quinidine, salicylates, or tetracyclines.

FOOD INTERACTIONS
Taking an aluminum salt with food can decrease its activity. Wait at least 60 minutes after eating before taking it.

DISEASE INTERACTIONS
Do not take aluminum salts if you have any symptoms of appendicitis or an inflamed bowel (abdominal pain, cramps, soreness, bloating, nausea, vomiting). Aluminum salts are not recommended for Alzheimer's patients. Consult your doctor if you have chronic constipation, colitis, ileostomy, colostomy, intestinal or stomach blockage, bone fractures, diarrhea, kidney disease, hypophosphatemia, heart disease, liver disease, edema, stomach bleeding, intestinal bleeding.

≡ SIDE EFFECTS ≡

SERIOUS
Severe and continuing constipation, dizziness, lightheadedness, heartbeat irregularities. Bone loss may occur, especially with prolonged use in dialysis patients. Hypophosphatemia (too little phosphate in the blood) may occur with prolonged use and a low-phosphate diet; symptoms include bone pain, fractures, muscle weakness, loss of appetite, mood changes, a general feeling of discomfort, swelling of the wrists and ankles, unusual weight loss, and anemia (decreased number of red blood cells; symptoms include weakness and fatigue).

COMMON
Chalky taste.

LESS COMMON
Mild constipation, stomach cramps, speckling or whitish coloration of stools, increased thirst, nausea and vomiting.

ASPIRIN

Available in: Tablets, capsules
Available as Generic? Yes
Drug Class: Nonsteroidal antiinflammatory drug (NSAID); analgesic; anticoagulant

▼ USAGE INFORMATION

WHY IT'S TAKEN
For mild to moderate every-day pain and inflammation; to reduce fever; to prevent the formation of blood clots, a primary cause of heart attack, stroke, and other circulatory problems; and to ease the joint inflammation, pain, and stiffness of arthritis.

HOW IT WORKS
Nonsteroidal antiinflammatory drugs (NSAIDs) such as aspirin inhibit the release of chemicals in the body called prostaglandins, which play a role in inflammation, although it is unknown exactly how they exert their pain-relieving, fever-reducing, and anti-inflammatory effects.

▼ DOSAGE GUIDELINES

RANGE AND FREQUENCY
For pain or fever: 325 to 650 mg every 4 hours as needed. For prevention of blood clots: 80 to 100 mg daily or every other day. For arthritis: 3,600 to 5,400 mg daily in 2 or more divided doses.

ONSET OF EFFECT
30 minutes.

DURATION OF ACTION
For pain relief: Up to 4 hours.

DIETARY ADVICE
Swallow aspirin with food or a full glass of water to lessen stomach irritation.

STORAGE
Store it in a tightly sealed container away from heat and direct light.

MISSED DOSE
For pain and fever, take a missed dose as soon as you remember, then wait 4 hours for your next dose. For arthritis, take the aspirin as soon as you remember—up to 2 hours late—then return to your regular schedule.

STOPPING THE DRUG
For pain and fever, stop when relief is achieved. For arthritis and blood clotting, consult your doctor about stopping.

PROLONGED USE
Talk to your doctor about the need for medical examinations or laboratory tests if you must take aspirin regularly for a prolonged period.

▼ PRECAUTIONS

Over 60: Gastrointestinal bleeding and irritation are more likely to occur in older persons taking this drug.

Driving and Hazardous Work: The use of aspirin should not impair your ability to perform such tasks safely.

Alcohol: Alcohol intake should be limited because it increases the risk of stomach irritation and bleeding.

Pregnancy: Do not use this drug during the last 3 months of pregnancy unless it is prescribed by your doctor.

Breast Feeding: Aspirin passes into breast milk. Avoid it or do not nurse.

Infants and Children: Do not give aspirin to children under age 16 years unless your doctor instructs otherwise, because it may cause a very rare but life-threatening condition known as Reye's syndrome.

OVERDOSE
Symptoms: Nausea, disorientation, seizures, vomiting, rapid breathing, fever.

What to Do: Call your doctor, emergency medical services (EMS), or the nearest poison control center immediately.

▼ INTERACTIONS

DRUG INTERACTIONS
Consult your doctor before taking aspirin if you currently take blood pressure medication, a medication for gout, an arthritis drug, an anticoagulant such as warfarin, diabetes medication, a steroid, or an antiseizure medication.

FOOD INTERACTIONS
No known adverse food interactions. Taking aspirin with foods or beverages containing caffeine may actually enhance the medicine's pain-relieving effects.

DISEASE INTERACTIONS
Consult your doctor about taking aspirin if you have asthma, a bleeding disorder, congestive heart failure, diabetes mellitus, gout, hemophilia, high blood pressure, kidney disease, liver disease, thyroid disease, or a peptic ulcer.

SIDE EFFECTS

SERIOUS
Vomiting, agitation, extreme fatigue, confusion; allergic reaction causing trouble breathing, redness of face, itching, and swelling of face, lips, or eyelids. These are symptoms of Reye's syndrome, a rare but serious disorder that is most likely to affect patients under the age of 16 years. Seek emergency medical attention immediately.

COMMON
Stomach upset, rash, nausea, ringing in the ears.

LESS COMMON
Insomnia.

ASPIRIN/CAFFEINE

Available in: Tablets
Available as Generic? No
Drug Class: Nonsteroidal antiinflammatory drug (NSAID); analgesic; antirheumatic

▼ USAGE INFORMATION

WHY IT'S TAKEN
For mild to moderate everyday pain and inflammation; to reduce fever; and to ease the joint inflammation, pain, and stiffness associated with arthritis.

HOW IT WORKS
Aspirin appears to interfere with the production of prostaglandins, naturally occurring substances in the body that cause inflammation and make nerves more sensitive to pain impulses. Caffeine may enhance the effectiveness of pain relievers.

▼ DOSAGE GUIDELINES

RANGE AND FREQUENCY
Adults—For pain or fever: 325 to 650 mg every 4 hours as needed. For arthritis: 3,600 to 5,400 mg daily in divided doses. Children 9 years of age and older under a doctor's supervision—For arthritis: 80 to 100 mg per 2.2 lb (1 kg) of body weight a day in divided doses.

ONSET OF EFFECT
For pain, inflammation, or fever: Within 30 minutes. For arthritis: It may take 2 to 3 weeks of treatment to achieve maximum effect.

DURATION OF ACTION
For pain relief, up to 4 hours.

DIETARY ADVICE
Take it with food or a full glass of water to lessen risk of stomach irritation.

STORAGE
Store it in a tightly sealed container, away from heat, moisture, and direct light.

MISSED DOSE
For pain and fever, take a missed dose as soon as you remember, then wait 4 hours for your next dose. For arthritis, take it as soon as you remember—up to 2 hours late—then return to your regular dosing schedule.

STOPPING THE DRUG
For pain and fever, stop when relief is achieved. For arthritis, consult your doctor about stopping therapy.

PROLONGED USE
Talk to your doctor about the need for regular medical examinations or laboratory tests if you must take this medication regularly for a prolonged period.

▼ PRECAUTIONS

Over 60: Gastrointestinal bleeding and irritation are more likely to occur in older persons taking aspirin.

Driving and Hazardous Work: No special precautions are necessary.

Alcohol: Alcohol intake should be limited because it increases the risk of stomach irritation and bleeding.

Pregnancy: Do not use this drug during the last 3 months of pregnancy unless it is prescribed by your doctor.

Breast Feeding: Aspirin passes into breast milk. Avoid it or do not nurse.

Infants and Children: Do not give products containing aspirin to children under age 16 years unless your doctor instructs otherwise, because it may cause a very rare but life-threatening condition known as Reye's syndrome.

OVERDOSE
Symptoms: Nausea, disorientation, seizures, vomiting, rapid breathing, fever.

What to Do: Call your doctor or contact the nearest emergency medical services (EMS) or poison control center immediately.

▼ INTERACTIONS

DRUG INTERACTIONS
Consult your doctor before taking this drug if you currently take blood pressure medication, medication for gout, an arthritis drug, an anticoagulant such as warfarin, diabetes medication, a steroid, or medication to control seizures.

FOOD INTERACTIONS
No known interactions.

DISEASE INTERACTIONS
Consult your doctor about taking this drug if you have asthma, a bleeding disorder, congestive heart failure, diabetes mellitus, gout, hemophilia, high blood pressure, kidney disease, liver disease, thyroid disease, or a peptic ulcer.

 SIDE EFFECTS

SERIOUS
Vomiting, agitation, extreme fatigue, confusion; allergic reaction causing trouble breathing, redness of face, itching, and swelling of face, lips, or eyelids. These are symptoms of Reye's syndrome, a rare but serious disorder that is most likely to affect patients under the age of 16 years. Seek emergency medical attention immediately.

COMMON
Stomach upset, rash, nausea, ringing in the ears.

LESS COMMON
Insomnia.

ATTAPULGITE

BRAND NAMES

Diar-Aid, Diarrest, Diasorb, Diatrol, Donnagel, K-Pek, Kaopectate, Kaopectate Advanced Formula, Kaopectate Maximum Strength, Kaopek, Parepectolin, Rheaban

Available in: Oral suspension, tablets, chewable tablets
Available as Generic? Yes
Drug Class: Antidiarrheal

▼ USAGE INFORMATION

WHY IT'S TAKEN
To treat diarrhea.

HOW IT WORKS
Attapulgite is believed to bind to and remove large volumes of bacteria and toxins from the digestive tract. It may also reduce the fluidity of the stool associated with diarrhea. There is some debate regarding attapulgite's effectiveness.

▼ DOSAGE GUIDELINES

RANGE AND FREQUENCY
Adults and teenagers—Suspension and tablets: 1,200 to 1,500 mg taken after each loose bowel movement; take no more than 9,000 mg in 24 hours. Chewable tablets: 1,200 mg after each loose bowel movement; take no more than 8,400 mg in 24 hours. Children ages 6 to 12 years— Suspension and chewable tablets: 600 mg after each loose bowel movement; take no more than 4,200 mg in 24 hours. Tablets: 750 mg after each loose bowel movement; take no more than 4,500 mg in 24 hours. Children ages 3 to 6 years—Suspension and chewable tablets: 300 mg after each loose bowel movement; take no more than 2,100 mg in 24 hours. Nonchewable tablets should not be taken by children in this age group.

ONSET OF EFFECT
Unknown.

DURATION OF ACTION
Unknown.

DIETARY ADVICE
A mild diet is recommended when recovering from diarrhea. Bananas, rice, applesauce, and plain toast are good choices. Be sure to get plenty of fluids.

STORAGE
Store it in a tightly sealed container protected from heat, moisture, and direct light.

MISSED DOSE
Take it as soon as you remember. However, if it is near the time for the next dose, skip the missed dose and resume your regular dosage schedule. Do not double the next dose.

STOPPING THE DRUG
You may stop taking the drug if you feel better before the scheduled end of therapy.

PROLONGED USE
If diarrhea has not improved or has gotten worse in 2 days, or if you develop a fever, call your doctor.

▼ PRECAUTIONS

Over 60: Older persons with diarrhea are more likely to experience excessive loss of body fluid and therefore are advised to increase their fluid intake accordingly.

Driving and Hazardous Work: The use of attapulgite should not impair your ability to perform such tasks safely.

Alcohol: Avoid alcohol.

Pregnancy: Attapulgite is not absorbed by the body and is not expected to cause problems during pregnancy.

Breast Feeding: Attapulgite is not absorbed by the body and is not expected to cause problems while nursing.

Infants and Children: It should not be given to children under age 3 years without consulting your doctor. Be sure your child drinks a sufficient amount of fluids.

Special Concerns: In addition to taking attapulgite, it is important to replace the body fluids lost because of diarrhea. During the first day, you should drink ample amounts of clear liquids, such as decaffeinated colas, ginger ale, and decaffeinated tea, and eat gelatin desserts, such as Jell-O. On the following day, you should continue your fluid intake and eat bland foods, such as applesauce, cooked cereals, and bread. Do not take attapulgite if your diarrhea is accompanied by blood or mucus in the stools.

OVERDOSE
Symptoms: No cases of overdose have been reported.

What to Do: An overdose is unlikely to be life-threatening. However, if someone takes a much larger dose than prescribed, seek medical assistance immediately.

▼ INTERACTIONS

DRUG INTERACTIONS
Other drugs may interact with attapulgite. If you are taking any other medication, do not take it within 2 to 3 hours before or after taking a dose of attapulgite.

FOOD INTERACTIONS
Eating fried or spicy foods, bran, fruits, vegetables, or drinking caffeinated or alcoholic beverages can make diarrhea worse.

DISEASE INTERACTIONS
Consult your doctor if you have an intestinal illness or any other medical condition.

SIDE EFFECTS

SERIOUS
No serious side effects are associated with attapulgite. However, loss of body water caused by diarrhea can cause dry mouth, increased thirst, dizziness, lightheadedness, decreased urination, and wrinkling of skin. Call your doctor immediately if these symptoms develop.

COMMON
Constipation.

LESS COMMON
There are no less common side effects associated with the use of attapulgite.

BACITRACIN

Available in: Ophthalmic ointment and solution; dermatologic (skin) ointment
Available as Generic? Yes
Drug Class: Antibiotic

▼ USAGE INFORMATION

WHY IT'S TAKEN
Dermatologic (skin) ointment is available over the counter for application to minor cuts and abrasions to prevent infection. Ophthalmic preparations are prescribed by a doctor for application to the eyelids or in the eye to treat early minor bacterial infections of the eyelids or conjunctiva (the mucous membranes that line the inner surface of the eyelids).

HOW IT WORKS
It hinders the ability of bacteria to manufacture cell walls, which causes cell death.

▼ DOSAGE GUIDELINES

RANGE AND FREQUENCY
Dermatologic ointment: Apply to a small cut or abrasion 2 times daily. Ophthalmic preparations: Apply to the eye 1 or more times daily.

ONSET OF EFFECT
Unknown.

DURATION OF ACTION
Unknown.

DIETARY ADVICE
No special restrictions.

STORAGE
Store it in a tightly sealed container away from heat and direct light.

MISSED DOSE
Apply it as soon as you remember and resume your regular dosage schedule.

STOPPING THE DRUG
You can stop using the dermatologic ointment as soon as the cut or abrasion is sufficiently healed. The decision to stop using the ophthalmic preparation should be made by your doctor.

PROLONGED USE
Ongoing observation to detect any possible over-growth of bacterial organisms that are not susceptible to the drug (a complication known as superinfection) is needed when the ointment is used.

▼ PRECAUTIONS

Over 60: No special problems are expected.

Driving and Hazardous Work: Ophthalmic ointment may cloud vision; caution is advised during use.

Alcohol: No special precautions required.

Pregnancy: Before using bacitracin, tell your doctor if you are pregnant or plan to become pregnant.

Breast Feeding: Bacitracin may pass into breast milk. Consult your doctor for specific advice.

Infants and Children: No special problems are expected in this group.

Special Concerns: Bacitracin preparations should not be used if you have a history of sensitivity or allergy to bacitracin or any of the other components in the ointment.

OVERDOSE
Symptoms: Severe eye pain, headache, rapid change in vision, sudden appearance of floating spots, acute redness of eye, pain on exposure to light, double vision, itching, burning, inflammation.

What to Do: Call your doctor, emergency medical services (EMS), or the nearest poison control center immediately.

▼ INTERACTIONS

DRUG INTERACTIONS
No other drugs should be applied topically when using bacitracin unless otherwise instructed by your doctor. Bacitracin has not been shown to have any significant interactions with medications taken orally.

FOOD INTERACTIONS
No known food interactions.

DISEASE INTERACTIONS
Caution is advised when using bacitracin. Consult your doctor so other appropriate treatment can be started immediately if superinfection (see Prolonged Use) with nonsusceptible bacteria occurs during therapy.

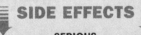

SIDE EFFECTS

SERIOUS
Dermatologic and ophthalmic ointment: Rare severe allergic reaction that may cause hives, breathing difficulty, or, at the extreme, total closure of the airways with potentially fatal anaphylactic shock. Contact emergency medical services (EMS) immediately. Ophthalmic preparations: Severe eye pain, headache, rapid change in vision, sudden appearance of floating spots, acute redness of eye, pain on exposure to light, double vision, itching, burning, inflammation. Call your doctor or ophthalmologist immediately.

COMMON
No common side effects have been reported.

LESS COMMON
Dermatologic ointment: Irritation or skin allergy at the site of application marked by redness, burning, itching, or development of a rash.

BENZOCAINE

Available in: Cream, ointment, aerosol spray, dental paste, lozenges, solution
Available as Generic? Yes
Drug Class: Anesthetic

▼ USAGE INFORMATION

WHY IT'S TAKEN
To relieve minor pain and itching of the skin caused by mild burns, bites, cuts, abrasions, and contact dermatitis (skin inflammation caused by contact with an irritant such as poison ivy or by an allergic response to certain metals or other substances). Dental forms of benzocaine are used to treat pain caused by toothache, teething, cold sores, canker sores, dentures, or other dental appliances.

HOW IT WORKS
Benzocaine interferes with the ability of certain nerves to conduct electrical signals, which blocks the transmission of nerve impulses that carry pain messages.

▼ DOSAGE GUIDELINES

RANGE AND FREQUENCY
Skin cream, ointment, aerosol spray: Apply to affected area 3 or 4 times a day as needed. Dental paste: Apply as needed. Lozenges: 1 lozenge dissolved in the mouth every 2 hours as needed. Aerosol dental solution: 1 or 2 sprays of at least 1 second each taken as needed.

ONSET OF EFFECT
Within minutes.

DURATION OF ACTION
Unknown.

DIETARY ADVICE
Forms applied to skin can be taken without regard to diet. Do not eat or drink anything for 1 hour after using oral and dental forms.

STORAGE
Store it in a tightly sealed container away from heat and direct light.

MISSED DOSE
Take it as soon as you remember. If it is near the time for the next dose, skip the missed dose and resume your regular dosage schedule. Do not double the next dose.

STOPPING THE DRUG
It is advisable to take the medication as prescribed for the full treatment period. However, you may stop taking the drug before the scheduled end of therapy if you are feeling better.

PROLONGED USE
For skin pain or discomfort: Check with your doctor if the condition does not improve within 7 days. For dental pain: If used temporarily for a toothache, arrange for proper dental treatment as soon as possible. For sore throat: Check with your doctor if pain lasts more than 2 days.

▼ PRECAUTIONS

Over 60: Skin: No information is available. Dental use: Adverse reactions may be more likely and more severe in older patients.

Driving and Hazardous Work: No special warnings.

Alcohol: No special precautions are necessary.

Pregnancy: Benzocaine has not been reported to cause problems in pregnancy.

Breast Feeding: No problems are expected.

Infants and Children: Dental paste can be used for teething babies 4 months and older. Other forms of benzocaine are not recommended for use by children under 2 years unless prescribed by your doctor.

Special Concerns: Do not swallow the dental form unless your doctor has instructed you to do so.

OVERDOSE
Symptoms: Both skin and dental forms: Blurred or double vision; confusion; convulsions; dizziness or lightheadedness; drowsiness; feeling hot, cold, or numb; headache; increased sweating; ringing or buzzing in ears; shivering or trembling; slow or irregular heartbeat; trouble breathing; anxiety, nervousness, or restlessness; pale skin; unusual fatigue.

What to Do: Call your doctor, emergency medical services (EMS), or the nearest poison control center immediately.

▼ INTERACTIONS

DRUG INTERACTIONS
With dental benzocaine, consult your doctor for specific advice if you are taking cholinesterase inhibitors or sulfonamides.

FOOD INTERACTIONS
No known food interactions.

DISEASE INTERACTIONS
Consult your doctor if you have any other condition affecting the mouth or skin.

 ≡ SIDE EFFECTS ≡

SERIOUS
Skin: Severe allergic reaction, producing large, red, hive-like swellings on the skin. Dental use: Large swellings in the mouth or throat. Call your doctor immediately.

COMMON
No common side effects are associated with the skin product or the dental product.

LESS COMMON
Contact dermatitis (skin irritation) causing mild burning, stinging, swelling, itching, redness, or tenderness not present before treatment; hives in or around the mouth.

BENZOYL PEROXIDE

Available in: Lotion, cream, gel, pads, cleansing bar, facial mask, stick
Available as Generic? Yes
Drug Class: Acne drug

BRAND NAMES

Benzac W, Benzagel, Benzashave, Clear By Design, Clearasil, Cuticura Acne Cream, Del-Aqua, Desquam, Fostex, Neutrogena Acne Mask, Noxzema Clear-ups, Oxy 10, Oxy 5, PanOxyl, Stri-Dex Maximum Strength, Theroxide

▼ USAGE INFORMATION

WHY IT'S TAKEN
To treat mild to moderate acne. In more severe cases, benzoyl peroxide may be used in conjunction with other acne treatments, such as antibiotics, retinoic acid preparations, and medications containing sulfur or salicylic acid. It may also be used to treat pressure sores and other skin disorders.

HOW IT WORKS
Benzoyl peroxide slowly releases oxygen, which has an antibacterial effect (bacteria are a primary cause of acne). It also causes peeling and drying of skin, which helps eliminate blackheads and whiteheads.

▼ DOSAGE GUIDELINES

RANGE AND FREQUENCY
For the cream, gel, lotion, or stick form of benzoyl, first wash the affected area of skin with medicated soap and water. Pat dry gently with a towel; apply enough medicine to cover the affected area and rub in gently once or twice a day. For the shave cream form, wet the area to be shaved, apply a small amount of the cream, rub over the entire area, shave, then rinse the area and pat it dry. Check with your doctor about using aftershave lotions. If you have a fair complexion, start with a single daily application at bedtime. Keep the medicine away from eyes, nose, and mouth.

ONSET OF EFFECT
1 to several weeks.

DURATION OF ACTION
Up to 24 hours.

DIETARY ADVICE
This medication may be used without regard to diet.

STORAGE
Store it in a tightly sealed container away from heat and direct light.

MISSED DOSE
If you miss a scheduled application, apply it as soon as you remember and then resume regular use.

STOPPING THE DRUG
Benzoyl peroxide can be discontinued when acne improves, but stopping usually leads to a recurrence of acne.

PROLONGED USE
Check with your doctor if you do not see improvement within 4 to 6 weeks. Other medications may be necessary to control acne and to prevent permanent scarring.

▼ PRECAUTIONS

Over 60: No special problems are expected.

Driving and Hazardous Work: No special warnings.

Alcohol: No special warnings.

Pregnancy: Problems during pregnancy have not been documented, but the manufacturer recommends that this drug not be used by pregnant women unless it is considered essential.

Breast Feeding: Benzoyl peroxide may pass into breast milk. Ask your doctor about its use during breast feeding.

Infants and Children: Studies on this medicine have been done only with teenagers and adults, so there is no specific information about its use with other age groups. Nonetheless, no special side effects or problems are expected for children over 12 years. No studies have been done on children under 12 years. Use and dose must be determined by a doctor.

OVERDOSE
Symptoms: Overapplication to the skin may cause burning, itching, scaling, swelling, or redness.

What to Do: Discontinue the drug and consult your doctor. If this drug is accidentally ingested, call your doctor, emergency medical services (EMS), or the nearest poison control center immediately.

▼ INTERACTIONS

DRUG INTERACTIONS
Use of this medicine with skin-peeling agents such as salicylic acid, sulfur, tretinoin, or resorcinol can cause excessive skin irritation. Consult your doctor if you take an oral contraceptive, if you are using any other prescription or nonprescription medication for acne, or if you use medicated cosmetics or abrasive skin cleaners.

FOOD INTERACTIONS
See below.

DISEASE INTERACTIONS
A history of allergy to cinnamon and foods containing benzoic acid increases the chances of developing an allergic skin rash to benzoyl peroxide. Be sure to notify your doctor if you have either of these allergies. Consult your doctor before you use benzoyl peroxide if you have any skin condition other than acne.

≡ SIDE EFFECTS ≡

SERIOUS
Allergic reaction causing burning, blistering, crusting, itching, severe redness, and swelling of skin. Contact your doctor immediately.

COMMON
Mild dryness and peeling of skin.

LESS COMMON
Excessive dryness, unusual feeling of warmth or heat, mild stinging, redness, irritation. This medicine may cause a rash or intensify sunburn in areas of the skin exposed to sunlight or ultraviolet light; avoid excessive sun exposure and tell your doctor if a skin reaction occurs.

BISACODYL

Available in: Tablets, powder, suppositories
Available as Generic? Yes
Drug Class: Stimulant laxative

▼ USAGE INFORMATION

WHY IT'S TAKEN
To relieve short-term constipation or to clear the bowel before rectal or bowel examination, surgery, or childbirth.

HOW IT WORKS
Bisacodyl increases the volume of fluid in the intestines to stimulate passage of the stool. It also acts on the smooth muscle of the intestine to increase contractions.

▼ DOSAGE GUIDELINES

RANGE AND FREQUENCY
For constipation–Adults and teenagers: Tablets: 10 to 15 mg at bedtime. Children age 6 years and older: 5 mg before breakfast. Do not chew tablets. For medical examination–Adults and teenagers: Up to 30 mg orally or 10 mg given rectally before examination. Children age 6 years and older: 5 mg orally or rectally before breakfast.

ONSET OF EFFECT
Tablets: Within 6 to 12 hours. Suppositories: Within 15 to 60 minutes.

DURATION OF ACTION
Variable.

DIETARY ADVICE
Take the tablet on an empty stomach for rapid effect. Increase intake of fluids and dietary fiber.

STORAGE
Store it in a tightly sealed container and keep it away from heat, moisture, and direct light.

MISSED DOSE
Take the missed dose as soon as you remember, unless it is almost time for your next dose. In that case, skip the missed dose and resume your regular dosage schedule. Do not double the next dose.

STOPPING THE DRUG
Take it as prescribed for the full treatment period. However, you may stop taking the drug if you are feeling better before the scheduled end of the therapy.

PROLONGED USE
Do not use this medicine for more than 1 week unless your doctor prescribes it.

▼ PRECAUTIONS

Over 60: Excessive use of this drug by an older person can cause loss of body fluid leading to weakness and lack of coordination.

Driving and Hazardous Work: Do not drive or engage in hazardous work until you determine how the medicine affects you.

Alcohol: Avoid alcohol while taking this drug.

Pregnancy: Bisacodyl is not usually used during pregnancy except immediately before delivery. Consult your doctor for advice.

Breast Feeding: Bisacodyl may pass into breast milk. Consult your doctor for specific advice.

Infants and Children: Do not give this medicine to a child younger than 6 years without your doctor's approval. Do not give this medicine to a child who refuses to have a bowel movement. It may result in a painful bowel movement, which will make the child resist even more.

Special Concerns: Remember that chronic use of bisacodyl or any laxative can lead to laxative dependence. You should consume adequate amounts of fiber in your diet, sources of which include bran and whole-grain cereals, fruit, and vegetables.

OVERDOSE
Symptoms: Weakness, increased sweating, lower abdominal pain, muscle cramps, irregular heartbeat.

What to Do: An overdose of bisacodyl is unlikely to be life-threatening. However, if someone takes a much larger dose than prescribed, seek medical assistance immediately.

▼ INTERACTIONS

DRUG INTERACTIONS
Be sure to tell your doctor about any other drugs you are taking, especially antacids. Do not take an antacid within 2 hours of taking this drug.

FOOD INTERACTIONS
Do not drink milk within 2 hours of taking this drug.

DISEASE INTERACTIONS
Caution is advised when taking bisacodyl. Consult your doctor if you have very severe constipation, severe pain in the stomach or lower abdomen, cramping, bloating, nausea, or unexplained rectal bleeding. Failure to produce a bowel movement or the presence of rectal bleeding may indicate a serious medical condition.

SIDE EFFECTS

SERIOUS
Severe stomach pain, laxative dependence. Call your doctor immediately.

COMMON
Abdominal cramping, burning sensation in the rectum (with suppository), diarrhea.

LESS COMMON
Nausea; vomiting; muscle weakness; rectal pain, bleeding, burning, or itching. If you have a sudden change in bowel habits that lasts longer than 2 weeks, consult your doctor.

BISMUTH SUBSALICYLATE

BRAND NAMES

Available in: Tablets, oral suspension
Available as Generic? Yes
Drug Class: Antidiarrheal/antacid

Bismatrol, Pepto-Bismol, Pink Bismuth

▼ USAGE INFORMATION

WHY IT'S TAKEN
To treat heartburn, acid indigestion, diarrhea, and duodenal ulcers and to help prevent traveler's diarrhea.

HOW IT WORKS
Bismuth subsalicylate stimulates the passage of fluid and electrolytes across the wall of the intestinal tract and binds or neutralizes the toxins of some bacteria, rendering them nontoxic. It decreases intestinal inflammation and increases the activity of intestinal muscles and lining.

▼ DOSAGE GUIDELINES

RANGE AND FREQUENCY
Adults—For acid indigestion or mild diarrhea: 2 tablets or 2 tbsp of liquid every 30 to 60 minutes, to a maximum of 16 doses daily of the regular-strength drug for no more than 2 days. Children ages 9 to 12 years: 1 tablet or 1 tbsp every 30 to 60 minutes, to a maximum of 8 doses daily of the regular-strength drug for no more than 2 days. Children ages 6 to 9

years: 2 tsp every 30 to 60 minutes, to a maximum of 16 doses daily of the regular-strength drug for no more than 2 days. Children under age 3 years: Consult your pediatrician. Tablets are not recommended for children under the age of 9 years.

ONSET OF EFFECT
Within 30 to 60 minutes.

DURATION OF ACTION
Unknown.

DIETARY ADVICE
A mild diet is recommended when you're recovering from diarrhea. Bananas, rice, applesauce, and plain toast are good choices. Be sure to get plenty of fluids.

STORAGE
Store it in a tightly sealed container away from heat and direct light. Keep liquid forms of bismuth subsalicylate refrigerated, but do not allow the medicine to freeze.

MISSED DOSE
Take it as soon as you remember. If it is near the time for the next dose, skip the missed dose and resume

your regular dosage schedule. Do not double the next dose.

STOPPING THE DRUG
Take it as recommended for the full treatment period. However, you may stop taking the drug if you feel better before the scheduled end of therapy.

PROLONGED USE
Prolonged use of this medicine may cause constipation. Consult your physician if relief is not achieved within 2 days.

▼ PRECAUTIONS

Over 60: Adverse reactions may be more likely and more severe in older patients.

Driving and Hazardous Work: Do not drive or engage in hazardous work until you determine how this medicine affects you.

Alcohol: Alcohol intake should be limited.

Pregnancy: Regular use of this medicine late in pregnancy may harm the fetus or cause delivery problems. Consult your doctor about taking it if you are pregnant or plan to become pregnant.

Breast Feeding: Bismuth subsalicylate passes into breast milk; avoid or discontinue use while nursing.

Infants and Children: Consult your doctor before giving this medicine to a child or teenager who has or is recovering from chicken pox or the flu.

Special Concerns: Do not take bismuth subsalicylate if

you are allergic to aspirin or another salicylate or if you are taking an anticoagulant or a medicine for diabetes or gout. Do not swallow tablets whole. Crush, chew, or allow the tablets to dissolve in your mouth.

OVERDOSE
Symptoms: Seizures, confusion, rapid or deep breathing, hearing loss or ringing or buzzing in the ears, severe excitability or nervousness, severe drowsiness, loss of consciousness.

What to Do: Call your doctor, emergency medical services (EMS), or the nearest poison control center immediately.

▼ INTERACTIONS

DRUG INTERACTIONS
Consult your doctor for specific advice if you are taking anticoagulants, aspirin and other salicylates, oral diabetes medicine, heparin, probenecid, thrombolytic agents, oral tetracycline, or sulfinpyrazone.

FOOD INTERACTIONS
No known food interactions.

DISEASE INTERACTIONS
Caution is advised when using bismuth subsalicylate. Before taking this drug, tell your doctor if you have diabetes, kidney disease, dehydration, stomach ulcers, dysentery, gout, a bleeding problem, or a history of allergies.

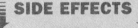

SIDE EFFECTS

SERIOUS
Ringing in the ears. Call your doctor immediately.

COMMON
Black stools, darkening of the tongue.

LESS COMMON
Nausea, vomiting (with high doses), abdominal pain, increased sweating, muscle weakness, hearing loss, thirst, confusion, dizziness, vision problems, trouble breathing. Discontinue the medicine and call your physician immediately.

BROMPHENIRAMINE MALEATE

Available in: Capsules, tablets, extended-release tablets, elixir
Available as Generic? Yes
Drug Class: Antihistamine

▼ USAGE INFORMATION

WHY IT'S TAKEN
To prevent or relieve symptoms of hay fever, allergies, itching skin, or hives.

HOW IT WORKS
The drug brompheniramine blocks the effects of histamine, a chemical substance released by the body that causes swelling, itching, sneezing, watery eyes, hives, and other symptoms of an allergic reaction.

▼ DOSAGE GUIDELINES

RANGE AND FREQUENCY
Capsules, tablets, elixir—Adults and teenagers: 4 mg every 4 to 6 hours. Children ages 6 to 12 years: 2 mg every 4 to 6 hours. Children ages 2 to 6 years: 1 mg every 4 to 6 hours. Extended-release tablets—Adults: 8 mg every 8 to 12 hours or 12 mg every 12 hours. Children age 6 years and older: 8 or 12 mg every 12 hours.

ONSET OF EFFECT
15 to 60 minutes.

DURATION OF ACTION
3 to 6 hours when taken in regular form; 8 to 12 hours for extended-release tablets.

DIETARY ADVICE
Take it with food or milk to minimize stomach upset.

STORAGE
Store it in a sealed container away from heat and light.

MISSED DOSE
Take it as soon as you remember. If it is near the time for the next dose, skip the missed dose and resume your regular dosage schedule. Do not double the next dose.

STOPPING THE DRUG
Take it as recommended for the full treatment period, but you may stop if you feel better before the scheduled end of therapy, or take it as needed.

PROLONGED USE
No special concerns.

▼ PRECAUTIONS

Over 60: Older persons are more sensitive to anti-histamine side effects, particularly confusion, dizziness, drowsiness, restlessness, irritability, nightmares, and dry mouth, nose, and throat.

Driving and Hazardous Work: Brompheniramine can make you feel tired and lessen your concentration. Do not drive or engage in hazardous work until you determine how the drug affects you.

Alcohol: Alcohol increases the likelihood and the severity of side effects such as drowsiness and confusion.

Pregnancy: Animal studies suggest that brompheniramine has no adverse effect on fetal development, but human studies have not been done. Before taking this drug, consult your doctor if you are pregnant or are planning to become pregnant.

Breast Feeding: Brompheniramine passes into breast milk; avoid or discontinue use while breast feeding.

Infants and Children: Brompheniramine should be given to children age 6 years and under only on a doctor's recommendation.

Special Concerns: Do not break, crush, or chew the capsules or the extended-release tablets.

OVERDOSE
Symptoms: Seizures, loss of consciousness, hallucinations, severe drowsiness.

What to Do: The patient should be made to vomit immediately using ipecac syrup. If he or she is unconscious, the patient should be taken to a hospital emergency room immediately.

▼ INTERACTIONS

DRUG INTERACTIONS
Monoamine oxidase (MAO) inhibitors can increase the sedative effects of brompheniramine. Central nervous system depressants such as alcohol, sedatives, or narcotics should be taken only if approved by a doctor.

FOOD INTERACTIONS
No known food interactions.

DISEASE INTERACTIONS
Before taking brompheniramine, consult your doctor if you wear contact lenses or if you have glaucoma, prostate enlargement, difficulty urinating, or dryness of the mouth or eyes.

SIDE EFFECTS

SERIOUS
Bleeding problems; small, red pinpoints on the skin; fever; extreme fatigue; bleeding ulcers in the rectum, mouth, and vagina; reduced white blood cell count (rare).

COMMON
Drowsiness; unusual excitability; dry mouth, nose, or throat. Symptoms of drowsiness tend to subside after a few days of use as your body adjusts to the drug.

LESS COMMON
Vision changes, loss of appetite, dizziness, painful or difficult urination, less tolerance for contact lenses.

BUTOCONAZOLE NITRATE

BRAND NAMES

Femstat 3

Available in: Vaginal cream
Available as Generic? No
Drug Class: Antifungal

▼ USAGE INFORMATION

WHY IT'S TAKEN
To treat fungal (yeast) infections of the vagina.

HOW IT WORKS
Butoconazole prevents fungal organisms from producing vital substances required for growth and function. This drug is effective only for infections caused by fungal organisms. It will not work for bacterial or viral infections.

▼ DOSAGE GUIDELINES

RANGE AND FREQUENCY
Nonpregnant women and teenagers: 5 g (1 applicatorful) of cream inserted with an applicator into the vagina at bedtime for 3 consecutive days. Pregnant women and teenagers: After the third month, 5 g (1 applicatorful) of cream inserted with an applicator into the vagina at bedtime for 6 consecutive days.

ONSET OF EFFECT
Unknown.

DURATION OF ACTION
Unknown.

DIETARY ADVICE
Butoconazole can be applied without regard to diet.

STORAGE
Store it in a tightly sealed container away from moisture, heat, and direct light. Do not allow it to freeze.

MISSED DOSE
Insert it as soon as you remember. If it is near the time for the next dose, skip the missed dose and resume your regular dosage schedule.

STOPPING THE DRUG
Use the medicine as directed for the full treatment period, even if you begin to feel better before the scheduled end of therapy. Recurrence of the infection is likely if you stop before the full treatment period is complete.

PROLONGED USE
Butoconazole is generally prescribed for short-term therapy (3 to 6 days).

▼ PRECAUTIONS

Over 60: No special problems are expected.

Driving and Hazardous Work: The use of butoconazole should not adversely affect your ability to perform such tasks safely.

Alcohol: No special precautions are necessary.

Pregnancy: Studies on the use of butoconazole during the first trimester of pregnancy have not been done. No adverse effects while using it during the second or third trimesters have been reported.

Breast Feeding: No problems are expected. Consult your doctor about using this medicine while nursing.

Infants and Children: Studies on the use of butoconazole for children have not been done. Consult your pediatrician for specific advice.

Special Concerns: The drug may be used with oral contraceptives and antibiotic therapy. Sanitary napkins should be used to prevent staining of clothing. The affected area should be kept cool and dry. The patient should wear loose-fitting cotton clothing and freshly laundered cotton underwear or pantyhose with a cotton crotch. Avoid underwear made from materials that block air. Do not sit for a long time in a wet bathing suit. Avoid feminine hygiene sprays. Wash the area daily with unscented soap and dry thoroughly with a clean towel. Tampons should not be used during therapy. The patient's sexual partner should wear a condom during intercourse and should consult a doctor if penile redness, itching, or discomfort occurs. Do not stop using this medicine during your menstrual period. After urination or a bowel movement, cleanse by wiping the area from front to back to prevent reinfection.

OVERDOSE
Symptoms: An overdose with butoconazole is unlikely.

What to Do: If someone swallows a large amount of butoconazole, call your doctor, emergency medical services (EMS), or the nearest poison control center immediately.

▼ INTERACTIONS

DRUG INTERACTIONS
Tell your doctor if you are using any other prescription or OTC vaginal medication.

FOOD INTERACTIONS
No food interactions have been reported.

DISEASE INTERACTIONS
No disease interactions have been reported.

 SIDE EFFECTS

SERIOUS
Vaginal itching, burning, discharge, or irritation not present prior to treatment. Call your doctor as soon as possible.

COMMON
No common side effects are associated with the use of butoconazole.

LESS COMMON
Headache, stomach cramps or pain, irritation or burning of sexual partner's penis.

CAFFEINE

Available in: Tablets, extended-release capsules
Available as Generic? Yes
Drug Class: Central nervous system stimulant

▼ USAGE INFORMATION

WHY IT'S TAKEN
To restore mental alertness.

HOW IT WORKS
Caffeine acts as a stimulant to all levels of the central nervous system.

▼ DOSAGE GUIDELINES

RANGE AND FREQUENCY
Tablets: 100 to 200 mg; repeat after 3 or 4 hours if needed. Extended-release capsules: 200 to 250 mg; can be repeated after 3 or 4 hours if needed. Citrated caffeine: 65 to 325 mg 3 times a day as needed. Take no more than 1,000 mg a day.

ONSET OF EFFECT
Unknown.

DURATION OF ACTION
Unknown.

DIETARY ADVICE
Take it with food to minimize stomach upset.

STORAGE
Store it in a tightly sealed container away from heat and direct light. Keep it away from moisture and extremes in temperature.

MISSED DOSE
Take it as soon as you remember. If it is near the time for the next dose, skip the missed dose and resume your regular dosage schedule. Do not double the next dose.

STOPPING THE DRUG
The decision to stop taking the drug should be made by your doctor.

PROLONGED USE
Caffeine is not intended for prolonged use.

▼ PRECAUTIONS

Over 60: No special problems are expected.

Driving and Hazardous Work: The use of caffeine should not impair your ability to perform such tasks safely.

Alcohol: No special precautions are necessary.

Pregnancy: Large doses can cause miscarriage, delay the growth of the fetus, or cause problems with the heart rhythm of the fetus. No more than 300 mg of caffeine (the amount in 3 cups of coffee) should be consumed daily during pregnancy.

Breast Feeding: Caffeine passes into breast milk; caution is advised. Consult your doctor for specific advice.

Infants and Children: Caffeine is not recommended for use by children under the age of 12 years.

Special Concerns: To prevent insomnia, do not take caffeine or drink beverages containing caffeine too close to bedtime. After you stop taking caffeine, especially if you stop abruptly, you may experience anxiety, dizziness, headache, irritability, muscle tension, nausea, nervousness, stuffy nose, and unusual fatigue. Consult your doctor if you suffer from any of these symptoms.

OVERDOSE

Symptoms: Stomach or abdominal pains, agitation, anxiety, excitement, restlessness, confusion, delirium, seizures. A very large overdose can cause an irregular heartbeat; seeing zigzag flashes of light; frequent urination; increased sensitivity to touch; muscle twitching; nausea and vomiting, sometimes with blood; insomnia; and ringing in the ears.

What to Do: An overdose of caffeine is unlikely to be life-threatening. However, if someone takes a much larger dose than directed, call your doctor, emergency medical services (EMS), or the nearest poison control center right away.

▼ INTERACTIONS

DRUG INTERACTIONS
Call your doctor for specific advice if you are also taking central nervous system stimulants; monoamine oxidase (MAO) inhibitors; amantadine; ciprofloxacin or norfloxacin (antibiotics); cold, sinus, hay fever, or allergy medications; asthma medicine; pemoline; amphetamines; nabilone; methylphenidate; or chlophedianol.

FOOD INTERACTIONS
Do not drink large amounts of beverages containing caffeine, such as coffee, tea, soft drinks, cocoa, or chocolate milk.

DISEASE INTERACTIONS
Caution is advised when taking caffeine. Consult your doctor if you have any of the following: anxiety, panic attacks, heart disease, high blood pressure, agoraphobia (fear of open places), or insomnia. Use of caffeine may cause complications in patients with liver disease, because this organ works to remove the medication from the body.

SIDE EFFECTS

SERIOUS
Diarrhea, insomnia, dizziness, rapid heartbeat, severe nausea, vomiting, irritability, unusual agitation, tremors. Call your doctor immediately.

COMMON
Mild nausea or jitters.

LESS COMMON
There are no less common side effects associated with the use of caffeine.

CALAMINE

Available in: Lotion, ointment
Available as Generic? Yes
Drug Class: Topical antiitching agent; astringent

▼ USAGE INFORMATION

WHY IT'S TAKEN
To relieve the itching, pain, and discomfort of skin irritations, such as those caused by poison ivy, poison oak, and poison sumac. Calamine will also dry the oozing and weeping of skin eruptions caused by poison ivy, poison oak, and poison sumac.

HOW IT WORKS
The exact mechanism of action is unknown; calamine appears to have natural soothing properties.

▼ DOSAGE GUIDELINES

RANGE AND FREQUENCY
Apply calamine to the affected area of skin as often as needed. To use the lotion, shake it well. Then moisten a wad of cotton with the lotion and use the cotton to apply the lotion to the affected area of skin. Allow the lotion to dry on the skin. To use the ointment, gently rub just enough ointment into the skin to lightly cover the affected area.

ONSET OF EFFECT
Within 1 hour.

DURATION OF ACTION
Unknown.

DIETARY ADVICE
Calamine can be used without regard to diet.

STORAGE
Store it in a tightly sealed container away from heat and direct light. Do not refrigerate calamine or allow it to freeze.

MISSED DOSE
If you are using calamine on a fixed schedule, apply the missed dose as soon as you remember. If it is close to the next dose, skip the missed dose and resume your regular dosage schedule. Do not use more lotion or ointment than necessary per application.

STOPPING THE DRUG
Apply calamine as recommended for as long as your symptoms last.

PROLONGED USE
Call your doctor if you have a skin condition that does not improve or gets worse after 7 days of treatment with calamine.

▼ PRECAUTIONS

Over 60: No special problems have been documented in older patients.

Driving and Hazardous Work: Use of calamine should not impair your ability to perform such tasks safely.

Alcohol: No special precautions are necessary.

Pregnancy: No problems during pregnancy have been documented.

Breast Feeding: Calamine may be used safely while nursing; no problems that affect the baby during breast feeding have been documented.

Infants and Children: Studies on the use of calamine on infants and children have not been done; however, no pediatric-specific problems have been documented.

Special Concerns: Calamine is for external use only. Do not swallow it. Do not use calamine on the eyes or mucous membranes, such as the inside of the mouth, nose, genitals, or anal area. Ingestion of calamine has been reported to cause gastritis (inflammation of the stomach lining) and vomiting. Milk or antacids may be used to treat these symptoms.

OVERDOSE
Symptoms: None.

What to Do: No emergency instructions are applicable, because no cases of overdose have been reported. However, if someone accidentally ingests calamine, seek medical assistance immediately.

▼ INTERACTIONS

DRUG INTERACTIONS
No drug interactions with calamine have been reported. However, you should tell your doctor if you are using any other prescription or over-the-counter medication to treat the same area of skin as calamine.

FOOD INTERACTIONS
No known food interactions.

DISEASE INTERACTIONS
No disease interactions with calamine have been documented. However, tell your doctor if you have any other skin condition.

≡ SIDE EFFECTS ≡
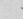

SERIOUS
No serious side effects are associated with calamine.

COMMON
No common side effects are associated with calamine.

LESS COMMON
Rash, irritation, or sensitivity of the treated area that was not present prior to beginning therapy. Call your doctor promptly if such symptoms persist.

CALCIUM

Available in: Capsules, oral suspension, tablets, chewable tablets, liquid
Available as Generic? Yes
Drug Class: Antihypocalcemic; dietary supplement; antacid

▼ USAGE INFORMATION

WHY IT'S TAKEN

To ensure adequate calcium intake in those who do not get sufficient amounts by diet alone. Calcium is essential to many body functions, including the transmission of nerve impulses, the regulation of muscle contraction and relaxation (including of the heart), blood clotting, and various metabolic activities. Calcium is also necessary for maintaining strong bones and is commonly recommended to prevent and treat postmenopausal osteoporosis (bone thinning). Vitamin D supplements, which aid in the absorption of calcium from the intestine, are often used along with calcium supplements to prevent or treat osteoporosis. (Indeed, some calcium supplement tablets contain vitamin D.) Calcium is also prescribed for individuals with persistently low levels of calcium in the blood (hypocalcemia) caused, for example, by low blood levels of parathyroid hormone (hypoparathyroidism).

HOW IT WORKS

Calcium supplements compensate for inadequate dietary intake of this essential mineral. Supplementary calcium is available in the form of calcium carbonate (the most common and inexpensive), calcium citrate (the best absorbed but relatively expensive), calcium phosphate, calcium lactate, or calcium gluconate. Because calcium carbonate and phosphate supplements are hard to absorb, other calcium products are preferable for individuals with low gastric (stomach) acid secretion.

▼ DOSAGE GUIDELINES

RANGE AND FREQUENCY

Optimal daily calcium intakes—Ages 0 to 6 months: 210 mg. Ages 6 months to 1 year: 270 mg. Ages 1 to 3 years: 500 mg. Ages 4 to 8 years: 800 mg. Ages 9 to 18 years: 1,300 mg. Ages 19 to 50 years: 1,000 mg. Age 51 and older: 1,200 mg. For pregnant or breast-feeding women, under 19 years: 1,300 mg. Ages 19 to 50 years: 1,000 mg. When you figure your calcium intake, be sure to include dietary calcium as well as the supplements. Calcium itself constitutes only a fraction of any pill containing calcium. For example, calcium accounts for only 40% of the weight of a calcium carbonate tablet. Thus, a 500-mg tablet of calcium carbonate provides only 200 mg of calcium.

ONSET OF EFFECT

Unknown.

DURATION OF ACTION

For as long as the supplement is taken.

DIETARY ADVICE

Calcium carbonate and calcium phosphate supplements are best absorbed if taken 60 to 90 minutes after meals. Take with 1 full glass (8 oz) of water or juice. Follow all special dietary guidelines your doctor recommends.

STORAGE

Store it in a tightly sealed container protected from heat, moisture, and direct light.

MISSED DOSE

If you are taking a calcium supplement on a regular basis and miss a dose, take it as soon as you remember, then resume your regular dosage schedule.

STOPPING THE DRUG

The decision to stop taking calcium supplements should be made in consultation with your doctor.

PROLONGED USE

Adverse effects are more likely to occur if supplements are taken in doses greater than 2,000 to 2,500 mg a day for a long period of time. Your doctor should regularly check your blood calcium levels if you are taking calcium supplements to treat low blood calcium (hypocalcemia).

▼ PRECAUTIONS

Over 60: No special problems are expected.

Driving and Hazardous Work: Calcium supplements should have no effect on your ability to perform such tasks safely.

Alcohol: To ensure proper absorption of calcium, consume alcohol in moderation only (2 drinks a day).

Pregnancy: It is crucial to take in enough calcium during pregnancy and to maintain those levels throughout pregnancy, preferably through diet alone. However, excessive calcium intake during pregnancy may be harmful to the mother or fetus and should be avoided.

 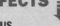

SIDE EFFECTS

SERIOUS

Serious side effects are associated with excessively high doses (see Overdose).

COMMON

No common side effects are associated with recommended doses of calcium.

LESS COMMON

Constipation, diarrhea, drowsiness, loss of appetite, dry mouth, and muscle weakness are some of the symptoms that could result if blood levels of calcium are too high (hypercalcemia).

Breast Feeding: Excessive amounts of this supplement taken while nursing may be harmful to the mother or infant and should be avoided.

Infants and Children: No special problems are expected.

OVERDOSE

Symptoms: Early symptoms: Constipation (especially in children), diarrhea, dry mouth, increased thirst and increased frequency of urination, loss of appetite, persistent headache, metallic taste, nausea and vomiting, unusual fatigue.

Advanced symptoms: Bone and muscle pain, irregular heartbeat, persistent itching, extreme drowsiness, mental changes. Severe calcium toxicity may be fatal.

What to Do: Call your doctor, emergency medical services (EMS), or the nearest poison control center immediately.

▼ INTERACTIONS

DRUG INTERACTIONS

Consult your doctor for specific advice if you are taking other preparations containing calcium, cellulose sodium phosphate, digitalis drugs, etidronate, gallium nitrate, phenytoin, or tetracycline antibiotics. Combined use of calcium supplements and thiazide diuretics or vitamin D may lead to excessively high calcium levels.

FOOD INTERACTIONS

Excessive protein consumption can increase the excretion of calcium in the urine. In meals preceding calcium consumption, avoid spinach and rhubarb (high in oxalic acid) and bran and whole cereals (high in phytic acid), because these substances may interfere with calcium absorption.

DISEASE INTERACTIONS

Consult your doctor if you have frequent episodes of diarrhea, any stomach or intestinal problems, heart disease, sarcoidosis, kidney disease, or kidney stones.

CAPSAICIN

Available in: Cream
Available as Generic? Yes
Drug Class: Analgesic

▼ USAGE INFORMATION

WHY IT'S TAKEN
To relieve neuralgia—pain in the nerve endings near the surface of the skin. Capsaicin is commonly recommended for neuralgia associated with shingles, an acutely painful condition caused by infection with the varicella zoster virus, the same organism that causes chicken pox. Capsaicin is also a treatment for mild to moderate arthritis, diabetic neuropathy (pain caused by nerve cell damage that occurs as a complication of diabetes), and postoperative pain.

HOW IT WORKS
When applied topically, capsaicin (a derivative of hot peppers) appears to reduce the amount of a natural chemical known as substance P, which is present in painful joints. Substance P is believed to be involved in two processes central to arthritis: the release of enzymes that produce inflammation and the transmission of pain impulses from the joints to the central nervous system. By blocking the production and release of substance P, capsaicin can reduce the pain associated with arthritis as well as dampen the transmission of pain messages to the brain.

▼ DOSAGE GUIDELINES

RANGE AND FREQUENCY
Apply a small amount to the affected area up to 4 times a day. Do not apply to broken or irritated skin. If the use of a bandage is recommended, do not apply it too tightly.

ONSET OF EFFECT
Therapeutic pain response is usually achieved in 1 to 2 weeks but may take as long as 4 weeks.

DURATION OF ACTION
Up to 6 hours.

DIETARY ADVICE
This medication can be used without regard to diet.

STORAGE
Store it in a tightly sealed container away from heat and direct light.

MISSED DOSE
Apply it as soon as you remember. If it is near the time for the next dose, skip the missed dose and resume your regular dosage schedule. Do not double the next dose.

STOPPING THE DRUG
Pain relief will last only as long as capsaicin is used regularly. If you stop using the medication and the pain returns, it is safe to resume treatment.

PROLONGED USE
No special problems are expected. Burning and stinging sensations on application frequently subside with prolonged use. If your condition worsens or does not improve after 1 month, discontinue use of capsaicin and consult your doctor.

▼ PRECAUTIONS

Over 60: No special problems are expected.

Driving and Hazardous Work: No problems are expected.

Alcohol: No special precautions are necessary.

Pregnancy: No problems have been reported.

Breast Feeding: No problems are expected.

Infants and Children: Not recommended for use on children under the age of 2 years. No problems are expected in older children.

Special Concerns: You may not be able to use capsaicin if you are allergic to it or if you have ever had an allergic reaction to hot peppers. Wash your hands thoroughly after applying the cream; if you are using it for arthritis of the hands, wait 30 minutes before washing. It can cause a burning sensation if even small amounts get into the eyes or on other sensitive areas of the body. If you wear contact lenses, be especially cautious. If it does get into your eyes, flush them with water. On other sensitive areas of the body, wash the area with warm (but not hot) soapy water. After applying capsaicin cream, avoid contact with children and pets until you have washed your hands thoroughly.

OVERDOSE
Symptoms: No cases of overdose have been reported.

What to Do: An overdose is unlikely to be life-threatening. However, if someone applies a much larger dose than prescribed, suffers adverse side effects, or accidentally ingests it, call your doctor or the nearest poison control center for advice.

▼ INTERACTIONS

DRUG INTERACTIONS
Capsaicin may alter the action of some drugs or trigger unwanted side effects. Consult your doctor about any other drugs that you take, including over-the-counter medications.

FOOD INTERACTIONS
None are known.

DISEASE INTERACTIONS
Consult your doctor if you have broken or irritated skin or conditions that may result in broken skin on the area to be treated.

≡ SIDE EFFECTS ≡

SERIOUS
No serious side effects are associated with capsaicin.

COMMON
Stinging or burning sensation when cream is applied. This should subside with regular use as your body adjusts to the medication.

LESS COMMON
Skin redness; coughing, sneezing, or shortness of breath if dried residue of the drug is inhaled.

CASTOR OIL

Available in: Oral solution
Available as Generic? Yes
Drug Class: Stimulant laxative

▼ USAGE INFORMATION

WHY IT'S TAKEN
For short-term relief of constipation.

HOW IT WORKS
Castor oil stimulates muscle contractions in the wall of the bowel. These contractions promote the passage of stool.

▼ DOSAGE GUIDELINES

RANGE AND FREQUENCY
The dose will be different for different products. A typical dose is 1 to 4 tbsp for adults and teenagers. Castor oil should be taken early in the day because the laxative effect is unpredictable and might interfere with a full night's sleep.

ONSET OF EFFECT
Within 2 to 6 hours.

DURATION OF ACTION
Variable.

DIETARY ADVICE
Laxatives may contain a large amount of sodium or sugar. Regular bowel movements are more likely with a diet that contains an adequate amount of liquid (6 to 8 full 8-oz glasses a day), whole-grain products and bran, fruit, and vegetables.

STORAGE
Store it in a tightly sealed container kept away from heat, moisture, and direct light. Refrigerate the liquid form, but do not allow it to freeze.

MISSED DOSE
If you are on a prescribed dosage schedule, take the missed dose as soon as you remember, unless the time for your next scheduled dose is within the next 2 hours. If so, do not take the missed dose. Take your next scheduled dose at the proper time and resume your regular dosage schedule. Do not double the next dose.

STOPPING THE DRUG
Take it as prescribed for the full treatment period. However, you may stop taking the drug if you are feeling better before the scheduled end of the therapy.

PROLONGED USE
Do not use castor oil for more than 3 to 5 days without informing your physician. Prolonged, excessive use of castor oil may be associated with an increased risk of side effects, including laxative dependence.

▼ PRECAUTIONS

Over 60: Adverse reactions may be more likely and more severe in older patients.

Driving and Hazardous Work: Do not drive or engage in hazardous work until you determine how the medicine affects you.

Alcohol: Avoid alcohol when using this medication.

Pregnancy: Castor oil may cause premature contractions and so should be avoided in pregnant women.

Breast Feeding: Castor oil may be used by nursing mothers.

Infants and Children: Do not give laxatives to children under 6 years of age unless prescribed by a physician.

Special Concerns: Occasional missed bowel movements do not constitute constipation; do not use castor oil under such circumstances. Persistent constipation or difficulty in passing stool is serious and requires evaluation.

OVERDOSE
Symptoms: No cases of overdose with castor oil have been reported.

What to Do: An overdose of castor oil is unlikely to be life-threatening. However, if someone takes a much larger dose than prescribed, contact a physician.

▼ INTERACTIONS

DRUG INTERACTIONS
Do not take a prescription medication within 2 hours of taking a laxative (either before or after), because this may diminish the effects of the prescription drug. Consult your doctor for specific advice if you are taking digitalis drugs or a diuretic.

FOOD INTERACTIONS
No known food interactions.

DISEASE INTERACTIONS
Caution is advised when taking castor oil. Do not use any laxative if you have any of the following: stomach or abdominal pain, especially if accompanied by fever; cramping; abdominal swelling or bloating; or nausea or vomiting. Consult your doctor if you are constipated and have any of the following problems: abdominal pain and fever, rectal bleeding, ostomy (an artificial surgical opening in the body to allow the release of urine or feces), diabetes mellitus, heart or kidney disease, or high blood pressure.

≡ SIDE EFFECTS ≡

SERIOUS
Confusion, irregular heartbeat, muscle cramps. Call your doctor immediately.

COMMON
Laxative dependence, skin rashes, stomach cramps, belching, diarrhea, nausea.

LESS COMMON
Fatigue or weakness.

CHARCOAL, ACTIVATED

Available in: Oral suspension, powder, tablets, capsules
Available as Generic? Yes
Drug Class: Antidote

▼ USAGE INFORMATION

WHY IT'S TAKEN
Used as an emergency anti-dote for treatment of poisonings by most drugs and chemicals; also used to relieve diarrhea or excess gas.

HOW IT WORKS
Activated charcoal prevents the absorption of certain kinds of drugs and chemicals by the body.

▼ DOSAGE GUIDELINES

RANGE AND FREQUENCY
For treatment of poisoning—Oral suspension and powder: Adults and teenagers: 25 to 100 g. Children: 1 g per 2.2 lb (1 kg) of body weight or 25 to 50 g. Mix powder with water. Take 1 time only. For treatment of diarrhea—Capsules: Adults and children age 3 years and older: 520 mg every 30 to 60 minutes as needed. Do not take more than 4.16 g per day. For treatment of excess gas—Tablets and capsules: Adults and teenagers: 975 mg to 3.9 g 3 times a day.

ONSET OF EFFECT
Immediate.

DURATION OF ACTION
Not applicable. Activated charcoal is not absorbed by the body.

DIETARY ADVICE
As an antidote: No special restrictions. To treat diarrhea: It is important to replace the fluid lost by your body and to eat a proper diet. During the first 24 hours, drink plenty of caffeine-free clear liquids, such as water, broth, ginger ale, and decaffeinated tea. During the second 24 hours, you may eat bland foods such as applesauce, bread, crackers, and oatmeal. Avoid caffeine, fried or spicy foods, bran, candy, fruits, and vegetables. These may worsen your condition.

STORAGE
Store it in a tightly sealed container away from heat, moisture, and direct light. The premixed suspension can be stored for up to 1 year. Do not allow the liquid form of activated charcoal to freeze.

MISSED DOSE
As an antidote: Not applicable. To treat diarrhea or excess gas: Take it as soon as you remember. If it is near the time for the next dose, skip the missed dose and resume your regular dosage schedule. Do not double the next dose.

STOPPING THE DRUG
As an antidote: Not applicable. To treat diarrhea or excess gas: Take it as directed for the full treatment period. However, you may stop taking the drug if you are feeling better before the scheduled end of therapy.

PROLONGED USE
As an antidote: Not applicable. To treat diarrhea: If your diarrhea has not improved or if you have developed a fever after 2 days, call your doctor. To treat excess gas: If your condition has not improved after 3 to 4 days, call your doctor.

▼ PRECAUTIONS

Over 60:
No special problems are expected.

Driving and Hazardous Work:
The use of activated charcoal should not impair your ability to perform such tasks safely.

Alcohol:
No special precautions are necessary.

Pregnancy:
Activated charcoal has not been reported to cause problems in an unborn child. Consult your doctor for specific advice.

Breast Feeding:
No problems have been reported.

Infants and Children:
May be used for infants and children only under strict supervision by a doctor.

Special Concerns:
Call your doctor, emergency medical services (EMS), or the nearest poison control center before administering activated charcoal. Charcoal will not be effective if you have been poisoned by swallowing alkalies (lye), petroleum products, strong acids, ethyl or methyl alcohol, iron, boric acid, or lithium. Activated charcoal will not prevent these poisons from being absorbed by the body. If inducing vomiting with ipecac syrup, do so 1 to 2 hours before administering activated charcoal.

OVERDOSE
Symptoms: None expected.

What to Do: Emergency procedures not applicable.

▼ INTERACTIONS

DRUG INTERACTIONS
Activated charcoal may decrease the absorption of any medicine taken within 2 hours of administration. Acetylcysteine and ipecac syrup can decrease the effectiveness of activated charcoal.

FOOD INTERACTIONS
Do not eat chocolate syrup, ice cream, or sherbet with activated charcoal. They will decrease the amount of poison the charcoal can absorb.

DISEASE INTERACTIONS
Caution is advised when taking activated charcoal if you also suffer from dysentery or dehydration.

SIDE EFFECTS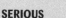

SERIOUS
Swelling or pain in stomach. If this symptom persists, call your doctor immediately.

COMMON
Black, tarry stools.

LESS COMMON
Nausea, constipation. Notify your doctor if any common or less common side effects persist.

CHLORPHENIRAMINE MALEATE ORAL

Available in: Tablets, sustained-release capsules, syrup
Available as Generic? Yes
Drug Class: Antihistamine

▼ USAGE INFORMATION

WHY IT'S TAKEN
To relieve the symptoms of hay fever and other allergies and for itching skin and hives.

HOW IT WORKS
Chlorpheniramine maleate works by blocking the effects of histamine, a naturally occurring substance that causes swelling, itching, sneezing, watery eyes, hives, and other symptoms of allergic reaction.

▼ DOSAGE GUIDELINES

RANGE AND FREQUENCY
Tablets–Adults: 4 mg 3 to 4 times a day as needed, for a maximum dose of 24 mg a day. Sustained-release capsules–8 mg every 8 hours or 12 mg every 12 hours as needed. Syrup–Children ages 6 to 12 years: 2 mg 3 to 4 times a day, not to exceed 12 mg a day. Children ages 2 to 6 years: 1 mg every 6 hours.

ONSET OF EFFECT
15 to 60 minutes.

DURATION OF ACTION
3 to 6 hours for regular form, 8 to 12 hours for sustained-release capsules.

DIETARY ADVICE
Chlorpheniramine maleate may be taken with food or milk to reduce stomach upset. Use sugar-free gum, sugar-free sour hard candy, or ice chips to ease dry mouth.

STORAGE
Store it in a tightly sealed container away from heat and direct light.

MISSED DOSE
Take it as soon as you remember, up to 2 hours late. If it is more than 2 hours late, skip the missed dose and resume your regular dosage schedule. Do not double the next dose.

STOPPING THE DRUG
You should take it as directed for the full treatment period, but you may stop if you are feeling better before the scheduled end of therapy. Chlorpheniramine may be taken as needed.

PROLONGED USE
No special concerns.

▼ PRECAUTIONS

Over 60: Older persons are more sensitive to antihistamine side effects, particularly confusion, dizziness, drowsiness, restlessness, irritability, nightmares, and dry mouth, nose, and throat.

Driving and Hazardous Work: Do not drive or engage in hazardous work until you determine how the medicine affects you. Use of this drug is a disqualification for piloting aircraft.

Alcohol: Alcohol increases the likelihood and the severity of side effects like drowsiness and confusion.

Pregnancy: In animal studies, no birth defects have been reported. Studies of pregnant women have not been undertaken. Before taking this drug, tell your doctor if you are pregnant or are planning to become pregnant.

Breast Feeding: Chlorpheniramine passes into breast milk; avoid or discontinue use while nursing.

Infants and Children: This drug is not recommended for children under the age of 2 years.

Special Concerns: Do not break, crush, or chew sustained-release capsules.

OVERDOSE
Symptoms: Marked drowsiness, dilated and sluggish pupils, combativeness, excessive excitability, confusion, loss of coordination, weak pulse, seizures, loss of consciousness.

What to Do: The patient should be made to vomit immediately using ipecac syrup. If the patient is unconscious, he or she should be taken to the nearest hospital emergency room right away.

▼ INTERACTIONS

DRUG INTERACTIONS
Consult your doctor for specific advice if you are taking anticholinergics, bepridil, medications containing alcohol, or monoamine oxidase (MAO) inhibitors.

FOOD INTERACTIONS
No known food interactions.

DISEASE INTERACTIONS
Before taking chlorpheniramine, consult your doctor if you wear contact lenses or if you have glaucoma, prostate enlargement, difficulty urinating, or dry mouth or eyes.

≡ SIDE EFFECTS ≡

SERIOUS
Bleeding problems; small red pinpoints on the skin; fever; extreme fatigue; bleeding ulcers in the rectum, mouth, and vagina; reduced white blood cell count (rare).

COMMON
Drowsiness; unusual excitability; dry mouth, nose, or throat. Symptoms of drowsiness tend to subside after a few days of use as your body adjusts to the drug.

LESS COMMON
Vision changes, loss of appetite, dizziness, painful or difficult urination, less tolerance for contact lenses.

CIMETIDINE

Available in: Tablets, oral solution, oral suspension
Available as Generic? Yes
Drug Class: Histamine (H2) blocker

▼ USAGE INFORMATION

WHY IT'S TAKEN
To treat ulcers of the stomach and duodenum as well as other conditions, such as esophagitis (chronic inflammation of the esophagus) and gastroesophageal reflux (backwash of stomach acid into the esophagus, resulting in heartburn).

HOW IT WORKS
Cimetidine blocks the action of histamine (a compound produced in the body's cells), which in turn decreases the stomach's secretion of hydrochloric acid. Once stomach acid production is decreased, the body is better able to heal itself.

▼ DOSAGE GUIDELINES

RANGE AND FREQUENCY
For treatment of acute (symptomatic, bothersome) duodenal or gastric ulcers— Adults and teenagers: Various dosage schedules are used, including 300 mg 4 times a day with meals and at bedtime, 400 or 600 mg 2 times a day, or 800 mg taken once daily at bedtime. For prevention of duodenal ulcers— Adults and teenagers: Usual dose is 300 mg 2 times a day; another common dosage schedule is 400 mg taken once daily at bedtime. For treatment as needed of heartburn and acid indigestion— Adults and teenagers: 200 mg with water when symptoms start; another 200 mg may be taken within the next 24 hours, for a maximum of 400 mg in a 24-hour period. For treatment of heartburn caused by gastroesophageal reflux disease—Adults: 800 to 1,600 mg a day in 2 to 4 divided doses for approximately 12 weeks.

ONSET OF EFFECT
Within 1 hour.

DURATION OF ACTION
At least 4 to 5 hours.

DIETARY ADVICE
Avoid foods that cause stomach irritation.

STORAGE
Store it away from heat and direct light. Keep the liquid form from freezing.

MISSED DOSE
Take it as soon as you remember. If it is near the time for the next dose, skip the missed dose and resume your regular dosage schedule. Do not double the next dose.

STOPPING THE DRUG
If your doctor has advised you to take it, continue until directed to stop, even if you begin to feel better before the scheduled end of therapy. Otherwise, take it as needed.

PROLONGED USE
Do not take cimetidine for more than 2 weeks unless told to do so by your doctor.

▼ PRECAUTIONS

Over 60: Adverse reactions may be more likely and more severe in older patients.

Driving and Hazardous Work: Do not drive or engage in hazardous work until you determine how the medicine affects you.

Alcohol: Avoid alcohol.

Pregnancy: Avoid or discontinue use if you are pregnant or trying to become pregnant.

Breast Feeding: Cimetidine passes into breast milk; avoid or discontinue use while breast feeding.

Infants and Children: Not recommended for use by children under age 16 years.

Special Concerns: Avoid cigarette smoking because it may increase stomach acid secretion and thus worsen the disease. Do not take cimetidine if you have ever had an allergic reaction to a histamine (H2) blocker. If stomach pain becomes worse while you are using the drug, tell your doctor immediately.

OVERDOSE
Symptoms: No symptoms have been reported.

What to Do: An overdose is unlikely to be life-threatening. However, if someone takes a much larger dose than recommended, seek medical assistance right away.

▼ INTERACTIONS

DRUG INTERACTIONS
Consult your doctor for specific advice before using cimetidine if you are taking aminophylline, anticoagulants, caffeine, metoprolol, oxtriphylline, phenytoin, propranolol, theophylline, tricyclic antidepressants, itraconazole, ketoconazole, or metronidazole.

FOOD INTERACTIONS
Carbonated drinks, citrus fruits and juices, beverages containing caffeine, and other acidic foods or liquids may irritate the stomach or interfere with the therapeutic action of cimetidine.

DISEASE INTERACTIONS
Patients with kidney or liver disease or weakened immune systems should not use cimetidine or should use it in smaller, limited doses under careful medical supervision.

⧯ SIDE EFFECTS ⧯

SERIOUS
Irregular heart rhythm (palpitations), slowed heartbeat, severe blood problems resulting in unusual bleeding, bruising, fever, chills, and increased susceptibility to infection. Call your doctor immediately.

COMMON
Headache, fatigue, drowsiness, dizziness, nausea, vomiting, abdominal pain, diarrhea.

LESS COMMON
Blurred vision, decreased sexual desire or function, swelling of breasts in males or females, temporary hair loss, hallucinations, depression, insomnia, skin rash, hives, or redness.

CLEMASTINE FUMARATE

BRAND NAMES

Contac 12 Hour Allergy, Tavist, Tavist-1, Tavist-D

Available in: Tablets, syrup, extended-release tablets and caplets
Available as Generic? Yes
Drug Class: Antihistamine

▼ USAGE INFORMATION

WHY IT'S TAKEN
To prevent or relieve symptoms of hay fever and other allergies and for itching skin and hives.

HOW IT WORKS
Clemastine blocks the effects of histamine, a naturally occurring substance within the body that causes swelling, itching, sneezing, watery eyes, hives, and other symptoms of allergic reactions.

▼ DOSAGE GUIDELINES

RANGE AND FREQUENCY
Adults and teenagers: 1.34 mg 2 times a day (for hay fever) or 2.68 mg 1 to 3 times a day (for hay fever or hives). Children ages 6 to 12 years: 0.67 mg (syrup) to 1.34 mg 2 times a day.

ONSET OF EFFECT
15 minutes to 60 minutes.

DURATION OF ACTION
At least 12 hours.

DIETARY ADVICE
Take it with food, water, or milk to avoid stomach irritation. Drinking coffee or tea will help reduce drowsiness. Use sugar-free gum, sugar-free sour hard candy, or ice chips to ease dry mouth.

STORAGE
Store it in a tightly sealed container away from heat and direct light.

MISSED DOSE
Take it as soon as you remember. If it is near the time for the next dose, skip the missed dose and resume your regular dosage schedule. Do not double the next dose.

STOPPING THE DRUG
You should take it as prescribed for the full treatment period, but you may stop if you are feeling better before the scheduled end of therapy. It may be taken as needed.

PROLONGED USE
No special problems are expected.

▼ PRECAUTIONS

Over 60: Adverse reactions may be more likely to occur and may be more severe in older patients.

Driving and Hazardous Work: The use of clemastine may impair your ability to perform such tasks safely. Do not drive or engage in hazardous work until you know how the medicine is going to affect you.

Alcohol: Alcohol increases the likelihood and the severity of side effects such as drowsiness and confusion.

Pregnancy: Animal studies with high doses of clemastine have found no birth defects. Human studies have not been done. Because the studies cannot rule out potential harm, the drug should be used during pregnancy only if it is clearly needed.

Breast Feeding: Clemastine passes into breast milk; do not use it while nursing.

Infants and Children: Children tend to be more sensitive to the effects of antihistamines. Symptoms of excitability, restlessness, and nightmares may occur.

OVERDOSE
Symptoms: Hallucinations, seizures, drowsiness, lethargy, coma.

What to Do: Call your doctor, emergency medical services (EMS), or the nearest poison control center immediately. A conscious patient should be induced to vomit using ipecac syrup.

▼ INTERACTIONS

DRUG INTERACTIONS
Sleeping pills, sedatives, tranquilizers, monoamine oxidase (MAO) inhibitors, and antidepressants can increase the sedative effects of clemastine. Anticholinergics may further increase the likelihood that drying of the mucous membranes and urinary obstruction will occur as side effects.

FOOD INTERACTIONS
No known food interactions.

DISEASE INTERACTIONS
Consult your doctor if you have any of the following: asthma, enlarged prostate, difficulty urinating, glaucoma, sleep apnea, or dry mouth or eyes.

 SIDE EFFECTS

SERIOUS
Confusion, hallucinations, convulsions, blurred vision, difficulty urinating (urinary obstruction).

COMMON
Drowsiness; nausea; thickening of mucus; dry mouth, nose, and throat; dizziness; disturbed coordination.

LESS COMMON
Chills, headache, fatigue, vomiting, restlessness, irritability, nasal congestion, profuse sweating, diarrhea, constipation.

CLOTRIMAZOLE

BRAND NAMES

FemCare, Femizole-7, Gyne-Lotrimin, Gyne-Lotrimin 3, Lotrimin, Mycelex, Mycelex Troche, Mycelex Twin Pack, Mycelex-7, Mycelex-G

Available in: Topical cream, lotion, solution, oral lozenges, vaginal cream, tablets
Available as Generic? Yes
Drug Class: Antifungal

▼ USAGE INFORMATION

WHY IT'S TAKEN
To treat fungal infections of the mouth and throat (thrush), vaginal area (yeast infection), and the skin, such as tinea corporis (ringworm), tinea cruris (jock itch), tinea pedis (athlete's foot), and pityriasis versicolor ("sun fungus," a fungal skin condition that is characterized by fine scaly patches of varying shapes, sizes, and colors).

HOW IT WORKS
Clotrimazole prevents fungal organisms from producing vital substances required for growth and function.

▼ DOSAGE GUIDELINES

RANGE AND FREQUENCY
Topical cream, lotion, solution (for skin infections)—Adults and children: Apply twice a day, in the morning and in the evening. Oral lozenges (to treat thrush)—Adults and children age 5 years and older: Dissolve 1 10-mg lozenge in mouth 5 times a day for 14 days. To prevent thrush: Adults and children age 5 years and older: Dissolve 1 10-mg lozenge in mouth 3 times a day. Vaginal cream (for yeast infections)—Adults and teenagers: At bedtime, insert vaginally with an applicator 50 mg of 1% cream for 6 to 14 nights, 100 mg of 2% cream for 3 nights, or 500 mg of 10% cream for 1 night. Vaginal tablets (for yeast infections)—Nonpregnant women and teenagers: At bedtime, insert 1 100-mg tablet for 6 to 7 nights, 1 200-mg tablet for 3 nights, or 1 500-mg tablet for 1 night only. Pregnant women and teenagers: At bedtime, insert 1 100-mg tablet for 7 nights.

ONSET OF EFFECT
Unknown.

DURATION OF ACTION
Lozenges: 3 hours. Other forms: Unknown.

DIETARY ADVICE
No special restrictions.

STORAGE
Store it in a tightly sealed container away from moisture, heat, and direct light. Do not allow it to freeze.

MISSED DOSE
Take it as soon as you remember. If it is near the time for the next dose, skip the missed dose and resume your regular dosage schedule. Do not double the next dose.

STOPPING THE DRUG
If you are using this drug by prescription, take it as prescribed for the full treatment period, even if you begin to feel better before the scheduled end of therapy. Recurrence of the infection is likely if you stop before the full treatment period is complete.

PROLONGED USE
Clotrimazole is generally prescribed for short-term therapy (1 to 14 days). Consult your doctor for further information.

▼ PRECAUTIONS

Over 60: No special problems are expected.

Driving and Hazardous Work: No special precautions are necessary.

Alcohol: No special precautions are necessary.

Pregnancy: Adequate studies on the use of clotrimazole during pregnancy have not been done; however, no problems have been reported. Consult your doctor for specific advice.

Breast Feeding: Clotrimazole may pass into breast milk; caution is advised. Consult your doctor for advice.

Infants and Children: Topical forms: No special warnings. Lozenges are not recommended for children younger than age 5 years. Vaginal forms: Not commonly prescribed for children under the age of 12 years.

Special Concerns: Do not chew or swallow lozenges. Clotrimazole lozenges may take 15 to 30 minutes to dissolve completely and are useless if swallowed.

OVERDOSE
Symptoms: An overdose with clotrimazole is unlikely.

What to Do: If someone swallows a large amount of the medicine, call your doctor, emergency medical services (EMS), or the nearest poison control center immediately.

▼ INTERACTIONS

DRUG INTERACTIONS
No drug interactions have been reported.

FOOD INTERACTIONS
No food interactions have been reported.

DISEASE INTERACTIONS
No disease interactions have been reported.

⬇ SIDE EFFECTS ⬇

SERIOUS
Topical: Hives, skin rash, itching, burning, peeling, stinging, redness, or other skin irritation not present prior to treatment. Lozenge and vaginal: None reported.

COMMON
Topical: None reported. Lozenge (when swallowed): Diarrhea, stomach cramping or pain, nausea or vomiting. Vaginal: Vaginal burning, itching, discharge, or other irritation not present prior to treatment.

LESS COMMON
Topical and lozenge: None reported. Vaginal: Headache, stomach cramps or pain, irritation or burning of sexual partner's penis.

COAL TAR

Available in: Cleansing bar, cream, gel, lotion, ointment, shampoo, liquid
Available as Generic? Yes
Drug Class: Antipsoriasis drug

▼ USAGE INFORMATION

WHY IT'S TAKEN
To treat skin conditions including dandruff, eczema, seborrheic dermatitis, and psoriasis.

HOW IT WORKS
Coal tar promotes softening, dissolution, and peeling of hard, scaly, roughened, or irregular surface skin. It also has antiseptic properties and fights fungal, bacterial, and parasitic organisms.

▼ DOSAGE GUIDELINES

RANGE AND FREQUENCY
Cleansing bar: Use 1 or 2 times a day as directed by your doctor. Cream: Apply to affected areas up to 4 times a day. Gel: Apply to affected areas 1 or 2 times a day. Lotion: Apply to affected areas as needed. Ointment: Apply to affected areas 2 or 3 times a day. Shampoo: Use once a day, once a week, or as directed by your doctor. Topical solution: Apply to skin or scalp or use in the bath, depending on product. Topical bath solution: Add appropriate amount to bath water; immerse yourself in the bath for 20 minutes. If you have any questions about its use, consult your doctor.

ONSET OF EFFECT
Unknown.

DURATION OF ACTION
Unknown.

DIETARY ADVICE
Coal tar can be used without regard to diet.

STORAGE
Store it in a tightly sealed container away from heat and direct light. Do not allow liquid forms to freeze.

MISSED DOSE
Apply it as soon as you remember. If it is near the time for the next dose, skip the missed dose and resume your regular dosage schedule. Do not apply a double dose.

STOPPING THE DRUG
If applying coal tar on medical order, the decision to stop using it should be made by your doctor. If you are using the drug on your own, you may stop treatment whenever you choose.

PROLONGED USE
Do not use coal tar for longer than the package specifies or your physician advises.

▼ PRECAUTIONS

Over 60: Coal tar is not expected to cause different side effects or problems in older patients than it does in younger persons.

Driving and Hazardous Work: The use of coal tar should not impair your ability to perform such tasks safely.

Alcohol: No special restrictions apply.

Pregnancy: Studies of coal tar use during pregnancy have not been done. Before you use coal tar, tell your doctor if you are pregnant or plan to become pregnant.

Breast Feeding: It is not known if coal tar passes into breast milk. Consult your doctor for specific advice.

Infants and Children: Use and dose for infants and children must be determined by your doctor.

Special Concerns: For external use only. Keep coal tar away from the eyes. If you accidentally get some of the medicine in your eyes, flush them thoroughly with water. After applying coal tar, protect the treated area from sunlight for 72 hours. Be sure to remove all coal tar before being exposed to sunlight or using a sunlamp. Do not apply coal tar to infected, blistered, raw, or oozing areas of the skin.

OVERDOSE
Symptoms: None reported.

What to Do: Emergency instructions not applicable.

▼ INTERACTIONS

DRUG INTERACTIONS
Consult your doctor for specific advice if you are using tetracyclines, psoralens, or retinoids. Also tell your doctor if you are using any other prescription or over-the-counter medication.

FOOD INTERACTIONS
No known food interactions.

DISEASE INTERACTIONS
You should not use coal tar if you have had a prior allergic reaction to it.

SIDE EFFECTS

SERIOUS
Skin irritation or rash not present before use of coal tar. Call your doctor immediately.

COMMON
Mild stinging, increased sensitivity to sunlight.

LESS COMMON
No less common side effects have been reported.

CROMOLYN SODIUM INHALANT AND NASAL

Available in: Nasal solution
Available as Generic? Yes
Drug Class: Respiratory inhalant

▼ USAGE INFORMATION

WHY IT'S TAKEN
To control, through regular use, chronic bronchial asthma. It may be used preventively just prior to exposure to certain conditions or substances (allergens such as pollen and dust mites, as well as cold air, chemicals, exercise, or air pollution) that can trigger an acute asthma attack (bronchospasm).

HOW IT WORKS
Cromolyn sodium inhibits the release of histamine, a naturally occurring substance that causes swelling, itching, sneezing, watery eyes, hives, and other symptoms of allergic reaction, including those that occur in association with an asthma attack.

▼ DOSAGE GUIDELINES

RANGE AND FREQUENCY
For hay fever: Adults and children age 6 years and older: 1 spray in each nostril 3 to 6 times a day.

ONSET OF EFFECT
Unknown.

DURATION OF ACTION
Unknown.

DIETARY ADVICE
This medication should be taken 30 minutes before meals.

STORAGE
Store it in a tightly sealed container away from heat and direct light.

MISSED DOSE
Take it as soon as you remember. If it is near the time for the next dose, skip the missed dose and resume your regular dosage schedule. Do not double the next dose.

STOPPING THE DRUG
The decision to stop taking cromolyn sodium should be made in consultation with your doctor.

PROLONGED USE
If your symptoms do not improve after 4 weeks, consult your doctor.

▼ PRECAUTIONS

Over 60: No special problems are expected in older patients.

Driving and Hazardous Work: No special problems are expected.

Alcohol: No special precautions are necessary.

Pregnancy: In studies done in animals, large doses of cromolyn sodium have caused a decrease in successful pregnancies and a decrease in fetal weight. Human studies have not yet been done. Before taking cromolyn sodium, tell your doctor if you are pregnant or if you plan to become pregnant.

Breast Feeding: It is not known whether cromolyn sodium passes into breast milk. Mothers who wish to breast-feed while using this drug should discuss the matter with their doctor.

Infants and Children: The nasal form of cromolyn has not been studied in children. Consult your pediatrician for specific advice.

Special Concerns: Clean the inhaler and other devices at least once a week.

OVERDOSE
Symptoms: None reported.

What to Do: An overdose of cromolyn sodium is unlikely to be life-threatening. However, if someone takes a much larger dose than recommended, call your doctor, emergency medical services (EMS), or the nearest poison control center immediately.

▼ INTERACTIONS

DRUG INTERACTIONS
Before taking cromolyn sodium, check with your doctor if you are using any other prescription or over-the-counter drug.

FOOD INTERACTIONS
No known food interactions.

DISEASE INTERACTIONS
Before taking cromolyn sodium, consult your physician if you are undergoing treatment for any other medical condition.

≡ SIDE EFFECTS ≡

SERIOUS
Difficulty swallowing; hives; itching; swelling of face, lips, or eyelids; rash; nosebleeds. Call your doctor immediately.

COMMON
Inhalation: Throat irritation or dryness. Nasal: Increased sneezing; burning, stinging, or irritation in nose.

LESS COMMON
Nasal: Cough, headache, postnasal drip, unpleasant taste.

DEXTROMETHORPHAN

Available in: Capsules, lozenges, tablets, oral suspension, syrup
Available as Generic? Yes
Drug Class: Cough suppressant

▼ USAGE INFORMATION

WHY IT'S TAKEN
To relieve a dry or minimally productive cough (that is, a mild cough that rids the lungs of modest amounts of phlegm or mucus) commonly associated with allergies, colds, influenza, and certain lung disorders. This medicine is ideally useful when a mild or hacking cough would interrupt sleep or interfere with your daily activities.

HOW IT WORKS
Dextromethorphan works by directly reducing the sensitivity of the cough center—the part of the brain that responds to stimuli in the lower respiratory passages that irritate and trigger the cough reflex.

▼ DOSAGE GUIDELINES

RANGE AND FREQUENCY
Adults: 10 to 20 mg every 4 hours or 30 mg every 6 to 8 hours; 30 to 60 mg of extended-release liquid twice a day. Children 6 to 12 years: 5 to 10 mg every 4 hours or 30 mg of extended-release liquid twice a day. Children 2 to 6 years: 2.5 to 5 mg every 4 hours, 7.5 mg every 6 to 8 hours, or 15 mg of the extended-release liquid twice a day. Children under 2 years: Dosage must be individualized.

ONSET OF EFFECT
15 to 30 minutes.

DURATION OF ACTION
Up to 6 hours.

DIETARY ADVICE
No special restrictions.

STORAGE
Store it in a tightly sealed container away from heat, moisture, and direct light.

MISSED DOSE
Take it as soon as you remember. However, if it is near the time for the next dose, skip the missed dose and resume your regular dosage schedule. Do not double the next dose.

STOPPING THE DRUG
Take it as prescribed for the full treatment period. However, you may stop taking the drug if you are feeling better before the scheduled end of therapy. If the cough does not improve after 7 days, consult your doctor.

PROLONGED USE
No problems are expected.

▼ PRECAUTIONS

Over 60: Side effects may be more frequent and severe than in younger persons. Smaller doses for shorter periods may be needed. If this drug is used to control coughing, other treatment measures may be needed to liquefy any accumulation of thick mucus that may form in the bronchial tubes.

Driving and Hazardous Work: Determine whether it causes drowsiness or dizziness before you drive or engage in hazardous work.

Alcohol: Avoid alcohol while using this drug; it may increase the risk of sedation.

Pregnancy: Ask your doctor whether the benefits of the drug justify the possible risk to the fetus.

Breast Feeding: Dextromethorphan may pass into breast milk; caution is advised. Consult your doctor for specific advice about taking dextromethorphan while you are nursing.

Infants and Children: Doses for children under 2 years must be individualized; consult your pediatrician.

Special Concerns: Do not take dextromethorphan to relieve a cough that is caused by asthma, emphysema, or smoking.

OVERDOSE
Symptoms: Nausea, vomiting, nervousness and agitation, extreme drowsiness or dizziness, extreme irritability or mood changes, hallucinations, blurred vision, uncontrollable eye movement, inability to urinate, confusion, loss of consciousness, or coma.

What to Do: Call your doctor, emergency medical services (EMS), or the nearest poison control center immediately.

▼ INTERACTIONS

DRUG INTERACTIONS
Taking it with a sedative or other depressant can increase the sedative effects of both drugs. Using doxepin increases the toxic effects of both drugs. Taking a monoamine oxidase (MAO) inhibitor can cause a high fever, disorientation, or loss of consciousness. Using quinidine increases the risk of experiencing side effects with dextromethorphan.

FOOD INTERACTIONS
No known food interactions.

DISEASE INTERACTIONS
Caution is advised when taking dextromethorphan. Consult your doctor before taking this drug if you have a history of asthma or impaired liver function.

 ≡ SIDE EFFECTS ≡

SERIOUS
Serious side effects occur only in cases of overdose (see Overdose).

COMMON
No common side effects are associated with this drug.

LESS COMMON
Mild dizziness or sedation, nausea or vomiting, abdominal pain. Such symptoms are more likely to occur at the beginning of therapy and tend to diminish as your body becomes accustomed to taking the drug. Consult your doctor if they persist or interfere with daily activities.

DIMENHYDRINATE

Available in: Capsules, tablets, elixir, syrup
Available as Generic? Yes
Drug Class: Antihistamine

▼ USAGE INFORMATION

WHY IT'S TAKEN
To relieve nausea and vomiting and to treat or prevent motion sickness.

HOW IT WORKS
Dimenhydrinate directly inhibits the stimulation of certain nerves in the brain and inner ear to suppress nausea, vomiting, dizziness, and vertigo.

▼ DOSAGE GUIDELINES

RANGE AND FREQUENCY
Adults: 50 to 100 mg every 4 to 6 hours. Children ages 6 to 12 years: 25 to 50 mg every 6 to 8 hours. Children ages 2 to 6 years: 12.5 to 25 mg every 6 to 8 hours. To prevent motion sickness, take this drug at least 30 minutes–preferably 1 to 2 hours–before you are planning to travel.

ONSET OF EFFECT
Within 20 to 30 minutes.

DURATION OF ACTION
3 to 6 hours.

DIETARY ADVICE
This drug can be taken with food or milk to minimize any gastrointestinal distress from occurring.

STORAGE
Store it in a tightly sealed container in a dry place away from heat and direct light.

MISSED DOSE
Take it as soon as you remember. However, if it is near the time for the next dose, skip the missed dose and resume your regular dosage schedule. Do not double the next dose.

STOPPING THE DRUG
You should take it according to package directions for the full treatment period, but you may stop if you are feeling better before the scheduled end of therapy.

PROLONGED USE
Take this drug only as long as it is needed.

▼ PRECAUTIONS

Over 60: Older persons are more sensitive to the effects of dimenhydrinate. Dizziness, drowsiness, confusion, difficult or painful urination, and other side effects are more likely to occur.

Driving and Hazardous Work: Do not drive or engage in hazardous work until you determine how the medicine affects you.

Alcohol: Avoid alcohol.

Pregnancy: Animal studies with high doses of dimenhydrinate have found no birth defects. Human studies have not been done. Because the studies cannot rule out harm, the drug should be used during pregnancy only if it is clearly needed.

Breast Feeding: Dimenhydrinate may pass into breast milk; caution is advised; avoid or discontinue use while breast feeding.

Infants and Children: The safety and efficacy of this drug for children under 2 years of age (6 years for the suppository form) have not been established. Older children are especially sensitive to the drug's side effects.

Special Concerns: Children should be observed carefully for signs of side effects; they are more likely to develop serious complications from these medications, and younger children are often unable to describe changes in the way they are feeling.

OVERDOSE
Symptoms: Seizures, hallucinations, drowsiness, difficulty breathing, unconsciousness.

What to Do: An overdose of dimenhydrinate is unlikely to be life-threatening. However, if someone takes a much larger dose than recommended, call your doctor, emergency medical services (EMS), or the nearest poison control center immediately.

▼ INTERACTIONS

DRUG INTERACTIONS
Consult your doctor for specific advice if you are taking any narcotic pain relievers, sedatives, tranquilizers, antidepressants, antibiotics, aspirin, barbiturates, cisplatin, diuretics, or theophylline.

FOOD INTERACTIONS
No known food interactions.

DISEASE INTERACTIONS
Caution is advised when taking dimenhydrinate. Consult your doctor if you have glaucoma or an enlarged prostate.

 SIDE EFFECTS

SERIOUS
No serious side effects are associated with this drug.

COMMON
Drowsiness.

LESS COMMON
Headache, blurred vision, palpitations, loss of coordination, dry mouth, low blood pressure causing dizziness and weakness, ringing in ears.

DIPHENHYDRAMINE HYDROCHLORIDE

BRAND NAMES

Benadryl, Benahist, Benylin Cough, Compoz, Diphenhist, Nytol, Phendry, Sleep-Eze 3, Sominex Formula 2, Unisom SleepGels Maximum Strength

Available in: Capsules, elixir, syrup, tablets
Available as Generic? Yes
Drug Class: Antihistamine

▼ USAGE INFORMATION

WHY IT'S TAKEN
To relieve hay fever symptoms, itching skin and hives, motion sickness, nonproductive cough caused by cold or hay fever, and sleeping difficulty; also used to treat symptoms of Parkinson's disease.

HOW IT WORKS
It blocks the effects of histamine, a naturally occurring substance that causes swelling, itching, sneezing, and watery eyes. In patients with Parkinson's disease, it decreases tremors and muscle stiffness.

▼ DOSAGE GUIDELINES

RANGE AND FREQUENCY
For hay fever symptoms—Capsules, elixir, syrup, tablets: Adults and teenagers: 25 to 50 mg every 4 to 6 hours. Children younger than age 6 years: 6.25 (½ tsp) to 12.5 (1 tsp) mg every 4 to 6 hours. Children ages 6 to 12 years: 12.5 (1 tsp) to 25 (2 tsp) mg every 4 to 6 hours. For nausea, vomiting, and dizziness—Capsules, elixir, syrup, tablets: Adults: 25 to 50 mg every 4 to 6 hours. Children: 1 to 1.5 mg per 2.2 lb (1 kg) every 4 to 6 hours. For Parkinson's disease—Capsules, elixir, syrup, tablets: Adults: 25 mg 3 times a day. Doctor may gradually increase dose. As a sedative—Capsules, elixir, syrup, tablets: Adults: 50 mg 20 to 30 minutes before bedtime. For cough—Liquid: Adults and teenagers: 25 mg every 4 to 6 hours. Children ages 2 to 6 years: 6.25 mg (½ tsp) every 4 to 6 hours. Children ages 6 to 12 (1 tsp): 12.5 mg (1 tsp) every 4 to 6 hours.

ONSET OF EFFECT
Capsules, elixir, syrup, or tablets: 15 minutes.

DURATION OF ACTION
6 to 8 hours.

DIETARY ADVICE
Take diphenhydramine with food or milk to reduce gastrointestinal distress, a possible side effect.

STORAGE
Store it in a dry place away from heat and direct light. Prevent liquid forms from freezing.

MISSED DOSE
Take it as soon as you remember. If it is near the time for the next dose, skip the missed dose and resume your regular dosage schedule. Do not double the next dose.

STOPPING THE DRUG
Stop taking this drug and call your doctor if it is not effective after 5 days.

PROLONGED USE
No special problems have been reported.

▼ PRECAUTIONS

Over 60: Adverse reactions may be more likely and more severe.

Driving and Hazardous Work: Do not drive or engage in hazardous work until you determine how the medicine affects you. Use of this drug is a disqualification for piloting aircraft.

Alcohol: Alcohol may increase the likelihood and severity of side effects such as drowsiness and mental confusion.

Pregnancy: No birth defects have been reported in animals. Studies of pregnant women have found no significant increase in birth defects.

Breast Feeding: Diphenhydramine passes into breast milk; avoid or discontinue use while nursing.

Infants and Children: This drug is not recommended for children under the age of 2 years.

Special Concerns: Children should be observed carefully for signs of side effects; they are more likely to develop serious complications, and younger children are often unable to describe changes in the way they are feeling.

OVERDOSE
Symptoms: Marked drowsiness, dilated and unreactive pupils, fever, excitability, breathing interruptions, combativeness, mental confusion, loss of coordination, weak pulse, seizures, loss of consciousness.

What to Do: Call your doctor, emergency medical services (EMS), or the nearest poison control center immediately.

▼ INTERACTIONS

DRUG INTERACTIONS
Consult your doctor for specific advice before using diphenhydramine if you are also taking anticholinergics, alcohol, disopyramide, central nervous system depressants, or monoamine oxidase (MAO) inhibitors.

FOOD INTERACTIONS
No known food interactions.

DISEASE INTERACTIONS
Consult your doctor if you have a history of severe respiratory disease, glaucoma, urinary obstruction, or prostate enlargement.

 ≡ **SIDE EFFECTS** ≡

SERIOUS
No serious side effects are associated with this drug.

COMMON
Drowsiness, dry mouth, nausea, thickening of mucus.

LESS COMMON
Confusion, difficult urination, blurred vision.

DOCUSATE

Available in: Capsules, tablets, liquid, syrup
Available as Generic? Yes
Drug Class: Stool softener

▼ USAGE INFORMATION

WHY IT'S TAKEN
To prevent constipation (but not to treat existing constipation). Recommended for persons who should not strain during defecation, such as those recovering from rectal or heart surgery or women who experience constipation after childbirth.

HOW IT WORKS
Docusate draws liquid into stools, forming a softer mass.

▼ DOSAGE GUIDELINES

RANGE AND FREQUENCY
Adults and teenagers: 50 to 500 mg once a day until bowel movements return to normal. Children ages 6 to 12 years: 40 to 140 mg once a day. Liquid forms should be mixed with milk or fruit juice.

ONSET OF EFFECT
Within 24 to 72 hours.

DURATION OF ACTION
Up to 72 hours.

DIETARY ADVICE
Add high-fiber foods such as bran and fresh fruits and vegetables to your diet. Drink at least 6 glasses (8 oz each) of water or other liquids a day to help soften stools.

STORAGE
Store it in a tightly sealed container kept away from heat, moisture, and direct light.

MISSED DOSE
Take it as soon as you remember. If it is near the time for the next dose, skip the missed dose and resume your regular dosage schedule. Do not double the next dose.

STOPPING THE DRUG
Take it as advised for the full treatment period. However, you may stop taking the drug if you are feeling better and normal bowel function has returned before the scheduled end of therapy.

PROLONGED USE
Docusate should not be taken for more than 1 week unless you are under your doctor's supervision. Be aware that overuse can make you dependent on it and may cause damage to the nerves, muscles, and other tissues of the bowel and lead to vitamin and mineral deficiency.

▼ PRECAUTIONS

Over 60: No special problems are expected.

Driving and Hazardous Work: The use of docusate should not impair your ability to perform such tasks safely.

Alcohol: No special precautions are necessary.

Pregnancy: Before taking docusate, tell your doctor if you are pregnant or plan to become pregnant.

Breast Feeding: No special problems are expected if you take docusate while nursing.

Infants and Children: Do not give docusate to children under age 6 years unless it is prescribed by your doctor.

Special Concerns: Do not take mineral oil while you are taking docusate.

OVERDOSE
Symptoms: Weakness, sweating, muscle cramps, irregular heartbeat.

What to Do: An overdose of docusate is unlikely to be life-threatening. However, if someone takes a much larger dose than prescribed, call your doctor, emergency medical services (EMS), or the nearest poison control center immediately.

▼ INTERACTIONS

DRUG INTERACTIONS
A number of drugs may interact with docusate if they are ingested at or near the time it is taken. Consult your doctor for specific advice if you are taking any other oral drug within 2 hours before or after taking docusate.

FOOD INTERACTIONS
No known food interactions.

DISEASE INTERACTIONS
This drug cannot be used by people with intestinal obstruction or appendicitis. The symptoms of these conditions include vomiting, abdominal rigidity and tenderness, and fever. Call your doctor or emergency medical services (EMS) immediately if you suspect that you may be suffering from intestinal obstruction or appendicitis.

≡ SIDE EFFECTS ≡

SERIOUS
Severe cramping. Stop taking the drug and call your doctor immediately.

COMMON
Diarrhea, mild abdominal cramps.

LESS COMMON
Throat irritation, laxative dependence. Consult your doctor if you cannot maintain normal bowel habits without docusate for more than 2 weeks.

EPHEDRINE

Available in: Capsules
Available as Generic? Yes
Drug Class: Adrenergic bronchodilator

▼ USAGE INFORMATION

WHY IT'S TAKEN
To relieve bronchial asthma, to decrease nasal and lower respiratory congestion, and to suppress allergic reactions. Ephedrine commonly appears in combination with other medications.

HOW IT WORKS
Ephedrine prevents cells from releasing histamine, a naturally occurring substance that causes swelling, itching, sneezing, watery eyes, hives, and other symptoms of allergic reaction. It also relaxes the smooth muscle surrounding the bronchial tubes, widening the airways, and causes constriction of blood vessels in the nose, which helps open the nasal passages.

▼ DOSAGE GUIDELINES

RANGE AND FREQUENCY
Adults: 25 to 50 mg every 3 or 4 hours if needed. Children: 3 mg per 2.2 lb (1 kg) of body weight per day in 4 to 6 divided doses.

ONSET OF EFFECT
15 to 60 minutes.

DURATION OF ACTION
3 to 5 hours.

DIETARY ADVICE
Swallow capsules with water and drink plenty of fluids.

STORAGE
Store it in a tightly sealed container away from heat, moisture, and direct light.

MISSED DOSE
Take it if you remember within 2 hours. If not, skip the missed dose and resume your normal dosage schedule. Do not double the next dose.

STOPPING THE DRUG
You may stop taking this drug at your own discretion. Consult your doctor.

PROLONGED USE
This drug may lose its effectiveness if taken steadily for 3 to 4 days. Men with an enlarged prostate gland may have difficulty urinating.

▼ PRECAUTIONS

Over 60: Adverse reactions may be more likely and more severe. Small doses are advisable until individual response has been evaluated.

Driving and Hazardous Work: Ephedrine may cause dizziness. Do not drive or engage in hazardous work until you determine how it affects you.

Alcohol: No special precautions are necessary.

Pregnancy: Consult your doctor; benefits must clearly outweigh risks.

Breast Feeding: Ephedrine passes into breast milk and may be harmful to the child; do not use it while nursing.

Infants and Children: Use caution. Ask your doctor if the benefits of ephedrine justify possible risk to the child.

Special Concerns: Ephedrine can cause insomnia. Take the last dose at least 2 hours before bedtime. Before you take ephedrine, tell your doctor if you will have surgery requiring general anesthesia, including dental surgery, within 2 months.

OVERDOSE
Symptoms: Severe anxiety, convulsions, coma, breathing difficulty, confusion, delirium, rapid and irregular pulse, muscle tremors.

What to Do: Call your doctor, emergency medical services (EMS), or the nearest poison control center immediately.

▼ INTERACTIONS

DRUG INTERACTIONS
Consult your doctor for specific advice if you are taking tricyclic antidepressants, high blood pressure medication, beta-blockers, dextrothyroxine, digitalis drugs, preparations containing ergot, furazolidone, guanadrel, guanethidine, heart medication, methyldopa, monoamine oxidase (MAO) inhibitors, nitrates, phenothiazines, pseudoephedrine, rauwolfia alkaloids, sympathomimetic drugs, terazosin, theophylline, or any nonprescription drug for a cough, cold, allergy, or asthma.

FOOD INTERACTIONS
No known food interactions.

DISEASE INTERACTIONS
Caution is advised when taking ephedrine. Consult your doctor if you have any of the following: enlarged prostate, high blood pressure, history of seizures, diabetes, an overactive thyroid gland, or Parkinson's disease.

≡ SIDE EFFECTS ≡

SERIOUS
Irregular heartbeat; hallucinations, with high doses, shortness of breath. Call your doctor.

COMMON
Nervousness, rapid heartbeat, paleness, insomnia.

LESS COMMON
Dizziness, loss of appetite, nausea, vomiting, muscle cramps, headache, difficult or painful urination.

EPINEPHRINE HYDROCHLORIDE

Available in: Inhalation aerosols and solutions, eye drops
Available as Generic? Yes
Drug Class: Bronchodilator/sympathomimetic; antiglaucoma agent

▼ USAGE INFORMATION

WHY IT'S TAKEN
To treat bronchial asthma, emphysema, and other lung diseases. Epinephrine is also a primary treatment for anaphylaxis—that is, hypersensitive (allergic) reaction to drugs or other substances. It may also be used to treat nasal congestion, to prolong the action of anesthetics, and to treat cardiac arrest. The ophthalmic form of the drug is used to treat glaucoma.

HOW IT WORKS
Epinephrine widens constricted airways in the lungs by relaxing smooth muscles that surround bronchial passages. It also raises blood pressure by constricting small blood vessels, increases the heart rate and strength of heart contractions, and decreases fluid pressure in the eye.

▼ DOSAGE GUIDELINES

RANGE AND FREQUENCY
It may be used when needed to relieve breathing difficulty. For adults and children 4 years of age or older with asthma—Inhaled aerosol: 200 micrograms (µg) to 275 µg (1 puff), repeated if needed after 1 or 2 minutes, with doses taken at least 3 hours apart. Inhalation solution: 1 puff of 1% solution repeated after 1 or 2 minutes, if needed. For open-angle glaucoma: 1 or 2 drops of 1% or 2% solution once or twice daily.

ONSET OF EFFECT
Within 5 minutes.

DURATION OF ACTION
1 to 3 hours.

DIETARY ADVICE
No special concerns.

STORAGE
Store in a tightly sealed container, away from moisture, heat, and direct light.

MISSED DOSE
Take your missed dose as soon as you remember, unless the time for your next scheduled dose is within the next 2 hours, in which case skip the missed dose. Take your next scheduled dose at the proper time and resume your regular dosage schedule. Do not take a double dose.

STOPPING THE DRUG
Take the drug exactly as prescribed. Contact your doctor if you do not respond to the strength of the dosage you have been given.

PROLONGED USE
Tolerance to epinephrine may develop with prolonged use.

▼ PRECAUTIONS

Over 60: Adverse reactions may be more likely and more severe in older patients.

Driving and Hazardous Work: Do not drive or engage in hazardous work until you determine how the medicine affects you.

Alcohol: It may increase the excretion of epinephrine in the urine.

Pregnancy: Benefits of taking the drug must outweigh the potential risks; consult your doctor for specific advice.

Breast Feeding: Epinephrine passes into the breast milk. Consult your doctor for specific advice.

Infants and Children: They may be especially sensitive to epinephrine; fainting by children with asthma taking the drug has been reported.

Special Concerns: Do not use it without a prescription, unless your problem has been diagnosed as asthma. Take aerosol doses exactly as directed; overuse has caused sudden death.

OVERDOSE
Symptoms: Chest discomfort, chills or fever, dizziness, seizures, irregular heartbeat, trouble breathing.

What to Do: Call your doctor, emergency medical services (EMS), or the nearest poison control center immediately.

▼ INTERACTIONS

DRUG INTERACTIONS
Consult your doctor for specific advice if you are taking anesthetics, tricyclic antidepressants, antidiabetic agents, antihypertensives or diuretics, beta-blockers, digitalis drugs, ergoloid mesylates, maprotiline, ergotamine, or monoamine oxidase (MAO) inhibitors.

FOOD INTERACTIONS
Avoid any foods that have previously triggered an allergic reaction or asthma attack.

DISEASE INTERACTIONS
The benefits of taking the drug need to be weighed against the potential risks if you have any of the following conditions: organic brain damage, diabetes mellitus, Parkinson's disease, heart or blood vessel disease, or overactive thyroid.

≡ SIDE EFFECTS ≡

SERIOUS
Bluish color of skin, severe dizziness, flushing, and difficulty breathing may indicate an allergic reaction to sulfites in the medication. Contact your doctor immediately.

COMMON
Dry mouth and throat, trembling, headaches. Check with your doctor if these symptoms continue or become bothersome.

LESS COMMON
Eye pain or headache from using eye drops.

FAMOTIDINE

BRAND NAMES

Pepcid, Pepcid AC, Pepcid RPD

Available in: Tablets, powder for suspension, orally disintegrating and chewable tablets
Available as Generic? Yes
Drug Class: Histamine (H2) blocker

▼ USAGE INFORMATION

WHY IT'S TAKEN
To treat heartburn, ulcers of the stomach and duodenum, conditions that cause excess production of stomach acid (such as Zollinger-Ellison syndrome), and gastroesophageal reflux (backwash of stomach acid into the esophagus, resulting in heartburn). The chewable tablets are taken for prevention or treatment of heartburn.

HOW IT WORKS
Famotidine blocks the action of histamine (a compound that is produced in the body's cells), which in turn decreases the stomach's secretion of hydrochloric acid. Once the production of stomach acid is decreased, the body is better able to heal itself.

▼ DOSAGE GUIDELINES

RANGE AND FREQUENCY
To prevent heartburn: 10 mg 1 hour before meals. For excess stomach acid: 20 to 160 mg every 6 hours. For acid reflux disease: 20 mg twice a day for up to 6 weeks. For stomach ulcers: 40 mg once a day for 8 weeks. For duodenal ulcers: To start, 40 mg once a day at bedtime or 20 mg twice a day; later, 20 mg once a day. Chewable tablets—For treatment of heartburn: Chew one tablet. For prevention of heartburn: Chew 1 tablet 15 to 60 minutes before eating.

ONSET OF EFFECT
The nonprescription form may take 45 minutes to relieve heartburn.

DURATION OF ACTION
Up to 12 hours.

DIETARY ADVICE
Take it after meals or with milk to minimize stomach irritation. Avoid foods that cause stomach irritation. Take chewable tablet with a glass of water.

STORAGE
Store tablets in a tightly sealed container away from heat, moisture, and direct light. After powder vials are reconstituted, store the medicine in the refrigerator, but keep it from freezing. Discard it after 30 days.

MISSED DOSE
Take it as soon as you remember. If it is near the time for the next dose, skip the missed dose and resume your regular dosage schedule. Do not double the next dose.

STOPPING THE DRUG
If your doctor advises you to take it, do not stop without consulting him or her.

PROLONGED USE
Do not take the prescription drug for more than 8 weeks unless your doctor orders it. Do not take the over-the-counter drug for more than 2 weeks unless otherwise instructed by your doctor.

▼ PRECAUTIONS

Over 60: Adverse reactions may be more likely and more severe in older patients.

Driving and Hazardous Work: Do not drive or engage in hazardous work until you determine how the medicine affects you.

Alcohol: Avoid alcohol while taking this drug; it may slow recovery. Also, this drug increases blood alcohol levels.

Pregnancy: Risks vary depending on patient and dosage. Consult your physician for advice.

Breast Feeding: Famotidine passes into breast milk; you should avoid or discontinue use while breast feeding.

Infants and Children: Famotidine is rarely recommended for infants and children.

Special Concerns: If necessary, famotidine may be given with antacids. Avoid cigarette smoking because it may increase secretion of stomach acid and thus worsen the disease.

OVERDOSE
Symptoms: Confusion, slurred speech, rapid heartbeat, difficulty breathing, delirium.

What to Do: Call your doctor, emergency medical services (EMS), or the nearest poison control center immediately.

▼ INTERACTIONS

DRUG INTERACTIONS
None reported.

FOOD INTERACTIONS
Carbonated drinks, citrus fruits and juices, beverages containing caffeine, and other acidic foods or liquids may irritate the stomach or interfere with the therapeutic action of famotidine.

DISEASE INTERACTIONS
Patients with kidney disease should use famotidine in smaller, limited doses under careful supervision by a physician.

≡ SIDE EFFECTS ≡

SERIOUS
Irregular heart rhythm (palpitations), slowed heartbeat, severe blood problems resulting in unusual bleeding, bruising, fever, chills, and increased susceptibility to infection. Call your doctor immediately.

COMMON
Headache, fatigue, drowsiness, dizziness, nausea, vomiting, abdominal pain, diarrhea, constipation.

LESS COMMON
Blurred vision, decreased sexual desire or function, temporary hair loss, hallucinations, depression, insomnia, skin rash, hives, or redness.

FERROUS SALTS

Available in: Capsules, drops, elixir, solution, tablets
Available as Generic? Yes
Drug Class: Dietary supplement

▼ USAGE INFORMATION

WHY IT'S TAKEN
To help increase the body's stores of iron, a mineral essential to the manufacture of red blood cells. An insufficient number of red blood cells results in anemia.

HOW IT WORKS
Ferrous salts are required for the production of hemoglobin in developing red blood cells. Hemoglobin is a complex iron-based protein in the red cell that carries oxygen to the body's tissues and carries carbon dioxide gas away from the tissues to be exhaled by the lungs.

▼ DOSAGE GUIDELINES

RANGE AND FREQUENCY
For iron deficiency–Adults: 325 mg 3 times a day. Children: 5 to 10 mg for every 2.2 lb (1 kg) of body weight 3 times a day.

ONSET OF EFFECT
From 5 to 7 days. Depending on the extent of the deficiency, more than 3 months of therapy may be needed for maximum benefit.

DURATION OF ACTION
Depends on the body's ability to utilize it.

DIETARY ADVICE
Take it 1 hour before or 2 hours after eating.

STORAGE
Store it in a tightly sealed container away from heat and direct light. Keep the liquid form from freezing.

MISSED DOSE
Take it as soon as you remember. If it is near the time for the next dose, skip the missed dose and resume your regular dosage schedule. Do not double the next dose.

STOPPING THE DRUG
If it was prescribed, the decision to stop taking this supplement should be made by your doctor.

PROLONGED USE
Prolonged use may result in the accumulation of iron in the tissues, the effects of which can include liver damage, heart problems, diabetes, erectile dysfunction, and unusually bronzed skin. Do not take iron supplements without consulting your doctor.

▼ PRECAUTIONS

Over 60: Problems in older adults have not been reported with intake of normal daily recommended amounts.

Driving and Hazardous Work: No problems expected.

Alcohol: Avoid alcohol while taking this medication because it may cause excess absorption of iron.

Pregnancy: This medication should be taken during pregnancy only if your doctor so advises.

Breast Feeding: No problems are expected during breast feeding; however, consult your doctor before taking ferrous salts.

Infants and Children: No unusual problems have been reported in infants and children. Close medical supervision is nonetheless recommended, and iron tablets should be stored out of reach of small children to avoid accidental ingestion, which can be severely toxic.

Special Concerns: The genetic disorder called hemochromatosis, in which the body accumulates excess iron, is very common. Iron deficiency may also be the first indication of a gastrointestinal malignancy. Therefore, iron should only be used on the advice of a physician. Liquid forms of iron can stain the teeth. To prevent stains, mix each dose in water, fruit juice, or tomato juice and drink it through a straw. When using a dropper, place the dose on the back of the tongue and drink a glass of water or juice. Tooth stains can be removed by brushing with baking soda or 3% hydrogen peroxide.

OVERDOSE
Symptoms: Lethargy, nausea, vomiting, weak and rapid pulse, dehydration, loss of consciousness.

What to Do: Call your doctor, emergency medical services (EMS), or the nearest poison control center immediately.

▼ INTERACTIONS

DRUG INTERACTIONS
The following drugs may interact with ferrous salts and prevent their absorption: antacids, antibiotics, fluoroquinolones, levodopa, cholestyramine, or vitamin E. Consult your doctor for specific advice.

FOOD INTERACTIONS
Some foods can reduce the effect of this drug. The following foods should be avoided or taken in small amounts for at least 1 hour before and 2 hours after iron is taken: eggs, milk, spinach, cheese, yogurt, tea, coffee, whole-grain bread, cereal, and bran.

DISEASE INTERACTIONS
Consult your doctor if you have any of the following: a history of alcoholism; kidney disease; liver disease; porphyria; rheumatoid arthritis; asthma; allergies; heart disease; or a stomach ulcer, colitis, or other intestinal problem.

 ## SIDE EFFECTS

SERIOUS
No serious side effects are associated with ferrous salts except for iron overload caused by prolonged, inappropriate use of the mineral.

COMMON
Nausea, constipation, black stools.

LESS COMMON
Stained teeth (with liquid forms), stomach pain, vomiting, diarrhea.

FOLIC ACID (FOLACIN; FOLATE)

Available in: Tablets
Available as Generic? Yes
Drug Class: Vitamin

▼ USAGE INFORMATION

WHY IT'S TAKEN
The vitamin folic acid (also known as folacin and folate) is prescribed for treatment or prevention of certain types of anemia that result from folic acid deficiency. Such deficiencies may occur because of insufficient intake of folic acid (a result of poor diet or malnutrition), an inability to absorb the vitamin (such as occurs in gastrointestinal disease), impaired ability to utilize the vitamin (caused by excessive alcohol intake or the use of the anticonvulsant drug phenytoin), or as a result of conditions requiring increased amounts of folic acid (such as pregnancy, breast feeding, hemodialysis, hemolytic anemia, and bone marrow failure).

HOW IT WORKS
Folic acid enhances chemical reactions within the body that contribute to the production of red blood cells, the manufacture of DNA needed for cell replication, and the metabolism of amino acids (compounds necessary for the manufacture of proteins).

▼ DOSAGE GUIDELINES

RANGE AND FREQUENCY
For severe deficiency—Adults and children regardless of age: 1 mg daily. For daily supplementation after correction of severe deficiency—Adults and adolescents: 1 mg once daily. During pregnancy: 400 micrograms (µg) once daily. While breast feeding: 260 to 280 µg once daily. Children, newborn to 3 years of age: 25 to 50 µg once daily. Children 4 to 6 years of age: 75 µg once daily. Children 7 to 10 years of age: 100 µg once daily.

ONSET OF EFFECT
Folic acid is used immediately by the body for a number of vital chemical functions.

DURATION OF ACTION
Folic acid is required by your body on a daily basis throughout your lifetime.

DIETARY ADVICE
Maintain your usual food and fluid intake. Increase fluids if you have a fever or diarrhea, in hot weather, or during exercise. Follow your doctor's dietary advice (such as low-cholesterol, low-fat, and low-salt recommendations) to improve control over high blood pressure and heart disease.

STORAGE
Store it in a tightly sealed container away from heat and direct light. Keep it away from moisture and extremes in temperature.

MISSED DOSE
Take it as soon as you remember. If it is near the time for the next dose, skip the missed dose and resume your regular dosage schedule. Do not double the next dose.

STOPPING THE DRUG
The decision to stop taking the drug should be made by your doctor.

PROLONGED USE
Therapy with folacin may require weeks or months.

▼ PRECAUTIONS

Over 60: No special problems are expected in older patients.

Driving and Hazardous Work: The use of folic acid should not impair your ability to perform such tasks safely.

Alcohol: Alcohol impairs the body's utilization of folic acid; avoid it completely if you are taking folic acid.

Pregnancy: Folic acid supplementation is recommended during pregnancy.

Breast Feeding: Folic acid supplementation is recommended while nursing.

Infants and Children: Folic acid may be used regardless of age.

Special Concerns: Folic acid ingestion can mask vitamin B_{12} deficiency and lead to irreversible neurological damage; therefore, folic acid should be taken only on the recommendation of your doctor. Folic acid deficiency should not occur and supplementation is not necessary in healthy individuals who consume a normal balanced diet.

OVERDOSE
Symptoms: No specific ones have been reported.

What to Do: An overdose of folic acid is not life-threatening. No emergency procedures are necessary.

▼ INTERACTIONS

DRUG INTERACTIONS
Consult your doctor for advice if you are taking pain relievers, antibiotics, anticonvulsants, epoetin, estrogens, oral contraceptives, methotrexate, pyrimethamine, triamterene, sulfasalazine, or zinc supplements.

FOOD INTERACTIONS
No known food interactions.

DISEASE INTERACTIONS
Consult your doctor if you have pernicious anemia.

≡ SIDE EFFECTS ≡

SERIOUS
Wheezing, breathing difficulty, chest pain, swelling, tightness in throat or chest, dizziness, rash, itching. Such symptoms may indicate a serious allergic reaction, although this is extremely rare.

COMMON
The are no known common side effects associated with the use of folic acid.

LESS COMMON
Mild allergic reactions.

GLYCERIN RECTAL

Available in: Rectal solution, rectal suppositories
Available as Generic? Yes
Drug Class: Hyperosmotic laxative

▼ USAGE INFORMATION

WHY IT'S TAKEN
To treat constipation.

HOW IT WORKS
Glycerin attracts and retains water in the intestine, softening stools and inducing the urge to defecate.

▼ DOSAGE GUIDELINES

RANGE AND FREQUENCY
Adults and children age 6 years and older: Insert 1 suppository or 1 tsp to 1 tbsp of solution as rectal enema and retain for 15 minutes. Do not lubricate suppositories with anything other than water.

ONSET OF EFFECT
Within 15 to 60 minutes.

DURATION OF ACTION
Only while the solution or suppository is in the rectum.

DIETARY ADVICE
Maintain your usual food and fluid intake. Increase your intake of fluids if you have a fever or diarrhea, during hot weather, or during exercise.

STORAGE
Store solutions and suppositories away from moisture, heat, and direct light. Suppositories may be refrigerated, but do not allow them to freeze.

MISSED DOSE
Laxatives are usually prescribed for use only on an as-needed basis and are not meant to be taken regularly or for a prolonged period.

STOPPING THE DRUG
Take rectal glycerin only as needed. However, you may stop using it if you are feeling better before the scheduled end of therapy.

PROLONGED USE
Prolonged, excessive use of glycerin may be associated with an increased risk of side effects, including laxative dependence. Therefore, do not use glycerin for more than 3 to 5 days unless your doctor instructs you to do otherwise.

≡ SIDE EFFECTS ≡

SERIOUS
There are no serious side effects associated with the use of glycerin rectal.

COMMON
Cramping.

LESS COMMON
Rectal pain, itching, or burning sensation. This is thought to be more common with dosage forms that require an applicator. If you notice increased pain or bleeding from the rectum after use of glycerin products, call your doctor. Weakness, sweating, and symptoms of dehydration (thirst, dizziness) also may occur.

▼ PRECAUTIONS

Over 60: Adverse reactions may be more likely and more severe in older patients.

Driving and Hazardous Work: Do not drive or engage in hazardous work until you determine how the medicine affects you.

Alcohol: No special precautions are required.

Pregnancy: Adequate human studies have not been done. Before taking glycerin, tell your doctor if you are or plan to become pregnant.

Breast Feeding: Glycerin suppositories may be used safely by nursing mothers.

Infants and Children: Not recommended for use by children under age 6 years.

Special Concerns: A single missed bowel movement does not constitute constipation; do not use glycerin under such circumstances. Prolonged constipation or persistent rectal pain and discomfort should be evaluated by your doctor. Remember that chronic use of glycerin or any laxative can lead to laxative dependence. You should be sure to consume adequate amounts of fiber in your diet; good sources include bran or other cereals, fresh fruit, and vegetables.

OVERDOSE
Symptoms: No specific symptoms have been reported.

What to Do: An overdose of glycerin is unlikely to be life-threatening. However, if someone takes a much larger dose than prescribed, call your doctor.

▼ INTERACTIONS

DRUG INTERACTIONS
No significant drug interactions have been reported.

FOOD INTERACTIONS
No known food interactions.

DISEASE INTERACTIONS
Caution is advised when taking glycerin laxatives. Consult your doctor if you have any of the following: abdominal pain and fever, rectal bleeding, ostomy (an artificial surgical opening in the body to allow the release of urine or feces), diabetes mellitus, heart or kidney disease, or high blood pressure.

GUAIFENESIN

Available in: Capsules, tablets, oral solution, syrup, extended-release forms
Available as Generic? Yes
Drug Class: Expectorant

▼ USAGE INFORMATION

WHY IT'S TAKEN
Guaifenesin is classified as an expectorant; that is, it is designed to reduce the thickness of mucus and phlegm, making it easier to cough up and out of the lungs and so improve breathing. It is used to treat minor upper respiratory infections and related conditions, such as bronchitis, colds, and sinus or throat infections. Guaifenesin is not a cough suppressant, and despite its popularity and its FDA approval as an expectorant, there is little scientific evidence that it is truly effective at reducing the thickness of mucus.

HOW IT WORKS
Guaifenesin supposedly increases the production of fluids in the respiratory tract and helps liquefy and thin mucus secretions.

▼ DOSAGE GUIDELINES

RANGE AND FREQUENCY
Adults—Capsules, tablets, oral solution, syrup: 200 to 400 mg every 4 hours, to a maximum of 2,400 mg a day. Extended-release capsules and tablets: 600 to 1,200 mg every 12 hours, to a maximum of 2,400 mg a day. Children 2 to 12 years of age: Consult your doctor.

ONSET OF EFFECT
Usually within several hours.

DURATION OF ACTION
The exact duration of action is not known.

DIETARY ADVICE
Maintain your usual food and fluid intake. Increase fluids if you have a fever or diarrhea. Coughing also increases your daily fluid requirements.

STORAGE
Store it in a tightly sealed container away from heat and direct light. Keep liquid forms of guaifenesin refrigerated, but do not allow them to freeze. Keep it away from moisture and extremes in temperature.

MISSED DOSE
Take it as soon as you remember. If it is near the time for the next dose, skip the missed dose and resume your regular dosage schedule. Do not double the next dose.

STOPPING THE DRUG
You may stop taking guaifenesin before the scheduled end of therapy if you are feeling better; otherwise, take it as prescribed for the full treatment period.

PROLONGED USE
Therapy with guaifenesin is usually completed within 7 to 10 days. If you have a persistent cough, you may need special evaluation. Do not take nonprescription guaifenesin for more than 7 days without your doctor's approval.

▼ PRECAUTIONS

Over 60: Adverse reactions may be more likely and more severe in this group.

Driving and Hazardous Work: Do not drive or engage in hazardous work until you determine how the medicine affects you.

Alcohol: No special warnings.

Pregnancy: Thorough studies have not been done, although no serious problems have been reported; consult your doctor for advice.

Breast Feeding: Guaifenesin may pass into breast milk, although no problems have been documented. Consult your doctor for advice.

Infants and Children: Generally, it should not be given to children under 2 years unless directed otherwise by a pediatrician; children under 12 years who have a persistent cough should be examined by a doctor before they are given guaifenesin.

Special Concerns: Guaifenesin is present in numerous nonprescription cough and cold remedies, so ask your pharmacist if you are unsure whether a product you are buying contains it. Do not treat a persistent cough on your own for more than a week or so without seeking medical advice. Avoid giving capsules or tablets to young children, because it is difficult to rely on children to swallow these dosage forms in one piece. Capsules and tablets should not be chewed.

OVERDOSE
Symptoms: No specific symptoms have been reported.

What to Do: An overdose of guaifenesin is unlikely to be life-threatening. However, if someone takes a much larger dose than prescribed, call your doctor, emergency medical services (EMS), or the nearest poison control center.

▼ INTERACTIONS

DRUG INTERACTIONS
None reported.

FOOD INTERACTIONS
None reported.

DISEASE INTERACTIONS
None reported.

SIDE EFFECTS

SERIOUS
No serious side effects are associated with guaifenesin.

COMMON
No common side effects are associated with guaifenesin.

LESS COMMON
Diarrhea; dizziness; headache; abdominal pain, nausea, or vomiting; skin rash; itching; hives.

HYDROCORTISONE TOPICAL

Available in: Cream, lotion, ointment, topical solution, dental paste
Available as Generic? Yes
Drug Class: Topical corticosteroid

BRAND NAMES

Acticort 100, Aeroseb-HC, Ala-Cort, Ala-Scalp HP, Allercort, Alphaderm, Anusol, Anusol-HC, Bactine, Beta HC, CaldeCORT Anti-Itch, Cetacort, Cort-Dome, Cortaid, Cortifair, Cortril, Delacort, Dermacort, DermiCort, Dermtex HC, Gly-Cort, Gynecort, Hi-Cor 2.5, Hydro-Tex, Hytone, LactiCare-HC, Lanacort, Lemoderm, Locoid, My Cort, Nutracort, Orabase-HCA, Pentacort, Rederm, S-T Cort, Synacort, Texacort, Westcort

▼ USAGE INFORMATION

WHY IT'S TAKEN
To treat certain skin conditions that are associated with itching, redness, scaling and peeling, pain, and other signs of inflammation. It is also used to treat inflammatory conditions in the mouth.

HOW IT WORKS
Topical hydrocortisone appears to interfere with the formation of natural substances within the body that are directly responsible for the process of inflammation, which produces swelling, redness, and pain.

▼ DOSAGE GUIDELINES

RANGE AND FREQUENCY
Adults—Dental paste: Apply at bedtime to affected areas of the mouth. Cream, lotion, ointment, solution: Apply sparingly to affected areas of the skin 1 to 2 (sometimes 3) times daily. Children: Consult your pediatrician for specific dosage and other advice.

ONSET OF EFFECT
Steroids begin to exert their effect soon after application. However, recognizable changes in your condition may take several days or more to develop.

DURATION OF ACTION
Unknown.

DIETARY ADVICE
Maintain your usual food and fluid intake.

STORAGE
Store it in a tightly sealed container away from heat and direct light. Keep it away from moisture and extremes in temperature.

MISSED DOSE
Apply it as soon as you remember. If it is near the time for the next dose, skip the missed dose and resume your regular dosage schedule. Do not double the next dose.

STOPPING THE DRUG
Use it as prescribed for the full treatment period, even if you begin to feel better before the scheduled end of therapy.

PROLONGED USE
Therapy with this medication may require weeks or months; long-term therapy requires monitoring by your physician even with a low-potency product.

▼ PRECAUTIONS

Over 60: Adverse reactions to this medication may be more likely and more severe; therapy with topical corticosteroids therefore should be brief and infrequent.

Driving and Hazardous Work: The use of a hydrocortisone topical preparation should not impair your ability to perform such tasks safely.

Alcohol: No special precautions are necessary.

Pregnancy: It should not be used for prolonged periods by pregnant women or by those trying to become pregnant.

Breast Feeding: Although problems have not been documented, caution is advised. Do not apply it to the breasts prior to nursing. Consult your doctor for specific advice.

Infants and Children: Not recommended for prolonged use. Consult your pediatrician.

Special Concerns: Avoid use of this medication around the eyes. Hydrocortisone is not a treatment for acne, burns, infections, or disorders of pigmentation. Do not bandage or wrap the medicated area of skin with any special dressings or coverings unless specifically told to do so by your doctor.

OVERDOSE
Symptoms: No specific symptoms have been reported.

What to Do: An overdose is unlikely to be life-threatening. However, in the event of accidental ingestion or apparent overdose, call your doctor, emergency medical services (EMS), or the nearest poison control immediately.

▼ INTERACTIONS

DRUG INTERACTIONS
None reported.

FOOD INTERACTIONS
None reported.

DISEASE INTERACTIONS
Consult your doctor before taking this medication if you have any of the following medical conditions: diabetes, skin infection or skin sores and ulcers, infection at another site in your body, tuberculosis, unusual bleeding or bruising, glaucoma, or cataracts.

⌰ SIDE EFFECTS ⌰

SERIOUS
Serious side effects from the use of topical hydrocortisone are very rare.

COMMON
Burning, itching, irritation, redness, dryness, acne, stinging and cracking of skin, numbness or tingling in the extremities (in 0.5% to 1% of patients).

LESS COMMON
Blistering and pus near hair follicles, unusual bleeding or easy bruising, darkening or prominence of small surface veins, increased susceptibility to infection.

IBUPROFEN

Available in: Tablets, oral solution, chewable tablets
Available as Generic? Yes
Drug Class: Nonsteroidal antiinflammatory drug (NSAID)

▼ USAGE INFORMATION

WHY IT'S TAKEN
To treat mild to moderate pain and inflammation caused by tendinitis, arthritis, bursitis, gout, soft tissue injuries, migraine and other vascular headaches, menstrual cramps, and other conditions. It is also used to reduce fever.

HOW IT WORKS
NSAIDs work by interfering with the formation of prostaglandins, substances that cause inflammation and make nerves more sensitive to pain impulses. NSAIDs also have other modes of action that are not as well understood.

▼ DOSAGE GUIDELINES

RANGE AND FREQUENCY
Adults—For mild to moderate pain, arthritis, and menstrual pain: 200 to 400 mg every 4 to 6 hours. For fever: 200 to 400 mg every 4 to 6 hours, to a maximum of 1,200 mg a day. Children ages 6 months to 12 years— For fevers below 102.5°F: 5 mg for every 2.2 lb (1 kg) of body weight every 6 to 8 hours. For higher fevers: 10 mg per 2.2 lb every 6 to 8 hours, to a maximum of 40 mg per 2.2 lb a day.

ONSET OF EFFECT
For pain and fever: 30 minutes. For arthritis: up to 3 weeks.

DURATION OF ACTION
4 hours or more.

DIETARY ADVICE
Take ibuprofen with food.

STORAGE
Store in a tightly sealed container away from moisture, heat, and direct light.

MISSED DOSE
Take it as soon as you remember. However, if it is near the time for the next dose, skip the missed dose and resume your regular dosage schedule. Do not double the next dose.

STOPPING THE DRUG
If your doctor has told you to take this drug, do not stop without consulting him or her.

PROLONGED USE
Prolonged use can cause gastrointestinal problems, which may include ulceration and bleeding, kidney dysfunction, and liver inflammation. See your doctor regularly for laboratory tests and examinations.

▼ PRECAUTIONS

Over 60: Because of the potentially greater consequences of gastrointestinal side effects, the dose of NSAIDs for older patients, especially those over age 70, is often cut in half.

Driving and Hazardous Work: Do not drive or engage in hazardous work until you determine how the medicine affects you.

Alcohol: Avoid alcohol, because it may increase the risk of stomach irritation.

Pregnancy: Avoid or discontinue this drug if you are pregnant or are planning to become pregnant.

Breast Feeding: Ibuprofen passes into breast milk; avoid use while nursing.

Infants and Children: It may be used in exceptional circumstances; consult your doctor.

Special Concerns: Because NSAIDs can interfere with blood coagulation, this drug should be stopped at least 3 days before any surgery.

▼ OVERDOSE

Symptoms: Severe nausea, vomiting, headache, confusion, seizures.

What to Do: Call your doctor, emergency medical services (EMS), or the nearest poison control center immediately.

▼ INTERACTIONS

DRUG INTERACTIONS
Do not take this drug with aspirin or any other NSAIDs without your doctor's approval. In addition, consult your doctor if you are taking antihypertensives, steroids, anticoagulants, antibiotics, itraconazole or ketoconazole, plicamycin, penicillamine, valproic acid, phenytoin, cyclosporine, digitalis drugs, lithium, methotrexate, probenecid, triamterene, or zidovudine.

FOOD INTERACTIONS
No known food interactions.

DISEASE INTERACTIONS
Consult your doctor if you have any of the following: bleeding problems, gastrointestinal inflammation or ulcers, diabetes mellitus, systemic lupus erythematosus (SLE, lupus), anemia, asthma, epilepsy, Parkinson's disease, kidney stones, or a history of heart disease or alcohol abuse. Use of ibuprofen may cause complications in patients with liver or kidney disease, because these organs work together to remove the medication from the body.

≡ SIDE EFFECTS ≡

SERIOUS
Shortness of breath or wheezing with or without swelling of legs or other signs of heart failure; chest pain; peptic ulcer disease with vomiting of blood; black, tarry stools; decreasing kidney function. Call your doctor immediately.

COMMON
Nausea, vomiting, heartburn, diarrhea, constipation, headache, dizziness, sleepiness.

LESS COMMON
Ulcers or sores in mouth, depression, rashes or blistering of skin, ringing sound in the ears, unusual tingling or numbness of the hands or feet, seizures, blurred vision. Also, elevated potassium levels and decreased blood cell counts; such problems can be detected by your doctor.

INSULIN (INTERMEDIATE-ACTING, NPH, LENTE)

Available in: Injection
Available as Generic? No
Drug Class: Antidiabetic agent

▼ USAGE INFORMATION

WHY IT'S TAKEN
For long-term treatment of diabetes mellitus. All patients with type 1 diabetes require lifelong insulin treatment. Patients with type 2 diabetes may require insulin if they are unable to control their blood glucose (sugar) levels with diet and oral medications.

HOW IT WORKS
Insulin, a hormone secreted by the beta cells of the pancreas, plays an essential role in controlling the metabolism and storage of carbohydrates, fat, and protein. Insulin is secreted in response to a rise in blood sugar (glucose). Insulin lowers blood glucose by increasing its uptake by body cells, especially muscle, and by reducing the release of glucose from the liver between meals.

▼ DOSAGE GUIDELINES

RANGE AND FREQUENCY
Injected 1 or 2 times a day. Doses and frequency are determined by your doctor. Intermediate-acting (NPH or Lente) insulin can be mixed in the same syringe with rapid-acting insulin; draw up the rapid-acting insulin first. Intermediate-acting insulin solutions are cloudy (insulin settles to the bottom of the bottle) and must be rolled or gently shaken to distribute the insulin evenly in the solution before drawing it up into the syringe.

ONSET OF EFFECT
Within 1 hour; peak effect occurs within 8 to 12 hours.

DURATION OF ACTION
From 12 to 18 hours.

DIETARY ADVICE
All patients with diabetes should follow the general dietary recommendations of the American Diabetes Association. Intake of simple sugars is not forbidden, but consuming a large amount of sugary foods at one time may trigger a rapid rise in blood glucose that can increase urination and thirst. In addition, patients who take insulin must remain consistent from day to day in the timing and caloric content of their meals. Depending on the timing, dose, and types of insulin prescribed, snacks may be recommended in the late afternoon, before bedtime, or prior to unusual physical activity. Patients with diabetes must always have available juice, food, or tablets that can raise their blood glucose levels rapidly to counteract an episode of hypoglycemia.

STORAGE
Refrigerate insulin but do not allow it to freeze. Insulin does not have to be kept refrigerated when you're traveling for short periods, but exposure to high temperatures must be avoided.

MISSED DOSE
Timing of insulin doses is extremely important. The best approach is to measure blood glucose and add a dose of regular insulin if your glucose levels are too high. Otherwise, wait for the next dose on your schedule.

STOPPING THE DRUG
Do not stop taking insulin injections unless ordered by your doctor. Patients with diabetes are often given general instructions for modifying their insulin doses based on repeated home blood glucose measurements.

PROLONGED USE
After many years with diabetes, some patients become insensitive to the symptoms of hypoglycemia and are at risk for serious brain complications caused by prolonged, unrecognized hypoglycemia.

▼ PRECAUTIONS

Over 60: No special warnings. Some older people may have vision problems that may make it difficult to draw up the correct dose of insulin.

Driving and Hazardous Work: Patients taking insulin must be very careful to avoid hypoglycemia when driving or engaging in hazardous work.

Alcohol: Moderate alcohol intake, especially when taken with large meals, does not adversely affect control of diabetes or alter the dose of insulin. However, large amounts of alcohol increase the risk of hypoglycemia.

Pregnancy: Strict metabolic control—using insulin injections in most women—must be maintained during pregnancy to reduce the risk of

▼ SIDE EFFECTS

SERIOUS
Symptoms of hypoglycemia can be caused by the release of adrenaline or by an inadequate supply of glucose to the brain. In severe hypoglycemia, lack of sufficient glucose to the brain may cause slurred speech, impaired concentration, confusion, seizures, coma, irreversible brain damage, and death. Mild hypoglycemia may cause restless sleep, nightmares, or a cold sweat that awakens patients at night.

COMMON
Symptoms resulting from the release of adrenaline are common with mild to moderate hypoglycemia. They include cold sweats, anxiety, shakiness, hunger, rapid heartbeat, and headache. Weight gain is also common when taking insulin.

LESS COMMON
Allergic reactions, lipoatrophy (depressions in the skin caused by loss of fat tissue), and lipohypertrophy (excessive accumulation of fat tissue).

INSULIN (INTERMEDIATE-ACTING, NPH, LENTE)

(continued)

birth defects, fetal complications, or death at the time of delivery. In women who had diabetes before pregnancy, the dose of insulin is often smaller during the first trimester of pregnancy and then higher during the final two trimesters. When women first develop diabetes during pregnancy (gestational diabetes), insulin requirements drop rapidly after delivery and most do not need to continue with insulin treatment.

Breast Feeding: Insulin requirements tend to be lower during breast feeding. Home glucose monitoring is important to avoid hypoglycemia. Insulin is not present in breast milk.

Infants and Children: Insulin treatment for children is the same as for older people with diabetes.

Special Concerns: Inadequate amounts of insulin in type 1 diabetes may lead to the serious complication of diabetic ketoacidosis, characterized by loss of appetite, excessive thirst and urination, nausea, vomiting, deep breathing, fruity breath odor, drowsiness, confusion, and loss of consciousness.

OVERDOSE

Symptoms: Insulin overdose results in hypoglycemia (see Side Effects for symptoms).

What to Do: For mild to moderate hypoglycemia, ingest drinks or food containing sugar. For more severe hypoglycemia, administer injections of glucagon or call emergency medical services (EMS) immediately.

▼ INTERACTIONS

DRUG INTERACTIONS
A large number of drugs can promote either elevated blood glucose levels or hypoglycemia. Be sure that your doctor knows about all of the medications you take and is informed before you start taking any new drugs, either prescription or over the counter. Corticosteroids in particular are likely to raise blood glucose levels and insulin requirements. Beta-blockers (commonly used for hypertension) may cause either high blood glucose levels or hypoglycemia; in addition, because these drugs may dampen the symptoms of hypoglycemia that are caused by adrenaline release, mild degrees of hypoglycemia may progress unnoticed to more serious hypoglycemia affecting the brain.

FOOD INTERACTIONS
Insulin requirements are increased when larger amounts of calories, especially simple sugars and carbohydrates, are ingested.

DISEASE INTERACTIONS
Insulin requirements are increased by infections, psychological stress, or an uncontrolled overactive thyroid, and often at a time of surgery. Requirements may diminish with kidney disease or an underactive adrenal or pituitary gland.

INSULIN (LONG-ACTING, ULTRALENTE)

Available in: Injection
Available as Generic? No
Drug Class: Antidiabetic agent

▼ USAGE INFORMATION

WHY IT'S TAKEN
For long-term treatment of diabetes mellitus. All patients with type 1 diabetes require lifelong insulin treatment. Patients with type 2 diabetes may require insulin if they are unable to control their blood glucose (sugar) levels with diet and oral medications.

HOW IT WORKS
Insulin, a hormone secreted by the beta cells of the pancreas, plays an essential role in controlling the metabolism and storage of carbohydrates, fat, and protein. Insulin is secreted in response to a rise in blood sugar (glucose). Insulin lowers blood glucose by increasing its uptake by body cells, especially muscle, and by reducing the release of glucose from the liver between meals.

▼ DOSAGE GUIDELINES

RANGE AND FREQUENCY
Injected 1 or 2 times a day. Doses and frequency are determined by your doctor. Long-acting (Ultralente) insulin can be mixed in the same syringe with rapid-acting insulin; draw up the rapid-acting insulin first. Long-acting insulin solutions are cloudy (insulin settles to the bottom of the bottle) and must be rolled or gently shaken to distribute the insulin evenly in the solution before drawing it up into the syringe.

ONSET OF EFFECT
It begins to take effect within 6 to 8 hours; the peak effect occurs within 10 to 20 hours of injection.

DURATION OF ACTION
From 24 to 36 hours.

DIETARY ADVICE
All patients with diabetes should follow the general dietary recommendations of the American Diabetes Association. Intake of simple sugars is not forbidden, but consuming a large amount of sugary foods at one time may trigger a rapid rise in blood glucose that can increase urination and thirst. In addition, patients who take insulin must remain consistent from day to day in the timing and caloric content of their meals. Depending on the timing, dose, and types of insulin prescribed, snacks may be recommended in the late afternoon, before bedtime, or prior to unusual physical activity. Patients with diabetes must always have available juice, food, or tablets that can raise their blood glucose levels rapidly to counteract an episode of hypoglycemia.

STORAGE
Refrigerate insulin but do not allow it to freeze. Insulin does not have to be kept refrigerated when you're traveling for short periods, but exposure to high temperatures makes it unusable.

MISSED DOSE
Timing of insulin doses is extremely important. The best approach is to measure blood glucose and add a dose of regular insulin if your glucose levels are too high. Otherwise, wait for the next dose on your schedule.

STOPPING THE DRUG
Do not stop taking insulin injections unless ordered by your doctor. Patients with diabetes are often given general instructions for modifying their insulin doses based on repeated home blood glucose measurements.

PROLONGED USE
After many years with diabetes, some patients become insensitive to the symptoms of hypoglycemia and are at risk for serious brain complications caused by prolonged, unrecognized hypoglycemia.

▼ PRECAUTIONS

Over 60: No special warnings. Some older people may have vision problems that may make it difficult to draw up the correct dose of insulin.

Driving and Hazardous Work: Patients taking insulin must be very careful to avoid hypoglycemia when driving or engaging in hazardous work.

Alcohol: Moderate alcohol intake, especially when taken with large meals, does not adversely affect control of diabetes or alter the dose of insulin. However, large amounts of alcohol increase the risk of hypoglycemia.

Pregnancy: Strict metabolic control—using insulin injections in most women—must be maintained during pregnancy to reduce the risk of birth defects, fetal complications, or death at the time of delivery. In women who had diabetes before pregnancy, the dose of insulin is often smaller during the first trimester of pregnancy and then higher during the final two trimesters. When women first develop diabetes during pregnancy (gestational dia-

---

≣ SIDE EFFECTS ≣

SERIOUS
Symptoms of hypoglycemia can be caused by the release of adrenaline or by an inadequate supply of glucose to the brain. In severe hypoglycemia, lack of sufficient glucose to the brain may cause slurred speech, impaired concentration, confusion, seizures, coma, irreversible brain damage, and death. Mild hypoglycemia may cause restless sleep, nightmares, or a cold sweat that awakens patients at night.

COMMON
Symptoms resulting from release of adrenaline are common manifestations of mild to moderate hypoglycemia. They include cold sweats, anxiety, shakiness, hunger, rapid heartbeat, headache, and nervousness. Weight gain is common when taking insulin.

LESS COMMON
Allergic reactions, lipoatrophy (depressions in the skin caused by loss of fat tissue), and lipohypertrophy (excessive accumulation of fat tissue).

betes), insulin requirements drop rapidly after delivery and most do not need to continue with insulin treatment.

Breast Feeding: Insulin requirements tend to be lower during breast feeding. Home glucose monitoring is important to avoid hypoglycemia. Insulin is not present in breast milk.

Infants and Children: Insulin treatment for young patients is the same as that for older people with diabetes.

Special Concerns: Inadequate amounts of insulin in type 1 diabetes may lead to the serious complication of diabetic ketoacidosis, characterized by loss of appetite, excessive thirst and urination, nausea, vomiting, deep breathing, fruity breath odor, drowsiness, confusion, and loss of consciousness.

OVERDOSE

Symptoms: Insulin overdose results in hypoglycemia (see Side Effects for symptoms).

What to Do: For mild to moderate hypoglycemia, ingest drinks or food containing sugar. For more severe hypoglycemia, administer injections of glucagon or call emergency medical services (EMS) immediately.

▼ INTERACTIONS

DRUG INTERACTIONS

A large number of drugs can promote either elevated blood glucose levels or hypoglycemia. Be sure that your doctor knows about all of the medications you take and is informed before you start taking any new drugs, either prescription or over the counter. Corticosteroids in particular are likely to raise blood glucose levels and insulin requirements. Beta-blockers (commonly used for hypertension) may cause either high blood glucose levels or hypoglycemia; in addition, because these drugs may dampen the symptoms of hypoglycemia that are caused by adrenaline release, mild degrees of hypoglycemia may progress unnoticed to more serious hypoglycemia affecting the brain.

FOOD INTERACTIONS

Insulin requirements are increased when larger amounts of calories, especially simple sugars and carbohydrates, are ingested.

DISEASE INTERACTIONS

Insulin requirements are increased by infections, psychological stress, or an uncontrolled overactive thyroid, and often at a time of surgery. Requirements may diminish with kidney disease or an underactive adrenal or pituitary gland.

INSULIN (REGULAR, RAPID-ACTING, OR SEMILENTE)

Available in: Injection
Available as Generic? No
Drug Class: Antidiabetic agent

▼ USAGE INFORMATION

WHY IT'S TAKEN
For long-term treatment of diabetes mellitus. All patients with type 1 diabetes require lifelong insulin treatment. Patients with type 2 diabetes may require insulin if they are unable to control their blood glucose (sugar) levels with diet and oral medications.

HOW IT WORKS
Insulin, a hormone secreted by the beta cells of the pancreas, plays an essential role in controlling the metabolism and storage of carbohydrates, fat, and protein. Insulin is secreted in response to a rise in blood sugar (glucose). Insulin lowers blood glucose by increasing its uptake by body cells, especially muscle, and by reducing the release of glucose from the liver between meals.

▼ DOSAGE GUIDELINES

RANGE AND FREQUENCY
It may be taken 1 to 4 times daily, before meals and possibly at bedtime. Doses and frequency are determined by your doctor. Regular (or rapid-acting or semilente) insulin should be administered 30 to 45 minutes before a meal. It can be mixed in the same syringe with intermediate-acting insulins. Draw up the regular insulin first.

ONSET OF EFFECT
It begins to take effect within 45 minutes; peak effect occurs within 2 to 4 hours.

DURATION OF ACTION
From 4 to 6 hours.

DIETARY ADVICE
All patients with diabetes should follow the general dietary recommendations of the American Diabetes Association. Intake of simple sugars is not forbidden, but consuming a large amount of sugary foods at one time may trigger a rapid rise in blood glucose that can increase urination and thirst. In addition, patients who take insulin must remain consistent from day to day in the timing and caloric content of their meals. Depending on the timing, dose, and types of insulin prescribed, snacks may be recommended in the late afternoon, before bedtime, or prior to unusual physical activity. Patients with diabetes must always have available juice, food, or tablets that can raise their blood glucose levels rapidly to counteract an episode of hypoglycemia.

STORAGE
Refrigerate insulin but do not allow it to freeze. Insulin does not have to be kept refrigerated when you're traveling for short periods, but exposure to high temperatures must always be avoided.

MISSED DOSE
Timing of insulin doses is extremely important. The best approach is to measure blood glucose and add a dose of regular insulin if glucose levels are too high. Otherwise, wait for the next scheduled dose.

STOPPING THE DRUG
Do not stop taking insulin injections unless ordered by your doctor. Patients with diabetes are often given general instructions for modifying their insulin doses based on home blood glucose measurements.

PROLONGED USE
After many years with diabetes, some patients become insensitive to the symptoms of hypoglycemia and are at risk for serious brain complications caused by prolonged, unrecognized hypoglycemia.

▼ PRECAUTIONS

Over 60: No special warnings. Some older people may have vision problems that may make it difficult to draw up the correct dose of insulin.

Driving and Hazardous Work: Patients taking insulin must be very careful to avoid hypoglycemia when driving or engaging in hazardous work.

Alcohol: Moderate alcohol intake, especially when taken with large meals, does not adversely affect control of diabetes or alter the dose of insulin. However, large amounts of alcohol increase the risk of hypoglycemia.

Pregnancy: Strict metabolic control—using insulin injections in most women—must be maintained during pregnancy to reduce the risk of birth defects, fetal complications, or death at the time of delivery. In women who had diabetes before pregnancy,

---

▼ SIDE EFFECTS

SERIOUS
Symptoms of hypoglycemia can be caused by the release of adrenaline or by an inadequate supply of glucose to the brain. In severe hypoglycemia, lack of sufficient glucose to the brain may cause slurred speech, impaired concentration, confusion, seizures, coma, irreversible brain damage, and death. Mild hypoglycemia may cause restless sleep, nightmares, or a cold sweat that awakens patients at night.

COMMON
Symptoms resulting from release of adrenaline are common manifestations of mild to moderate hypoglycemia. They include cold sweats, anxiety, shakiness, hunger, rapid heartbeat, headache, and nervousness. Weight gain is common when taking insulin.

LESS COMMON
Allergic reactions, lipoatrophy (depressions in the skin caused by loss of fat tissue), and lipohypertrophy (excessive accumulation of fat tissue).

the dose of insulin is often smaller during the first trimester of pregnancy and then higher during the final two trimesters. When women first develop diabetes during pregnancy (gestational diabetes), insulin requirements drop rapidly after delivery and most do not need to continue with insulin treatment.

Breast Feeding: Insulin requirements tend to be lower during breast feeding. Home glucose monitoring is important to avoid hypoglycemia. Insulin is not present in breast milk.

Infants and Children: Insulin treatment for young patients is the same as that for older people with diabetes.

Special Concerns: Inadequate amounts of insulin in type 1 diabetes may lead to the serious complication of diabetic ketoacidosis, characterized by loss of appetite, excessive thirst and urination, nausea, vomiting, deep breathing, fruity breath odor, drowsiness, confusion, and loss of consciousness.

OVERDOSE

Symptoms: Insulin overdose results in hypoglycemia (see Side Effects for symptoms).

What to Do: For mild to moderate hypoglycemia, ingest drinks or food containing sugar. For more severe hypoglycemia, inject glucagon or call emergency medical services (EMS) immediately.

▼ INTERACTIONS

DRUG INTERACTIONS

A large number of drugs can promote either elevated blood glucose levels or hypoglycemia. Be sure that your doctor knows about all of the medications you take and is informed before you start taking any new drugs, either prescription or over the counter. Corticosteroids in particular are likely to raise blood glucose levels and insulin requirements. Beta-blockers (commonly used to treat hypertension) may cause either high blood glucose levels or hypoglycemia; in addition, because these medications may dampen the symptoms of hypoglycemia that are caused by adrenaline release, mild degrees of hypoglycemia may progress unnoticed to more serious hypoglycemia affecting the brain.

FOOD INTERACTIONS

Insulin requirements are increased when larger amounts of calories, especially simple sugars and carbohydrates, are ingested.

DISEASE INTERACTIONS

Insulin requirements are increased by infections, psychological stress, or an uncontrolled overactive thyroid, and often at a time of surgery. Requirements may diminish with kidney disease or an underactive adrenal or pituitary gland.

IODINE TOPICAL

BRAND NAMES

Iodine Tincture, Iodopen

Available in: Topical solution
Available as Generic? Yes
Drug Class: Antibacterial (topical); antiseptic

▼ USAGE INFORMATION

WHY IT'S TAKEN
Iodine is a very effective disinfectant used for prevention and treatment of minor skin infections caused by bacteria. It is also used to disinfect the skin before needle procedures and minor surgeries (such as blood drawing, dialysis, and injections).

HOW IT WORKS
Iodine poisons bacteria on contact by causing the proteins comprising the organism to congeal.

▼ DOSAGE GUIDELINES

RANGE AND FREQUENCY
Adults: Apply to affected site as directed by a physician or according to manufacturer's instructions on the label. Children 1 month of age and older: Consult a pediatrician.

ONSET OF EFFECT
Immediate.

DURATION OF ACTION
Unknown.

DIETARY ADVICE
Maintain your usual food and fluid intake. Increase fluids if you have a fever or diarrhea, in hot weather, or during exercise.

STORAGE
Store it in a tightly sealed container away from heat and direct light. Keep iodine away from moisture and extremes in temperature.

MISSED DOSE
Apply it as soon as you remember. If it is near the time for the next dose, skip the missed dose and resume your regular dosage schedule.

STOPPING THE DRUG
Use it as prescribed for the full treatment period, even if you begin to feel better before the scheduled end of therapy.

PROLONGED USE
Therapy with this medication should be concluded within 7 to 10 days. Consult your physician if your condition has not improved—and especially if it has worsened—at any time after starting therapy with iodine.

▼ PRECAUTIONS

Over 60: No special problems are expected.

Driving and Hazardous Work: The use of iodine should not impair your ability to perform such tasks safely.

Alcohol: No special precautions are necessary.

Pregnancy: Avoid or discontinue using iodine if you are pregnant or trying to become pregnant.

Breast Feeding: Iodine passes into breast milk; avoid or discontinue use while nursing.

Infants and Children: Iodine is not recommended for use on children younger than 1 month of age.

Special Concerns: Iodine has serious side effects if it is absorbed into your blood in large amounts. Therefore, do not apply excessive amounts to affected skin. Do not swallow iodine solutions. Above all, never apply this medication to open wounds, deep cuts, or bleeding or ulcerated skin. Do not use this medication near your eyes and be careful when applying iodine to the skin of your forehead or cheeks. Use small quantities and apply them carefully instead of pouring on a large volume. If iodine gets into your eyes, wash them with water immediately.

OVERDOSE
Symptoms: Overdose with topical iodine is unlikely when used as directed. Swallowing this medication may cause such symptoms as diarrhea, abdominal pain, nausea, vomiting, fever, excessive thirst, and decreased passage of urine.

What to Do: Call your doctor, emergency medical services (EMS), or the nearest poison control center immediately.

▼ INTERACTIONS

DRUG INTERACTIONS
No specific drug interactions have yet been documented. If you are concerned about whether a prescription or nonprescription medication you are taking may interact with topical iodine, consult your doctor or pharmacist for current information.

FOOD INTERACTIONS
No known food interactions.

DISEASE INTERACTIONS
Consult your doctor if you have any of the following: animal bites; large sores, blisters, ulcerations, or broken skin at the application site; severe injury at the application site; puncture wounds or other deep wounds; serious burns; or allergies to shellfish.

≡ SIDE EFFECTS ≡

SERIOUS
When used as directed, topical iodine is not expected to produce any serious side effects.

COMMON
Momentary burning or tingling at the site of application.

LESS COMMON
Irritation or skin allergy with blistering, crusting, itching, or reddening of skin at site of application.

IPECAC SYRUP

Available in: Syrup
Available as Generic? Yes
Drug Class: Emetic

▼ USAGE INFORMATION

WHY IT'S TAKEN
To cause vomiting in persons who have ingested certain toxic substances or have taken an overdose of a drug.

HOW IT WORKS
Ipecac induces vomiting because it chemically irritates the stomach lining, which triggers the body's vomiting reflex.

▼ DOSAGE GUIDELINES

RANGE AND FREQUENCY
Adults and teenagers: 1 to 2 tbsp, followed by 1 full glass of water. Children ages 1 to 12 years: 1 tbsp followed by ½ to 1 full glass of water. Children ages 6 months to 1 year: 1 to 2 tsp, followed by ½ to 1 full glass of water. If vomiting does not occur, the first dose may be repeated one time after 20 minutes.

ONSET OF EFFECT
Within 20 to 30 minutes.

DURATION OF ACTION
20 to 25 minutes.

DIETARY ADVICE
Drink water immediately after taking ipecac syrup.

STORAGE
Store it in a tightly sealed container away from moisture, heat, and direct light.

MISSED DOSE
Not applicable. It should be used more than once only if clearly necessary.

STOPPING THE DRUG
Do not give more than 2 doses. If not effective, consult your doctor, emergency medical services (EMS), or local poison control center.

PROLONGED USE
Ipecac is not intended for prolonged use.

▼ PRECAUTIONS

Over 60: No special problems are expected.

Driving and Hazardous Work: Do not drive or engage in hazardous work until you determine how the drug affects you.

Alcohol: Avoid alcohol.

Pregnancy: No studies of the use of ipecac syrup during pregnancy have been done. Discuss with your doctor the relative risks and benefits of using it while pregnant.

Breast Feeding: Ipecac syrup may pass into breast milk; caution is advised. Consult your doctor for advice.

Infants and Children: Use by children should be under strict supervision. There is an increased risk of children under 1 year of age swallowing the vomited substance. Consult your doctor before using ipecac syrup.

Special Concerns: Before giving ipecac syrup, consult your doctor, emergency medical services (EMS), or the nearest poison control center. Ipecac syrup should not be given to anyone who has ingested gasoline, paint thinner, kerosene, or a caustic substance such as lye. Do not give ipecac syrup to anyone who is unconscious or very drowsy, because of an increased risk that the vomited substance can enter the lungs. If you have a child older than 1 year of age in the house, keep 1 oz (2 tbsp) of ipecac syrup on hand for emergencies. Ipecac syrup should not be used to induce vomiting as a means of losing weight. It can be toxic to the heart.

OVERDOSE
Symptoms: Breathing difficulty, muscle stiffness, diarrhea.

What to Do: Call your doctor, emergency medical services (EMS), or the nearest poison control center immediately.

▼ INTERACTIONS

DRUG INTERACTIONS
Do not give any other medicines, including OTC drugs, with ipecac unless you first consult your doctor. Antiemetics can decrease the syrup's effect and increase its toxicity. If you are also using activated charcoal, wait until the ipecac-induced vomiting has stopped before administering it.

FOOD INTERACTIONS
Ipecac syrup should not be taken with milk, milk products, or carbonated drinks. Milk and milk products prevent ipecac syrup from working properly. Carbonated beverages can cause the stomach to swell.

DISEASE INTERACTIONS
You should not take ipecac syrup if you suffer from or have heart disease, a history of seizures, shock, reduced gag reflex, drowsiness, or unconsciousness.

SIDE EFFECTS

SERIOUS
Heartbeat irregularities; nausea or vomiting lasting for more than 30 minutes; excessive diarrhea; weakness or stiffness of the muscles in the neck, arms, and legs; stomach pain or cramps; unusual fatigue; difficulty breathing. Call your doctor immediately.

COMMON
Drowsiness and mild diarrhea.

LESS COMMON
There are no less common side effects associated with the use of ipecac syrup.

KAOLIN WITH PECTIN

BRAND NAMES

K-P, Kao-Spen, Kapectolin

Available in: Oral suspension
Available as Generic? Yes
Drug Class: Antidiarrheal

▼ USAGE INFORMATION

WHY IT'S TAKEN
To treat diarrhea.

HOW IT WORKS
Kaolin with pectin absorbs fluids and binds to and removes bacteria and toxins from the digestive tract.

▼ DOSAGE GUIDELINES

RANGE AND FREQUENCY
Adults: 4 to 8 tbsp after each loose bowel movement. Children age 12 years and older: 3 to 4 tbsp after each loose bowel movement. Children ages 6 to 12 years: 2 to 4 tbsp after each loose bowel movement. Children ages 3 to 6 years: 1 to 2 tbsp after each loose bowel movement.

ONSET OF EFFECT
Unknown.

DURATION OF ACTION
Unknown.

DIETARY ADVICE
A mild diet is recommended when recovering from diarrhea. Bananas, rice, applesauce, and plain toast are good choices. Be sure to drink plenty of fluids.

STORAGE
Store it in a tightly sealed container away from moisture, heat, and direct light.

MISSED DOSE
Take it as soon as you remember. If it is nearly time for another dose, skip the missed dose. Do not double the next dose.

STOPPING THE DRUG
Do not use this drug for more than 2 days without consulting your doctor.

PROLONGED USE
This drug is not intended for prolonged use. Consult your doctor if diarrhea continues for more than 2 days.

▼ PRECAUTIONS

Over 60: Adverse reactions associated with diarrhea may be more severe in older patients. They should be sure to consume enough liquids to replace body fluids lost because of diarrhea.

Driving and Hazardous Work: The use of kaolin with pectin should not impair your ability to perform such tasks safely.

Alcohol: Avoid alcohol.

Pregnancy: It is not absorbed into the body and is not expected to cause problems during pregnancy.

Breast Feeding: It is not absorbed into the body and is not expected to cause problems during breast feeding.

Infants and Children: Kaolin with pectin should be used for children younger than 3 years of age only under the supervision of a doctor.

Special Concerns: In addition to taking medicine for diarrhea, it is important to replace the fluid lost by your body and to eat a proper diet. During the first 24 hours, drink plenty of caffeine-free clear liquids such as water, broth, ginger ale, and decaffeinated tea. During the second 24 hours, you may eat bland foods such as applesauce, bread, crackers, and oatmeal. Avoid caffeine, fried or spicy foods, bran, candy, fruits, and vegetables. They can make your condition worse.

OVERDOSE
Symptoms: Constipation.

What to Do: An overdose of kaolin with pectin is unlikely to be life-threatening. However, if someone takes a much larger dose than recommended or prescribed, call your doctor, emergency medical services (EMS), or the nearest poison control center immediately.

▼ INTERACTIONS

DRUG INTERACTIONS
Consult your doctor for specific advice if you are taking anticholinergics, antidyskinetics, digitalis drugs, lincomycins, loxapine, phenothiazines, thioxanthenes, or any other oral medication. Do not take any medication within 2 to 3 hours of taking kaolin with pectin.

FOOD INTERACTIONS
Fruits, fried or spicy foods, bran, candy, and beverages containing caffeine can make diarrhea worse.

DISEASE INTERACTIONS
Caution is advised when taking kaolin with pectin. Consult your doctor if the diarrhea is suspected to be caused by parasites or dysentery.

≣ SIDE EFFECTS ≣

SERIOUS
No serious side effects have been reported.

COMMON
No common side effects have been reported.

LESS COMMON
Constipation.

KETOCONAZOLE TOPICAL

BRAND NAMES

Nizoral A-D,
Nizoral Cream

Available in: Cream, shampoo
Available as Generic? Yes
Drug Class: Topical antifungal

▼ USAGE INFORMATION

WHY IT'S TAKEN
Ketoconazole is used to treat fungal infections of the skin. These infections include tinea pedis (athlete's foot), tinea corporis (ringworm), tinea cruris (jock itch), yeast infections of the skin, seborrheic dermatitis, and others.

HOW IT WORKS
Ketoconazole prevents fungal organisms from manufacturing vital substances required for growth and function.

▼ DOSAGE GUIDELINES

RANGE AND FREQUENCY
Adults—For tinea and yeast: Apply once daily to affected skin. Treatment generally requires 2 to 6 weeks. For seborrheic dermatitis: Apply 2 times a day to affected skin. Treatment generally requires 4 weeks. Children: Consult your pediatrician.

ONSET OF EFFECT
Ketoconazole begins killing susceptible fungi shortly after contact. The effects may not be noticeable for several days or weeks.

DURATION OF ACTION
Unknown.

DIETARY ADVICE
Maintain your usual food and fluid intake. Increase fluid intake in hot weather, during exercise, or if you have a fever or diarrhea.

STORAGE
Store it in a tightly sealed container away from heat and direct light.

MISSED DOSE
Apply it as soon as you remember. If it is near the time for the next dose, skip the missed dose and resume your regular dosage schedule. Do not double the next dose or apply an excessively thick film of topical medication to compensate for a missed application.

STOPPING THE DRUG
Apply ketoconazole as recommended for the full treatment period, even if you notice marked improvement before the scheduled end of the therapy.

PROLONGED USE
Therapy with this medication should not exceed 4 weeks.

▼ PRECAUTIONS

Over 60: Adverse reactions may be more likely and more severe in older patients.

Driving and Hazardous Work: The use of ketoconazole cream should not impair your ability to perform such tasks safely.

Alcohol: No special precautions are necessary.

Pregnancy: Avoid or discontinue use of ketoconazole if you are pregnant or planning to become pregnant.

Breast Feeding: Ketoconazole may pass into breast milk; avoid or discontinue use while nursing. Consult your doctor for specific advice.

Infants and Children: Not recommended for use by young children.

Special Concerns: Avoid contact with your eyes and wash your hands thoroughly after application. Tell your doctor if your condition has not improved within a few days of starting ketoconazole. As with any other antifungal, ketoconazole is useful only against organisms that are vulnerable to its effects. Therefore, it is important to tell your doctor if your condition has not improved—or has worsened—within a few days of starting ketoconazole. The particular organism causing your illness may be resistant to this medication.

OVERDOSE
Symptoms: No specific symptoms have been reported.

What to Do: An overdose of ketoconazole is unlikely to be life-threatening. However, if someone applies a much larger dose than prescribed or ingests the medication, call your doctor, emergency medical services (EMS), or the nearest poison control center.

▼ INTERACTIONS

DRUG INTERACTIONS
No specific drug interactions are known. If you are concerned about whether a prescription or over-the-counter medication you are taking may interact with ketoconazole, consult your physician or pharmacist for current information.

FOOD INTERACTIONS
No known food interactions.

DISEASE INTERACTIONS
Consult your physician if you have had previous allergies or an undesirable reaction to any other topical medication.

SIDE EFFECTS

SERIOUS
Blistering or ulceration of the skin; blistering of the lips, nose, and mouth.

COMMON
Brief burning, itching, or irritation after application of cream; peeling.

LESS COMMON
Severe burning, itching, swelling, increased redness, or any discomfort at the application site not present before therapy (as a result of allergic reaction).

KETOPROFEN

Available in: Tablets and capsules (also extended-release forms), rectal suppositories
Available as Generic? Yes
Drug Class: Nonsteroidal antiinflammatory drug (NSAID)

▼ USAGE INFORMATION

WHY IT'S TAKEN
To treat mild to moderate pain and inflammation caused by tendinitis, arthritis, bursitis, gout, soft tissue injuries, migraine and other vascular headaches, menstrual cramps, and other conditions. When patients fail to respond to one NSAID, another may be tried. The greatest effectiveness often requires trial and error of several different NSAIDs.

HOW IT WORKS
NSAIDs work by interfering with the formation of prostaglandins, naturally occurring substances in the body that cause inflammation and make nerves more sensitive to pain impulses. NSAIDs also have other modes of action that are less well understood.

▼ DOSAGE GUIDELINES

RANGE AND FREQUENCY
Adults—Tablets or capsules: 50 mg 4 times a day or 75 mg 3 times a day. Extended-release tablets or capsules: 200 mg once a day. Suppositories: 50 to 100 mg inserted twice a day (morning and evening). Sometimes, suppositories may be used only at night by people who take an oral dose during the day. Maximum dosage for all forms is 300 mg per day.

ONSET OF EFFECT
1 to 2 hours.

DURATION OF ACTION
3 to 4 hours.

DIETARY ADVICE
Take oral forms with food.

STORAGE
Store it in a tightly sealed container away from moisture, heat, and direct light.

MISSED DOSE
Take it as soon as you remember. If it is near the time for the next dose, skip the missed dose and resume your regular dosage schedule. Do not double the next dose.

STOPPING THE DRUG
If your doctor has advised you to take this drug, do not stop without consulting him or her.

PROLONGED USE
Prolonged use can cause gastrointestinal ulceration and bleeding, kidney dysfunction, and liver inflammation. Consult your doctor about the need for medical examinations and laboratory studies.

▼ PRECAUTIONS

Over 60: Because of the potentially greater consequences of gastrointestinal side effects, the dose of NSAIDs for older patients, especially those over age 70, is often cut in half.

Driving and Hazardous Work: Do not drive or engage in hazardous work until you determine how the medicine affects you.

Alcohol: Avoid alcohol when using this medication because it increases the risk of stomach irritation.

Pregnancy: Do not use ketoprofen during pregnancy.

Breast Feeding: Ketoprofen passes into breast milk; avoid use while nursing.

Infants and Children: Ketoprofen may be used in exceptional circumstances; consult your doctor.

Special Concerns: Because NSAIDs can interfere with blood coagulation, this drug should be stopped at least 3 days before any surgery.

OVERDOSE
Symptoms: Severe nausea, vomiting, headache, confusion, seizures.

What to Do: Call your doctor, emergency medical services (EMS), or the nearest poison control center immediately.

▼ INTERACTIONS

DRUG INTERACTIONS
Do not take this drug with aspirin or any other NSAIDs without your doctor's approval. In addition, consult your doctor if you are taking antihypertensives, steroids, anticoagulants, antibiotics, itraconazole or ketoconazole, plicamycin, penicillamine, valproic acid, phenytoin, cyclosporine, digitalis drugs, lithium, methotrexate, probenecid, triamterene, or zidovudine.

FOOD INTERACTIONS
No known food interactions.

DISEASE INTERACTIONS
Consult your doctor if you have any of the following: bleeding problems, gastrointestinal inflammation or ulcers, diabetes mellitus, systemic lupus erythematosus (SLE, lupus), anemia, asthma, epilepsy, Parkinson's disease, kidney stones, or a history of heart disease or alcohol abuse. Use of ketoprofen may cause complications in patients with liver or kidney disease, because these organs work together to remove the medication from the body.

≣ SIDE EFFECTS ≣

SERIOUS
Shortness of breath or wheezing with or without swelling of legs or other signs of heart failure; chest pain; peptic ulcer disease with vomiting of blood; black, tarry stools; decreasing kidney function. Call your doctor immediately.

COMMON
Nausea, vomiting, heartburn, diarrhea, constipation, headache, dizziness, sleepiness.

LESS COMMON
Ulcers or sores in mouth, depression, rashes or blistering of skin, ringing in the ears, unusual tingling or numbness of the hands or feet, seizures, blurred vision. Also, elevated potassium levels, decreased red and white blood cell counts; such problems can be detected by your doctor.

LOPERAMIDE HYDROCHLORIDE

Available in: Capsules, oral solution, tablets
Available as Generic? Yes
Drug Class: Antidiarrheal

▼ USAGE INFORMATION

WHY IT'S TAKEN
To treat diarrhea.

HOW IT WORKS
Loperamide relieves diarrhea by slowing the activity of the intestines.

▼ DOSAGE GUIDELINES

RANGE AND FREQUENCY
Capsules—Adults and teenagers: 4 mg after the first loose bowel movement, 2 mg after each subsequent loose bowel movement. Take no more than 16 mg every 24 hours. Children ages 9 to 12 years: 2 mg 3 times a day. Children ages 6 to 8 years: 2 mg 2 times a day. Oral solution—Adults and teenagers: 4 mg (4 tsp) after the first loose bowel movement, 2 mg after each subsequent loose bowel movement. No more than 8 mg every 24 hours. Children ages 9 to 11 years: 2 mg after the first loose bowel movement, 1 mg after each subsequent loose bowel movement. No more than 6 mg every 24 hours. Children ages 6 to 8 years: 2 mg after the first loose bowel movement, 1 mg after each subsequent loose bowel movement. No more than 4 mg every 24 hours. Tablets—Adults and teenagers: 4 mg after the first loose bowel movement, 1 mg after each subsequent loose bowel movement. No more than 8 mg every 24 hours. Children ages 9 to 11 years: 2 mg after the first loose bowel movement, 1 mg after each subsequent loose bowel movement. No more than 6 mg every 24 hours. Children ages 6 to 8 years: 2 mg after the first loose bowel movement, 1 mg after each subsequent loose bowel movement. No more than 4 mg every 24 hours.

ONSET OF EFFECT
Unknown.

DURATION OF ACTION
Up to 24 hours.

DIETARY ADVICE
Take it on an empty stomach 1 hour before or 2 hours after eating. A mild diet is recommended when recovering from diarrhea. Bananas, rice, applesauce, and plain toast are good choices. Be sure to drink plenty of fluids.

STORAGE
Store this medication in a tightly sealed container away from heat, moisture, and direct light.

MISSED DOSE
Skip the missed dose and resume your regular dosage schedule. Do not double the next dose.

STOPPING THE DRUG
You may stop taking the drug whenever you choose.

PROLONGED USE
Loperamide should not be used for more than 2 days unless otherwise directed by your doctor.

▼ PRECAUTIONS

Over 60: Diarrhea may easily lead to dehydration, especially in older patients, and loperamide may mask the effects of dehydration. When using loperamide, older persons should be sure to get plenty of fluids.

Driving and Hazardous Work: Avoid such activities until you determine how the medicine affects you.

Alcohol: Avoid alcohol.

Pregnancy: Discuss with your doctor the relative risks and benefits of using loperamide while pregnant.

Breast Feeding: It is not known whether loperamide passes into breast milk; caution is advised. Consult your doctor for specific advice.

Infants and Children: Do not give this drug to children under 6 years of age unless directed by your doctor.

Special Concerns: During the first 24 hours, drink plenty of caffeine-free clear liquids such as water, broth, ginger ale, and decaffeinated tea. During the second 24 hours, eat bland foods such as applesauce, bread, crackers, and oatmeal.

OVERDOSE
Symptoms: Constipation, central nervous system depression, gastrointestinal irritation.

What to Do: An overdose of loperamide is unlikely to be life-threatening. However, if someone takes a much larger dose than prescribed, call your doctor, emergency medical services (EMS), or the nearest poison control center.

▼ INTERACTIONS

DRUG INTERACTIONS
Consult your doctor for specific advice if you are taking any narcotic pain medication or antibiotics such as cephalosporin, erythromycin, and tetracycline.

FOOD INTERACTIONS
Fruits, fried or spicy foods, bran, candy, and beverages containing caffeine can make diarrhea worse.

DISEASE INTERACTIONS
Consult your doctor if you have an intestinal illness, severe colitis, or liver disease.

 SIDE EFFECTS

SERIOUS
Bloating, skin rash, constipation, loss of appetite, stomach pains, nausea, vomiting. Call your doctor immediately.

COMMON
No common side effects are associated with loperamide.

LESS COMMON
Dizziness or drowsiness, dry mouth.

LOPERAMIDE/SIMETHICONE

Available in: Chewable tablet
Available as Generic? No
Drug Class: Antidiarrheal/antigas combination

▼ USAGE INFORMATION

WHY IT'S TAKEN
To treat diarrhea and to relieve bloating, pain, pressure, and cramps caused by excess gas in the stomach and intestines.

HOW IT WORKS
Loperamide eases diarrhea by slowing the activity of the intestines. Simethicone disperses and prevents the formation of gas bubbles in the gastrointestinal tract.

▼ DOSAGE GUIDELINES

RANGE AND FREQUENCY
Adults and teenagers: Chew 2 tablets and drink a full glass of water after the first loose stool. If needed, chew 1 tablet and drink more water after the next loose stool. Take no more than 4 tablets a day. Children ages 6 to 11 years: Chew 1 tablet after the first loose stool. If needed, chew half a tablet after the next loose stool. Children ages 9 to 11 years (or weighing 60 to 95 lb) should take no more than 3 tablets a day. Children ages 6 to 8 (or weighing 48 to 59 lb) should take no more than 2 tablets a day. Follow each dose with plenty of clear liquids.

ONSET OF EFFECT
Unknown.

DURATION OF ACTION
Unknown.

DIETARY ADVICE
A mild diet is recommended when recovering from diarrhea. Bananas, rice, applesauce, and plain toast are good choices. Be sure to drink plenty of fluids.

STORAGE
Store it in a tightly sealed container away from moisture, heat, and direct light.

MISSED DOSE
Not applicable: the drug is taken only when necessary.

STOPPING THE DRUG
You may stop taking the drug whenever you choose.

PROLONGED USE
This drug should not be used for more than 2 days unless otherwise directed by your doctor.

▼ PRECAUTIONS

Over 60: Diarrhea may easily lead to dehydration, especially in older patients, and this drug may mask the symptoms of dehydration. When using this drug, older persons should be sure to get plenty of fluids.

Driving and Hazardous Work: No special precautions are necessary.

Alcohol: Avoid alcohol, because it may irritate the lining of the gastrointestinal tract and promote dehydration.

Pregnancy: Discuss with your doctor the relative risks and benefits of using this drug during pregnancy.

Breast Feeding: This drug may pass into breast milk; caution is advised. Consult your doctor for specific advice.

Infants and Children: Not recommended for use by children younger than 6 years or who weigh less than 48 lb.

Special Concerns: Chew the tablets thoroughly before swallowing for quicker and more complete relief. You should change position frequently and walk around to help eliminate gas. During the first 24 hours, drink plenty of caffeine-free clear liquids, such as water, broth, ginger ale, and decaffeinated tea. During the second 24 hours, you may eat bland foods such as applesauce, bread, crackers, and oatmeal. Tell your doctor if you have diarrhea while on a low-sodium, low-sugar, or other special diet. Do not smoke before meals.

OVERDOSE
Symptoms: Constipation, gastrointestinal irritation, drowsiness, confusion.

What to Do: An overdose of this drug is unlikely to be life-threatening. However, if someone takes a much larger dose than prescribed, call your doctor.

▼ INTERACTIONS

DRUG INTERACTIONS
Consult your doctor for specific advice if you are taking any narcotic pain medication or antibiotics such as cephalosporin, erythromycin, and tetracycline.

FOOD INTERACTIONS
Fruits, fried or spicy foods, bran, candy, and beverages containing caffeine can make diarrhea worse. Avoid any foods that increase gas formation. Chew your food slowly and thoroughly.

DISEASE INTERACTIONS
Do not use this drug if you have a high fever (over 101°F) or stools containing blood or mucus. Consult your physician before using this drug if you have an intestinal illness, severe colitis, or liver disease.

SIDE EFFECTS

SERIOUS
Skin rash, bloating, constipation, loss of appetite, stomach pain, nausea, vomiting. Call your doctor immediately.

COMMON
Expulsion of excess gas, causing belching and flatulence.

LESS COMMON
Dizziness or drowsiness, dry mouth.

LORATADINE

Available in: Tablets, syrup
As Generic? Yes
Drug Class: Antihistamine

▼ USAGE INFORMATION

WHY IT'S TAKEN
To prevent or relieve symptoms of hay fever and other allergies, such as watery or itchy eyes, sneezing, runny nose, or itchy skin. The drug loratadine is also used sometimes to treat chronic (or persistent) hives.

HOW IT WORKS
Loratadine blocks the effects of histamine, a naturally occurring substance that causes swelling, itching, sneezing, watery eyes, hives, and other symptoms of allergic reaction.

▼ DOSAGE GUIDELINES

RANGE AND FREQUENCY
Tablets and syrup—Adults and children age 10 years and older: 10 mg once a day. Children ages 2 to 9 years: 5 mg once a day. Do not increase the dose in an attempt to achieve quicker relief of symptoms.

ONSET OF EFFECT
Within 1 hour.

DURATION OF ACTION
24 hours or more.

DIETARY ADVICE
Loratadine can be taken without regard to diet, but taking this medicine with food may be beneficial because it can increase absorption of the drug from the gastrointestinal tract by up to 40%.

STORAGE
Store it in a tightly sealed container at room temperature, away from heat, moisture, and direct light.

MISSED DOSE
Take it as soon as you remember. However, if it is near the time for the next dose, skip the missed dose and resume your regular dosage schedule. Do not double the next dose.

STOPPING THE DRUG
The decision to stop taking the drug should be made in consultation with your doctor.

PROLONGED USE
Loratadine can be taken safely for extended periods. Long-term use is not linked to decreased effectiveness of the drug (a problem with certain allergy medications and other drugs).

▼ PRECAUTIONS

Over 60: Adverse reactions may be more likely and more severe in older patients.

Driving and Hazardous Work: The use of loratadine at recommended doses should not impair your ability to perform such tasks safely.

Alcohol: No special precautions are necessary.

Pregnancy: Before you take loratadine, tell your doctor if you are pregnant or plan to become pregnant.

Breast Feeding: Loratadine passes into breast milk; avoid or discontinue use while breast feeding.

Infants and Children: Adverse reactions may be more likely and more severe in children.

Special Concerns: Stop taking loratadine 4 to 7 days before you have an allergy skin test.

OVERDOSE
Symptoms: Rapid heartbeat, headache, drowsiness.

What to Do: An overdose of loratadine is unlikely to be life-threatening. However, if someone takes a much larger dose than prescribed, call your doctor, emergency medical services (EMS), or the nearest poison control center.

▼ INTERACTIONS

DRUG INTERACTIONS
Be sure to consult your doctor for advice if you are taking clarithromycin, erythromycin, troleandomycin, itraconazole, or ketoconazole.

FOOD INTERACTIONS
There are no known interactions between loratadine and specific foods.

DISEASE INTERACTIONS
There are no known disease interactions.

≣ SIDE EFFECTS ≣

SERIOUS
No serious side effects are associated with the use of loratadine.

COMMON
No common side effects are associated with the use of loratadine.

LESS COMMON
In rare cases, adverse reactions have been reported in persons taking loratadine, but none of these reactions is clearly linked to use of the drug.

MAGALDRATE

BRAND NAMES

Losopan, Riopan

Available in: Oral suspension
Available as Generic? Yes
Drug Class: Antacid

▼ USAGE INFORMATION

WHY IT'S TAKEN
To relieve symptoms of heartburn, acid indigestion, sour stomach, and gastroesophageal reflux. Also used to treat hyperacidity associated with peptic ulcers, gastritis, and esophagitis.

HOW IT WORKS
Magaldrate neutralizes stomach acid and reduces the action of pepsin, a digestive enzyme. This provides symptomatic relief from excess stomach acid.

▼ DOSAGE GUIDELINES

RANGE AND FREQUENCY
Adults: 540 to 1,080 mg (5 to 10 ml). Children: 5 to 10 mg. Take it between meals and at bedtime.

ONSET OF EFFECT
Within 20 minutes.

DURATION OF ACTION
20 to 60 minutes in fasting patients; 3 hours when taken after meals.

DIETARY ADVICE
Eat a balanced diet.

STORAGE
Store it in a tightly sealed container away from moisture, heat, and direct light.

MISSED DOSE
Take it as soon as you remember. If it is near the time for the next dose, skip the missed dose and resume your regular dosage schedule. Do not double the next dose.

STOPPING THE DRUG
Take it as directed for the full treatment period.

PROLONGED USE
Do not take magaldrate for more than 2 weeks unless your doctor advises you to do otherwise.

≡ SIDE EFFECTS ≡

SERIOUS
Severe and continuing constipation, dizziness, lightheadedness, and heartbeat irregularities. Bone loss (osteomalacia) may occur, especially with prolonged use in dialysis patients. Hypophosphatemia (too little phosphate in the blood) may occur with prolonged use and a low-phosphate diet; symptoms include bone pain, fractures (caused by bone loss), muscle weakness, loss of appetite, mood changes, a general feeling of discomfort, swelling of the wrists and ankles, unusual weight loss, and anemia (decreased number of red blood cells; symptoms include weakness and fatigue). Call your doctor immediately.

COMMON
Chalky taste.

LESS COMMON
Increased thirst, speckling or whitish color of stools, stomach cramps, diarrhea, mild constipation.

▼ PRECAUTIONS

Over 60: Constipation and intestinal trouble are more common in older persons. Older patients who have or who are at high risk for osteoporosis or other bone disorders should avoid frequent use of magaldrate.

Driving and Hazardous Work: No special precautions.

Alcohol: Avoid alcohol.

Pregnancy: Adequate studies have not been done. Before taking magaldrate, tell your doctor if you are pregnant or plan to become pregnant.

Breast Feeding: Magaldrate may pass into breast milk but has not been reported to cause problems in nursing babies. Consult your doctor for advice.

Infants and Children: Do not give antacids and other medicines containing magnesium to young children unless prescribed by a physician.

Special Concerns: Use over-the-counter antacids only occasionally unless otherwise directed by your doctor. Persistent heartburn not readily relieved by antacids may be signaling a heart attack or other serious disorder. Seek medical help promptly.

OVERDOSE
Symptoms: Diarrhea, nausea, vomiting, constipation, confusion, palpitations, weakness, fatigue, bone pain, stupor.

What to Do: An overdose of magaldrate is unlikely to be life-threatening. However, if someone takes a much larger dose than prescribed, call your doctor, emergency medical services (EMS), or the nearest poison control center.

▼ INTERACTIONS

DRUG INTERACTIONS
Magaldrate and other antacids containing magnesium may interact with vitamin D (including calcitediol and calcitriol), and may decrease the effectiveness of pancrelipase. Note that other medications may lose their effectiveness when taken within 1 hour of antacids. Consult your doctor for specific advice if you are taking amphetamines, bisacodyl, cellulose sodium phosphate, citrates, chenodiol, digoxin, enteric-coated medications, fluoroquinolones, isoniazid, ketoconazole, mecamylamine, methenamine, nitrofurantoin, penicillamine, phosphates, sodium polystyrene sulfonate resin, tetracyclines, or quinidine.

FOOD INTERACTIONS
No known food interactions.

DISEASE INTERACTIONS
Do not take magaldrate if you have any symptoms of appendicitis or an inflamed bowel (abdominal pain, cramps, soreness, bloating, nausea, and vomiting). Magaldrate is not recommended for Alzheimer's patients. Consult your doctor if you have any of the following: broken bones, colitis, diarrhea, intestinal blockage or bleeding, colostomy or ileostomy, edema, hypophosphatemia, heart disease, liver disease, toxemia of pregnancy, or kidney disease.

MAGNESIUM CITRATE

BRAND NAMES

Citrate of Magnesia, Citro-Nesia, Citroma

Available in: Oral solution
Available as Generic? Yes
Drug Class: Hyperosmotic laxative

▼ USAGE INFORMATION

WHY IT'S TAKEN
To treat short-term constipation and for rapid emptying of the colon for rectal and bowel examinations.

HOW IT WORKS
Magnesium citrate attracts and retains water in the intestine, softening stools and inducing the urge to defecate.

▼ DOSAGE GUIDELINES

RANGE AND FREQUENCY
Adults and teenagers: 11 to 25 g daily in 1 or more doses. Children ages 6 to 12 years: 5.5 to 12.5 g daily in 1 or more doses.

ONSET OF EFFECT
30 minutes to 3 hours.

DURATION OF ACTION
Variable.

DIETARY ADVICE
Take it on an empty stomach with a full glass of cold water or juice.

STORAGE
Store it in a tightly sealed container away from moisture, heat, and direct light.

MISSED DOSE
If you are taking this drug on a fixed schedule, take the missed dose as soon as you remember. If it is near the time for the next dose, skip the missed dose and resume your regular dosage schedule. Do not double the next dose.

STOPPING THE DRUG
Take it as directed for the full treatment period. However, you may stop taking the drug if you are feeling better before the scheduled end of the therapy.

PROLONGED USE
Magnesium citrate is intended for short-term therapy only.

▼ PRECAUTIONS

Over 60: No special problems are expected.

Driving and Hazardous Work: This medication should not impair your ability to perform such tasks safely.

Alcohol: Avoid alcohol.

Pregnancy: Pregnant women with impaired kidney function should avoid taking magnesium citrate.

Breast Feeding: Magnesium citrate may pass into breast milk; caution is advised. Consult your doctor for advice.

Infants and Children: Do not give magnesium citrate and other laxatives to children under 6 years of age unless prescribed by a doctor.

Special Concerns: Chilling the medication, taking it with ice, or following it with citrus fruit juice or citrus-flavored carbonated beverages may make it more palatable. Remember that chronic use of magnesium citrate or any laxative can lead to laxative dependence. You should consume adequate amounts of fiber in your diet, such as bran, whole-grain cereals, fruit, and vegetables. Magnesium citrate should be taken on a schedule that doesn't interfere with activities or sleep, because it produces watery stools in 3 to 6 hours. It should not be taken within 2 hours of taking other medications.

OVERDOSE
Symptoms: Severe or protracted diarrhea.

What to Do: An overdose of magnesium citrate is unlikely to be life-threatening. However, if someone takes a much larger dose than prescribed, call your doctor, emergency medical services (EMS), or the nearest poison control center right away.

▼ INTERACTIONS

DRUG INTERACTIONS
Consult your doctor for specific advice if you are taking cellulose sodium phosphate; other medications containing magnesium, such as antacids; other laxatives; sodium polystyrene sulfonate; and oral tetracycline antibiotics.

FOOD INTERACTIONS
No known food interactions.

DISEASE INTERACTIONS
Caution is advised when taking magnesium citrate. Consult your doctor if you have kidney problems, symptoms of appendicitis (abdominal pain, nausea, vomiting), heart damage, intestinal obstruction or perforation, heart block, or rectal fissures.

☰ SIDE EFFECTS ☰

SERIOUS
Confusion, dizziness or lightheadedness, intestinal blockage, skin rash or itching, difficulty swallowing. Call your doctor immediately.

COMMON
Cramping, diarrhea, gas, increased thirst.

LESS COMMON
Sweating, weakness.

MAGNESIUM OXIDE

Available in: Capsules, tablets
Available as Generic? Yes
Drug Class: Antacid

▼ USAGE INFORMATION

WHY IT'S TAKEN
To treat low magnesium in the blood (hypomagnesemia). Also used to replace or prevent magnesium loss caused by other medications or conditions. It is used as an antacid to relieve heartburn, sour stomach, and acid indigestion.

HOW IT WORKS
Magnesium oxide neutralizes stomach acid and reduces the action of pepsin, a digestive enzyme. This provides symptomatic relief from excess stomach acid and heartburn.

▼ DOSAGE GUIDELINES

RANGE AND FREQUENCY
Capsules: 140 mg 3 to 4 times a day. Tablets: 400 to 800 mg a day in evenly divided doses.

ONSET OF EFFECT
Within 20 minutes.

DURATION OF ACTION
For 20 minutes in fasting patients; 3 hours when taken after meals.

DIETARY ADVICE
Take this medication at least 1 hour after meals.

STORAGE
Store it in a tightly sealed container away from moisture, heat, and direct light.

MISSED DOSE
Take it as soon as you remember. If it is near the time for the next dose, skip the missed dose and resume your regular dosage schedule. Do not double the next dose.

STOPPING THE DRUG
Take it as directed for the full treatment period. However, when magnesium oxide is used as an antacid, it may be taken as needed.

PROLONGED USE
You should see your doctor regularly for tests and examinations if you must take this drug for a prolonged period.

▼ PRECAUTIONS

Over 60: Adverse reactions may be more likely and more severe.

Driving and Hazardous Work: Do not drive or engage in hazardous work until you determine how the medicine affects you.

Alcohol: Avoid alcohol.

Pregnancy: Adequate studies have not been done. Be sure to tell your doctor if you are pregnant or planning to become pregnant.

Breast Feeding: Magnesium oxide may pass into breast milk; consult your doctor for advice.

Infants and Children: Not recommended for use by children under 6 years unless prescribed by a doctor.

Special Concerns: Using magnesium oxide in large amounts or for prolonged periods may have a laxative effect; the drug should not be used regularly for this purpose. In general, do not take other medicines within 2 hours of taking antacids containing magnesium. Upper abdominal pain or heartburn not readily relieved by antacids may signal a heart attack or other serious disorder. In such cases, seek medical help promptly.

OVERDOSE
Symptoms: Diarrhea, bloating, change in mental state, muscle pain or twitching, slowed or shallow breathing, coma.

What to Do: An overdose of magnesium oxide is unlikely to be life-threatening. However, if someone takes a much larger dose than prescribed, call your doctor, emergency medical services (EMS), or the nearest poison control center immediately.

▼ INTERACTIONS

DRUG INTERACTIONS
Consult your doctor if you are taking fluoroquinolones, ketoconazole, methenamine, mecamylamine, sodium polystyrene sulfonate, tetracyclines, urinary acidifiers, digitalis drugs, misoprostol, pancrelipase, iron salts, phosphates, salicylates, or vitamin D (including calcifediol and calcitriol). Also, certain medications may lose their effectiveness or cause unexpected side effects when taken within 2 hours of magnesium oxide. These include enteric-coated medicines, folic acid, penicillamine, phenothiazines, and phenytoin. Take them at least 2 hours apart (and 3 hours before or after phenytoin).

FOOD INTERACTIONS
No known food interactions.

DISEASE INTERACTIONS
Do not take magnesium oxide if you have any symptoms of appendicitis or an inflamed bowel (abdominal pain, cramps, soreness, bloating, nausea, and vomiting). Antacids containing magnesium should not be taken by patients with kidney disease. Consult your doctor if you have any of the following: bone fractures, colitis, severe and continuing constipation, hemorrhoids, intestinal or rectal bleeding, a colostomy or ileostomy, persistent diarrhea, edema, heart disease, liver disease, preeclampsia, sarcoidosis, or underactive parathyroid glands.

≡ SIDE EFFECTS ≡

SERIOUS
Dizziness, lightheadedness, continuing feeling of discomfort, irregular heartbeat, loss of appetite, mental or mood changes, muscle weakness, unusual fatigue or weakness, unusual weight loss. Call your doctor immediately.

COMMON
Chalky taste, laxative effect.

LESS COMMON
Diarrhea, increased thirst, speckling or discoloration of stools, stomach cramps, nausea or vomiting, elevated magnesium in the blood (detectable by your doctor).

MAGNESIUM SULFATE

Available in: Crystals, tablets
Available as Generic? Yes
Drug Class: Laxative/dietary supplement

▼ USAGE INFORMATION

WHY IT'S TAKEN
Magnesium sulfate is used to evacuate the bowel before surgery and as a dietary supplement for people with a magnesium deficiency caused by illness or as a result of the use of certain medications.

HOW IT WORKS
As a laxative, magnesium sulfate attracts and retains water in the intestine, softening stools and inducing the urge to defecate.

▼ DOSAGE GUIDELINES

RANGE AND FREQUENCY
As a laxative–Adults and teenagers: 10 to 30 g daily in 1 or more doses. Children ages 6 to 12 years: 5 to 10 g daily in 1 or more doses. To treat magnesium deficiency: The dose is determined by your doctor according to the severity of the deficiency.

ONSET OF EFFECT
Within 30 minutes to 3 hours.

DURATION OF ACTION
Variable.

DIETARY ADVICE
Take it on an empty stomach with a full glass of cold water or juice.

STORAGE
Store it in a tightly sealed container away from heat, moisture, and direct light.

MISSED DOSE
If you are taking this drug on a fixed schedule, take the missed dose as soon as you remember. If it is near the time for the next dose, skip the missed dose and resume your regular dosage schedule. Do not double the next dose.

STOPPING THE DRUG
You should not take magnesium sulfate for more than 1 week unless your physician directs otherwise.

PROLONGED USE
You should see your doctor regularly for tests and examinations if you must take this drug for a prolonged period.

▼ PRECAUTIONS

Over 60: No special problems are expected.

Driving and Hazardous Work: The use of magnesium sulfate should not impair your ability to perform such tasks safely.

Alcohol: Avoid alcohol.

Pregnancy: Magnesium sulfate is used as a treatment, in the hospital only, for certain symptoms of preeclampsia. If necessary, pregnant women can take magnesium sulfate as a dietary supplement.

Breast Feeding: Magnesium sulfate passes into breast milk; caution is advised. Consult your doctor for advice.

Infants and Children: Magnesium sulfate and other laxatives should not be given to children under 6 years of age unless prescribed by your pediatrician.

Special Concerns: Taking magnesium sulfate with ice or following it with citrus fruit juice or a citrus-flavored carbonated beverage may make it more palatable. Remember that chronic use of magnesium sulfate or any laxative can lead to laxative dependence. Consume adequate amounts of fiber, such as bran, fruit, whole-grain cereals, and vegetables, in your diet. It should be taken on a schedule that does not interfere with activities or sleep, because it produces watery stools within 3 to 6 hours. It should not be taken within 2 hours of taking other drugs.

OVERDOSE
Symptoms: Blurred or double vision, dizziness or fainting, severe drowsiness, increased or decreased urination, slow heartbeat, trouble breathing.

What to Do: Call your doctor, emergency medical services (EMS), or the nearest poison control center immediately.

▼ INTERACTIONS

DRUG INTERACTIONS
Consult your doctor for specific advice if you are taking oral tetracycline, other preparations containing magnesium, cellulose sodium phosphate, sodium polystyrene sulfonate, or digitalis drugs.

FOOD INTERACTIONS
No known food interactions.

DISEASE INTERACTIONS
Use caution when taking magnesium sulfate. Consult your doctor if you have any of the following: myasthenia gravis, severe kidney disease, heart blockage, intestinal obstruction or perforation, or any respiratory disease.

▼ SIDE EFFECTS

SERIOUS
Abdominal cramps, nausea, diarrhea. Call your doctor immediately.

COMMON
There are no common side effects associated with the use of magnesium sulfate.

LESS COMMON
There are no less common side effects associated with the use of magnesium sulfate.

MECLIZINE

Available in: Capsules, tablets, chewable tablets
Available as Generic? Yes
Drug Class: Antiemetic; antivertigo agent

▼ USAGE INFORMATION

WHY IT'S TAKEN
To treat and prevent nausea, vomiting, and dizziness caused by motion sickness, as well as to treat vertigo (dizziness) associated with other medical problems.

HOW IT WORKS
Meclizine acts on the brain centers that control nausea, vomiting, and dizziness.

▼ DOSAGE GUIDELINES

RANGE AND FREQUENCY
To prevent and treat motion sickness—Adults and teenagers: 25 to 50 mg 1 hour before travel. The dose may be repeated every 24 hours. To prevent and treat vertigo—Adults and teenagers: 25 to 100 mg a day as needed in divided doses.

ONSET OF EFFECT
Within 1 hour.

DURATION OF ACTION
Up to 24 hours.

DIETARY ADVICE
It can be taken with food.

STORAGE
Store it in a tightly sealed container protected from heat, moisture, and direct light.

MISSED DOSE
Take it as soon as you remember. If it is near the time for the next dose, skip the missed dose and resume your regular dosage schedule. Do not double the next dose.

STOPPING THE DRUG
Take it as prescribed for the full treatment period. However, you may stop taking the medication if you are feeling better before the scheduled end of therapy.

PROLONGED USE
See your doctor regularly for tests and examinations if you must use this drug for a prolonged period.

▼ PRECAUTIONS

Over 60: Adverse reactions may be more likely and more severe in older patients.

Driving and Hazardous Work: Do not drive or engage in hazardous work until you determine how the medicine affects you.

Alcohol: Avoid alcohol when using this medication.

Pregnancy: Adequate human studies have not been completed. Before taking meclizine, tell your doctor if you are pregnant or plan to become pregnant.

Breast Feeding: Meclizine may pass into breast milk, but it has not been reported to cause problems in nursing babies. It may reduce the flow of breast milk. Consult your doctor for advice.

Infants and Children: Meclizine is not recommended for use by children younger than 12 years.

Special Concerns: If dry mouth occurs, use sugar-free candy or gum or ice chips for temporary relief. If constipation occurs, a high-fiber diet and drinking plenty of fluids can help relieve the problem. Meclizine can cause false-negative results in allergy skin testing.

OVERDOSE
Symptoms: Extreme excitability, seizures, drowsiness, hallucinations.

What to Do: Call your doctor, emergency medical services (EMS), or the nearest poison control center immediately.

▼ INTERACTIONS

DRUG INTERACTIONS
Consult your doctor for specific advice if you are taking medications that can depress the central nervous system, such as tranquilizers, sleep medications, antihistamines, medicines for hay fever, prescription pain medicines, or muscle relaxants, or if you are taking any additional OTC medication.

FOOD INTERACTIONS
No known food interactions.

DISEASE INTERACTIONS
Caution is advised when taking meclizine. Consult your doctor if you have any of the following: urinary tract blockage, glaucoma, asthma, bronchitis, emphysema or any other chronic lung disease, enlarged prostate, heart failure, or intestinal blockage.

 ≣ SIDE EFFECTS ≣

SERIOUS
No serious side effects are associated with the use of meclizine.

COMMON
Drowsiness.

LESS COMMON
Blurred or double vision; upset stomach; constipation or diarrhea; insomnia; painful or difficult urination; dizziness; dry mouth, nose, and throat; headache; loss of appetite; fast heartbeat; nervousness; restlessness; skin rash.

MICONAZOLE

BRAND NAMES

M-Zole 3, Miconazole-7, Monistat 3, Monistat 7

Available in: Vaginal cream and suppositories
Available as Generic? Yes
Drug Class: Antifungal

▼ USAGE INFORMATION

WHY IT'S TAKEN
To treat severe fungal infections, particularly vaginal yeast infections.

HOW IT WORKS
Miconazole prevents fungal organisms from producing vital substances required for growth and function. This medication is effective only for infections caused by fungal organisms. It will not be effective against bacterial or viral infections.

▼ DOSAGE GUIDELINES

RANGE AND FREQUENCY
Adults and teenagers—Vaginal cream: At bedtime, insert into the vagina 1 applicatorful for 7 to 14 nights. Vaginal suppositories: At bedtime, insert 1 100-mg suppository into the vagina for 7 nights or 1 200-mg or 1 400-mg suppository for 3 nights.

ONSET OF EFFECT
Unknown.

DURATION OF ACTION
Unknown.

DIETARY ADVICE
No special restrictions.

STORAGE
Store it in a tightly sealed container away from moisture, heat, and direct light. Refrigerate the suppositories, and do not allow the medication to freeze.

MISSED DOSE
Take it as soon as you remember. This will help keep a constant level of medication in your system. If it is near the time for the next dose, skip the missed dose and resume your regular dosage schedule. Do not double the next dose.

STOPPING THE DRUG
Take it as directed for the full treatment period, even if you begin to feel better before the scheduled end of therapy. Stopping prematurely increases the risk of reinfection. Some fungal infections take many months to clear up, and some may require continuous treatment.

PROLONGED USE
Therapy with this medication may require months. Prolonged use may increase the risk of adverse effects.

▼ PRECAUTIONS

Over 60:
Adverse reactions may be more likely and more severe in older patients.

Driving and Hazardous Work:
Do not drive or engage in hazardous work until you determine how the medicine affects you.

Alcohol:
Avoid alcohol.

Pregnancy:
Adequate studies of miconazole use during pregnancy have not been done. Consult your doctor for advice if you are pregnant or plan to become pregnant.

Breast Feeding:
Miconazole passes into breast milk; caution is advised. Consult your doctor for advice.

Infants and Children:
Not recommended for use by children younger than 1 year of age.

Special Concerns:
Sanitary napkins should be used to prevent staining of clothing. The affected area should be kept cool and dry. Do not sit for a long time in a wet bathing suit. Avoid feminine hygiene sprays. Wash daily with unscented soap and dry thoroughly with a clean towel. Tampons should not be used during therapy. The patient's sexual partner should wear a condom during intercourse. Do not stop using this medicine during your menstrual period. After urination or a bowel movement, cleanse by wiping the area from front to back to prevent reinfection.

OVERDOSE
Symptoms: An overdose with miconazole is unlikely.

What to Do: Emergency instructions not applicable.

▼ INTERACTIONS

DRUG INTERACTIONS
Tell your doctor if you are using any other vaginal prescription or OTC medicine when using the vaginal forms of miconazole. Do not take medications containing alcohol, such as cough syrups, elixirs, and tonics. Consult your doctor for specific advice if you are taking cyclosporine, phenytoin, or warfarin.

FOOD INTERACTIONS
No known food interactions.

DISEASE INTERACTIONS
Consult your doctor if you have a history of alcohol abuse. Use of miconazole can cause complications in patients with liver or kidney disease, because these organs work together to remove the medication from the body.

 SIDE EFFECTS

SERIOUS
Skin rash or itching; fever or chills; pain at site of injection; vaginal burning, itching, discharge, or irritation not present before treatment. Call your doctor immediately.

COMMON
No common side effects are associated with miconazole.

LESS COMMON
Diarrhea, nausea, vomiting, constipation, dizziness, headache, redness or flushing of skin, stomach cramps or pain, burning or irritation of sexual partner's penis.

MILK OF MAGNESIA (MAGNESIA; MAGNESIUM HYDROXIDE)

Available in: Oral suspension, chewable tablets
Available as Generic? Yes
Drug Class: Antacid; hyperosmotic laxative

▼ USAGE INFORMATION

WHY IT'S TAKEN
To relieve symptoms of upset stomach; sometimes used for short-term treatment of constipation.

HOW IT WORKS
As an antacid, milk of magnesia neutralizes stomach acid. As a laxative, it attracts and retains water in the intestine, increasing intestinal movement (peristalsis) and inducing the urge to defecate.

▼ DOSAGE GUIDELINES

RANGE AND FREQUENCY
As an antacid—Adults and teenagers: 1 tsp to 1 tbsp of liquid form or 650 mg to 1.3 g of tablets 3 or 4 times a day. To relieve constipation—Adults and teenagers: 2.4 to 4.8 g (2 tsp to 4 tbsp) daily in 1 or more doses. Children ages 6 to 12 years: 1.2 to 2.4 g (1 to 2 tbsp) daily in 1 or more doses.

ONSET OF EFFECT
30 minutes to 3 hours.

DURATION OF ACTION
Variable.

DIETARY ADVICE
Take it 1 to 3 hours after meals or at bedtime with a full glass of water.

STORAGE
Store milk of magnesia in a tightly sealed container away from heat, moisture, and direct light.

MISSED DOSE
Take it as soon as you remember. If it is near the time for the next dose, skip the missed dose and resume your regular dosage schedule. Do not double the next dose.

STOPPING THE DRUG
You may stop taking the drug whenever you choose.

PROLONGED USE
Do not take milk of magnesia for more than 2 weeks unless your doctor prescribes it.

▼ PRECAUTIONS

Over 60: No special advice.

Driving and Hazardous Work: This medicine should not impair your ability to perform such tasks safely.

Alcohol: Avoid alcohol.

Pregnancy: Extensive human studies have not been done. There have been reports of side effects in babies whose mothers took high doses of antacids for a long time during pregnancy. Before you take milk of magnesia, consult your doctor if you are pregnant or you plan to become pregnant.

Breast Feeding: Milk of magnesia may pass into breast milk but has not been reported to cause problems in nursing babies. Consult your doctor for advice.

Infants and Children: Antacids and other medications containing magnesium should not be given to children under age 6 years unless prescribed by a doctor.

Special Concerns: Take milk of magnesia on a schedule that does not interfere with activities or sleep, because it produces watery stools in 3 to 6 hours. Remember that frequent or protracted use can lead to laxative dependence. Do not take milk of magnesia within 2 hours of taking other medications. Before swallowing, chew tablets well to allow the medicine to work more quickly and effectively.

OVERDOSE

Symptoms: Severe or protracted diarrhea, painful or difficult urination, muscle weakness, continued loss of appetite, irregular heartbeat, difficulty breathing.

What to Do: An overdose of milk of magnesia is unlikely to be life-threatening. However, if someone takes a much larger dose than prescribed, call your doctor, emergency medical services (EMS), or the nearest poison control center immediately.

▼ INTERACTIONS

DRUG INTERACTIONS
Consult your physician for specific advice if you are taking other antacids or laxatives or any of the following medications: cellulose sodium phosphate, fluoroquinolones, isoniazid, ketoconazole, sodium polystyrene sulfonate resin, methenamine, mecamylamine, salicylates, or tetracyclines.

FOOD INTERACTIONS
None are known.

DISEASE INTERACTIONS
Do not use this medication if you have any symptoms of appendicitis or inflamed bowel such as lower abdominal or stomach pain, nausea or vomiting, cramping, soreness, or bloating. Consult your physician if you have any of the following: broken bones, colitis, hemorrhoids, intestinal blockage or bleeding, a recent colostomy or ileostomy, swelling of feet or lower legs, heart disease, toxemia of pregnancy, liver disease, or kidney disease.

≡ SIDE EFFECTS ≡

SERIOUS
Dizziness or lightheadedness, continuing feeling of discomfort, irregular heartbeat, loss of appetite, mood or mental changes, muscle weakness, unusual fatigue, unusual weight loss, rectal bleeding. Call your doctor immediately.

COMMON
Nausea, diarrhea.

LESS COMMON
Increased thirst, speckling or whitish color of stools, abdominal cramps.

MINOXIDIL TOPICAL

BRAND NAME

Rogaine

Available in: Topical solution
Available as Generic? Yes
Drug Class: Hair growth stimulant

▼ USAGE INFORMATION

WHY IT'S TAKEN
Minoxidil topical solution is prescribed to stimulate hair growth in men and women with the type of baldness known as androgenetic alopecia, a condition popularly known as male pattern baldness or female pattern baldness.

HOW IT WORKS
It is not known how minoxidil works. Although it increases the flow of blood, nutrients, and other important substances to hair follicles, other or additional poorly understood actions are believed responsible for hair growth.

▼ DOSAGE GUIDELINES

RANGE AND FREQUENCY
Adults: Apply ⅛ tsp (1 ml) regardless of the size of the balding area under treatment.

ONSET OF EFFECT
At least 4 months with twice-daily therapy.

DURATION OF ACTION
New hair resulting from minoxidil treatments will likely be lost approximately 3 to 4 months after the discontinuation of the medication.

DIETARY ADVICE
No special restrictions.

STORAGE
Store it in a tightly sealed container away from heat and direct light. Keep it away from moisture and extremes in temperature.

MISSED DOSE
Apply it as soon as you remember. If it is near the time for the next dose, skip the missed dose and resume your regular dosage schedule. Do not double the next dose.

STOPPING THE DRUG
Use it until you are able to assess changes, if any, in hair growth and cosmetic appearance. This may take at least 4 months. If you decide to abandon efforts to achieve hair regrowth, you may stop the medication at any time.

PROLONGED USE
Ongoing therapy with this medication is required for continued results. Prolonged use may increase the risk of undesirable side effects.

▼ PRECAUTIONS

Over 60: Adverse reactions may be more likely and more severe in older patients.

Driving and Hazardous Work: Do not drive or engage in hazardous work until you determine how the medicine affects you.

Alcohol: No special warnings.

Pregnancy: Avoid or discontinue topical minoxidil if you are pregnant or are trying to become pregnant. Consult your physician.

Breast Feeding: Minoxidil passes into breast milk; do not use it while nursing.

Infants and Children: Not recommended for children.

Special Concerns: Anyone with a history of allergy to minoxidil or other components of the product should not use this medication. Minoxidil has potentially serious side effects if absorbed in large amounts into the body. Persons with a history of heart disease should consult their doctor before using this product. Do not apply it to irritated, blistered, bleeding, or broken skin. Do not use more than the recommended dose, and do not apply it more frequently than twice a day. Do not use hair dryers to accelerate drying of the medication.

OVERDOSE
Symptoms: Symptoms are similar to those listed under Serious Side Effects: rapid pulse; weakness, dizziness, or a lightheaded feeling; chest pain.

What to Do: If the above symptoms occur or someone ingests the medication, call your doctor, emergency medical services (EMS), or the nearest poison control center immediately.

▼ INTERACTIONS

DRUG INTERACTIONS
Consult your doctor for specific advice if you are taking oral minoxidil, steroids, petrolatum, or acne preparations such as tretinoin. Persons using heart or blood pressure medications should discuss minoxidil use with their doctor before starting treatment.

FOOD INTERACTIONS
No known food interactions.

DISEASE INTERACTIONS
Consult your doctor if you have any disorders affecting your skin or scalp, including rashes, sunburn, or other types of skin eruption or inflammation; heart disease; or high blood pressure.

 SIDE EFFECTS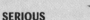

SERIOUS
Rapid pulse; weakness, dizziness, or lightheaded feeling; chest pain. Notify your doctor immediately. If chest pain is present, call emergency medical services (EMS).

COMMON
Burning, tingling, or mild redness of scalp at application site; mild dryness or flaking of skin; itching.

LESS COMMON
Significant irritation or allergy with redness, itching, flaking, or rash; tingling of hands or feet; water retention (swelling of face, hands, fingers, or legs); flushing; headache. Stop the drug and notify your doctor immediately.

NAPROXEN

Available in: Tablets, oral suspension, gelcaps
Available as Generic? Yes
Drug Class: Nonsteroidal antiinflammatory drug (NSAID)

▼ USAGE INFORMATION

WHY IT'S TAKEN
To relieve minor pain or inflammation associated with headaches, the common cold, toothache, muscle aches, backache, arthritis, gout, tendinitis, bursitis, or menstrual cramps; also, to reduce fever. When patients fail to respond to one NSAID, several others may be tried.

HOW IT WORKS
NSAIDs work by interfering with the formation of prostaglandins, naturally occurring substances in the body that cause inflammation and make nerves more sensitive to pain impulses. NSAIDs also have other modes of action that are not as well understood.

▼ DOSAGE GUIDELINES

RANGE AND FREQUENCY
Adults: 440 to 1,500 mg daily. Maximum dose is 1,500 mg a day taken in 2 or 3 evenly divided doses.

ONSET OF EFFECT
Rapid; relieves pain within 1 hour. It may take up to 2 weeks to suppress inflammation.

DURATION OF ACTION
Up to 12 hours.

DIETARY ADVICE
Take with food; maintain your usual food and fluid intake.

STORAGE
Store tablets in a tightly sealed container away from heat, moisture, and direct light. Store the oral suspension in the refrigerator, but do not freeze it.

MISSED DOSE
Take it as soon as you remember. However, if it is near the time for the next dose, skip the missed dose and resume your regular dosage schedule. Do not double the next dose.

STOPPING THE DRUG
If you are taking this drug by prescription, do not stop taking it without first consulting your doctor.

PROLONGED USE
Prolonged use can cause gastrointestinal problems such as ulceration and bleeding, kidney dysfunction, and liver inflammation. Consult your doctor about the need for medical examinations and lab studies.

▼ PRECAUTIONS

Over 60: Because of the potentially greater consequences of gastrointestinal side effects, the dose of NSAIDs for older patients, especially those over age 70, is often cut in half.

Driving and Hazardous Work: Avoid such activities until you determine how the medication affects you.

Alcohol: Avoid alcohol when taking this drug; the combination of naproxen and alcoholic beverages can be highly toxic to the liver.

Pregnancy: Avoid this drug if you are pregnant or plan to become pregnant.

Breast Feeding: Naproxen passes into breast milk; avoid use while nursing.

Infants and Children: Naproxen may be used in exceptional circumstances; consult your pediatrician for advice.

Special Concerns: Because NSAIDs can interfere with blood coagulation, this drug should be stopped at least 3 days prior to any surgery.

OVERDOSE
Symptoms: Severe nausea, vomiting, headache, confusion, seizures.

What to Do: Call your doctor, emergency medical services (EMS), or the nearest poison control center immediately.

▼ INTERACTIONS

DRUG INTERACTIONS
Do not take this drug with aspirin or any other NSAIDs without your doctor's approval. In addition, consult your doctor if you are taking antihypertensives, steroids, anticoagulants, antibiotics, itraconazole or ketoconazole, plicamycin, penicillamine, valproic acid, phenytoin, cyclosporine, digitalis drugs, lithium, methotrexate, probenecid, triamterene, or zidovudine.

FOOD INTERACTIONS
No known food interactions.

DISEASE INTERACTIONS
Consult your doctor if you have any of the following: bleeding problems, inflammation or ulcers of the stomach and intestines, diabetes mellitus, systemic lupus erythematosus (SLE, lupus), anemia, asthma, epilepsy, Parkinson's disease, kidney stones, or a history of heart disease or alcohol abuse. Use of naproxen may cause complications in patients with liver or kidney disease, because these organs work together to remove the medication from the body.

▤ SIDE EFFECTS ▤

SERIOUS
 Shortness of breath or wheezing with or without swelling of legs or other signs of heart failure; chest pain; peptic ulcer disease with vomiting of blood; black, tarry stools; decreasing kidney function. Call your doctor immediately.

COMMON
Nausea, vomiting, heartburn, diarrhea, constipation, headache, dizziness, sleepiness.

LESS COMMON
Ulcers or sores in mouth, depression, rashes or blistering of skin, ringing in the ears, unusual tingling or numbness of the hands or feet, seizures, blurred vision. Also elevated potassium levels and decreased red and white blood cell counts; such problems can be detected by your doctor.

NEOMYCIN/POLYMYXIN B/BACITRACIN TOPICAL

BRAND NAMES

Bactine First Aid Antibiotic, Foille, Mycitracin, Neosporin Maximum Strength Ointment, Neosporin Ointment, Topisporin

Available in: Ointment
Available as Generic? Yes
Drug Class: Antibiotic combination

▼ USAGE INFORMATION

WHY IT'S TAKEN
To help prevent bacterial skin infections after minor cuts, abrasions, or burns.

HOW IT WORKS
This is a combination drug that contains three distinct antibiotics. Each of these drugs attacks and kills bacteria in a different way. Their combined effect is capable of warding off infection by a variety of bacterial organisms.

▼ DOSAGE GUIDELINES

RANGE AND FREQUENCY
The usual treatment is to apply the ointment 2 to 5 times a day to areas of the skin that have suffered a minor injury. If you are using the prescription-strength form of the medication, follow your doctor's orders carefully; for over-the-counter forms, follow the directions.

ONSET OF EFFECT
Unknown.

DURATION OF ACTION
Unknown.

DIETARY ADVICE
This medication can be used without regard to diet.

STORAGE
Store it in a tightly sealed container away from heat and direct light. Keep it away from moisture and extremes in temperature.

MISSED DOSE
Apply it as soon as you remember. However, if it is near the time for the next dose, skip the missed dose and resume your regular dosage schedule. Do not apply a double dose.

STOPPING THE DRUG
Use it as prescribed for the full treatment period, even if the affected area begins to look and feel better before the scheduled end of therapy. If you stop treatment prematurely, the heartier strains of bacteria are likely to survive, reproduce, and cause a worse infection later (known as a rebound infection).

PROLONGED USE
Consult your physician if you must use this medicine for a prolonged period.

▼ PRECAUTIONS

Over 60: No special precautions for older patients.

Driving and Hazardous Work: No special precautions are necessary.

Alcohol: No special precautions are necessary.

Pregnancy: Clinical studies of the use of this medication during pregnancy have not been done. Consult your doctor if you are or plan to become pregnant.

Breast Feeding: It is not known whether this combination antibiotic passes into breast milk; caution is advised. Consult your doctor for specific advice.

Infants and Children: There is no information about use of this combination antibiotic for infants and children. However, no special problems are expected in this group.

Special Concerns: Do not use this medication if you have a history of allergic reaction to any of the active or inactive ingredients in the ointment. If you're applying this medicine without a prescription, do not use it to treat puncture wounds, deep wounds, serious burns, or raw areas unless you first have consulted your doctor. Do not use this medicine in your eyes. Before you apply the medication, wash the affected area with soap and water and dry thoroughly. You may cover the treated area with a gauze bandage if you desire.

OVERDOSE
Symptoms: No specific ones have been reported.

What to Do: No cases of overdose have been reported, but if someone accidentally ingests this medicine, call your doctor, emergency medical services (EMS), or the nearest poison control center.

▼ INTERACTIONS

DRUG INTERACTIONS
Do not use other topical medications with this preparation unless otherwise instructed by your doctor.

FOOD INTERACTIONS
No known food interactions.

DISEASE INTERACTIONS
No disease interactions have been reported with the use of this combination antibiotic.

≡ SIDE EFFECTS ≡

SERIOUS
Rare, severe allergic reaction that may cause breathing difficulty or, at the extreme, total closure of the airways with potentially fatal anaphylactic shock. Contact emergency medical services (EMS) immediately. In very rare cases, hearing loss may occur; if so, call your doctor immediately.

COMMON
No common side effects are associated with this medicine.

LESS COMMON
Irritation or skin allergy with burning, stinging, itching, redness, or rash. Contact your doctor as soon as possible if such side effects persist.

NICOTINE

Available in: Chewing gum, inhaler, nasal spray, skin patch
Available as Generic? Yes
Drug Class: Smoking deterrent

▼ USAGE INFORMATION

WHY IT'S TAKEN
To reduce nicotine withdrawal symptoms as part of a comprehensive program for smoking cessation.

HOW IT WORKS
It replaces the nicotine that would otherwise be taken in by tobacco use.

▼ DOSAGE GUIDELINES

RANGE AND FREQUENCY
Used when you have the desire to smoke. Chewing gum: 20 to 24 mg a day, not to exceed 24 pieces of gum a day. The number of sticks is gradually reduced. Skin patch: To start, 1 patch supplying 22 to 24 mg a day. Dose is gradually reduced over 2 to 5 months. Inhaler and nasal spray: Ask your doctor.

ONSET OF EFFECT
30 minutes to 2 hours.

DURATION OF ACTION
3 to 6 hours.

DIETARY ADVICE
Gum should be chewed slowly over 30 minutes. Other forms can be used without regard to diet.

STORAGE
Store it in a tightly sealed container away from heat and direct light.

MISSED DOSE
If you are on a specific regimen, take a missed dose as soon as you remember. If it is near the time for the next dose, skip the missed dose and resume your regular dosage schedule. Otherwise, nicotine is taken as needed.

STOPPING THE DRUG
The decision to stop taking the drug should be made in consultation with your doctor. Dose for the patch should be tapered as directed.

PROLONGED USE
Treatment should generally not exceed 2 to 6 months. If relapse of smoking occurs, treatment may be repeated.

▼ PRECAUTIONS

Over 60: Adverse reactions are not expected to be more severe in older patients than in younger persons.

Driving and Hazardous Work: The use of nicotine should not impair your ability to perform such tasks safely.

Alcohol: No special warnings.

Pregnancy: Nicotine should not be used during pregnancy. Before you use this drug, tell your doctor if you are pregnant or plan to become pregnant.

Breast Feeding: Nicotine passes into breast milk; do not use it while nursing.

Infants and Children: It should not be used. Even small amounts of nicotine can cause serious problems in infants and children.

Special Concerns: When disposing of patches or gum, be sure to use a method that keeps them out of the reach of children and animals. You should not smoke while being treated with nicotine. Do not apply a patch in the same place for at least a week.

OVERDOSE
Symptoms: Nausea, vomiting, increased salivation, severe abdominal or stomach pain, diarrhea, severe headache, cold sweats, severe dizziness, hearing and vision disturbances, confusion, weakness, breathing difficulty, heartbeat irregularities, seizures, loss of consciousness.

What to Do: Call your doctor, emergency medical services (EMS), or the nearest poison control center immediately.

▼ INTERACTIONS

DRUG INTERACTIONS
Other drugs may interact with nicotine. Consult your doctor for specific advice if you are taking aminophylline, insulin, oxtriphylline, propoxyphene, or theophylline.

FOOD INTERACTIONS
No known food interactions.

DISEASE INTERACTIONS
Caution is advised when taking nicotine. Consult your doctor if you have a history of diabetes, dental problems (with gum), heart or blood vessel disease, inflamed mouth or throat (with gum), skin allergies (with patch), an overactive thyroid, pheochromocytoma, or stomach ulcer.

≣ SIDE EFFECTS ≣

SERIOUS
With gum: Injury to mouth, dental work, or teeth. Call your dentist. With patch: Hives, itching, skin rash, or swelling. Call your doctor immediately.

COMMON
Mild headache, rapid heartbeat, increased appetite, increased salivation (with gum), sore mouth or throat, pain in jaw or neck, tooth problems (with gum and inhaler), belching (with gum), redness, burning, or itching at site of application (with patch), stinging in the nose (nasal spray).

LESS COMMON
Constipation, diarrhea, lightheadedness, dry mouth, hiccups (with gum), coughing (with inhaler), hoarseness (with gum and nasal spray), nervousness, irritability, loss of appetite, menstrual pain, joint or muscle pain, stomach upset, sweating, insomnia, unusual dreams, runny nose (with inhaler).

NIZATIDINE

BRAND NAMES

Axid, Axid AR

Available in: Capsules, tablets
Available as Generic? Yes
Drug Class: Histamine (H2) blocker

▼ USAGE INFORMATION

WHY IT'S TAKEN
To treat and prevent the return of ulcers of the stomach and duodenum, as well as conditions that cause increased stomach acid production (such as Zollinger-Ellison syndrome), gastroesophageal reflux (backwash of stomach acid into the esophagus, resulting in heartburn), andminor episodes of heartburn.

HOW IT WORKS
Nizatidine blocks the action of histamine (a compound produced in the body's cells), which in turn decreases the stomach's secretion of hydrochloric acid. Once stomach acid production has been decreased, the body is better able to heal itself.

▼ DOSAGE GUIDELINES

RANGE AND FREQUENCY
Adults and teenagers—To treat stomach ulcers: 300 mg once a day at bedtime or 150 mg twice a day. To prevent duodenal ulcer recurrence: 150 mg once a day at bedtime. To treat gastroesophageal reflux: 150 mg 2 times a day. To prevent minor cases of heartburn, acid indigestion, and sour stomach: 75 mg taken 30 to 60 minutes before a meal once a day.

ONSET OF EFFECT
Within 30 minutes.

DURATION OF ACTION
Up to 12 hours.

DIETARY ADVICE
If you are taking 2 doses of nizatidine a day, the first dose can be taken after breakfast. Avoid foods that can cause stomach irritation.

STORAGE
Store it in a tightly sealed container away from heat and direct light.

MISSED DOSE
Take it as soon as you remember. If it is near the time for the next dose, skip the missed dose and resume your regular dosage schedule. Do not double the next dose.

STOPPING THE DRUG
Take the prescription-strength form for the full treatment period, even if you begin to feel better before the scheduled end of therapy.

PROLONGED USE
Do not take the maximum daily dosage continually for more than 2 weeks unless directed by your doctor.

▼ PRECAUTIONS

Over 60: Adverse reactions may be more likely and more severe in older patients.

Driving and Hazardous Work: Do not drive or engage in hazardous work until you determine how the medicine affects you.

Alcohol: Avoid alcohol.

Pregnancy: Risks vary depending on patient and dosage. Consult your doctor.

Breast Feeding: Nizatidine passes into breast milk and may pose harm to the child; avoid or discontinue use while nursing.

Infants and Children: Nizatidine is not recommended for young patients, although it has not been shown to cause side effects or problems different from those in adults when used for short periods of time.

Special Concerns: Avoid cigarette smoking because it may increase stomach acid secretion and thus worsen the disease. Do not take nizatidine if you have ever had an allergic reaction to a histamine H2 blocker. If your stomach pain becomes worse while using the drug, be sure to tell your doctor immediately.

OVERDOSE
Symptoms: No cases of overdose have been reported.

What to Do: Although an overdose is unlikely, if someone takes a much larger dose than prescribed, call your doctor, emergency medical services (EMS), or the nearest poison control center immediately.

▼ INTERACTIONS

DRUG INTERACTIONS
No significant drug interactions have been identified. However, nizatidine may increase blood levels of aspirin. Consult your doctor for specific advice if you are taking aspirin.

FOOD INTERACTIONS
Tomato-based mixed vegetable juices, carbonated drinks, citrus fruits and juices, beverages containing caffeine, and other acidic foods or liquids may irritate the stomach or interfere with the therapeutic action of nizatidine.

DISEASE INTERACTIONS
Patients with kidney disease should not use nizatidine or should use it in smaller, limited doses under careful supervision by a physician.

≡ SIDE EFFECTS ≡

SERIOUS
Irregular heart rhythm (palpitations), slowed heartbeat, severe blood problems, resulting in unusual bleeding, bruising, fever, chills, and increased susceptibility to infection. Call your doctor immediately.

COMMON
Headache, fatigue, drowsiness, dizziness, nausea, vomiting, abdominal pain, diarrhea, constipation.

LESS COMMON
Blurred vision, decreased sexual desire or function, swelling of breasts in males and females, temporary hair loss, hallucinations, depression, insomnia, skin rash, hives, or redness.

OMEPRAZOLE

BRAND NAME

Prilosec

Available in: Capsules
As Generic? Yes
Drug Class: Antacid/proton pump inhibitor

▼ USAGE INFORMATION

WHY IT'S TAKEN
To treat duodenal (intestinal) ulcers, as well as conditions that cause increased stomach acid production (such as Zollinger-Ellison syndrome), erosive esophagitis (severe, chronic inflammation of the esophagus), and gastro-esophageal reflux (backwash of stomach acid into the esophagus, resulting in heartburn).

HOW IT WORKS
Omeprazole blocks the action of a specific enzyme in the cells that line the stomach, thereby decreasing the production of stomach acid. Reduction of stomach acid promotes healing of ulcers.

▼ DOSAGE GUIDELINES

RANGE AND FREQUENCY
For duodenal ulcer, esophagitis, or gastroesophageal reflux: 20 mg a day. For Zollinger-Ellison syndrome or similar conditions: 60 mg a day.

ONSET OF EFFECT
Within 1 to 3 hours.

DURATION OF ACTION
At least 72 hours.

DIETARY ADVICE
Take omeprazole immediately before a meal. Capsules should be swallowed whole.

STORAGE
Store it in a tightly sealed container away from heat and direct light.

MISSED DOSE
Take it as soon as you remember. If it is near the time for the next dose, skip the missed dose and resume your regular dosage schedule. Do not double the next dose.

STOPPING THE DRUG
Take it as prescribed for the full treatment period, even if you begin to feel better before the scheduled end of therapy. The decision to stop taking the drug should be made in consultation with your doctor.

PROLONGED USE
Omeprazole should not be used indefinitely as mainte-nance therapy for duodenal ulcer or esophagitis; it is generally taken for a limited period of 4 to 8 weeks. Do not take it for a longer period unless instructed to do so by your doctor. See your doctor regularly for tests and exami-nations if you must take this drug for an extended period of time.

▼ PRECAUTIONS

Over 60: No specific prob-lems for older people have been reported.

Driving and Hazardous Work: Do not drive or engage in hazardous activities until you determine how the drug affects you.

Alcohol: Avoid alcohol while taking this medication, because it may aggravate your condition.

Pregnancy: In animal tests, omeprazole has not caused problems. Human tests have not been done. Before you take omeprazole, tell your doctor if you are pregnant or plan to become pregnant.

Breast Feeding: Omeprazole may pass into breast milk; caution is advised. Consult your doctor for advice.

Infants and Children: Use and dose for anyone younger than 18 years of age should be determined by your doctor or pediatrician.

Special Concerns: Tell any doctor or dentist you see for

treatment that you are taking omeprazole. Do not chew the capsules. If you have trouble swallowing them, you may open them and sprinkle the contents on applesauce or similar food. If your doctor directs, you may take an antacid along with omeprazole.

OVERDOSE
Symptoms: Blurred vision, confusion, profuse sweating, drowsiness, dry mouth, flush-ing of the face, headache, nausea, palpitations or an unusually rapid heartbeat.

What to Do: Call your doctor, emergency medical services (EMS), or the nearest poison control center immediately.

▼ INTERACTIONS

DRUG INTERACTIONS
The following drugs may interact with omeprazole. Consult your doctor for specific advice if you are taking: ampicillin, sucralfate, iron salts or supplements, cyclosporine, diazepam, disulfiram, ketoconazole, phenytoin, or theophylline.

FOOD INTERACTIONS
No significant food interac-tions have been reported.

DISEASE INTERACTIONS
Caution is advised when tak-ing omeprazole. Consult your doctor if you have liver dis-ease, because it may increase the risk of side effects.

≡ SIDE EFFECTS ≡

SERIOUS
No serious side effects are associated with this medication.

COMMON
Diarrhea, constipation, vomiting, headache, dizziness, stomach pain. Consult your physician if such side effects persist or interfere with daily activities.

LESS COMMON
Bloody or cloudy urine, persistent or recurring sores or ulcers in the mouth, painful or very frequent urination, sore throat, fever, unusual bruising or bleeding, unusual weakness or tiredness, muscle pain, chest pain, nausea. Consult your doctor if such symptoms occur.

OXYMETAZOLINE NASAL

Available in: Nasal drops, nasal spray
Available as Generic? Yes
Drug Class: Decongestant

▼ USAGE INFORMATION

WHY IT'S TAKEN
To relieve nasal congestion caused by allergies, colds, or sinus conditions.

HOW IT WORKS
Oxymetazoline constricts blood vessels to reduce the blood flow to swollen nasal passages and other upper-airway tissues, which reduces nasal secretions and improves nasal airflow.

▼ DOSAGE GUIDELINES

RANGE AND FREQUENCY
Adults and children 6 years of age and older: 2 or 3 drops or sprays of 0.05% solution in each nostril 2 times a day, in the morning and evening. Children ages 2 to 6 years: 2 or 3 drops of 0.025% solution in each nostril 2 times a day, in the morning and evening.

ONSET OF EFFECT
Rapid.

DURATION OF ACTION
Unknown.

DIETARY ADVICE
Drink plenty of fluids.

STORAGE
Store it in a tightly sealed container away from heat and direct light.

MISSED DOSE
Take it as soon as you remember. If it is near the time for the next dose, skip the missed dose and resume your regular dosage schedule. Do not double the next dose.

STOPPING THE DRUG
Do not use this medicine for more than 3 days without consulting your doctor.

PROLONGED USE
Using this medicine for more than 3 days may lead to rebound congestion (more severe congestion caused by the body's adaptation to the drug) when you stop.

▼ PRECAUTIONS

Over 60: Although no studies have specifically examined the use of this drug in older patients, no special problems are expected.

Driving and Hazardous Work: Do not drive or engage in hazardous work until you determine how the medicine affects you.

Alcohol: Avoid alcohol.

Pregnancy: Oxymetazoline has not been shown to cause birth defects or any other problems when taken during pregnancy.

Breast Feeding: It is not known whether oxymetazoline passes into breast milk; caution is advised. Consult your doctor for advice.

Infants and Children: This drug is not recommended for children under the age of 2 years.

Special Concerns: Each container of medicine should be used by only one person to avoid spread of infection. Blow your nose gently before using this medicine. To use the nose drops, tilt your head back or lie down on a bed and hang your head over the side. Keep your head tilted back for a few minutes after instilling the drops. To use the nasal spray, keep your head upright and sniff briskly while spraying. For best results, spray again in 3 to 5 minutes.

OVERDOSE
Symptoms: Rapid, irregular, or pounding heartbeat; headache or dizziness; increased sweating; nervousness; trembling; paleness; insomnia. Such symptoms are more likely to be seen in young children.

What to Do: If someone takes a much larger dose than recommended, call your doctor, emergency medical services (EMS), or the nearest poison control center immediately.

▼ INTERACTIONS

DRUG INTERACTIONS
Before you take oxymetazoline, tell your doctor if you are taking maprotiline or tricyclic antidepressants.

FOOD INTERACTIONS
No known food interactions.

DISEASE INTERACTIONS
Consult your doctor if you have a history of any of the following: high blood pressure, diabetes mellitus, heart disease, blood vessel disease, or an overactive thyroid gland.

SIDE EFFECTS

SERIOUS
No serious side effects have been reported.

COMMON
Burning, dryness, or stinging inside the nose. An increase in nasal discharge or congestion may occur after 3 to 5 days of continuous use.

LESS COMMON
Headache, rapid or irregular heartbeat, unusual excitability, restlessness.

OXYMETAZOLINE OPHTHALMIC

Available in: Ophthalmic solution
Available as Generic? No
Drug Class: Ophthalmic decongestant

▼ USAGE INFORMATION

WHY IT'S TAKEN
To reduce redness of the eye caused by minor irritation.

HOW IT WORKS
Ophthalmic oxymetazoline reduces redness by constricting the superficial blood vessels in the whites (sclera) of the eye.

▼ DOSAGE GUIDELINES

RANGE AND FREQUENCY
Adults and children age 6 years and older: 1 drop in the affected eye every 6 hours as needed.

ONSET OF EFFECT
Rapid, within 5 minutes.

DURATION OF ACTION
About 6 hours.

DIETARY ADVICE
No special restrictions.

STORAGE
Store it in a tightly sealed container away from moisture, heat, and direct light. Do not allow the medicine to freeze.

MISSED DOSE
Apply it as soon as you remember. However, if it is near the time for the next dose, skip the missed dose and resume your regular dosage schedule. Do not double the next dose.

STOPPING THE DRUG
Do not use this medicine for more than 3 days without consulting your doctor.

PROLONGED USE
Consult your doctor if you intend to use this medicine for more than 3 days.

▼ PRECAUTIONS

Over 60: Although no studies have specifically examined the use of this drug in older patients, no special problems are expected.

Driving and Hazardous Work: Do not drive or engage in hazardous work until you determine how the medicine affects you.

Alcohol: No special warnings.

Pregnancy: No problems are expected, but studies of effects in pregnancy have not been done in humans. Consult your physician.

Breast Feeding: No problems are expected, but studies of effects in breast feeding have not been done in humans. Consult your doctor.

Infants and Children: Dosage for children under the age of 6 years should be determined by a pediatrician.

Special Concerns: To use the eye drops, first wash your hands. Tilt your head back. Gently apply pressure to the inside corner of the eyelid and with the index finger of the same hand, pull downward on the lower eyelid to make a space. Drop the medicine into this space and close your eye. Apply pressure for 1 or 2 minutes while keeping the eye closed without blinking. Then wash your hands again. To avoid contamination, be sure the tip of the dropper does not touch your eye, finger, or any other surface.

OVERDOSE
Symptoms: Dizziness; headache; rapid, irregular, or pounding heartbeat; trembling; insomnia.

What to Do: Call your doctor, emergency medical services (EMS), or the nearest poison control center immediately.

▼ INTERACTIONS

DRUG INTERACTIONS
Before you take oxymetazoline, tell your doctor if you are taking maprotiline or tricyclic antidepressants.

FOOD INTERACTIONS
No known food interactions.

DISEASE INTERACTIONS
Caution is advised when taking oxymetazoline. Consult your doctor if you have a history of any of the following: high blood pressure; eye disease, infection, or injury; narrow-angle glaucoma; heart disease; blood vessel disease; or an overactive thyroid gland.

 SIDE EFFECTS

SERIOUS
No serious side effects have been reported.

COMMON
No common side effects have been reported.

LESS COMMON
Headache, rapid or irregular heartbeat, excitability, restlessness, increase in redness of the eye.

PERMETHRIN

Available in: Lotion
Available as Generic? Yes
Drug Class: Topical antiparasitic

▼ USAGE INFORMATION

WHY IT'S TAKEN
To treat head lice infestations.

HOW IT WORKS
Permethrin is absorbed into the bodies of lice, where it blocks nerve activity, ultimately causing paralysis and death of the lice. (The drug does not have this toxic effect on humans.)

▼ DOSAGE GUIDELINES

RANGE AND FREQUENCY
For treatment of head lice (*Pediculus humanus capitis*): After the hair has been washed with shampoo, rinsed with water, and dried with a towel, apply a sufficient amount (approximately 5 tsp) of liquid. Allow it to remain on the hair for 10 minutes, then rinse off with water. Rinse thoroughly and dry with a clean towel. Use a fine-toothed comb to remove any remaining nits or nit shells. If lice are found after 7 days, repeat the treatment.

ONSET OF EFFECT
Within 10 minutes.

DURATION OF ACTION
Up to 10 days.

DIETARY ADVICE
Permethrin can be used without regard to diet.

STORAGE
Store it in a tightly sealed container away from heat and direct light.

MISSED DOSE
If a second dose is needed and you do not apply it after 7 days, do so as soon as you remember.

STOPPING THE DRUG
You do not need to apply the second dose if no lice are found after 7 days.

PROLONGED USE
If lice recur, consult your doctor.

▼ PRECAUTIONS

Over 60: No special problems are expected.

Driving and Hazardous Work: The use of permethrin should not impair your ability to perform such tasks safely.

Alcohol: No special warnings.

Pregnancy: In animal studies, permethrin has not caused problems or birth defects. Human studies have not been done. Before you use permethrin, tell your doctor if you are pregnant or plan to become pregnant.

Breast Feeding: Permethrin may pass into breast milk; caution is advised. Consult your doctor for advice.

Infants and Children: Use and dosage for children up to 2 years of age must be determined by your doctor.

Special Concerns: All members of your household should be examined for lice and given treatment if necessary. Any sexual partner should be examined and treated if necessary. Clothing, household linen, hairbrushes, combs, and bedding should be thoroughly cleaned by machine washing with hot water and machine drying for at least 20 minutes on the hottest setting. Seal nonwashable items in a plastic bag for at least 2 weeks or spray them with a product designed to eliminate lice and their nits. You should not use this drug if you are hypersensitive to chrysanthemums. Treatment with permethrin may temporarily worsen the itching and other symptoms of head lice infestation.

OVERDOSE
Symptoms: No cases of overdose have been reported.

What to Do: Overdose is unlikely, but if someone accidentally ingests the drug, call your doctor, emergency medical services (EMS), or the nearest poison control center immediately.

▼ INTERACTIONS

DRUG INTERACTIONS
Before you use this medicine, tell your doctor if you are using any other prescription or over-the-counter medication that is to be applied to the scalp.

FOOD INTERACTIONS
No known food interactions.

DISEASE INTERACTIONS
Consult your doctor if you have severe inflammation of the skin.

 ## SIDE EFFECTS

SERIOUS
No serious side effects have been reported.

COMMON
Burning, itching, numbness, rash, redness, stinging, swelling, or tingling of scalp. In most cases, such symptoms are mild and temporary; notify your doctor if they are more troublesome or if they persist.

LESS COMMON
No less common side effects have been reported.

PHENAZOPYRIDINE HYDROCHLORIDE

Available in: Tablets
Available as Generic? Yes
Drug Class: Urinary analgesic

▼ USAGE INFORMATION

WHY IT'S TAKEN
For short-term relief of symptoms caused by irritation of the urinary tract. Such symptoms include burning, pain, and discomfort during urination, as well as an increased urge to urinate with only small amounts of urine passed on each occasion. Irritation of the urinary tract commonly occurs as a result of bladder infection; phenazopyridine can ease symptoms but will not cure such an infection.

HOW IT WORKS
Phenazopyridine passes through—and has a local anesthetic effect on the lining of—the urinary tract, thus relieving the discomfort associated with urinary infection or inflammation.

▼ DOSAGE GUIDELINES

RANGE AND FREQUENCY
Adults: 200 mg 3 times a day. Children: 1.8 mg per lb of body weight 3 times a day.

ONSET OF EFFECT
Unknown.

DURATION OF ACTION
Unknown.

DIETARY ADVICE
This medication is best taken with or after meals to minimize stomach upset.

STORAGE
Store in a tightly sealed container away from moisture, heat, and direct light.

MISSED DOSE
Take it as soon as you remember. If it is near the time for the next dose, skip the missed dose and resume your regular dosage schedule. Do not double the next dose.

STOPPING THE DRUG
The decision to stop taking the drug should be made by your doctor. If it is being taken with an antibiotic, it should be taken for only 2 days (6 doses).

PROLONGED USE
Phenazopyridine is intended only for short-term use.

▼ PRECAUTIONS

Over 60: No special problems are expected.

Driving and Hazardous Work: Do not drive or engage in hazardous work until you determine how the medicine affects you.

Alcohol: No special precautions are necessary.

Pregnancy: Adequate human studies have not been done. Before taking phenazopyridine, tell your doctor if you are pregnant or plan to become pregnant.

Breast Feeding: Phenazopyridine may pass into breast milk; caution is advised. Consult your doctor for advice.

Infants and Children: No special problems are expected.

Special Concerns: Phenazopyridine causes the urine to turn reddish orange. This is harmless, but it may stain clothing. The drug may also cause permanent staining or discoloration of soft contact lenses; it is best to wear glasses while taking the drug. For diabetic patients, phenazopyridine may cause false-positive test results with sugar and urine ketone tests. Do not chew the tablets; chewing may cause permanent discoloration of teeth. Do not use any leftover medicine for future urinary tract infections without consulting your doctor.

OVERDOSE
Symptoms: Fatigue, paleness, shortness of breath, heart palpitations, bloody or cloudy urine, decreased urine output, swelling of the ankles and calves, lower back or flank pain, nausea or vomiting.

What to Do: An overdose is unlikely, but call your doctor, emergency medical services (EMS), or the nearest poison control center immediately if any symptoms of overdose occur.

▼ INTERACTIONS

DRUG INTERACTIONS
Some drugs may interact with phenazopyridine. Consult your doctor for specific advice if you are taking any prescription or over-the-counter medication.

FOOD INTERACTIONS
No known food interactions.

DISEASE INTERACTIONS
Caution is advised when taking phenazopyridine. Consult your doctor if you have any of the following: hepatitis, glucose-6-phosphate dehydrogenase deficiency (G6PD) uremia, pyelonephritis (kidney infection) during pregnancy, or other kidney disease.

≡ SIDE EFFECTS ≡

SERIOUS
Serious side effects are rare. Call your doctor immediately if you experience any of the following: difficulty breathing; swelling of the face, fingers, feet, or lower legs; blue or purple-blue skin color; unusual fatigue; fever; confusion; sudden decrease in urine output; shortness of breath; tightness in the chest; skin rash; yellow discoloration of the eyes or skin; or unusual weight gain.

COMMON
Reddish orange urine.

LESS COMMON
Indigestion, dizziness, stomach cramps or pain, headache.

PHENYLEPHRINE HYDROCHLORIDE OPHTHALMIC

Available in: Ophthalmic solution
Available as Generic? Yes
Drug Class: Adrenergic agent

▼ USAGE INFORMATION

WHY IT'S TAKEN
The 2.5% and 10% solutions are used to dilate the pupil of the eye (prior to eye examinations or ophthalmologic procedures) and to treat certain eye conditions. The 0.12% solution is recommended to reduce redness of the eye that is caused by minor irritation.

HOW IT WORKS
Ophthalmic phenylephrine affects the muscles that control the pupils, causing them to dilate, which helps the doctor view the interior structures of the eye. The drug reduces redness by constricting the superficial blood vessels in the whites of the eye.

▼ DOSAGE GUIDELINES

RANGE AND FREQUENCY
For redness—Adults and children: 1 drop of 0.12% solution every 3 or 4 hours as needed.

ONSET OF EFFECT
Rapid.

DURATION OF ACTION
From 2 to 7 hours depending on the strength of the solution used.

DIETARY ADVICE
No special precautions.

STORAGE
Store it in a tightly sealed container away from moisture, heat, and direct light. Do not allow it to freeze.

MISSED DOSE
Apply it as soon as you remember. If it is near the time for the next dose, skip the missed dose and resume your regular dosage schedule. Do not double the next dose.

STOPPING THE DRUG
The decision to stop using the drug should be made by your doctor.

PROLONGED USE
You should see your doctor regularly if you must use this drug for an extended period of time.

▼ PRECAUTIONS

Over 60: No special advice.

Driving and Hazardous Work: Do not drive or engage in hazardous work until you determine how the medicine affects your vision.

Alcohol: No special precautions are necessary.

Pregnancy: No problems are expected, but studies of effects in pregnancy have not been done in humans. Consult your physician.

Breast Feeding: No problems are expected, but studies of effects in breast feeding have not been done in humans. Consult your doctor.

Infants and Children: Adverse reactions may be more likely and more severe in infants and children. The 10% solution should not be used on infants. The other strengths should not be used on low-birth-weight infants.

Special Concerns: To use the eye drops, first wash your hands. Tilt your head back. Gently apply pressure to the inside corner of the eyelid and with the index finger of the same hand, pull downward on the lower eyelid to make a space. Drop the medicine into this space and close your eye. Apply pressure for 1 or 2 minutes while keeping the eye closed without blinking. Then wash your hands again. Make sure the tip of the dropper does not touch your eye, finger, or any other surface. Phenylephrine will make your eyes more sensitive to sunlight. If this occurs, wear sunglasses or avoid bright light as comfort dictates. If this effect continues for more than 12 hours after you have stopped the medicine, consult your doctor.

OVERDOSE
Symptoms: Dizziness; paleness; rapid, irregular, or pounding heartbeat; trembling; profuse sweating; vomiting; coma; shock.

What to Do: Call your doctor, emergency medical services (EMS), or the nearest poison control center immediately.

▼ INTERACTIONS

DRUG INTERACTIONS
Be sure to tell your doctor if you are using any other prescription or OTC medication.

FOOD INTERACTIONS
No known food interactions.

DISEASE INTERACTIONS
Consult your doctor if you have a history of heart disease, blood vessel disease, diabetes mellitus, high blood pressure, or idiopathic orthostatic hypotension (low blood pressure). This drug should not be used by those with a history of closed-angle glaucoma.

≡ SIDE EFFECTS ≡

SERIOUS
Dizziness; paleness; rapid, irregular, or pounding heartbeat; trembling; increased sweating. Call your doctor immediately.

COMMON
Unusually large pupils; burning, stinging, or watering of eyes; sensitivity of eyes to light; headache or brow ache.

LESS COMMON
Eye irritation not present prior to therapy.

PHENYLEPHRINE HYDROCHLORIDE SYSTEMIC

Available in: Nasal jelly, nasal drops, nasal spray
Available as Generic? Yes
Drug Class: Decongestant

▼ USAGE INFORMATION

WHY IT'S TAKEN
To relieve nasal congestion caused by allergies, colds, or sinus conditions and to relieve congestion associated with ear infections.

HOW IT WORKS
Phenylephrine constricts blood vessels to reduce blood flow to swollen nasal passages, which reduces nasal secretions and improves airflow.

▼ DOSAGE GUIDELINES

RANGE AND FREQUENCY
Adults and children 12 years and older: 2 to 3 drops of 0.25% to 0.5% solution 1 to 2 sprays, or a small amount of jelly in each nostril every 4 hours. Children 6 to 12 years of age: 2 to 3 drops or 1 to 2 sprays of a 0.25% solution in each nostril every 4 hours. Children under 6 years of age: 2 to 3 drops of 0.125% solution every 4 hours.

ONSET OF EFFECT
Rapid.

DURATION OF ACTION
From 30 minutes to 4 hours.

DIETARY ADVICE
Drink plenty of fluids.

STORAGE
Store it in a tightly sealed container away from heat and direct light.

MISSED DOSE
Take it as soon as you remember. If it is near the time for the next dose, skip the missed dose and resume your regular dosage schedule. Do not double the next dose.

STOPPING THE DRUG
Do not take this medicine for more than 3 days without consulting your doctor about its use.

PROLONGED USE
Using this medicine for more than 3 days may lead to rebound congestion (more severe congestion caused by the body's adaptation to the drug).

▼ PRECAUTIONS

Over 60: Although no studies have specifically examined the use of this drug in older patients, no special problems are expected.

Driving and Hazardous Work: Do not drive or engage in hazardous work until you determine how the medicine affects you.

Alcohol: Avoid alcohol.

Pregnancy: Phenylephrine hydrochloride has not been shown to cause birth defects or other problems if taken during pregnancy.

Breast Feeding: It is not known whether phenylephrine passes into breast milk; caution is advised. Consult your doctor for advice.

Infants and Children: Adverse reactions may be more likely and more severe in infants and children.

Special Concerns: Each container of medicine should be used by only one person to avoid spread of infection. Blow your nose gently before using this medicine. To use the nose drops, tilt your head back or lie down on a bed and hang your head over the side. Keep your head tilted back for a few minutes after instilling the drops. To use the nasal spray, keep your head upright and sniff briskly while spraying. For best results, spray again in 3 to 5 minutes. To use the nasal jelly, first wash your hands, then place an amount of jelly about the size of a pea into each nostril and sniff it well back into the nose.

OVERDOSE
Symptoms: Rapid, irregular, or pounding heartbeat; headache or dizziness; increased sweating; nervousness; trembling; paleness; insomnia.

Such symptoms are more likely to be seen in young children.

What to Do: If someone takes a much larger dose than recommended, call your doctor, emergency medical services (EMS), or the nearest poison control center immediately.

▼ INTERACTIONS

DRUG INTERACTIONS
Before you take phenylephrine, tell your doctor if you are taking any other prescription or OTC drug.

FOOD INTERACTIONS
No known food interactions.

DISEASE INTERACTIONS
Consult your doctor if you have a history of any of the following: high blood pressure, diabetes mellitus, heart disease, blood vessel (vascular) disease, or an overactive thyroid gland.

 SIDE EFFECTS

SERIOUS
No serious side effects have been reported.

COMMON
Burning, dryness, or stinging inside the nose. An increase in nasal discharge or congestion may occur after 3 to 5 days of continuous use.

LESS COMMON
Headache, rapid or irregular heartbeat, excitability, restlessness.

PSEUDOEPHEDRINE

Available in: Extended-release capsules, oral solution, syrup, tablets
Available as Generic? Yes
Drug Class: Decongestant/cough drug

▼ USAGE INFORMATION

WHY IT'S TAKEN
To relieve nasal or sinus congestion caused by colds, sinus infection, hay fever, or other respiratory allergies.

HOW IT WORKS
Pseudoephedrine narrows and constricts blood vessels to reduce the blood flow to swollen nasal passages and other tissues, which reduces nasal secretions, shrinks swollen nasal mucous membranes, and improves airflow in nasal passages.

▼ DOSAGE GUIDELINES

RANGE AND FREQUENCY
Short-acting forms—Adults and teenagers: 60 mg every 4 to 6 hours; not more than 240 mg in 24 hours. Children 6 to 12 years of age: 30 mg every 4 to 6 hours; not more than 120 mg in 24 hours. Children 2 to 6 years of age: 15 mg every 4 hours; not more than 60 mg in 24 hours. Extended-release form—Adults and teenagers: 120 mg every 12 hours or 240 mg every 24 hours.

ONSET OF EFFECT
15 to 30 minutes.

DURATION OF ACTION
3 to 4 hours for short-acting forms, 8 to 12 hours for extended-release form.

DIETARY ADVICE
Drink plenty of fluids.

STORAGE
Store it in a tightly sealed container away from heat and direct light. Do not allow the liquid form to freeze.

MISSED DOSE
Take it as soon as you remember. If it is near the time for the next dose, skip the missed dose and resume your regular dosage schedule. Do not double the next dose.

STOPPING THE DRUG
Do not take this drug longer than recommended on the label unless directed to do so by your doctor.

PROLONGED USE
Consult your doctor about taking pseudoephedrine for more than 5 to 7 days.

▼ PRECAUTIONS

Over 60: Side effects may be more likely and more severe in older patients.

Driving and Hazardous Work: Avoid such activities until you determine how the medicine affects you.

Alcohol: No special precautions are necessary.

Pregnancy: Safety has not been established; it should be used only if clearly necessary. Consult your doctor for specific advice.

Breast Feeding: Pseudoephedrine passes into breast milk; avoid or discontinue use while nursing.

Infants and Children: Use of extended-release forms of pseudoephedrine is not recommended for children under the age of 12 years.

Special Concerns: If your symptoms do not improve within 7 days, check with your doctor. To help prevent insomnia, take the last dose of the day at least 2 hours before bedtime.

OVERDOSE

Symptoms: Drowsiness, sedation, profuse sweating, pale or clammy skin, low blood pressure, diminished urine output, dizziness, changes in mental state, hallucinations, seizures, loss of consciousness.

What to Do: In some cases, an overdose can be fatal, especially among older patients. At the first sign of overdose, call your doctor, emergency medical services (EMS), or the nearest poison control center immediately.

▼ INTERACTIONS

DRUG INTERACTIONS
Consult your doctor for specific advice before using pseudoephedrine if you are taking beta-blockers or monoamine oxidase (MAO) inhibitors.

FOOD INTERACTIONS
No known food interactions.

DISEASE INTERACTIONS
Caution is advised when taking pseudoephedrine. Consult your doctor if you have any of the following: diabetes, enlarged prostate, heart disease, blood vessel disease, high blood pressure, or an overactive thyroid gland.

SIDE EFFECTS

SERIOUS
Seizures, irregular or slowed heartbeat, shortness of breath, breathing difficulty, hallucinations. Stop taking the medication and call your doctor immediately.

COMMON
Nervousness, restlessness, insomnia.

LESS COMMON
Difficult or painful urination, dizziness or lightheadedness, rapid or pounding heartbeat, increased sweating, nausea or vomiting, trembling, trouble breathing, paleness, weakness.

PSEUDOEPHEDRINE/GUAIFENESIN

Available in: Capsules, oral solution, syrup, tablets, extended-release forms
Available as Generic? No
Drug Class: Decongestant/cough drug

▼ USAGE INFORMATION

WHY IT'S TAKEN
To relieve nasal or sinus congestion caused by colds, influenza (flu), hay fever, and other respiratory allergies. Also intended to break up congestion in the lungs to promote better breathing.

HOW IT WORKS
Pseudoephedrine narrows and constricts blood vessels to reduce the blood flow to swollen nasal passages and other tissues, which reduces nasal secretions, shrinks swollen nasal mucous membranes, and improves airflow. Guaifenesin purportedly breaks up, liquefies, and loosens mucus secretions in the respiratory tract, making it easier to cough up phlegm and thus breathe easier. (There is some debate, however, as to whether the medication is actually effective in this regard.)

▼ DOSAGE GUIDELINES

RANGE AND FREQUENCY
Take the drug as directed to relieve symptoms.

ONSET OF EFFECT
Within 1 hour.

DURATION OF ACTION
Unknown.

DIETARY ADVICE
No special restrictions.

STORAGE
Store in a tightly sealed container away from heat and direct light.

MISSED DOSE
Take it as soon as you remember. If it is near the time for the next dose, skip the missed dose and resume your regular dosage schedule. Do not double the next dose.

STOPPING THE DRUG
The decision to stop taking the drug should be made by your doctor or when you note improvement.

PROLONGED USE
Check with your doctor if symptoms do not improve within 5 days.

▼ PRECAUTIONS

Over 60: Adverse reactions may be more likely and more severe in older patients.

Driving and Hazardous Work: Do not drive or engage in hazardous work until you determine how the medicine affects you.

Alcohol: Avoid alcohol.

Pregnancy: Before taking pseudoephedrine and guaifenesin, tell your doctor if you are pregnant or plan to become pregnant.

Breast Feeding: Pseudoephedrine passes into breast milk; avoid or discontinue use while nursing.

Infants and Children: Check the package label or with your doctor before giving it to infants or children.

Special Concerns: If you have trouble sleeping, take the last dose of pseudoephedrine and guaifenesin a few hours before bedtime. Before having any surgery, tell your doctor or dentist that you are taking this drug. Be sure your doctor knows if you have high blood pressure.

OVERDOSE
Symptoms: Rapid, pounding, or irregular heartbeat; contin-

uing and severe headache; severe nausea or vomiting; severe nervousness or restlessness; severe shortness of breath or troubled breathing.

What to Do: Call your doctor, emergency medical services (EMS), or the nearest poison control center immediately.

▼ INTERACTIONS

DRUG INTERACTIONS
Consult your doctor if you are taking any prescription or nonprescription medication. Do not take any drug for diet or appetite control unless you have checked with your doctor first.

FOOD INTERACTIONS
No known food interactions.

DISEASE INTERACTIONS
Caution is advised when taking pseudoephedrine and guaifenesin. Consult your doctor if you have any of the following: anemia, gout, hemophilia, stomach problems, brain disease, colitis, seizures, diarrhea, gallbladder disease or gallstones, cystic fibrosis, diabetes mellitus, any chronic lung disease, enlarged prostate, difficulty urinating, glaucoma, heart or blood vessel disease, thyroid disease, or high blood pressure. Use of pseudoephedrine and guaifenesin may cause complications in persons with liver or kidney disease, because these organs work together to remove the medication from the body.

≡ SIDE EFFECTS ≡

SERIOUS
Skin rash, hives, itching, rapid or irregular heartbeat, persistent headache, nervousness or restlessness, shortness of breath or breathing difficulty, seizures, unusual fear and anxiety. Call your doctor or emergency medical services (EMS) immediately.

COMMON
Constipation; decreased sweating; difficulty urinating; dizziness or lightheadedness; drowsiness; dry mouth, nose, or throat; increased sensitivity of skin to sun; thickened mucus; nausea or vomiting; nightmares; stomach pain; insomnia; unusual excitement or restlessness; unusual tiredness or weakness. Contact your doctor if these symptoms persist or interfere with your daily activities.

LESS COMMON
There are no less common side effects associated with the use of this drug.

PYRANTEL PAMOATE

Available in: Oral suspension
Available as Generic? Yes
Drug Class: Anthelmintic

▼ USAGE INFORMATION

WHY IT'S TAKEN
To treat various worm infections, including ascariasis (common roundworm) and enterobiasis or oxyuriasis (pinworm). It may be used to treat more than one worm infection at a time. It may also be used for other types of infection as determined by your doctor.

HOW IT WORKS
Pyrantel paralyzes the worm. While it is paralyzed, the worm is expelled from the body in the stool.

▼ DOSAGE GUIDELINES

RANGE AND FREQUENCY
Adults and children age 2 years and older—For roundworms: 1 dose of 11 mg per 2.2 lb (1 kg) of body weight. Maximum dose is 1,000 mg. If necessary, the dose may be repeated in 2 to 3 weeks. For pinworms: 1 dose of 11 mg per 2.2 lb of body weight. Maximum dose is 1,000 mg. Repeat the dose in 2 to 3 weeks.

ONSET OF EFFECT
Variable.

DURATION OF ACTION
Variable.

DIETARY ADVICE
Pyrantel can be taken with fruit juice, milk, or food.

STORAGE
Store it in a tightly sealed container away from moisture, heat, and direct light. Do not allow it to freeze.

MISSED DOSE
Take a missed dose as soon as you remember.

STOPPING THE DRUG
The decision to stop taking the drug should be made in consultation with your doctor.

PROLONGED USE
Pyrantel is generally recommended for one-time use (two-time use for pinworms).

▼ PRECAUTIONS

Over 60: Adverse reactions may be more likely and more severe in older patients.

Driving and Hazardous Work: Do not drive or engage in hazardous work until you determine how the medicine affects you.

Alcohol: No special precautions are necessary.

Pregnancy: Pyrantel is not recommended for use by pregnant women. Consult your doctor for specific advice if you are pregnant or plan to become pregnant.

Breast Feeding: Pyrantel may pass into breast milk; caution is advised. Consult your doctor for advice.

Infants and Children: Use and dosage for children under the age of 2 years should be determined by your doctor. Not recommended for use by children under the age of 1 year.

Special Concerns: To prevent reinfection, wash clothing, bedding, and towels every day. All members of the family may have to be treated to eradicate the infestation. A second treatment for all household members may be necessary after 2 or 3 weeks. All bedding and nightclothes should be washed again after treatment. To prevent reinfection, you should wash your anal region daily, change your underwear and bedding every day, and wash your hands and fingernails before each meal and after bowel movements. Consult your doctor if your condition has not improved on completion of therapy.

OVERDOSE
Symptoms: An overdose of pyrantel is unlikely.

What to Do: If someone takes a much larger dose than directed, call your doctor, emergency medical services (EMS), or the nearest poison control center right away.

▼ INTERACTIONS

DRUG INTERACTIONS
Do not take piperazine when taking pyrantel. The effectiveness of both drugs may be reduced. Consult your doctor for specific advice. Also tell your doctor if you are taking any other prescription or OTC medication.

FOOD INTERACTIONS
No known food interactions.

DISEASE INTERACTIONS
Caution is advised when taking pyrantel. Consult your doctor for specific advice if you have any other medical condition.

≡ SIDE EFFECTS ≡

SERIOUS
Skin rash. Stop using the drug and call your doctor as soon as possible.

COMMON
No common side effects are associated with the use of pyrantel.

LESS COMMON
Pain or cramps in abdomen or stomach, headache, dizziness, diarrhea, drowsiness, insomnia, nausea or vomiting, loss of appetite.

PYRETHRINS/PIPERONYL BUTOXIDE

Available in: Gel, solution shampoo, topical solution
Available as Generic? Yes
Drug Class: Topical antiparasitic

▼ USAGE INFORMATION

WHY IT'S TAKEN
To treat head, body, and pubic lice infestations. Although this drug is available without a prescription, your doctor may have special instructions regarding its proper use.

HOW IT WORKS
Pyrethrins and piperonyl butoxide are a combination of active ingredients. The medication is absorbed into the bodies of lice, where it blocks nerve activity, ultimately causing paralysis and death of the lice. (The drug has no such toxic effect on humans.)

▼ DOSAGE GUIDELINES

RANGE AND FREQUENCY
Use 1 time, then repeat 1 more time in 7 to 10 days. Gel or solution: Apply enough medicine to thoroughly wet hair, scalp, or skin. Allow the medicine to remain on the affected areas for 10 minutes, then wash with warm water and soap or regular shampoo. Rinse thor-oughly and dry with a clean towel. Shampoo: Apply enough medicine to wet the hair, scalp, or skin. Allow the medicine to remain on the affected areas for 10 minutes, then use a small amount of water to work shampoo more thoroughly into affected area. Rinse and dry with a clean towel. With either method, use a nit removal comb to remove dead lice and eggs from hair.

ONSET OF EFFECT
Within 10 minutes.

DURATION OF ACTION
Up to 10 days.

DIETARY ADVICE
This medication can be used without regard to diet.

STORAGE
Store it in a tightly sealed container away from heat, direct light, and children.

MISSED DOSE
If you do not apply the second dose within 10 days after the initial dose, do so as soon as you remember.

STOPPING THE DRUG
Apply both recommended doses, even if you are feeling better before the scheduled end of therapy.

PROLONGED USE
If lice recur, consult your doctor.

▼ PRECAUTIONS

Over 60: No special problems are expected to occur in older patients.

Driving and Hazardous Work: The use of pyrethrins and piperonyl butoxide should not impair your ability to perform such tasks safely.

Alcohol: No special precautions are necessary.

Pregnancy: This drug has not been shown to cause birth defects or other problems during pregnancy. Before you use pyrethrins and piperonyl butoxide, tell your doctor if you are pregnant or plan to become pregnant.

Breast Feeding: Pyrethrins and piperonyl butoxide may pass into breast milk; caution is advised. Consult your doctor for specific information.

Infants and Children: No special problems are expected in younger patients.

Special Concerns: All members of your household should be examined for lice and given treatment if necessary. Clothing, household linen, hairbrushes, combs, and bedding should be thoroughly cleaned. Furniture, rugs, and floors should be vacuumed thoroughly. Toilet seats should be scrubbed often. If you use this medicine for pubic lice, your sexual partner may also need to be treated. Keep this medicine away from the mouth and do not inhale it. Apply it in a well-ventilated room to help prevent inhalation. Keep the medicine away from the eyes and other mucous membranes, such as the inside of the nose or vagina.

OVERDOSE
Symptoms: If accidentally ingested, pyrethrins and piperonyl butoxide can cause nausea, vomiting, muscle paralysis, and central nervous system depression.

What to Do: Call your doctor, emergency medical services (EMS), or the nearest poison control center immediately.

▼ INTERACTIONS

DRUG INTERACTIONS
Before you use this medicine, tell your doctor if you are using any other prescription or over-the-counter drugs.

FOOD INTERACTIONS
No known food interactions.

DISEASE INTERACTIONS
Consult your doctor if you have any severe inflammation of the skin.

SIDE EFFECTS

SERIOUS
Skin irritation not present before use of the medicine, skin rash or infection, sudden attacks of sneezing, stuffy or runny nose, wheezing or difficulty breathing. Call your doctor immediately.

COMMON
No common side effects are associated with pyrethrins and piperonyl butoxide.

LESS COMMON
No less common side effects are associated with pyrethrins and piperonyl butoxide.

RANITIDINE

BRAND NAMES

Zantac 75

Available in: Capsules, tablets, syrup, granules
Available as Generic? Yes
Drug Class: Histamine (H2) blocker

▼ USAGE INFORMATION

WHY IT'S TAKEN
To treat ulcers of the stomach and duodenum, conditions that cause increased stomach acid production (such as Zollinger-Ellison syndrome), erosive esophagitis (severe, chronic inflammation of the esophagus), and gastro-esophageal reflux (backwash of stomach acid into the esophagus, causing heartburn).

HOW IT WORKS
Ranitidine blocks the action of histamine (a compound produced in the body's cells), which in turn decreases the stomach's secretion of hydrochloric acid. Once stomach acid production is decreased, the body is better able to heal itself.

▼ DOSAGE GUIDELINES

RANGE AND FREQUENCY
Adults: 150 mg 2 times a day, in the morning and at bedtime, or 300 mg once daily before bedtime.

Patients with Zollinger-Ellison syndrome may require up to 6 g per day (and the medication should be taken orally). For treatment of heartburn with the OTC form: 75 mg as needed, not to exceed 150 mg a day. Children: Consult your pediatrician for the appropriate dosage for your child.

ONSET OF EFFECT
30 to 60 minutes.

DURATION OF ACTION
Up to 13 hours.

DIETARY ADVICE
Avoid foods that cause stomach irritation.

STORAGE
Store it away from heat and direct light. Keep the liquid form from freezing.

MISSED DOSE
Take it as soon as you remember. If it is near the time for the next dose, skip the missed dose and resume your regular dosage schedule. Do not double the next dose.

STOPPING THE DRUG
Take the prescription-strength medication for the full treatment period, even if you begin to feel better before the scheduled end of therapy.

PROLONGED USE
Do not take the OTC non-prescription-strength drug for more than 2 weeks unless you have been instructed otherwise by your doctor.

▼ PRECAUTIONS

Over 60: Adverse reactions may be more likely and more severe in older patients.

Driving and Hazardous Work: Do not drive or engage in hazardous work until you determine how the medicine affects you.

Alcohol: Avoid alcoholic beverages. Ranitidine may increase blood alcohol levels.

Pregnancy: Risks vary depending on the patient and dosage. Consult your doctor.

Breast Feeding: Ranitidine passes into breast milk and may pose harm to the child; avoid or discontinue use while nursing.

Infants and Children: Ranitidine is not recommended for young patients, although it has not been shown to cause any side effects or problems different from those in adults when used for short periods of time.

Special Concerns: Avoid cigarette smoking because it may increase stomach acid secretion and thus worsen

the disease. Do not take ranitidine if you have ever had an allergic reaction to a histamine (H2) blocker. If stomach pain becomes worse while using the drug, be sure to tell your doctor right away.

OVERDOSE
Symptoms: Vomiting, diarrhea, breathing problems, slurred speech, rapid heartbeat, delirium.

What to Do: Call your doctor, emergency medical services (EMS), or the nearest poison control center immediately.

▼ INTERACTIONS

DRUG INTERACTIONS
Consult your doctor for specific advice if you are taking antacids, antidepressants, aspirin, beta-blockers, caffeine, diazepam, glipizide, ketoconazole, lidocaine, phenytoin, procainamide, theophylline, or warfarin.

FOOD INTERACTIONS
Carbonated drinks, citrus fruits and juices, beverages containing caffeine, and other acidic foods or liquids may irritate the stomach or interfere with the therapeutic action of ranitidine.

DISEASE INTERACTIONS
Patients with kidney disease should not use ranitidine or should use it in smaller, limited doses under careful supervision by a physician.

≡ SIDE EFFECTS ≡

SERIOUS
Irregular heart rhythm (palpitations), slowed heartbeat, severe blood problems resulting in unusual bleeding, bruising, fever, chills, and increased susceptibility to infection. Call your doctor immediately.

COMMON
Headache, fatigue, drowsiness, dizziness, nausea, vomiting, abdominal pain, diarrhea, constipation.

LESS COMMON
Blurred vision, decreased sexual desire or function, swelling of breasts in males or females, temporary hair loss, hallucinations, depression, insomnia, skin rash, hives, or redness.

RESORCINOL

Available in: Lotion, cream, stick
Available as Generic? Yes
Drug Class: Acne drug

▼ USAGE INFORMATION

WHY IT'S TAKEN
To treat acne and seborrheic dermatitis. Resorcinol is also infrequently used to treat eczema, psoriasis, corns, calluses, warts, and other similar skin conditions.

HOW IT WORKS
Resorcinol fights fungal and bacterial organisms that can cause infection and promotes the softening, dissolution, and peeling of the skin.

▼ DOSAGE GUIDELINES

RANGE AND FREQUENCY
For acne and seborrheic dermatitis: Apply once or twice daily as recommended or as tolerated. Wash your hands thoroughly after each application of resorcinol.

ONSET OF EFFECT
Unknown.

DURATION OF ACTION
Unknown.

DIETARY ADVICE
No special restrictions.

STORAGE
Store it in a tightly sealed container away from heat and direct light.

MISSED DOSE
Skip the missed application and resume your regular dosage schedule. Do not double the next dose.

STOPPING THE DRUG
If you are using resorcinol on doctor's orders, the decision to stop using the drug should be made by your doctor. If you are using the drug without a prescription, you may stop using it whenever your acne clears; however, it is likely that discontinuing use of the drug will lead to a recurrence of acne.

PROLONGED USE
Do not use resorcinol for longer than prescribed.

▼ PRECAUTIONS

Over 60: No special advice.

Driving and Hazardous Work: No special precautions are necessary.

Alcohol: No special precautions are necessary.

Pregnancy: Resorcinol has not been shown to cause birth defects or other problems during pregnancy. It may, however, be absorbed through the skin. Consult your doctor for specific advice if you are pregnant or plan to become pregnant.

Breast Feeding: Resorcinol may be absorbed into the body through the skin; caution is advised. Consult your doctor for advice.

Infants and Children: Children should not use resorcinol on large areas of the body.

Special Concerns: Anyone with a history of allergy to resorcinol or any other ingredients in the specific product should not use this medication. Resorcinol should not be used on wounds, because it may cause methemoglobinemia, a blood disorder. It should not be applied over large areas of the body, especially when it is used in high concentrations. Avoid contact of resorcinol with the eyes. This medication is generally not recommended for blacks, because it may significantly darken treated areas of skin. Resorcinol may darken light-colored hair.

OVERDOSE
Symptoms: If ingested, diarrhea, nausea, abdominal pain, vomiting, drowsiness, dizziness, severe or persistent headache, breathing difficulty, unusual tiredness or weakness, slow heartbeat, and profuse sweating may occur.

What to Do: In case of resorcinol ingestion, call your doctor, emergency medical services (EMS), or the nearest poison control center.

▼ INTERACTIONS

DRUG INTERACTIONS
The following drugs or other products may irritate the skin and therefore should not be used with resorcinol unless recommended by your doctor: abrasive cleansers or soaps; preparations containing alcohol (including astringents, aftershave lotions, other perfumed toiletries); any other acne agent; any preparation containing a peeling agent such as benzoyl peroxide, salicylic acid, alpha-hydroxy acids, sulfur, or vitamin A; and soaps, medicated cosmetics, or other cosmetics that dry the skin.

FOOD INTERACTIONS
No known food interactions.

DISEASE INTERACTIONS
You should not use resorcinol if you have had a prior allergic reaction to it.

 ≡ SIDE EFFECTS ≡

SERIOUS
No serious side effects are associated with resorcinol during normal use (as prescribed).

COMMON
Mild redness and peeling of the skin. Such side effects tend to occur at the beginning of therapy and diminish as your body adjusts to the medication; notify your doctor if such symptoms persist or interfere with daily activities.

LESS COMMON
More severe irritation or allergy with redness, peeling, burning, stinging, itching, or rash. Call your doctor.

SENNA

Available in: Tablets, granules, oral solution, syrup
Available as Generic? Yes
Drug Class: Laxative

▼ USAGE INFORMATION

WHY IT'S TAKEN
For short-term treatment of constipation.

HOW IT WORKS
Senna stimulates water and electrolyte (mineral salt) secretion in the intestine to induce defecation.

▼ DOSAGE GUIDELINES

RANGE AND FREQUENCY
Adults and teenagers: 2 tablets, 1 tsp of granules, or 2 to 3 tsp of syrup. Children ages 6 to 12 years: 1 tablet or ½ tsp of granules. Take at bedtime.

ONSET OF EFFECT
Within 6 to 10 hours.

DURATION OF ACTION
Variable.

DIETARY ADVICE
Each dose of senna should be taken on an empty stomach with 8 oz of water or fruit juice.

STORAGE
Store it in a tightly sealed container away from moisture, heat, and direct light.

MISSED DOSE
Take it as soon as you remember. If it is near the time for the next dose, skip the missed dose and resume your regular dosage schedule. Do not double the next dose.

STOPPING THE DRUG
Take senna as directed for the full treatment period. You may stop taking the drug if you are feeling better before the scheduled end of therapy.

PROLONGED USE
If regular bowel movement does not resume in 1 week, discontinue use of senna and consult your doctor.

▼ PRECAUTIONS

Over 60: Adverse reactions may be more likely and more severe in older patients.

Driving and Hazardous Work: Do not drive or engage in hazardous work until you determine how the medicine affects you.

Alcohol: Avoid alcohol.

Pregnancy: Senna may cause unwanted effects during pregnancy if not used properly. Consult your doctor.

Breast Feeding: Senna may pass into breast milk; caution is advised. Consult your doctor for advice.

Infants and Children: Senna is not recommended for use by children under the age of 6 years unless it has been prescribed by a doctor.

Special Concerns: You should increase your intake of foods containing vitamin D, such as milk products, and maintain an adequate intake of foods containing folic acid, such as fresh vegetables, fruits, whole grains, and liver, while taking senna. Senna is one of the most effective laxatives for relieving the severe constipation caused by narcotic analgesics such as morphine and codeine.

OVERDOSE
Symptoms: Sudden vomiting, nausea, diarrhea, or cramping.

What to Do: An overdose of senna is unlikely to be life-threatening. However, if someone takes a much larger dose than prescribed, call your doctor, emergency medical services (EMS), or the nearest poison control center immediately.

▼ INTERACTIONS

DRUG INTERACTIONS
Do not take any other medicine within 2 hours of taking senna. Consult your doctor for specific advice if you are taking anticoagulants, digitalis drugs, ciprofloxacin, etidronate, sodium polystyrene sulfonate, or oral tetracycline antibiotics.

FOOD INTERACTIONS
No known food interactions.

DISEASE INTERACTIONS
Use caution when taking senna. Consult your doctor if you have a history of any of the following: appendicitis, rectal bleeding of unknown cause, colostomy, intestinal blockage, ileostomy, diabetes, heart disease, high blood pressure, kidney disease, or difficulty swallowing.

SIDE EFFECTS

SERIOUS
Confusion, irregular heartbeat, muscle cramps, pink to red or yellow to brown coloration of urine and stools, unusual tiredness or weakness, laxative dependence. Call your doctor immediately.

COMMON
Belching, cramping, diarrhea, nausea.

LESS COMMON
No less common side effects have been reported.

SIMETHICONE

Available in: Tablets, chewable tablets, capsules, drops
Available as Generic? Yes
Drug Class: Antacid; antiflatulant

▼ USAGE INFORMATION

WHY IT'S TAKEN
To relieve pain caused by excess gas in the stomach and intestines. It may also be employed in a clinical setting to decrease gas before diagnostic radiography of the stomach or intestines or prior to endoscopy.

HOW IT WORKS
Simethicone disperses throughout the gastrointestinal tract and prevents the formation of gas bubbles.

▼ DOSAGE GUIDELINES

RANGE AND FREQUENCY
Tablets or capsules: 60 to 125 mg 4 times a day, after meals and at bedtime. Chewable tablets: 40 to 125 mg 4 times a day, after meals and at bedtime, or 150 mg 3 times a day, after meals. Drops: Take 40 to 95 mg by mouth, 4 times a day, after meals and at bedtime. The dose should not exceed 500 mg a day for all forms unless your doctor advises otherwise.

ONSET OF EFFECT
Immediate.

DURATION OF ACTION
Unknown.

DIETARY ADVICE
This medicine should be taken after meals and at bedtime for optimal results.

STORAGE
Store it in a tightly sealed container away from heat, moisture, and direct light. Store the liquid form at room temperature.

MISSED DOSE
Take it as soon as you remember. However, if it is near the time for the next dose, skip the missed dose and resume your regular dosage schedule. Do not double the next dose.

STOPPING THE DRUG
Take simethicone as recommended for the full treatment period. However, you may stop taking the drug if you are feeling better before the scheduled end of therapy.

PROLONGED USE
Consult your doctor if you take simethicone for a prolonged period.

▼ PRECAUTIONS

Over 60: There is no specific information comparing use of simethicone in older persons with use in younger persons.

However, no special problems are expected.

Driving and Hazardous Work: The use of simethicone should not impair your ability to perform such tasks safely.

Alcohol: No special problems are expected.

Pregnancy: Simethicone is not absorbed into the body and is not expected to cause problems during pregnancy.

Breast Feeding: Simethicone has not been reported to cause problems in babies who are nursed.

Infants and Children: Use of simethicone for the treatment of infant colic is not recommended because of limited information on its safety in infants. Simethicone should be given to children only under a doctor's instructions.

Special Concerns: If you take the chewable tablets, chew them thoroughly before swallowing for more complete and faster results. Shake the liquid form well before using. You should change position frequently and walk around to help eliminate gas. Tell your doctor if you are on a low-sodium, low-sugar, or other special diet. You should exercise regularly and develop regular bowel habits. Do not smoke before meals.

OVERDOSE
Symptoms: No specific ones have been reported.

What to Do: An overdose of simethicone is not life-threatening. However, if someone takes a much larger dose than recommended, call your doctor or the nearest poison control center.

▼ INTERACTIONS

DRUG INTERACTIONS
None known.

FOOD INTERACTIONS
Avoid any foods that increase gas formation. Chew your food slowly and thoroughly. Avoid carbonated drinks.

DISEASE INTERACTIONS
None known.

 SIDE EFFECTS

SERIOUS
No serious side effects have been reported.

COMMON
Expulsion of excess gas causing belching and flatulence.

LESS COMMON
No less common side effects have been reported.

SODIUM BICARBONATE

BRAND NAMES

Alka-Seltzer, Arm and Hammer Pure Baking Soda, Bell/ans, Citrocarbonate, Soda Mint

Available in: Effervescent powder, powder, tablets
Available as Generic? Yes
Drug Class: Antacid

▼ USAGE INFORMATION

WHY IT'S TAKEN
To relieve heartburn, sour stomach, or acid indigestion. It may also be prescribed to treat metabolic acidosis (excess acid buildup in the body fluids), to prevent urinary stones, and as part of the treatment of gout.

HOW IT WORKS
Sodium bicarbonate neutralizes stomach acid and reduces the action of pepsin, a digestive enzyme. This provides symptomatic relief from excess stomach acid. Also, the bicarbonate is a base, so it can help correct the pH balance (reduce the acidity) of blood and urine.

▼ DOSAGE GUIDELINES

RANGE AND FREQUENCY
Effervescent powder—For heartburn or sour stomach: 3.9 to 10 g (1 to 2½ tsp) in a glass of cold water. Usually not more than 19.5 g (5 tsp) a day. Children ages 6 to 12 years: 1 to 1.9 g (¼ to ½ tsp) in a glass of cold water. Powder—For heartburn or sour stomach: ½ tsp in a glass of water every 2 hours. Dose may be changed if needed. To make the urine less acidic: 1 tsp (1.9 g) in a glass of water every 4 hours; usually not more than 4 tsp a day. Dose may be changed by your doctor. Tablets—For heartburn or sour stomach: 325 mg to 2 g 1 to 4 times a day. Children ages 6 to 12 years: 520 mg. Dose may be repeated in 30 minutes. To make the urine less acidic—To start, 4 g, then 1 to 2 g every 4 hours. Maximum adult dose usually not more than 16 g a day. Children: 23 to 230 mg per 2.2 lb (1 kg) of body weight a day. The dose may be changed if needed.

ONSET OF EFFECT
Rapid when used as an antacid for heartburn and sour stomach.

DURATION OF ACTION
Unknown.

DIETARY ADVICE
Sodium bicarbonate should be taken after meals. Be sure to account for the large amount of sodium in this medication if you are on a salt-restricted diet.

STORAGE
Store it in a tightly sealed container away from moisture, heat, and direct light.

MISSED DOSE
Take it as soon as you remember. If it is near the time for the next dose, skip the missed dose and resume your regular dosage schedule. Do not double the next dose.

STOPPING THE DRUG
Take as directed if taking it by prescription.

PROLONGED USE
Do not take sodium bicarbonate for more than 2 weeks or on a routine basis without consulting your physician about its use.

▼ PRECAUTIONS

Over 60: See Dietary Advice.

Driving and Hazardous Work: No special precautions are necessary.

Alcohol: Avoid alcohol.

Pregnancy: No problems have been reported.

Breast Feeding: No problems have been reported.

Infants and Children: Use and dosage for infants and children under 6 years of age should be determined by your doctor.

OVERDOSE
Symptoms: See Serious Side Effects.

What to Do: An overdose of sodium bicarbonate is unlikely to be life-threatening. However, if someone takes a much larger dose than recommended, call your doctor, emergency medical services (EMS), or the nearest poison control center immediately.

▼ INTERACTIONS

DRUG INTERACTIONS
Do not take more than one OTC medication containing sodium bicarbonate at a time. Consult your doctor for specific advice if you are taking ketoconazole, tetracyclines, mecamylamine, methenamine, urinary acidifiers, amphetamines, anticholinergics, quinidine, citrates, enteric-coated medications, ephedrine, flecainide, fluoroquinolones, iron, lithium, methotrexate, mexiletine, sucralfate, or salicylates.

FOOD INTERACTIONS
Do not take sodium bicarbonate with milk or milk products.

DISEASE INTERACTIONS
Do not take sodium bicarbonate if you are experiencing any sign of appendicitis (stomach pain, bloating, nausea, and vomiting). If you have any kidney problems, use sodium bicarbonate only on advice of your doctor. Consult your doctor if you have intestinal or rectal bleeding; edema (swelling of the hands or feet); heart, liver, or kidney disease; hypertension; urination problems; or preeclampsia during pregnancy.

≡ SIDE EFFECTS ≡

SERIOUS
Frequent urge to urinate, nervousness or restlessness, mental or mood changes, muscle twitching or pain, nausea or vomiting, slow breathing, continuing headache, loss of appetite, swelling of feet or lower legs, unpleasant taste, unusual fatigue. Call your doctor immediately.

COMMON
No common side effects have been reported.

LESS COMMON
Stomach cramps, increased thirst.

SODIUM PHOSPHATE/SODIUM BIPHOSPHATE

BRAND NAMES

Fleet, Fleet Phospho-Soda

Available in: Oral solution, effervescent powder, enema
Available as Generic? Yes
Drug Class: Hyperosmotic laxative

▼ USAGE INFORMATION

WHY IT'S TAKEN
To treat short-term constipation or for rapid emptying of the colon prior to bowel or rectal examination.

HOW IT WORKS
This medication attracts and retains water in the intestine, increasing peristalsis (bowel activity) and producing the urge to defecate.

▼ DOSAGE GUIDELINES

RANGE AND FREQUENCY
Oral—Adults and teenagers: 4 to 6 tsp mixed with ½ glass cool water. Children ages 10 to 12 years: 2 tsp. Children ages 6 to 10 years: 1 tsp. Enema—Adults and teenagers: ½ cup (contents of 1 disposable adult enema) given rectally. Children over 2 years: ½ adult dose (entire contents of 1 disposable pediatric enema).

ONSET OF EFFECT
30 minutes to 3 hours after oral administration, 3 to 5 minutes after enema.

DURATION OF ACTION
Variable with oral use; on evacuation with enema.

DIETARY ADVICE
Sodium phosphate/sodium biphosphate should not be used with food. The unpleasant taste that may occur when you take the medicine can be lessened by taking it with citrus fruit juice or a citrus-flavored soft drink.

STORAGE
Store it in a tightly sealed container away from heat and direct light.

MISSED DOSE
Oral forms: If you are taking this laxative on a fixed schedule, take the missed dose as soon as you remember. If it is near the time for the next dose, skip the missed dose and resume your regular dosage schedule. Do not double the next dose. Enema: Not applicable.

STOPPING THE DRUG
Take the medicine as directed for the full treatment period. However, you may stop taking the drug if you feel better before the scheduled end of therapy.

PROLONGED USE
Do not use any laxative for longer than 2 weeks without consulting your doctor.

▼ PRECAUTIONS

Over 60: Adverse reactions may be more likely and more severe in older patients.

Driving and Hazardous Work: Do not drive or engage in hazardous work until you determine how the medicine affects you.

Alcohol: Avoid alcohol.

Pregnancy: This laxative contains a large amount of sodium, which may have unwanted effects, such as higher blood pressure, during pregnancy. If you have to take a laxative during pregnancy, consult your doctor for specific advice.

Breast Feeding: Sodium phosphate may pass into breast milk; caution is advised. Consult your doctor for specific advice.

Infants and Children: Do not give sodium phosphate/sodium biphosphate to a child under the age of 6 years without consulting your doctor.

Special Concerns: Chilling the oral form of the medication or taking it with ice or following it with citrus fruit juice or citrus-flavored carbonated beverages may make it more palatable. Remember that chronic use of sodium phosphate or any laxative can lead to laxative dependence. You should consume adequate amounts of bulk (fiber), such as bran, whole-grain cereals, fruit, and vegetables, in your diet. This laxative should be taken on a schedule that does not interfere

with activities or sleep; it produces watery stools within 3 to 6 hours. It should not be taken within 2 hours of taking other medications.

OVERDOSE
Symptoms: Excessive bowel activity, dehydration causing low blood pressure and abnormal heartbeat, metabolic acidosis, blood chemistry abnormalities.

What to Do: An overdose of sodium phosphate/sodium biphosphate is unlikely to be life-threatening. However, if someone takes a much larger dose than prescribed, call your doctor, emergency medical services (EMS), or the nearest poison control center immediately.

▼ INTERACTIONS

DRUG INTERACTIONS
Consult your doctor for advice if you are taking anticoagulants, digitalis drugs, ciprofloxacin, etidronate, sodium polystyrene sulfonate, or oral tetracyclines.

FOOD INTERACTIONS
No known food interactions.

DISEASE INTERACTIONS
Consult your doctor if you have a history of appendicitis, rectal bleeding of unknown cause, colostomy, intestinal blockage, ileostomy, diabetes mellitus, heart disease, high blood pressure, kidney disease, or any difficulties in swallowing.

≣ SIDE EFFECTS ≣

SERIOUS
Confusion, dizziness or lightheadedness, irregular heartbeat, muscle cramps, unusual tiredness or weakness. Call your doctor immediately.

COMMON
Cramping, diarrhea, gas, increased thirst.

LESS COMMON
No less common side effects have been reported.

SULFUR TOPICAL

BRAND NAMES

Cuticura Ointment, Finac, Fostex Regular Strength Medicated Cover-Up, Fostril Lotion, Lotio-Asulfa, Sulpho-Lac

Available in: Cream, lotion, ointment, bar soap
Available as Generic? Yes
Drug Class: Acne drug

▼ USAGE INFORMATION

WHY IT'S TAKEN
To treat skin conditions including acne, seborrheic dermatitis, and scabies.

HOW IT WORKS
Topical sulfur is lethal to various strains of bacteria (which are a primary cause of acne), fungus, parasites, and other types of microorganisms. It also promotes softening, dissolution, and peeling of hard, scaly, roughened, or irregular surface skin.

▼ DOSAGE GUIDELINES

RANGE AND FREQUENCY
For acne, lotion, cream, or bar soap: Use on skin as needed. To use the soap, work up a rich lather using warm water. Wash the affected area, rinse thoroughly, apply again, and rub in gently for a few minutes. Remove excess lather with a towel or tissue without rinsing. Lotion: Apply 2 or 3 times a day. Ointment: Apply the 0.5% ointment as needed. Wash the affected area with soap and water and dry thoroughly before application. For seborrheic dermatitis: Use 1 or 2 times a day as directed on the package instructions. For scabies: Apply the 6% ointment every night for 3 nights. The ointment should be applied to the entire body from the neck down. You may bathe before each application and should bathe 24 hours after the last (third) application.

ONSET OF EFFECT
Unknown.

DURATION OF ACTION
Unknown.

DIETARY ADVICE
Topical sulfur can be used without regard to diet.

STORAGE
Store it in a tightly sealed container away from heat and direct light. Keep the cream, lotion, and ointment forms from freezing.

MISSED DOSE
Resume your regular dosage schedule with the next application. Do not double the next dose.

STOPPING THE DRUG
If you are using sulfur by prescription, the decision to stop taking the drug should be made by your doctor. If you are using it without a prescription, you may stop taking the drug when your skin has cleared; however, it is likely that the condition will recur.

PROLONGED USE
If your doctor recommends sulfur, use it no longer than directed.

▼ PRECAUTIONS

Over 60: No special precautions are necessary.

Driving and Hazardous Work: No special precautions are necessary.

Alcohol: No special precautions are necessary.

Pregnancy: Sulfur has not been shown to cause birth defects or other problems during pregnancy. Before you use sulfur, tell your doctor if you are pregnant or plan to become pregnant.

Breast Feeding: Topical sulfur has not been reported to cause problems in nursing infants. Consult your doctor for specific advice.

Infants and Children: Use and dosage for children must be determined by your pediatrician.

Special Concerns: Anyone with a history of allergy to sulfur and other ingredients in the medication should not use this product. Keep sulfur away from the eyes. If you accidentally get some of the medicine in your eyes, flush them thoroughly with water.

OVERDOSE
Symptoms: Excessive application of topical sulfur may lead to more severe irritation of the skin.

What to Do: If topical sulfur is accidentally ingested, call your doctor, emergency medical services (EMS), or the nearest poison control center immediately.

▼ INTERACTIONS

DRUG INTERACTIONS
Consult your doctor for specific advice if you are using abrasive soaps or cleansers; preparations containing alcohol; any other acne agent; any preparation containing a peeling agent such as benzoyl peroxide, salicylic acid, alpha-hydroxy acids, sulfur, or vitamin A; or soaps, medicated cosmetics, or other cosmetics that dry the skin. Also tell your doctor if you are using any other prescription or over-the-counter drug for a skin condition.

FOOD INTERACTIONS
No known food interactions.

DISEASE INTERACTIONS
You should not use sulfur if you have had a prior allergic reaction to it.

 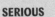
SIDE EFFECTS

SERIOUS
No serious side effects have been reported.

COMMON
Mild redness and peeling of skin.

LESS COMMON
Skin irritation or allergy with redness, peeling, burning, stinging, itching, or rash. Contact your doctor.

TERBINAFINE HYDROCHLORIDE

BRAND NAME

Lamisil

Available in: Topical cream
Available as Generic? No
Drug Class: Antifungal

▼ USAGE INFORMATION

WHY IT'S TAKEN
The cream is used to treat fungal infections of the skin, such as tinea corporis (ringworm), tinea cruris (jock itch), and tinea pedis (athlete's foot).

HOW IT WORKS
Terbinafine inhibits an enzyme essential for the production of substances vital for the reproduction and survival of some types of fungal organisms.

▼ DOSAGE GUIDELINES

RANGE AND FREQUENCY
Apply a thin film of medicine to the affected area 1 to 2 times a day for ringworm or jock itch, 2 times a day for athlete's foot. Apply the cream for at least 1 week but no longer than 4 weeks.

ONSET OF EFFECT
Unknown.

DURATION OF ACTION
Unknown.

DIETARY ADVICE
Terbinafine can be applied without regard to meals.

STORAGE
Store it in a tightly sealed container away from moisture, heat, and direct light. Do not allow the cream to freeze.

MISSED DOSE
It is important to not miss any doses. Apply it as soon as you remember. If you do not remember until the next day, skip the missed dose and resume your regular dosage schedule. Do not use excessive amounts of the cream.

STOPPING THE DRUG
Use it for as long as directed or until infection clears.

PROLONGED USE
Side effects are more likely to occur with prolonged use.

▼ PRECAUTIONS

Over 60: No special advice.

Driving and Hazardous Work: No special precautions.

Alcohol: No special warnings.

Pregnancy: Not recommended for pregnant women.

Breast Feeding: Avoid it while nursing.

Infants and Children: Terbinafine is not recommended for children under the age of 18 years.

Special Concerns: Wash your hands before and after applying the cream. Avoid allowing topical terbinafine to come into contact with your eyes, nose, and mouth. If using terbinafine for ringworm, wear loose-fitting, well-ventilated clothing and avoid excess heat and humidity. It is also recommended to use a bland, absorbent powder such as talcum once or twice a day after the cream has been applied and absorbed by the skin. If using the medication for jock itch, do not wear underwear that is tight or made from synthetic materials; wear loose-fitting cotton underwear. If using terbinafine for athlete's foot, dry your feet carefully after bathing and wear clean cotton socks with sandals or well-ventilated shoes. Before applying the medication, wash the affected area with soap and warm water and dry thoroughly.

OVERDOSE
Symptoms: An overdose with terbinafine cream is unlikely.

What to Do: Call your doctor as soon as possible.

▼ INTERACTIONS

DRUG INTERACTIONS
Consult your doctor if you are using any other preparation that is to be applied to the same area of skin as terbinafine cream.

FOOD INTERACTIONS
No known food interactions.

DISEASE INTERACTIONS
No disease interactions have been reported.

≡ SIDE EFFECTS ≡

SERIOUS
Serious side effects with terbinafine are rare. However, terbinafine tablets may cause liver dysfunction; severe skin reactions such as Stevens-Johnson syndrome; severe blood disorders, potentially resulting in increased susceptibility to infection, uncontrolled bleeding, or other problems; or severe allergic reactions. Seek emergency medical assistance immediately.

COMMON
Headache, diarrhea, rash, stomach pain, indigestion, nausea.

LESS COMMON
Tablets may cause flatulence, itching, skin eruptions, loss of taste, weakness, fatigue, vomiting, joint and muscle pain, or hair loss. Terbinafine cream may cause redness, itching, burning, blistering, swelling, oozing, or other signs of skin irritation not present before using the drug.

TIOCONAZOLE

Available in: Vaginal ointment
Available as Generic? No
Drug Class: Antifungal

▼ USAGE INFORMATION

WHY IT'S TAKEN
To treat fungal (yeast) infections of the vagina.

HOW IT WORKS
Tioconazole prevents the growth and function of some fungal organisms by interfering with the production of substances needed to preserve the cell membrane. This drug is effective only for infections caused by fungal organisms. It will not work for bacterial or viral infections.

▼ DOSAGE GUIDELINES

RANGE AND FREQUENCY
A single 300-mg (1 applicatorful) dose of ointment inserted with an applicator into the vagina at bedtime.

ONSET OF EFFECT
Some relief may be felt within 1 day. Complete relief of symptoms generally occurs within 7 days.

DURATION OF ACTION
Unknown.

DIETARY ADVICE
Tioconazole may be used without regard to diet.

STORAGE
Store it in a tightly sealed container away from moisture, heat, and direct light. Do not allow it to freeze.

MISSED DOSE
Not applicable. Tioconazole is usually effective with a single, 1-time use.

STOPPING THE DRUG
Tioconazole is generally used on a 1-time basis. If needed, a second dose may be applied 1 to 2 weeks after the first dose.

PROLONGED USE
Tioconazole is for short-term use only.

▼ PRECAUTIONS

Over 60: No special problems are expected.

Driving and Hazardous Work: This drug should not impair your ability to perform such tasks safely.

Alcohol: No special warnings.

Pregnancy: Adequate studies on the use of tioconazole during pregnancy have not been done; however, there are no reports of adverse effects while using it. Consult your doctor before using.

Breast Feeding: No problems are expected. Consult your doctor before using this medicine while nursing.

Infants and Children: No studies have been done on the use of tioconazole by children. Consult a pediatrician for specific advice.

Special Concerns: Tioconazole may be used with oral contraceptives and antibiotic therapy. Sanitary napkins should be used to prevent staining of clothing. The affected area should be kept cool and dry. The patient should wear loose-fitting cotton clothing and freshly laundered cotton underwear or pantyhose with a cotton crotch. Avoid underwear made from nonventilating materials. Do not sit for a long time in a wet bathing suit. Avoid feminine hygiene sprays. Wash daily with unscented soap and dry thoroughly with a clean towel. Tampons should not be used during therapy. Do not have sex for 3 days after treatment and wait an additional 3 days before relying on a condom or diaphragm, because the medication may weaken latex. After this time, the patient's sexual partner should wear a condom during intercourse and should consult a doctor if penile redness, itching, or discomfort occurs. You may use this medicine during your menstrual period. After urination or a bowel movement, cleanse by wiping the area from front to back to prevent reinfection by yeast.

OVERDOSE
Symptoms: An overdose with tioconazole is unlikely.

What to Do: If someone swallows a large amount of the medicine, call your doctor.

▼ INTERACTIONS

DRUG INTERACTIONS
Tell your doctor if you are using any other OTC or prescription vaginal medication.

FOOD INTERACTIONS
No food interactions have been reported.

DISEASE INTERACTIONS
No disease interactions have been reported.

 SIDE EFFECTS

SERIOUS
Vaginal itching, burning, discharge, or irritation not present prior to treatment. Call your doctor as soon as possible.

COMMON
No common side effects have been reported.

LESS COMMON
Headache, stomach cramps or pain, irritation or burning of sexual partner's penis.

TOLNAFTATE

Available in: Cream, gel, powder, solution
Available as Generic? Yes
Drug Class: Topical antifungal

▼ USAGE INFORMATION

WHY IT'S TAKEN
To treat a variety of fungal infections of the skin, including tinea corporis (ringworm), tinea cruris (jock itch), and tinea pedis (athlete's foot).

HOW IT WORKS
Tolnaftate prevents fungi from manufacturing vital substances required for growth and function. This medication is effective only for infections caused by ringworm fungal organisms. It will not work for bacterial or viral infections.

▼ DOSAGE GUIDELINES

RANGE AND FREQUENCY
Apply to the affected area 2 times a day. All forms should be used immediately after the affected area is washed and dried. Wash your hands before and after application.

ONSET OF EFFECT
Unknown.

DURATION OF ACTION
Unknown.

DIETARY ADVICE
No special restrictions.

STORAGE
Store it in a tightly sealed container away from moisture, heat, and direct light.

MISSED DOSE
Apply it as soon as you remember. If it is near the time for the next dose, skip the missed dose and resume your regular dosage schedule. Do not double the next dose.

STOPPING THE DRUG
Use of tolnaftate should continue for 2 weeks after symptoms disappear. This helps ensure eradication of the fungus.

PROLONGED USE
You should consult your doctor if symptoms do not improve within 10 days of beginning therapy.

▼ PRECAUTIONS

Over 60: No special problems are expected.

Driving and Hazardous Work: The use of tolnaftate should not impair your ability to perform such tasks safely.

Alcohol: No special warnings.

Pregnancy: Tolnaftate has not been shown in studies to cause problems when used during pregnancy.

Breast Feeding: Tolnaftate may pass into breast milk, but no problems have been reported. Consult your doctor for specific advice.

Infants and Children: Children younger than age 2 years should use tolnaftate only under the close supervision of a pediatrician.

Special Concerns: Do not allow tolnaftate to come in contact with your eyes. If your skin condition does not improve or instead gets worse after 10 days of treatment, consult your doctor. Tolnaftate should not be used alone to treat fungal infections of the hair or nails; your doctor can prescribe an additional medication for this condition. If you are using tolnaftate for an infection of the feet, be sure to wear well-fitting and well-ventilated shoes and to change your shoes and put on clean socks every day. Do not cover the treated area of skin with bandages unless your doctor specifically instructs you to do so.

OVERDOSE
Symptoms: None are known; no cases of overdose have been reported.

What to Do: An overdose of tolnaftate is unlikely to occur. However, if someone accidentally ingests some of the medication, call your doctor, emergency medical services (EMS), or the nearest poison control center immediately.

▼ INTERACTIONS

DRUG INTERACTIONS
Some drugs may interact adversely with tolnaftate. Consult your doctor for specific advice if you are using any other prescription or OTC medication that is applied to the same area of skin being treated by tolnaftate.

FOOD INTERACTIONS
No known food interactions.

DISEASE INTERACTIONS
Caution is advised when taking tolnaftate. Consult your doctor for specific advice if you have a history of any other skin condition.

 SIDE EFFECTS

SERIOUS
Skin irritation that was not present before use of tolnaftate. Call your doctor immediately.

COMMON
No common side effects are associated with the use of tolnaftate.

LESS COMMON
No less common side effects are associated with the use of tolnaftate.

TRIPROLIDINE HYDROCHLORIDE

Available in: Syrup
Available as Generic? Yes
Drug Class: Antihistamine

▼ USAGE INFORMATION

WHY IT'S TAKEN
To relieve symptoms of hay fever and other allergies.

HOW IT WORKS
Triprolidine blocks the effects of histamine, a naturally occurring substance that causes swelling, itching, sneezing, watery eyes, hives, and other symptoms of allergic reaction.

▼ DOSAGE GUIDELINES

RANGE AND FREQUENCY
Adults and children age 12 years and older: 2.5 mg every 4 to 6 hours. The maximum dose is 10 mg a day. Children ages 6 to 12 years: 1.25 mg (1 tsp) every 4 to 6 hours. The maximum dose is 5 mg a day. Children ages 4 to 6 years: 0.938 mg (¾ tsp) every 4 to 6 hours. The maximum dose is 3.744 mg a day. Children ages 2 to 4 years: 0.625 mg (½ tsp) every 4 to 6 hours. The maximum dose is 2.5 mg a day. Children ages 4 months to 2 years: 0.313 mg (¼ tsp) every 4 to 6 hours. The maximum dose is 1.25 mg a day.

ONSET OF EFFECT
15 to 60 minutes.

DURATION OF ACTION
4 to 6 hours.

DIETARY ADVICE
Take with food or milk to reduce stomach upset.

STORAGE
Store in a tightly sealed container away from heat and direct light. Do not allow the drug to freeze.

MISSED DOSE
Take it as soon as you remember. If it is near the time for the next dose, skip the missed dose and resume your regular dosage schedule. Do not double the next dose.

STOPPING THE DRUG
The decision to stop taking the drug should be made by your doctor.

PROLONGED USE
Tolerance, or decreased responsiveness to the drug, usually does not develop with prolonged use. If it does, consult your doctor.

▼ PRECAUTIONS

Over 60: Adverse reactions may be more likely and more severe in older patients.

Driving and Hazardous Work: Do not drive or engage in hazardous work until you determine how the medicine affects you.

Alcohol: Avoid alcohol.

Pregnancy: Before you take triprolidine, tell your doctor if you are pregnant or plan to become pregnant.

Breast Feeding: Triprolidine passes into breast milk; avoid or discontinue use while nursing. Flow of breast milk may be reduced.

Infants and Children: Adverse effects may be more likely to occur and be more severe in children.

Special Concerns: Stop taking triprolidine 4 days before you have an allergy skin test. Drink water frequently or use ice chips, sugar-free candy, or sugar-free gum if dry mouth occurs. Coffee or tea may reduce the common side effect of drowsiness.

OVERDOSE

Symptoms: Central nervous system depression or, paradoxically, nervous system stimulation; very low blood pressure; breathing difficulty; seizures; loss of consciousness; severe dryness of the mouth, nose, or throat.

What to Do: Call your doctor, emergency medical services (EMS), or the nearest poison control center immediately.

▼ INTERACTIONS

DRUG INTERACTIONS
Consult your doctor for advice if you are taking anticholinergics, clarithromycin, erythromycin, itraconazole, ketoconazole, bepridil, disopyramide, maprotiline, phenothiazines, pimozide, procainamide, quinidine, tricyclic antidepressants, central nervous system depressants, monoamine oxidase (MAO) inhibitors, or quinine.

FOOD INTERACTIONS
No known food interactions.

DISEASE INTERACTIONS
Caution is advised when taking triprolidine. Consult your doctor if you have an enlarged prostate, urinary tract blockage, difficulty urinating, or glaucoma. Use of triprolidine may cause complications in patients with liver disease, because this organ works to remove the medication from the body.

SIDE EFFECTS

SERIOUS
Sore throat and fever, unusual tiredness or weakness, unusual bleeding or bruising. Call your doctor immediately.

COMMON
Drowsiness, thickening of mucus.

LESS COMMON
Blurred vision; rapid heartbeat; skin rash; stomach upset; nervousness; increased sensitivity of skin to sunlight; confusion; difficult or painful urination; dizziness; dry mouth, nose, or throat; loss of appetite; nightmares; ringing or buzzing in ears; restlessness; irritability.

UNDECYLENIC ACID

Available in: Aerosol foam, aerosol powder, cream, ointment, powder, solution
Available as Generic? Yes
Drug Class: Topical antifungal

▼ USAGE INFORMATION

WHY IT'S TAKEN
To treat fungal infections of the skin. (Note: Undecylenic acid generally has been replaced by newer and more effective topical antifungal medications; however, your doctor may find it worthwhile to recommend undecylenic acid under certain circumstances—for example, if you have a history of allergic reaction to other antifungal preparations.)

HOW IT WORKS
Undecylenic acid prevents the growth and reproduction of fungus cells.

▼ DOSAGE GUIDELINES

RANGE AND FREQUENCY
Aerosol foam, aerosol powder, ointment, powder, or solution: Apply to the affected area of the skin 2 times a day. The aerosol powder and aerosol spray form of the medicine should be sprayed on the affected area from a distance of 4 to 6 inches. The powder may also be sprayed in socks and shoes. If the powder is used on the feet, sprinkle it between the toes, on the feet, and in shoes and socks. Cream: Apply to the affected area of the skin as often as necessary.

ONSET OF EFFECT
Unknown.

DURATION OF ACTION
Unknown.

DIETARY ADVICE
No special restrictions.

STORAGE
Store it in a tightly sealed container away from heat and direct light. Keep aerosol, cream, ointment, and liquid solution forms of undecylenic acid from freezing. Do not puncture, rupture, or incinerate the aerosol container.

MISSED DOSE
Apply a missed dose as soon as you remember. If it is close to the time for the next dose, skip the missed dose and resume your regular dosage schedule. Do not apply a double dose.

STOPPING THE DRUG
Apply it as recommended for the full treatment period, even if you begin to feel better before the scheduled end of therapy. Discontinuing the drug prematurely may result in an even worse fungal infection later (known as rebound infection). In general, keep using this medication for 2 weeks after burning, itching, and other symptoms have cleared up.

PROLONGED USE
If your skin problem does not improve or becomes worse after 4 weeks of treatment, consult your doctor.

▼ PRECAUTIONS

Over 60: There is no specific information comparing use of undecylenic acid in older persons with use in patients in other age groups.

Driving and Hazardous Work: No special precautions are necessary.

Alcohol: No special precautions are necessary.

Pregnancy: Undecylenic acid has not been shown to cause birth defects or other problems in humans.

Breast Feeding: Undecylenic acid may pass into breast milk; caution is advised. Consult your doctor for specific advice.

Infants and Children: Not recommended for use on children younger than 2 years of age.

Special Concerns: Keep this medicine away from the eyes, nose, and mouth. To help prevent reinfection, the powder or spray form of undecylenic acid may be used every day after bathing and careful drying. Do not use it on pus-producing sores or on badly broken skin.

OVERDOSE

Symptoms: No specific ones have been reported.

What to Do: An overdose of undecylenic acid is unlikely. However, if someone accidentally ingests the drug, call your doctor, emergency medical services (EMS), or the nearest poison control center.

▼ INTERACTIONS

DRUG INTERACTIONS
Consult your doctor for specific advice if you are taking any other topical prescription or over-the-counter medication that is to be applied to the same area of the skin.

FOOD INTERACTIONS
No known food interactions.

DISEASE INTERACTIONS
Caution is advised when taking undecylenic acid. Consult your doctor if you have any other medical condition that affects the skin.

⧨ SIDE EFFECTS ⧨

SERIOUS
No serious side effects have been reported.

COMMON
No common side effects have been reported.

LESS COMMON
Skin irritation that was not present before use of this medicine. Call your doctor promptly.

YOHIMBINE

Available in: Tablets
Available as Generic? Yes
Drug Class: Alpha-adrenergic blocking agent

▼ USAGE INFORMATION

WHY IT'S TAKEN
To aid in the treatment of male erectile dysfunction (impotence).

HOW IT WORKS
The exact way that yohimbine works has not been determined. It is believed to block certain chemical receptors that cause constriction of blood vessels. In doing so, yohimbine theoretically improves blood flow into (and inhibits blood flow out of) the spongy columns of tissue in the penis involved in the mechanics of erection. Yohimbine may also have a mild stimulant effect and may promote the release of brain chemicals that control mood, relaxation, and sex drive, among other functions.

▼ DOSAGE GUIDELINES

RANGE AND FREQUENCY
Adult males: 5.4 mg 3 times a day.

ONSET OF EFFECT
Within 2 to 3 weeks in most cases.

DURATION OF ACTION
Unknown.

DIETARY ADVICE
No special restrictions.

STORAGE
Store it in a tightly sealed container away from moisture, heat, and direct light. Do not refrigerate the medication or allow it to freeze.

MISSED DOSE
Take it as soon as you remember. If it is near the time for the next dose, skip the missed dose and resume your regular dosage schedule. Do not double the next dose.

STOPPING THE DRUG
If your doctor has recommended yohimbine, consult him or her before stopping.

PROLONGED USE
See your doctor regularly for tests and examinations if you take this drug for a prolonged period of time.

▼ PRECAUTIONS

Over 60: No special problems are expected.

Driving and Hazardous Work: Do not drive or engage in hazardous work until you determine how the medicine affects you.

Alcohol: There are no special restrictions; however, excess alcohol consumption may impair sexual function.

Pregnancy: Yohimbine is generally not prescribed for women and should not be used during pregnancy.

Breast Feeding: Not applicable to female patients.

Infants and Children: Not applicable to children.

Special Concerns: This drug should be used only by men who have been diagnosed with and are being medically treated for erectile dysfunction.

OVERDOSE
Symptoms: Agitation, restlessness, dizziness, and rapid or irregular heartbeat.

What to Do: An overdose with yohimbine is unlikely. However, if someone takes a much larger dose than prescribed, call your doctor, emergency medical services (EMS), or the nearest poison control center.

▼ INTERACTIONS

DRUG INTERACTIONS
Consult your doctor for specific advice if you are taking antidepressants (especially monoamine oxidase (MAO) inhibitors) or any other mood-modifying medications, including selective serotonin reuptake inhibitors (SSRIs) such as fluoxetine. Before you take yohimbine, tell your doctor if you are taking any other prescription or OTC drugs, especially cold remedies or weight loss aids.

FOOD INTERACTIONS
Because yohimbine is a mild MAO inhibitor, it should not be taken with any food or drink containing tyramines, including cheese, chocolate, beer, aged meats, and nuts, and particularly not with the amino acids tyrosine or phenylalanine. The combination may cause a dangerous rise in blood pressure.

DISEASE INTERACTIONS
Caution is advised when taking yohimbine. Consult your doctor if you have a history of angina pectoris, mental depression or any other psychiatric illness, heart disease, high blood pressure, or impaired kidney function. Use of yohimbine may cause complications in patients with liver disease, because this organ works to remove the medication from the body.

≡ SIDE EFFECTS ≡

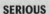

SERIOUS
Rapid heartbeat; increased blood pressure, possibly causing symptoms such as persistent headaches or ringing in the ears. Call your doctor immediately.

COMMON
No common side effects have been reported.

LESS COMMON
Headache, dizziness, irritability, nervousness, restlessness, flushing of skin, shakiness, increased sweating.

ZINC OXIDE

BRAND NAMES

Ken Tox

Available in: Cream, ointment
Available as Generic? Yes
Drug Class: Sunscreen

▼ USAGE INFORMATION

WHY IT'S TAKEN
To prevent sunburn.

HOW IT WORKS
Zinc oxide blocks ultraviolet radiation in sunlight from reaching the skin.

▼ DOSAGE GUIDELINES

RANGE AND FREQUENCY
Apply as needed before exposure to sunlight. A sunscreen should be applied uniformly to all exposed skin surfaces, including the lips.

ONSET OF EFFECT
Immediate.

DURATION OF ACTION
Keeps working until removed or worn off by perspiration or swimming.

DIETARY ADVICE
Zinc oxide can be used without regard to diet.

STORAGE
Store it in a tightly sealed container away from heat and direct light.

MISSED DOSE
If you forget to apply zinc oxide before exposure to sunlight, apply as soon as you think of it.

STOPPING THE DRUG
No special warnings.

PROLONGED USE
No problems are expected.

▼ PRECAUTIONS

Over 60: Studies suggest that frequent use of sunscreens such as zinc oxide may increase the risk of vitamin D deficiency, which may promote osteoporosis or bone fractures later in life. Oral vitamin D supplements and consumption of foods rich in vitamin D may be recommended.

Driving and Hazardous Work: The use of zinc oxide should not impair your ability to perform such tasks safely.

Alcohol: No special precautions are necessary.

Pregnancy: No problems have been reported.

Breast Feeding: No problems have been reported.

Infants and Children: Zinc oxide should not be used on children (especially infants under 6 months of age) who have shown signs of allergic skin reaction (hypersensitivity). Otherwise, it is safe for use in children. To prevent accidental ingestion, do not allow small children to apply sunscreens themselves. In general, children should be kept out of the sun during peak daylight hours (from 10 A.M. to 2 P.M.) and physically protected from direct sun exposure with clothing and other physical barriers (such as a beach umbrella). Infants over 6 months of age should be protected by a sunscreen with an SPF (sun protection factor) of 15 or higher. Older children should regularly use a sunscreen with an SPF of 15 or higher to protect against excess and repeated exposure to solar ultraviolet radiation, which can lead to skin cancer and other skin damage later in life.

Special Concerns: Zinc oxide sunscreen should be applied liberally before exposure to sunlight and reapplied every 1 to 2 hours, especially after swimming or heavy perspiration and after eating and drinking. Contact of zinc oxide with the eyes should be avoided. If skin rash or irritation develops, consult your doctor. Keep sun exposure to a minimum during peak daylight hours (10 A.M. to 2 P.M.), when the sun's rays are strongest. Extra precautions should be taken around reflective surfaces such as sand, water, and concrete.

OVERDOSE
Symptoms: No specific symptoms have been reported.

What to Do: Not applicable. However, if someone accidentally ingests zinc oxide, call a doctor, emergency medical services (EMS), or the nearest poison control center immediately.

▼ INTERACTIONS

DRUG INTERACTIONS
Consult your doctor for specific advice if you are using any other topical medications or skin preparations.

FOOD INTERACTIONS
No known food interactions.

DISEASE INTERACTIONS
Consult your doctor for advice if you have a history of any of the following: dermatitis (skin inflammation), herpes labialis (herpes simplex of the mouth and face), lichen planus (a rare nonmalignant skin condition causing chronic itching and a distinctive skin eruption), systemic lupus erythematosus (lupus), photosensitivity (heightened sensitivity to sunlight), phytophotodermatitis (dermatitis caused by contact with certain plants followed by exposure to sunlight), polymorphous light eruption (skin lesions occurring after exposure to sunlight), or xeroderma pigmentosum (a rare genetic disorder causing extreme sensitivity to ultraviolet light, abnormal skin growths including malignancies, and serious eye problems).

≣ SIDE EFFECTS ≣

SERIOUS
Acne, folliculitis (burning, pain, inflammation, and itching in hairy regions of the skin; pus in hair follicles), and skin rash may occur with zinc oxide and other physical sunscreens that block the pores. Notify your doctor if you experience such side effects.

COMMON
No common side effects have been reported.

LESS COMMON
No less common side effects have been reported.

ZINC SULFATE OPHTHALMIC

Available in: Ophthalmic solution
Available as Generic? Yes
Drug Class: Ophthalmic astringent/analgesic

▼ USAGE INFORMATION

WHY IT'S TAKEN
For the temporary relief of discomfort and redness from minor eye irritation. It is recommended in combination with other drugs such as phenylephrine, naphazoline, and tetrahydrozoline.

HOW IT WORKS
The mineral zinc is an integral component in the proper functioning of several important enzymes involved in wound healing and the general maintenance and proper hydration of certain body tissues. Zinc sulfate ophthalmic solution has a mild astringent effect (that is, it causes tissues to contract when applied topically), which can help shrink the tiny blood vessels in the whites of the eye (sclera) and thus relieve redness and irritation.

▼ DOSAGE GUIDELINES

RANGE AND FREQUENCY
Put 1 to 2 drops in the affected eye(s) up to 4 times a day.

ONSET OF EFFECT
Rapid.

DURATION OF ACTION
Up to several hours.

DIETARY ADVICE
No special restrictions.

STORAGE
Store it in a tightly sealed container away from heat and direct light. Do not allow the solution to freeze.

MISSED DOSE
Use the missed dose as soon as possible unless it is near the time for the next dose. In that case, skip the missed dose and go back to your regular schedule. Do not double the next dose.

STOPPING THE DRUG
You may stop applying this drug or resume using it after discontinuing as comfort dictates. No complications are expected.

PROLONGED USE
Eye drops containing zinc sulfate should generally not be used for self-medication for more than 3 days. If relief is not achieved in this time or if redness and irritation persist or worsen, discontinue use and contact your doctor or ophthalmologist right away.

▼ PRECAUTIONS

Over 60: No special problems are expected.

Driving and Hazardous Work: The use of this medication should not affect your ability to perform such tasks safely.

Alcohol: No special precautions are necessary.

Pregnancy: No problems are expected; however, if you are pregnant or plan to become pregnant and you have any concerns about the safe use of this or any other medication, consult your doctor.

Breast Feeding: Adequate studies on the use of ophthalmic zinc sulfate during breast feeding have not been done; however, no adverse consequences have been reported. Consult your doctor for specific advice.

Infants and Children: No specific information is available on children's use of this medication.

Special Concerns: Contact your ophthalmologist or general practitioner right away if you experience eye pain or changes in vision or if eye irritation persists for more than 72 hours. To use the eye drops, first wash your hands. Tilt your head back. Gently apply pressure to the inside corner of the lower eyelid and with the index finger of the same hand, pull downward on the eyelid to make a space. Drop the medicine into this space and close your eye. Apply pressure for 1 or 2 minutes while keeping the eye closed without blinking. Then wash your hands again. To avoid contamination, make sure that the tip of the dropper does not touch your eye, finger, or any other surface.

OVERDOSE
Symptoms: No cases of overdose have been reported.

What to Do: An overdose is unlikely to occur; in case of accidental ingestion, call your doctor, emergency medical services (EMS), or the nearest poison control center immediately.

▼ INTERACTIONS

DRUG INTERACTIONS
No drug interactions have been reported, although phenylephrine, naphazoline, and tetrahydrozoline (other medications prescribed in combination with zinc sulfate ophthalmic solution) may adversely affect the action of certain glaucoma drops. Consult your doctor first before taking any other prescription or OTC eye medications.

FOOD INTERACTIONS
No known food interactions.

DISEASE INTERACTIONS
If you have glaucoma, do not use this medication without first consulting your doctor. It is not an over-the-counter substitute for antibiotic or antiinflammatory drops. Consult your doctor for specific advice if you have any other eye disorders or a history of allergic reaction to any other ophthalmic preparations.

 SIDE EFFECTS

SERIOUS
No serious side effects have been reported.

COMMON
Overuse of this drug may cause increased eye irritation and redness.

LESS COMMON
No less common side effects have been reported.

A-to-Z
Supplement
Profiles

ACIDOPHILUS *(Lactobacillus acidophilus)*

The "friendly" bacteria called acidophilus help create a healthy environment in the gastrointestinal tract. For this reason, taking acidophilus supplements may combat a number of digestive disorders, control recurring vaginal yeast infections, and help the body resist assorted diseases caused by "unfriendly" bacteria.

COMMON USES

■ May treat chronic gastrointestinal tract disorders, such as irritable bowel syndrome, and recurrent gas and bloating caused by lactose intolerance.

■ Controls vaginal yeast infections.

■ May prevent and treat diarrhea.

FORMS

■ Capsule

■ Tablet

■ Liquid

■ Powder

■ Suppository

▼ WHAT IT IS

About 500 species of bacteria inhabit the digestive tract. Of these, the most beneficial are two strains of *Lactobacillus* bacteria, acidophilus and bifidus. Both are probiotics, meaning that they help provide a proper balance of health-promoting bacteria in the intestine. They also manufacture natural antibiotics that are able to kill dangerous microbes.

Yogurt, the traditional source of acidophilus, has been used as an elixir in folk medicine for hundreds, possibly thousands, of years. It can be difficult, however, to determine how much acidophilus is really in yogurt.

When using supplements, read labels carefully. A therapeutic form should contain at least 1 billion organisms in each pill; smaller amounts may not be potent enough to have beneficial effects. Acidophilus is sometimes sold in combination with bifidus or with another ingredient that promotes the growth of friendly bacteria called FOS (fructo-oligosaccharides).

▼ WHAT IT DOES

Acidophilus aids in restoring a normal balance of healthy bacteria in the gastrointestinal tract and vagina, thereby helping fight digestive disorders and control vaginal yeast infections. It may contain cancer-fighting agents and may lower serum cholesterol levels. Acidophilus also supplies certain vitamins, including B_{12}, K, thiamine, and folic acid.

MAJOR BENEFITS

Acidophilus may be especially useful for anyone taking antibiotics to treat an infection. A healthy colon should contain about 85% *Lactobacillus* (including acidophilus and bifidus) and 14% coliform bacteria (including healthy types of *Escherichia coli* and other bacterial strains). In many people (and particularly those on antibiotics) these counts can be upset, causing flatulence, diarrhea, constipation, and poor absorption of nutrients. Acidophilus creates an inhospitable environment for harmful types of *E. coli* bacteria,

ALERT

SIDE EFFECTS

• If ingested in large quantities, acidophilus may cause diarrhea or other gastrointestinal complaints.

• Prolonged douching with acidophilus can irritate the vagina.

• Acidophilus may interact with birth control pills, certain antianxiety drugs such as diazepam (Valium), and sulfasalazine (Azulfidine).

CAUTION

• If you have a vaginal infection for the first time, see your doctor before treating it yourself. Acidophilus is useful against the yeast *Candida albicans*, but it has little effect on other types of vaginal problems and may worsen symptoms.

• **Reminder:** If you have a medical condition, are pregnant, or have a weakened immune system, talk to your doctor before taking supplements.

as well as for salmonella, streptococcus, and many other strains of bacteria that can be dangerous.

Acidophilus may also be useful in preventing diarrhea in children.

ADDITIONAL BENEFITS
Along with a high-fiber diet, acidophilus contributes to overall colon health, which is necessary to help avert diverticulosis, a disorder in which the mucous lining of the colon bulges into the colon wall and creates small sacs (diverticula). Acidophilus may also relieve diarrhea triggered by irritable bowel syndrome and replenish beneficial intestinal microorganisms that diarrhea flushes out of the body.

Studies in animals suggest that acidophilus may help combat some cancers. When given to patients surgically treated for bladder cancer, acidophilus helped prevent the recurrence of single tumors, perhaps because acidophilus prevents harmful bacteria from creating cancer-causing substances when the bacteria react with foods. Acidophilus may also lower blood cholesterol levels. Certain strains of these bacteria absorb cholesterol in the intestine before it reaches the arteries.

Scientific studies have shown that acidophilus can improve the symptoms of asthma.

▼ HOW TO TAKE IT

DOSAGE
Doses of *Lactobacillus acidophilus* preparations are based on the number of live baceria.

For vaginal infections (adults 18 years or older):
Capsules/tablets/liquid: Take 1 to 10 billion live bacteria by tablet or capsule in divided doses daily by mouth. Vaginal suppositories: Insert 1 to 2 suppositories, each containing 10 million to 1 billion live bacteria, into the vagina once or twice daily.
Children (under 18 years): Capsules/liquid: ¼ tsp or ¼ capsule by mouth is likely safe for children to replace bacteria destroyed by antibiotics. You may apply liquid formulations to diaper area to treat yeast infections, although this use has not been proven in scientific studies..

GUIDELINES FOR USE
• When using acidophilus orally, take it 30 to 60 min before eating.

• If you are on antibiotics, do not take your prescription medication at the same time of day as the acidophilus. Continue the acidophilus even after you finish the antibiotics.

• Acidophilus is not to be taken with alcohol.

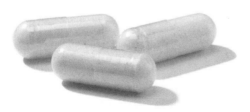

ALOE VERA *(Aloe vera, A. barbadensis, A. vulgaris)*

Since the reign of Cleopatra in ancient Egypt, the cool, soothing gel from inside the fleshy leaf of the aloe vera plant has been gently applied to treat skin problems ranging from burns and minor wounds to itchy insect bites. This clear gel is also the basis of aloe vera juice, which can calm digestive complaints.

COMMON USES

Applied topically

■ Useful in treating skin conditions, including dandruff, psoriasis, genital herpes, and canker sores.

■ May soothe skin burns and skin irritation caused by radiation therapy.

Taken internally

■ Treats constipation.

FORMS

■ Cream/Ointment ■ Capsule
■ Fresh herb/Gel ■ Softgel
■ Liquid/Juice

▼ WHAT IT IS

A succulent in the lily family, aloe vera has fleshy leaves that provide a gel widely used as a topical treatment for skin problems—a practice dating back to at least 1500 B.C., when Egyptian healers described it in their treatises.

The plant is native to the Cape of Good Hope and grows wild in much of Africa and Madagascar; commercial growers cultivate it in the Caribbean, the Mediterranean, Japan, and the United States.

▼ WHAT IT DOES

Scientists aren't exactly sure how aloe vera works, but they have identified many of its active ingredients. The gel contains a gummy material that acts as a soothing emollient, as well as brady-kininase, a compound that helps treat pain and reduce swelling, and magnesium lactate, which relieves itching.

Aloe vera also dilates the capillaries, allowing more blood to get to an injury and thus speeding healing. In addition, some studies show that it destroys or inhibits some bacteria, viruses, and fungi.

MAJOR BENEFITS

Aloe vera gel particularly helps damaged skin. It aids in the healing of first-degree burns, sunburn, minor skin wounds, and even painful shingles by relieving pain and reducing itching. Scientific evidence also supports use in the treatment of dandruff, psoriasis, and genital herpes. It may also help canker sores and treat skin irritation caused by radiation therapy. Aloe vera increases blood circula-

---

 ALERT

SIDE EFFECTS

• Topical aloe vera is very safe. In rare cases, some people get a mild allergic skin reaction with itching or rash; simply discontinue use.

• Aloe vera juice may contain small amounts of the laxative ingredient in aloe latex because of poor processing. If you experience cramping, diarrhea, or loose stools, stop taking the juice immediately. Never take aloe vera juice if you are pregnant or breast feeding.

CAUTION

• Don't confuse aloe vera with the bitter yellow aloe latex, which is sold as a laxative and can cause severe cramping and diarrhea. Pregnant or breast-feeding women in particular should avoid aloe latex.

• Do not apply to surgical wounds; it may increase the wound healing time.

• People with a history of irregular heartbeat (arrhythmia), diabetes, heart disease, or kidney diseases should not take aloe internally.

• Aloe may interact with certain medications, including those that affect blood sugar, some heart medications, diuretics ("water pills"), laxatives, oral or topical corticosteroids, some HIV medications, and herbs and supplements with similar effects.

• **Reminder:** If you have a medical condition, talk to your doctor before taking supplements.

tion, speeding the regeneration of skin and relieving mild cases of frostbite.

Although effective against minor cuts and abrasions, aloe vera may not be a good choice for more serious, infected woundsr. In a study of 21 new mothers hospitalized in Los Angeles with infected cesarean section wounds, applying the aloe vera increased the length of time—from 53 to 83 days—that it took for the abdominal wounds to heal.

ADDITIONAL BENEFITS
At this time there is insufficient evidence to recommend aloe vera to treat peptic ulcers. A U.S. commercial lab is currently conducting trials with an aloe-derived compound as a treatment for people with ulcerative colitis—a type of inflammatory bowel disease.

Other studies are exploring aloe vera's effectiveness as a possible antiviral and immune-boosting agent for people with AIDS, as a treatment for leukemia and other types of cancer, and as a therapy to help those with diabetes manage the demands of their disease.

▼ HOW TO TAKE IT

DOSAGE
For external use: Liberally apply aloe vera gel or cream to injured skin as needed or desired.
For internal use: Take ½ to ¾ cup of aloe vera juice 3 times a day or take 1 or 2 capsules as directed on the label.

GUIDELINES FOR USE
• Topically, aloe vera gel can be applied repeatedly, especially to burns. Just rub it on the affected area, let it dry, and reapply when needed. Fresh gel from a live leaf is the most potent (and economical) form. Cut off several inches from a leaf, then slice the cutting lengthwise. Spread the gel from the center of the leaf onto the affected area.

• Do not use aloe vera on deep or surgical wounds.

• For internal use, take aloe vera juice between meals. Another form of aloe called aloe latex, a yellow extract from the inner leaf, is a powerful laxative and should be used sparingly and only under a doctor's care.

SHOPPING HINTS
■ When buying aloe products, be sure aloe vera is near the top of the ingredients list. Creams and ointments should contain at least 20% aloe vera. For internal use, look for juice that contains at least 98% aloe vera and no aloin or aloe emodin.

■ The International Aloe Science Council, a voluntary certification program, provides the "IASC-certified" seal to products that use certified raw ingredients and process them according to standard guidelines. Look for this seal, especially when you are purchasing aloe vera juice.

LATEST FINDINGS
■ Add another potential use for aloe vera gel: treating the inflammatory skin condition psoriasis. A study of 60 people with long-standing psoriasis found that applying aloe to skin lesions 3 times a day for 8 months led to significant improvement in 83% of the patients, versus only 6% in those who used a placebo.

DID YOU KNOW?
Aloe vera makes a soothing bath, which is especially helpful for sunburn. Just add a cup or two of the juice to a tub of lukewarm water.

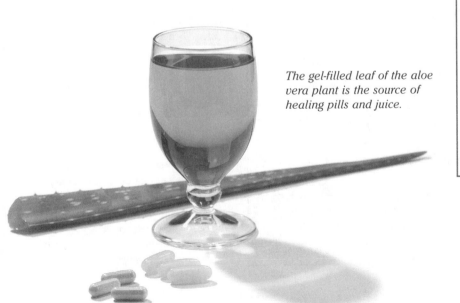

The gel-filled leaf of the aloe vera plant is the source of healing pills and juice.

ALPHA-LIPOIC ACID

This relatively recent addition to the supplement scene has shown great promise in treating nerve damage in people with diabetes. Alpha-lipoic acid also appears to protect the liver and brain cells, prevent cataracts, and serve as a powerful general antioxidant because it's easily absorbed by most tissues in the body.

COMMON USES

■ May help treat numbness, tingling, and other symptoms of nerve damage in people with diabetes or other nerve-related conditions.

■ May protect the liver from damage caused by hepatitis, alcohol abuse, or exposure to toxic chemicals.

■ May protect against glaucoma.

■ May treat memory loss associated with HIV infection.

■ May lower blood sugar in people with diabetes.

■ May protect against radiation damage.

FORMS

■ Tablet
■ Capsule

▼ WHAT IT IS

In the 1950s, scientists discovered that versatile alpha-lipoic acid (also known as thioctic acid or simply lipoic acid) worked with enzymes throughout the body to speed the processes involved in energy production. More recently, in the late 1980s, researchers found that alpha-lipoic acid can be a powerful antioxidant as well, neutralizing naturally occurring, highly reactive molecules called free radicals, which can damage cells.

Although the body manufactures it in minute amounts, alpha-lipoic acid is mainly present in foods such as spinach, meats (especially liver), and brewer's yeast. It's difficult, however, to obtain therapeutic amounts of this vitaminlike substance through diet alone. Instead, many nutritional experts recommend using supplements to get the full benefits of alpha-lipoic acid.

▼ WHAT IT DOES

Alpha-lipoic acid affects nearly every cell in the body. It assists all of the B vitamins (including thiamine, riboflavin, pantothenic acid, and niacin) in converting carbohydrates, protein, and fats found in foods into energy that the body can store and later use.

Alpha-lipoic acid is a cell-protecting antioxidant that may help the body recycle other antioxidants, such as vitamins C and E, boosting their potency. Thanks to its unique chemical properties, alpha-lipoic acid is easily absorbed by most tissues in the body, including the brain, nerves, and liver, making it valuable for treating a wide range of different ailments.

MAJOR BENEFITS
One of alpha-lipoic acid's primary uses is to treat nerve damage, including diabetic neuropathy, a dangerous long-term complication of diabetes that causes pain and loss of feeling in the limbs. The nerve condition may be caused in part by free-radical damage to nerve cells, in turn caused by runaway levels of sugar (glucose) in the blood. Alpha-lipoic acid may play a role in countering such nerve damage because of its antioxidant effects.

ALERT

SIDE EFFECTS
• Alpha-lipoic acid appears to be very safe, and there have been no reports of serious side effects in people taking it.

• Occasionally, the supplement may produce mild gastrointestinal upset, and in rare cases, allergic skin rashes have occurred. If side effects appear, lower the dose or discontinue using the supplement.

CAUTION
• For people with diabetes, the use of alpha-lipoic acid may require a change in insulin or other medications.

• **Reminder:** If you have a medical condition, especially a thyroid condition or thiamin deficiency; are pregnant or breast feeding; or are using herbs or other supplements that lower blood sugar levels, talk to your doctor before taking alpha-lipoic acid.

In addition, alpha-lipoic acid can help people with diabetes respond to insulin, the hormone that regulates glucose. In a study of 74 people with type 2 diabetes who were given 600 mg or more of alpha-lipoic acid daily, all benefited from lowered glucose levels.

Studies in animals also show that alpha-lipoic acid increases blood flow to the nerves and enhances the conduction of nerve impulses. These effects may make alpha-lipoic acid suitable for the treatment of numbness, tingling, and other symptoms of nerve damage from any cause, not just diabetes.

ADDITIONAL BENEFITS

Alpha-lipoic acid may have other potential uses, although more research is needed. Some scientific evidence shows that alpha-lipoic acid may treat glaucoma. Animal experiments suggest that it may improve memory (making it potentially beneficial against Alzheimer's disease, for example) and protect brain cells against damage caused by an insufficient blood supply to the brain (the result of surgery or stroke, for example).

Researchers have studied alpha-lipoic acid as a treatment for alcohol-related liver disease. However, no benefits have been observed, and there is not enough scientific evidence to recommend alpha-lipoic acid for this use at this time.

▼ HOW TO TAKE IT

DOSAGE

Capsules: A common dose for lowering blood sugar levels and treating diabetic nerve pain or damage (neuropathy) is 800 to 1,800 mg a day by mouth in divided doses. Experts believe that it is safe to use alpha-lipoic acid at recommended dosages for up to 2 years.

GUIDELINES FOR USE

• Alpha-lipoic acid can be taken with or without food. No major adverse effects have been reported.

• Single antioxidants such as alpha-lipoic acid are no longer recommended for use at high doses. Combination products are safer, more convenient, and less costly.

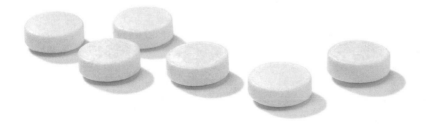

AMINO ACIDS

The protein in food and in your body is a combination of chemical units called amino acids. A diet lacking even one amino acid can have a negative effect on your health. Supplements may be needed to help your body work more efficiently and to treat medical conditions ranging from heart disease to cold sores.

COMMON USES
- Treat heart disease.
- Lower blood pressure.
- Boost immune function.
- Improve some nerve disorders.

FORMS
- Capsule
- Tablet
- Liquid
- Powder

▼ WHAT IT IS

Every cell in the body needs and uses amino acids. Your body breaks down the protein from foods into its individual amino acids, which are then recombined to create the specific types of proteins the body requires. (Each cell, in fact, is programmed to produce exactly the right combination for its particular needs.)

There are two types of amino acids: nonessential and essential. The body can manufacture nonessential amino acids but must obtain essential amino acids from the foods you eat.

Nonessential amino acids include alanine, arginine, asparagine, aspartic acid, cysteine, glutamic acid, glutamine, glycine, proline, serine, taurine, and tyrosine. Essential amino acids include histidine, isoleucine, leucine, lysine, methionine, phenylalanine, threonine, tryptophan, and valine.

▼ WHAT IT DOES

Amino acids are needed to maintain and repair muscles, tendons, skin, ligaments, organs, glands, nails, and hair. They also aid in the production of hormones (such as insulin), neurotransmitters (message-carrying chemicals within the brain), various body fluids, and enzymes that trigger bodily functions. When even one amino acid is lacking, serious health problems will eventually occur.

Though the major cause of an amino acid deficiency is a poor diet (particularly one low in protein), amino acids may also be affected by infection, trauma, stress, medications, age, and chemical imbalances within the body.

Nutritionally oriented doctors often give blood tests to determine whether a patient has a deficiency. Amino acid supplements can compensate for such deficiencies and can also be taken therapeutically (even when patients aren't deficient) for a wide variety of health problems.

MAJOR BENEFITS
Different amino acids (and their by-products) are very effective in the treatment of heart disease. Highly concentrated in the cells of the heart

---

 ALERT

SIDE EFFECTS
- Amino acid supplements have no side effects as long as they are taken in the recommended amounts. High doses of certain amino acids, however, may be toxic and can produce nausea, vomiting, or diarrhea.

CAUTION
- Pregnant women or anyone with liver or kidney disease should consult a doctor about using amino acid supplements.

- **Reminder:** If you have a medical condition, talk to your doctor before taking supplements.

muscle, carnitine—a substance similar to an amino acid that the body produces from lysine—strengthens the heart, helps those with congestive heart failure, and can improve the chances of surviving a heart attack. Because it is also involved in fat metabolism, carnitine may help lower high levels of triglycerides (blood fats related to cholesterol).

The nonessential amino acid arginine reduces the risk of heart attack and stroke by widening blood vessels and lowering blood pressure; it eases the symptoms and pains of angina as well. Taurine treats congestive heart failure and lowers high blood pressure by balancing the blood's ratio of sodium to potassium and by regulating excessive activity of the central nervous system.

N-acetylcysteine (NAC), a by-product of the amino acid cysteine that's better absorbed than cysteine, stimulates the body's production of antioxidants and may be an antioxidant itself. As such, it aids in repairing cell damage and boosting the immune system. NAC also thins the mucus of chronic bronchitis and has been used to protect the liver in overdoses of acetaminophen (Tylenol). It may also be of value for disorders involving damage to brain or nerve cells, such as multiple sclerosis.

ADDITIONAL BENEFITS

Concentrated in the cells of the digestive tract, glutamine can help heal ulcers and soothe irritable bowel syndrome and diverticulosis. By enhancing the production of certain brain chemicals, taurine may be a boon to people with epilepsy. It's also a key element in bile and may prevent gallstones. People with diabetes can also benefit from taurine because it facilitates the body's use of insulin.

Carnitine feeds the muscles by making it possible for them to burn fat for energy. Lysine is one of the most effective treatments for cold sores and is also useful for shingles and canker sores. (Arginine, on the other hand, can trigger cold sore or genital herpes outbreaks.)

▼ HOW TO TAKE IT

DOSAGE

For the recommended dosage of individual amino acids, follow label directions on the package.

When using any individual amino acid for longer than 1 month, take it with a mixed amino acid complex—a supplement that contains a variety of amino acids—to be sure you are receiving adequate, balanced amounts of all the amino acids.

GUIDELINES FOR USE

• Amino acid supplements are more effective when they don't have to compete with the amino acids in high-protein foods. Take the supplements at least an hour and a half before or after meals (first thing in the morning or at bedtime may be best).

• Individual amino acid supplements should not be used for longer than 3 months unless you are under the supervision of a doctor familiar with their use.

• Take mixed amino acid supplements on an empty stomach and not at the same time of day that you take the individual supplement.

ARNICA *(Arnica montana)*

Commonly called "leopard's bane or mountain tobacco," this bright yellow flower has been used in homeopathic medicine for hundreds of years. The plant is protected in parts of Europe, and the supplement is popular in Germany. It is often used to treat skin irritations, circulation problems, and sore muscles.

COMMON USES

- Reduces eye damage from diabetes.
- Relieves pain resulting from surgery.
- Counteracts the effects of stroke.
- Relieves muscle soreness caused by exercise.
- Treats hematoma after surgery.

FORMS

- Tablets
- Pearls
- Ointment
- Lotion
- Tincture

▼ WHAT IT IS

Arnica is a bright yellow flower with heart-shaped leaves growing to less than 2 feet height in high mountains of Europe, especially in Germany and the Swiss Alps. Arnica has been well tolerated in studies when used in very dilute (homeopathic) doses for up to 2 weeks under the supervision of a qualified health care provider.

The extract of the blossoms of the arnica plant is used in homeopathic preparations. Sesquiterpene lactones, which are thought to reduce inflammation and decrease pain, are one of the active components in arnica. Other active components include thymol (an essential oil), flavonoids, unulin, carotenoids, and tannins.

Arnica is thought to stimulate blood circulation and, theoretically, to raise blood pressure, especially in the coronary arteries. The plant is also thought to have antibacterial and antiinflammatory properties that can help reduce pain and swelling and can help heal wounds.

There are several species of arnica in addition to *Arnica montana*. Two that are native to the western United States and Canada are *Arnica cordifolia*, commonly known as heartleaf arnica, and *Arnica latifolia*, commonly known as broadleaf or mountain arnica. Healing properties of these plants are not popularly known.

 ALERT

SIDE EFFECTS

- Some people may experience stomach discomfort, including nausea and vomiting, after taking arnica internally. Liver and kidney damage has also been reported. Arnica may cause skin rashes, eczema, or lesions in the mouth. These side effects may be the result of arnica allergies.

- Arnica may also have serious side effects. It may cause muscle weakness, organ damage, coma, and death. It may cause irregular heart rhythms, rapid heartbeat, high blood pressure, or failure of heartbeat if you take it by mouth, especially in large doses. In theory, arnica may increase the risk of bleeding.

CAUTION

- Arnica is toxic when taken by mouth unless diluted in homeopathic preparations.

- People should avoid arnica if they have a known allergy to arnica or any member of the Asteraceae or Compositae plant families. Signs of allergy may include rash, itching, or shortness of breath.

- Do not use topical arnica on open wounds or near your eyes or mouth. Speak with your doctor before using arnica if you have diabetes or use blood thinners or antiplatelet drugs. It may be necessary to stop taking arnica before some surgeries. Arnica may decrease the effectiveness of drugs used to lower blood pressure.

- Arnica is not recommended for children because of potential side effects and a lack of scientific data.

Reminder: If you have a medical condition, or are pregnant or breast feeding, talk to your doctor before taking supplements.

▼ WHAT IT DOES

MAJOR BENEFITS

Some studies suggest that arnica in very dilute (homeopathic) doses may improve vision in people with eye damage caused by diabetes, may relieve pain after surgery, and may have beneficial effects for individuals who have suffered a stroke. Further studies comparing arnica with standard treatments are needed.

ADDITIONAL BENEFITS

Arnica has been used to treat the following conditions, but it's effectiveness for these uses has *absolutely not* been scientifically proven: abscesses, acne, fungal infections, aphthous ulcers, asthma, bad breath, bedsores, blindness, blood clots, boils, bronchitis, bruises, chest pain, clogged arteries, concussion, contusion, corns, coronary artery disease, cough, cramps, decongestant, dental pain, diabetes, diarrhea, fever, fibrositis, flu, gallstones, gum disease, hair loss, healing wounds, heart disorders, high cholesterol, immune system stimulation, inflammation, insect bites, joint pain,

kidney problems, miscarriage, pain, paralysis, phlebitis, pleural effusions, poor circulation, rheumatoid arthritis, sore throat, sweating, swelling after broken bones, thirst, tumors, and whooping cough. Arnica is also used as an antiseptic.

▼ HOW TO TAKE IT

DOSAGE

Adults: 2 to 3 tablets or pearls 2 to 3 times daily by mouth.

Ointment or lotion: Use ointments that consist of 20% to 25% arnica tincture or 15% arnica oil. Apply to sore areas 2 to 3 times daily.

GUIDELINES FOR USE

■ Some doctors recommend taking arnica more frequently before and after some surgeries.

■ You may swallow doses or dissolve them under your tongue.

■ Safety of use beyond 2 weeks has not been thoroughly studied.

■ Do not use arnica if you are pregnant or breast feeding. Studies indicate an increased risk of birth defects or spontaneous abortion.

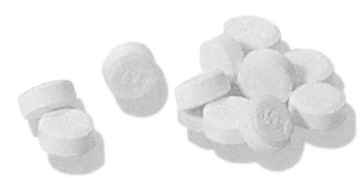

Arnica, shown here in tablet form, is made from the yellow blossoms of the plant.

ASTRAGALUS *(Astragalus membranaceous)*

For more than 2,000 years, astragalus has been an integral part of traditional medicine in China, where it is used to balance the life force, or *qi*. Because of its powerful effect on the immune system, this herb is particularly valuable for fighting disease and for dealing with the aftereffects of cancer treatments.

COMMON USES

■ Helps fight respiratory infections.

■ May fight cancer and reduce chemotherapy side effects.

■ May stimulate the immune system and increase white blood cell counts.

■ May be beneficial for certain diseases of the heart or kidneys, and may protect the liver.

FORMS

■ Tablet

■ Capsule

■ Liquid extract

■ Dried herb/Tea

▼ WHAT IT IS

Astragalus contains a variety of compounds that stimulate the body's immune system. In China, this native plant has long been used both to treat and to prevent disease.

Botanically, astragalus is related to licorice and the pea. Although its sweet-smelling pale yellow blossoms and delicate structure give the plant a frail appearance, it is actually a very hardy species.

Medicinally, the herb's most important part is its root. The plant is harvested when it is 4 to 7 years old; its flat, yellowish roots resemble wide popsicle sticks or tongue depressors. (The Chinese name for astragalus, *huang qi*, means "yellow leader," a testament both to its color and to its importance as a therapeutic herb.) Astragalus root is loaded with health-promoting substances, including polysaccharides, a class of carbohydrates that appear to be responsible for the herb's immune-boosting effects.

▼ WHAT IT DOES

A tonic in the truest sense of the word, astragalus seems to enhance overall health by improving a person's resistance to disease, increasing stamina and vitality, and by promoting general well-being. It also acts as an antioxidant, helping the body correct or prevent cell damage caused by free radicals. It may have antiviral and antibiotic properties as well.

PREVENTION

This herb is particularly effective in fighting off colds, the flu, bronchitis, and sinus infections because it keeps viruses from gaining a foothold in the respiratory system. Like echinacea, astragalus can kill germs at the first sign of symptoms.

If an illness does develop, astragalus can shorten its duration and often reduce its severity. People who frequently suffer from respiratory problems should consider using astragalus on a regular basis to prevent recurrences. It also appears to help minimize the health-damaging effects of excessive stress.

ADDITIONAL BENEFITS

Astragalus is widely used in China to rebuild the immune system of people undergoing radiation or chemotherapy for cancer; this practice is gaining popularity in the West as well. The herb is especially valuable because it increases the body's production of white blood cells. For this reason, it may be useful in treating patients with low white blood cell counts.

Some evidence shows that astragalus may be beneficial for treating conditions of the heart, including coronary artery disease, heart failure, and infections of the heart (myocarditis and endocarditis). It may also protect the liver and be useful in the treatment of kidney failure.

▼ HOW TO TAKE IT

DOSAGE

For strengthening the immune system: Take 250 to 500 mg of astragalus 4 times daily. Astralagus is often a component of multiherb mixtures. For proper dosage, follow directions on the label.
For acute bronchitis: Take 250 to 500 mg 4 times a day until the symptoms lessen. Always try to choose a product that contains a standardized extract of astragalus, with 0.5% glucosides and 70% polysaccharides.

GUIDELINES FOR USE

• The herb astragalus can be taken at any time during the day with or without food.

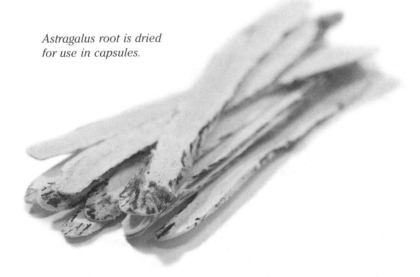

Astragalus root is dried for use in capsules.

BEE PRODUCTS

Many intriguing claims have been made for the natural healing powers of bee products over the years, but there is little scientific evidence to support most of them. Yet bee pollen, royal jelly, and propolis remain popular nutritional supplements, and they continue to be the subject of ongoing research studies.

COMMON USES

- May help hay fever symptoms.
- Aid in healing skin abrasions.
- May treat a variety of dental complaints.
- May treat certain viruses and bacterial and parisitic infections.
- May prevent colds.
- May treat rheumatic diseases.

FORMS

- Tablet
- Capsule
- Softgel
- Liquid
- Powder/Granules
- Cream
- Lozenge
- Dried and fresh pollen

▼ WHAT IT IS

There are three types of bee products available in health food stores: bee pollen, propolis, and royal jelly. The most familiar of these is bee pollen. After the bees gather pollen from plants, they compress it into pellets, which beekeepers then collect from the hives. (A second type of pollen, also sold as bee pollen, is collected directly from plants, not from bees at all.) Bee pollen contains protein, B vitamins, carbohydrates, and various enzymes.

Propolis (also called bee glue) is a sticky resin that bees collect from the buds of pine trees and use to repair cracks in their hives. Then there's royal jelly, a milky white substance produced by the salivary glands of worker bees as a food source for the queen bee.

The specialized nutritional content of royal jelly may account for the fertility, large size, and increased longevity of the queen.

▼ WHAT IT DOES

Bee products, especially bee pollen, have been touted as virtual cure-alls. Proponents assert that, among other things, these products slow aging, improve athletic performance, boost immunity, contribute to weight loss, fight bacteria, and alleviate the symptoms of allergies and hay fever.

Although bee pollen shows some promise in treating allergies and propolis may be an effective salve for cuts and bruises, the scant research that has been conducted does not support the extravagant claims generally made for bee products.

MAJOR BENEFITS

Bee pollen seems to help prevent the sneezing, runny nose, watery eyes, and other symptoms of seasonal pollen allergies. Some scientists believe that ingesting small amounts of pollen can desensitize an individual to its allergenic compounds, much as allergy shots do. Because your body produces antibodies when exposed to even a tiny amount of pollen, your immune system then "remembers" it, preventing an extreme reaction that causes classic allergy symptoms.

 ALERT

SIDE EFFECTS

- Because some individuals will have an allergic reaction to bee pollen, begin with a small amount so you can determine if it will have an adverse effect on you. Watch for hives, itchy throat, skin flushing, wheezing, or headache. Discontinue use immediately if any of these reactions occur.

CAUTION

- People with asthma or allergies to bee stings should be very careful when using bee products; they should avoid royal jelly entirely.

- **Reminder:** If you have a medical condition, talk to your doctor before taking supplements.

Testing of this theory is under way, and until results are available, there appears to be no harm for most people in trying bee pollen. Various advocates maintain that to get the full antiallergy benefit, you need to use bee pollen that comes from a local source, which will desensitize you to the specific pollens in your own environment.

ADDITIONAL BENEFITS

Bee propolis may play some role as a skin softener or wound healer. Research has shown that although propolis contains antibacterial compounds, these are not as effective as standard antibiotics or over-the-counter antibiotic ointments at fighting infection.

Propolis may also fight dental plaque and gingivitis, ease dental pain, speed dental wound healing, and fight bacterial and parasitic infections. It may also prevent colds and reduce inflammation in rheumatic diseases.

Because royal jelly enhances the growth, fertility, and longevity of queen bees, many people think that it will do the same thing for humans. There's no evidence to support this view, however, so there appears to be little reason to use royal jelly.

▼ HOW TO TAKE IT

DOSAGE

The amount of bee pollen needed to relieve allergy symptoms varies from person to person. In general, start with a few granules a day and increase the dose gradually until you're up to 1 to 3 rounded tsp a day.

Dental plaque: Swish 2 tsp of 0.2% to 10% propolis ethanol extract mouthwash in your mouth for 60 to 90 seconds, then spit. Do this once or twice daily.
Infections: Safety and effectiveness of particular dosages have not been established.

GUIDELINES FOR USE

• Prior to hay fever season, start taking very small amounts of bee pollen each day—a few granules or a portion of a tablet. If you don't suffer any adverse reaction (see Alert box, opposite), slowly increase your dosage every few days until you experience relief from your allergy symptoms.

• Take bee pollen supplements with plenty of water; you can also mix dried or fresh pollen with juice or sprinkle it over food.

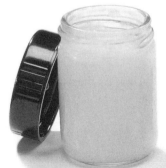
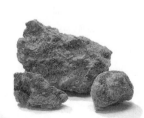
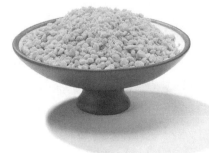

The three types of bee products on the market are royal jelly (left), propolis (center), and bee pollen (right).

BETA-CAROTENE

Once considered just a potent source of vitamin A, beta-carotene has recently gained prominence as a disease-fighting substance. Today, experts think that beta-carotene—along with a number of related nutrients called carotenoids—may protect against such serious illnesses as heart disease and cancer.

COMMON USES

■ Acts as a preventive for cancer and heart disease.

■ May reverse some precancerous conditions.

■ Has cell-protecting properties that may aid in the treatment of a wide variety of ailments, from Alzheimer's disease to male infertility.

FORMS

■ Capsule
■ Tablet
■ Softgel
■ Liquid

▼ WHAT IT IS

Beta-carotene is part of a larger team of nutrients known as carotenoids, which are the yellow-orange pigments found in fruits and vegetables (see page 350). Because the body converts it to vitamin A, beta-carotene is sometimes called provitamin A. However, beta-carotene provides many benefits in addition to supplying vitamin A.

▼ WHAT IT DOES

An immune system booster and powerful antioxidant, beta-carotene helps neutralize the free radicals that can damage cells and promote disease. By acting directly on cells, it combats—and may even reverse—some disorders. It appears to be most effective when combined with other carotenoids.

PREVENTION

Beta-carotene is a celebrated soldier in the war on heart disease. Results from a survey of more than 300 doctors enrolled in the Harvard University Physicians' Health Study revealed that taking 50 mg (85,000 IU) of beta-carotene a day cut the risk of heart attack, stroke, and all cardiovascular deaths in half. Other studies have shown that it can prevent LDL ("bad") cholesterol from damaging the heart and coronary vessels. High levels of beta-carotene may also offer protection against cancers of the lung, digestive tract, bladder, breast, and prostate.

MAJOR BENEFITS

Acting as an antioxidant, beta-carotene has reversed some precancerous conditions, particularly those affecting the skin, mucous membranes, lungs, mouth, throat, stomach, colon, prostate, cervix, and uterus. It also has been shown to inhibit the growth of abnormal cells, strengthen the immune system, fortify cell membranes, and increase communication among cells.

One hint of concern has come up, however, about beta-carotene's cancer-fighting benefits. In the early 1990s, landmark studies in Finland and the United States found that male smokers taking beta-carotene supplements had an increased risk of lung cancer. Although some found the studies flawed, many experts caution smokers

---

 ALERT

CAUTION

• Consult your physician before using beta-carotene if you have a sluggish thyroid (hypothyroidism), kidney or liver disease, or an eating disorder.

• Many experts recommend that smokers, particularly those who consume large amounts of alcohol, avoid beta-carotene supplements.

• Don't take more than 50,000 IU of beta-carotene daily.

• **Reminder:** If you have a medical condition, talk to your doctor before taking supplements.

to maintain adequate beta-carotene levels through natural food sources, not through dietary supplements.

ADDITIONAL BENEFITS

As an antioxidant, beta-carotene may be helpful for a wide range of additional ailments, including Alzheimer's disease, chronic fatigue syndrome, male infertility, fibromyalgia, psoriasis, and a number of vision disorders.

▼ HOW MUCH YOU NEED

There is no recommended daily allowance (RDA) for beta-carotene, although about 10,000 IU meets the RDA for vitamin A. Higher doses are needed, however, to provide the full antioxidant and immune-boosting effects. Some findings (including the Finnish smokers study), however, showed that megadoses may do more harm than good. For this reason, it's advisable to limit your upper daily intake to no more than 50,000 IU daily.

IF YOU GET TOO LITTLE

Signs of a beta-carotene deficiency are similar to those of inadequate vitamin A: poor night vision, dry skin, increased risk of infection, and the formation of precancerous cells. A deficiency may also increase your risk of cancer and heart disease. However, vitamin A deficiencies are rare. Even if you don't eat fruits and vegetables or take supplements, you can still meet your vitamin A needs with eggs, fortified milk, or other foods that supply it.

IF YOU GET TOO MUCH

For the most part, the body discards what beta-carotene it doesn't process. If you ingest high levels in foods or supplements (more than 100,000 IU a day), your palms and soles may acquire a harmless orange tone, which will disappear when you lower the dose.

▼ HOW TO TAKE IT

DOSAGE

Beta-carotene is probably most effective when combined with other carotenoids in a mixed carotenoid formula. Most people benefit from one dose daily of a mixed carotenoid supplement that provides 25,000 IU vitamin A activity. If you are at particularly high risk for cancer or heart disease, consider increasing your dose to two mixed carotenoid pills daily.

GUIDELINES FOR USE

• Take supplements with meals.

• No adverse effects have been noted in pregnant or nursing women taking up to 50,000 IU a day.

▼ OTHER SOURCES

Carrots are a rich source of beta-carotene, as are other yellow, orange, and red fruits and vegetables, from sweet potatoes to cantaloupe. Green vegetables, such as broccoli, spinach, or lettuce, are also beneficial—the darker the green, the more beta-carotene they contain.

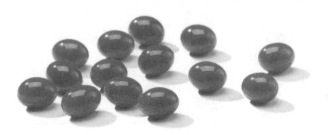

BILBERRY *(Vaccinium myrtillus)*

During World War II, British RAF pilots noted the curious fact that their night vision improved after they had eaten bilberry preserves. Their anecdotal reports sparked scientific research on this herb, which today is used to treat a wide range of visual disorders—from night blindness to cataracts—as well as other complaints.

COMMON USES

- May improve hardening of the arteries (atheroslerosis).
- May relieve painful menstruation and fibrocystic breast disease.
- May treat stomach ulcers and diarrhea.
- May improve a wide array of eye disorders, including diabetic retinopathy, cataracts, and macular degeneration, and may improve vision, in general.

FORMS

- Tablet
- Capsule
- Softgel
- Liquid extract
- Dried herb/Tea

▼ WHAT IT IS

Although the fruit of the bilberry bush has been enjoyed since prehistoric times, its first recorded medicinal use was in the sixteenth century. Historically, dried berry or leaf preparations were recommended for a variety of conditions, including scurvy (a disease caused by a severe vitamin C deficiency), urinary tract infections, and kidney stones.

A relative of the American blueberry, bilberry is a short, shrubby perennial that grows in the forests and wooded meadows of northern Europe. Bushes of these sweet blue-black berries are also found in western Asia and the Rocky Mountains of North America.

The medically active components in the ripe fruit consist primarily of flavonoid compounds known as anthocyanosides. Accordingly, the modern medicinal form of bilberry is an extract containing a highly concentrated amount of these compounds.

▼ WHAT IT DOES

Many of the medicinal qualities of bilberry derive from its major constituents, anthocyanosides, which are potent antioxidants. These compounds help counteract cell damage caused by unstable oxygen molecules called free radicals.

MAJOR BENEFITS

Bilberry extract is the leading herbal remedy for maintaining healthy vision and managing various eye disorders. In particular, bilberry helps the retina, the light-sensitive portion of the eye, adapt properly to both dark and light.

With its ability to strengthen tiny blood vessels (capillaries)—and, in turn, facilitate the delivery of oxygen-rich blood to the eyes—bilberry may also play a significant role in preventing and treating degenerative diseases of the retina (retinopathy). In one study, 31 patients were treated with bilberry extract daily for 4 weeks. Use of the extract fortified the capillaries and reduced hemorrhaging in the eyes, especially in cases of diabetes-related retinopathy.

Bilberry is useful for preventing macular degeneration (a progressive disor-

---

 ALERT

SIDE EFFECTS
- Possible side effects include bleeding, stomach upset, diarrhea, low blood sugar, poisoning (hydroquinone), and low blood pressure. It's a good idea to avoid taking more than 480 mg of bilberry a day.

CAUTION
- Use bilberry cautiously if you are allergic to members of the Ericaceae family or to anthocyanosides (a constituent of bilberry).

- **Reminder:** If you are taking medication for, or have a history of, low blood pressure, bleeding, diabetes, blood clots, or stroke, or are pregnant or breast feeding, talk to your doctor before taking supplements.

der affecting the central part of the retina) and cataracts (loss of transparency of the eye's lens)—two leading causes of vision loss in older people. A study of 50 patients with age-related cataracts found that bilberry extract combined with vitamin E supplements inhibited cataract formation in almost all of the participants.

Because it can strengthen collagen—the abundant protein that forms the "backbone" of healthy connective tissue—bilberry may also be valuable in preventing and treating glaucoma, a disease caused by excessive pressure within the eye.

ADDITIONAL BENEFITS

Because the anthocyanosides in bilberry improve blood flow in capillaries, as well as in larger blood vessels, bilberry in standardized extract form may be worthwhile for people with poor circulation in their extremities.

Although more study is needed, limited data indicate that bilberry may have other uses as well. One study showed that long-term use of bilberry extract improved the vision of normally nearsighted people—although how it produced this effect is unknown.

Preliminary results in women show that bilberry helps treat menstrual cramps because anthocyanosides relax smooth muscle, including the uterus. Studies have also shown that it may improve fibrocystic breast disease. Research studies done in animals suggest that bilberry anthocyanosides may fight stomach ulcers.

▼ HOW TO TAKE IT

DOSAGE

Normal dosages range from 40 mg to 160 mg of bilberry extract 2 or 3 times a day. The lower dose is generally recommended for long-term use, including prevention of macular degeneration; higher doses—up to 320 mg a day—may be needed to prevent retinal disease associated with diabetes.

GUIDELINES FOR USE

• Bilberry can be taken with or without food.

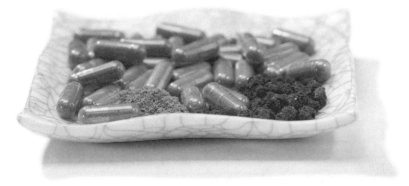

Bilberry, available in capsule form, is now a popular herbal remedy for treating a number of eye disorders.

BIOTIN AND PANTOTHENIC ACID

It's surprising that these two members of the B-vitamin family don't get more attention. They work together at the most basic level to produce enzymes that trigger many bodily functions. In addition, biotin promotes healthy hair and nails and pantothenic acid appears to play a valuable role in how the body deals with stress.

COMMON USES

Biotin

■ Promotes healthy nails and hair.

■ Helps the body use carbohydrates, fats, and protein.

Pantothenic acid

■ Promotes healthy function of the central nervous system.

■ Helps the body use carbohydrates, fats, and protein.

FORMS

■ Capsule

■ Tablet

■ Softgel

■ Liquid

▼ WHAT IT IS

The names of these two vitamins suggest their widespread presence in the body. Both words have Greek roots: *pantothenic* from *pantos*, which means "everywhere," and *biotin* from *bios,* which means "life."

Because these vitamins are in many foods, deficiencies are virtually nonexistent. Biotin is also produced by intestinal bacteria, although this form may be difficult for the body to use.

Multivitamins and B-complex vitamins usually include biotin and pantothenic acid (also called vitamin B_5), and both are also available as individual supplements. The main form of biotin is D-biotin. Pantothenic acid comes in two forms: pantethine and calcium pantothenate. The latter is suitable for most purposes and is less expensive than pantethine.

▼ WHAT IT DOES

Both biotin and pantothenic acid are involved in the breakdown of carbohydrates, fats, and protein from foods and in the production of enzymes. Biotin plays a special role in helping the body use glucose, its basic fuel, and it promotes healthy nails and hair. The body needs pantothenic acid to maintain proper communication between the brain and nervous system and to produce certain stress hormones.

MAJOR BENEFITS

Biotin improves the quality of weak and brittle fingernails and may help slow hair loss caused by biotin deficiency. Research suggests that the overproduction of stress hormones during long periods of emotional upset, depression, or anxiety increases the need for pantothenic acid, which is used to manufacture these hormones.

ADDITIONAL BENEFITS

In high doses, biotin may help people with diabetes, increasing the body's response to insulin so blood sugar (glucose) levels stay low. In addition, it may protect against the nerve damage that sometimes occurs in diabetes (called diabetic neuropathy).

▼ HOW MUCH YOU NEED

There is no RDA for biotin or pantothenic acid, but an adequate intake

 ALERT

SIDE EFFECTS

• Diarrhea can result from taking 10 (10,000 mg) or more of pantothenic acid a day.

CAUTION

• Very high doses of biotin (more than 8 mg a day) used to treat diabetes may alter insulin requirements.

• **Reminder:** If you have a medical condition, talk to your doctor before taking supplements.

(AI) has been established. For biotin it is 30 µg and for pantothenic acid 5 mg a day for both men and women. These amounts appear to be enough to maintain normal body functioning, but for treating specific diseases or disorders, higher doses may be needed.

IF YOU GET TOO LITTLE

Deficiencies of biotin or pantothenic acid are virtually unknown in adults. Long-term use of antibiotics or anti-seizure medications, however, can lead to less than optimal levels of biotin.

IF YOU GET TOO MUCH

There are no known serious adverse effects from high doses of biotin or pantothenic acid. Some people report diarrhea when taking doses of 10 g a day or more of pantothenic acid.

▼ HOW TO TAKE IT

DOSAGE

For hair and nails: Take 1,000 to 1,200 µg of biotin a day.

For diabetes: Talk with your doctor about taking high doses of biotin to help or even prevent diabetic neuropathy.

GUIDELINES FOR USE

• Most people will get enough biotin and pantothenic acid from a daily multivitamin or a B-complex supplement. Individual supplements are necessary only to treat a specific disorder.

• In most cases, take individual supplements with meals.

▼ OTHER SOURCES

Biotin is found in liver, soy products, nuts, oatmeal, rice, barley, legumes, cauliflower, egg yolks, milk, and whole wheat. Organ meats, fish, poultry, whole grains, yogurt, and legumes are the best sources of pantothenic acid.

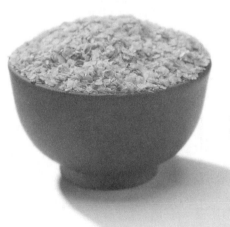

Wheat germ is a good food source of pantothenic acid, one of the B vitamins.

BLACK COHOSH *(Cimicifuga racemosa)*

Although baby boomers may claim black cohosh as the new "in" herb, its healing abilities were clearly recognized more than a century ago, when Native American and pioneer women singled out the root of this plant as one of the most useful natural medicines for treating menstrual and menopausal complaints.

COMMON USES

 Reduces menopausal symptoms, including hot flashes, mood disturbances, excessive sweating, palpitations, and vaginal dryness.

 Works as an antiinflammatory; relieves muscle pain.

FORMS

- Capsule
- Tablet
- Tincture
- Dried herb/Tea

▼ WHAT IT IS

Long used to treat "women's problems," black cohosh ("black" describes the dark color of the root; "cohosh" is derived from an Algonquian word for "rough") grows up to 8 feet high and is distinguished by its tall stalks of fluffy white flowers. This member of the buttercup family is also known as bugbane, squawroot, rattle root, or *Cimicifuga racemosa,* its botanical name.

This herb's most common nickname, black snakeroot, describes its gnarled root, the part of the plant that is used medicinally. Contained in the root is a complex network of natural chemicals, some of them as powerful as the most modern pharmaceuticals.

▼ WHAT IT DOES

Traditionally, black cohosh has long been prescribed to treat menstrual problems, pain after childbirth, nervous disorders, and joint pain. Today, the herb is recommended primarily for relief of the hot flashes that some women experience during menopause.

MAJOR BENEFITS

In Europe and increasingly in the United States, black cohosh is a popular remedy for hot flashes, vaginal dryness, and other menopausal symptoms. Scientific study has shown that black cohosh can reduce levels of LH (luteinizing hormone), which is produced by the brain's pituitary gland. The rise in LH that occurs during menopause is thought to be one cause of hot flashes.

In addition, black cohosh contains phytoestrogens, plant compounds that have an effect similar to that of estrogen produced by the body. Phytoestrogens bind to hormone receptors in the breast and uterus and elsewhere in the body, easing menopausal symptoms without increasing the risk of breast cancer, a possible side effect of

≡ ALERT ≡

SIDE EFFECTS

- Possible side effects include reduced pulse rate, headache, dizziness, sweating, visual disturbances, constipation, osteoporosis, nausea, and vomiting.

CAUTION

- Never use black cohosh while pregnant or breast feeding.

- The herb's safety and effectiveness remain unclear for women with estrogen-sensitive cancers.

- This herb may interfere with hormonal medications (birth control pills, estrogens, or antiestrogens), so check with your doctor.

- Be careful if you're on a hypertension medication; black cohosh may intensify the drug's blood pressure–lowering effect.

- If you are allergic to aspirin or members of the Ranunculaceae family, such as buttercups or crowfoot; if you have a history of blood clots, stroke, or seizures; or if you are taking medications to thin the blood, such as warfarin (Coumadin) or aspirin, you should not take black cohosh.

- **Reminder:** If you have a medical condition or are taking hormonal medications, talk to your doctor before taking this supplement.

hormone replacement therapy (HRT). In fact, some experts believe phytoestrogens may even help prevent breast cancer by keeping the body's own estrogen from locking onto breast cells.

ADDITIONAL BENEFITS

Although these effects are less frequently noted, black cohosh has demonstrated some mildly sedating and antiinflammatory capabilities, which may be particularly valuable in treating muscle aches as well as in relieving nerve-related pain such as sciatica or neuralgia.

▼ HOW TO TAKE IT

DOSAGE

For menopausal symptoms: Take 20 to 40 mg of black cohosh tablets twice daily or 40 drops of a liquid extract. If the dried root of the herb is used, 40 to 200 mg may be taken in divided doses, up to a maximum of 3 g of dried root a day.

GUIDELINES FOR USE

• Black cohosh can be taken at any time of day, but to reduce the chance of stomach upset, you may prefer to use it with meals.

• Allow 4 to 8 weeks to see its benefits. Many experts recommend a 6-month limit on taking black cohosh, although some studies have shown that longer use seems to be safe and free of significant side effects.

The root of black cohosh is dried, ground to a powder, and sold as a supplement in capsule form.

CALCIUM

Renowned for preventing—or at least minimizing—the devastating effects of osteoporosis (age-related bone thinning), calcium is now also thought to lower high blood pressure and help prevent colon cancer. Because this important mineral is often seriously lacking in the modern American diet, supplements may be needed.

COMMON USES

■ Maintains bones and teeth.

■ Helps prevent progressive bone loss and osteoporosis.

■ Aids heart and muscle contraction, nerve impulses, and blood clotting.

■ May help lower blood pressure in people with hypertension.

■ Eases heartburn.

FORMS

■ Tablet

■ Capsule

■ Softgel

■ Powder

■ Liquid

▼ WHAT IT IS

Although it's the most abundant mineral in the body, most adults get only half the calcium they need each day. Eating enough calcium-rich foods may be difficult, but you can prevent a deficiency by taking supplements.

A wide array of products line store shelves. The most common forms are calcium carbonate, calcium citrate, calcium citrate malate, calcium gluconate, calcium phosphate, and calcium lactate. A supplement's elemental (or pure) calcium depends on its accompanying compound. Calcium carbonate (useful in antacids to relieve heartburn) provides 40% elemental calcium, whereas calcium gluconate supplies 9%.

The lower the calcium content, the more pills you need to meet recommended amounts. The amount of elemental calcium you absorb (and use) differs too; for most people, the elemental calcium in calcium citrate is absorbed best.

▼ WHAT IT DOES

The majority of the body's calcium is stored in the bones and teeth, where it provides strength and structure. The small amount circulating in the bloodstream helps move nutrients across cell membranes and plays a role in producing the hormones and enzymes that regulate digestion and metabolism. Calcium is also needed for normal communication among nerve cells as well as for blood clotting, wound healing, and muscle contraction.

To have enough of this mineral available in the blood to perform vital functions, the body will steal it from the bones. Over time, too many calcium withdrawals leave bones porous and fragile. Only an adequate daily calcium intake will maintain healthy levels in the blood—and provide enough extra for the bones to absorb as a reserve.

PREVENTION
Getting enough calcium throughout life is a central factor in preventing osteoporosis, the bone-thinning disease that leads to a higher risk of hip and vertebral fractures, spinal deformities, and loss of height. The body is best equipped to absorb calcium and build up

bone mass before age 35, but it's never too late to increase your intake of it. Several studies show that even for people over age 65, taking calcium supplements and eating calcium-rich foods help maintain bone density and reduce the risk of fractures.

ADDITIONAL BENEFITS

By limiting the irritating effects of bile acids in the colon, calcium may reduce the incidence of colon cancer. Other research indicates that diets including plenty of calcium—as well as fruits and vegetables—may actually help lower blood pressure as much as some prescription medications.

▼ HOW MUCH YOU NEED

Official dietary guidelines, now called adequate intake (AI) levels, have been increased to reflect new findings about the body's daily calcium needs. The AI is currently 1,000 mg for men and women ages 19 to 50 and 1,200 mg for ages 51 to 70 and older.

IF YOU GET TOO LITTLE

A prolonged calcium deficiency can lead to bone abnormalities, such as osteoporosis. Muscle spasms can result from low levels of calcium in the blood.

IF YOU GET TOO MUCH

A daily calcium intake as high as 2,500 mg from a combination of food and supplements appears to be safe. However, taking calcium supplements may impair the body's absorption of zinc, iron, and magnesium. Very high doses of calcium from supplements might lead to kidney stones. Calcium carbonate may cause gas or constipation; if this becomes a problem, switch to calcium citrate.

▼ HOW TO TAKE IT

DOSAGE

Be sure to get the recommended amount of 1,000 to 1,200 mg of elemental calcium a day from foods, supplements, or both. It's often a good idea to add supplemental magnesium when taking calcium.

GUIDELINES FOR USE

• To enhance absorption, divide your supplement dose so that you don't consume more than 600 mg of calcium at any one time.

• Be sure to take the supplements with food.

▼ OTHER SOURCES

The most familiar and plentiful sources of calcium are dairy products, such as milk, yogurt, and cheese. Choose low-fat or nonfat varieties; they're better for you and also contain slightly more calcium, ounce for ounce.

Orange juice fortified with calcium malate, canned salmon and sardines (eaten with the soft bones), collard greens, arugula, broccoli, and almonds are good nondairy sources.

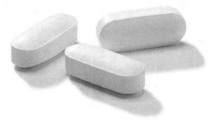

CALENDULA *(Calendula officinalis)*

Calendula, commonly called the marigold, is an annual with yellow to deep orange flower heads produced through a long blooming season. It was a popular garden flower in Shakespeare's time, as it is today. It has been used medicinally throughout central Europe and the Mediterranean since the twelfth century.

COMMON USES

- Aids in wound healing
- Relieves skin inflammation
- Relieves pain
- Treats ear infection

FORMS

- Ointment
- Ear drops
- Tincture

▼ WHAT IT IS

Calendula *(Calendula officinalis)*, also known as marigold, has been widely used topically to treat minor skin wounds, skin infections, burns, bee stings, sunburn, warts, and cancer. Most scientific evidence regarding its ability to heal wounds is based on animal and laboratory studies; there is virtually no evidence of its effects on humans.

Calendula is an annual flower in the daisy family that grows to a height of 12 to18 inches and is native to Asia and southern Europe. Calendula has been cultivated for centuries in ornamental gardens, where it readily grows in poor soils.

The principal active components of calendula are triterpenoids and flavonoids; these are often thought to have antiinflammatory, immunostimulating, antibacterial, antiviral, antiprotozoal, antineoplastic, and numerous other pharmacological properties. The reasons they act as they do are poorly understood.

▼ WHAT IT DOES

MAJOR BENEFITS

A few studies suggest that applying calendula to the skin speeds the healing of wounds caused by burns, ulcers, cuts, or skin irritation. It is

ALERT

SIDE EFFECTS

- Calendula may lower blood pressure.

- Based on the high doses of calendula used in animal studies, calendula may, in theory, increase the drowsiness caused by some drugs. It is not clear, however, if using calendula topically will have this effect.

CAUTION

- Calendula is thought to be safe when used externally or topically (on the skin); it should NOT be taken by mouth.

- People with allergies to plants in the Asteraceae or Compositae families (including ragweed, chrysanthemums, marigolds, and daisies) may be more likely to have allergic reactions to calendula. One case of anaphylactic shock (severe allergic reaction) was reported after gargling with calendula.

- Do not use calendula while pregnant or breast feeding. In animal studies, calendula has had effects on the uterus, and it has traditionally been thought to have harmful effects on sperm and to cause abortion. Topical applications may not be harmful; studies are not clear on this.

- If you are taking calendula, exercise caution when driving or operating machinery.

- If you have low blood pressure or are taking blood pressure medications or supplements that may cause drowsiness, exercise caution while using calendula.

Reminder: If you have a medical condition, talk to your doctor before taking supplements.

thought to heal by speeding cell growth and repair. These studies, however, have been small, low quality, and not fully convincing.

Animal studies suggest that calendula may have antiinflammatory properties if applied to irritated areas, but studies in humans are lacking.

Early evidence suggests that calendula may possess mild anesthetic (pain-relieving) properties and may be helpful in treating pain related to ear infections. Further studies are needed before a recommendation can be made.

ADDITIONAL BENEFITS

Calendula has been used to treat the following conditions, although its effects *are unproven:* abscesses, acne, anemia, anxiety, atherosclerosis (clogged arteries), athlete's foot, bladder irritation, blood clots, blood purification, bowel diseases, bruises, circulation problems, constipation, cough, cramps, diaper rash, diaphoresis (increased sweating), diarrhea, diuresis (increased urination), dizziness, eczema, eye inflammation, fatigue, fever, frostbite, gastrointestinal tract disorders, gout, headache, heart disease, hemorrhoids, herpes, HIV infection, immune stimulation, infections (bacterial, viral, fungal), various inflammations and swellings, influenza, insomnia, jaundice, lack of menstrual period, liver and gallbladder disease, metabolic disorders, mouth and throat infection and irritation, muscle spasms, muscular degeneration, nausea, nosebleeds, poor appetite, prostate enlargement, prostatitis, skin cancer, sore throat, spleen disorders, stomach ulcers, syphilis, tinnitus, toothache, tuberculosis, ulcerative colitis, urinary retention, uterus problems, varicose veins, warts, and yeast infections

▼ HOW TO TAKE IT

DOSAGE

Ointment: Apply 2% to 5% to the affected area of skin 3 to 4 times daily for wound healing or skin inflammation
Tincture: Use 1:1 in 40% alcohol or 1:5 in 90% alcohol, diluted to at least 1:3 with freshly boiled water; apply to the skin as a compress 3 to 4 times daily.
Ear drops: Calendula is one of several herbs in a commercially available product called Otikon Otic Solution. Use 5 drops in the affected ear 3 times daily. Consult your doctor if you experience ear pain.

GUIDELINES FOR USE

• The dosing for and safety of calendula use by children have not been studied thoroughly, so calendula cannot be recommended at this time.

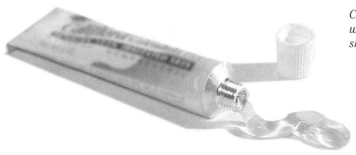

Calendula ointment aids in wound healing and relieves skin irritations.

CAROTENOIDS

The built-in pigments that give some fruits and vegetables their rich red, orange, and yellow colors are called carotenoids. Scientists are now discovering that these natural compounds are also potent disease fighters. If your diet doesn't contain enough of them, nutritional supplements can be a handy option.

COMMON USES

- May lower the risk of certain types of cancers, including prostate and lung cancers.
- May provide protection against heart disease.
- Slow the development of age-related macular degeneration.
- Enhance immunity.

FORMS

- Capsule
- Tablet
- Softgel

▼ WHAT IT IS

Although more than 600 carotenoid pigments have been identified in foods, it appears that only 6 of them are used in significant ways by the blood or tissues of the body. Besides beta-carotene (see page 338), which is probably the best-known carotenoid, these substances include alpha-carotene, lycopene, lutein, zeaxanthin, and cryptoxanthin.

Although carotenoids are found in various fruits and vegetables, the foods that represent the most concentrated sources may not be part of your daily fare. Alpha-carotene is found in carrots and pumpkin; lycopene is abundant in red fruits, such as watermelon, red grapefruit, guava, and especially processed tomatoes. Lutein and zeaxanthin are plentiful in dark green vegetables, pumpkin, and red peppers, and cryptoxanthin is present in mangoes, oranges, and peaches.

To prevent certain diseases, supplements providing a mix of the six key carotenoids may be in order.

▼ WHAT IT DOES

The primary benefit of carotenoids lies in their antioxidant potential. Antioxidants are compounds that in the body neutralize disease-causing unstable oxygen molecules called free radicals. Although the carotenoids are similar, each acts on a specific type of body tissue. In addition, alpha-carotene and cryptoxanthin can be converted into vitamin A in the body but not to the same extent as beta-carotene.

PREVENTION

Carotenoids may guard against certain types of cancer, apparently by limiting the abnormal growth of cells. Lycopene, for example, appears to inhibit prostate cancer formation. Researchers at Harvard University found that men who ate 10 or more servings a week of tomato-based foods—tomatoes are the richest dietary source of lycopene—cut their risk of prostate cancer by nearly 45%. Lycopene may also be effective against some cancers of the stomach and digestive tract.

Studies show that high intakes of alpha-carotene, lutein, and zeaxanthin

  ALERT

SIDE EFFECTS

- Large doses of carotenoids (through food or supplements) can turn your skin orange, especially the palms of your hands and the soles of your feet. This effect is harmless and will gradually go away if you reduce your intake of these pigments.

- Taking high doses of individual carotenoids may interfere with the workings of other carotenoids in your body and could even cause harm.

CAUTION

- **Reminder:** If you have a medical condition, talk to your doctor before taking supplements.

decrease the risk of lung cancer and that cryptoxanthin and alpha-carotene lower the risk of cervical cancer.

In addition, carotenoids may fight heart disease. In a survey of 1,300 elderly people, the ones who ate the most carotenoid-rich foods had half the risk of developing heart disease and a 75% lower chance of heart attack than did those who ate the least amount of these foods. This was true even after researchers adjusted for other heart disease risk factors, such as smoking and high cholesterol levels.

Scientists believe that all carotenoids, and particularly alpha-carotene and lycopene, block the formation of LDL ("bad") cholesterol. High LDL levels can lead to heart attacks and other cardiovascular problems.

ADDITIONAL BENEFITS

The carotenoids lutein and zeaxanthin promote clear vision by absorbing the sun's harmful ultraviolet rays and neutralizing free radicals in the retina (the light-sensitive portion of the eye). This may help reduce the risk of macular degeneration, an age-related vision disorder that is the leading cause of blindness in older adults. Other carotenoids may prevent damage to the lens of the eye and so decrease the risk of cataracts.

Preliminary studies also indicate that there may be a link between low levels of carotenoids and various menstrual disorders. In addition, other studies show that even after the onset of cancer, a diet that is high in carotenoids may improve the overall prognosis for the disease.

▼ HOW TO TAKE IT

DOSAGE

If you don't eat a wide variety of carotenoid-rich foods, take a supplement that contains mixed carotenoids—alpha-carotene, beta-carotene, lycopene, lutein, zeaxanthin, and cryptoxanthin—and supplies a minimum of 25,000 IU of vitamin A activity each day. Higher doses of mixed carotenoids may be recommended for the prevention of specific disorders.

GUIDELINES FOR USE

• Take carotenoid supplements with foods that contain a bit of fat, which helps the body absorb the carotenoids more effectively.

• Some experts also believe that your body will absorb more of these nutrients if you divide the total daily amount of carotenoids you plan to take in half and take them at two different times during the day.

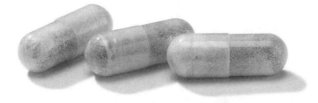

Although capsules for individual carotenoids such as lycopene (left) are available, it's best to take a mixed carotenoid supplement.

CAT'S CLAW *(Uncaria tomentosa, U. guianensis)*

Although Western researchers have studied cat's claw since the 1970s and European doctors have used it since the 1980s, popular interest in this herb has surged only recently. Studies suggest that it may give the immune system a needed boost, which may be particularly beneficial for people who are fighting cancer.

COMMON USES

- May enhance immunity, making it useful for sinusitis and other infections.
- Supports cancer treatment.
- May help relieve joint pain from osteoarthritis.
- Reduces pain and inflammation from gout or arthritis.

FORMS

- Tablet
- Capsule
- Softgel
- Liquid extract/Tincture
- Dried herb/Tea

▼ WHAT IT IS

In the Amazon basin, one woody tropical vine twining up trees in the rain forest features at the base of its leaves two curved thorns that resemble the claws of a cat. The herb derived from the inner bark or roots of this plant is known as cat's claw, or *uña de gato* (its Spanish name).

Although there are dozens of related species, two specific ones, *Uncaria tomentosa* and *U. guianensis,* are harvested in the wild (primarily in Peru and Brazil) for medicinal purposes. Large pieces of their bark are a common sight in South American farmers' markets; native Indians have long made tea from the bark and used it to treat wounds, stomach ills, arthritis, cancer, and other ailments.

▼ WHAT IT DOES

Modern scientific studies have identified several active ingredients in cat's claw that enhance the activity of the immune system and inhibit inflammation. Their presence may help explain why this herb traditionally has been employed to fight cancer, arthritis, dysentery, ulcers, and other infectious and inflammatory conditions.

MAJOR BENEFITS

In Germany and Austria, physicians prescribe cat's claw to stimulate the immune response in cancer patients, many of whom may be weakened by chemotherapy, radiation, or other conventional cancer treatments.

Several compounds in cat's claw—some of which have been studied for decades—may account for its cancer-fighting and immune-boosting effects. In the 1970s, researchers reported that the inner bark and root contain compounds called procyanidolic oligomers (PCOs), which inhibit tumors in animals. In the 1980s, German scientists identified other compounds in cat's claw that enhance the immune system, in part by stimulating immune cells called phagocytes. These engulf and devour viruses, bacteria, and other disease-causing microorganisms.

ALERT

SIDE EFFECTS
- Possible side effects include stomach discomfort, nausea, diarrhea, slow heartbeat or altered rhythm of heartbeat, kidney disease, decreases in estrogen or progesterone levels, and an increased risk of bleeding.

CAUTION
- If you are pregnant, considering pregnancy, or breast feeding; have a condition affecting the immune system; or are taking certain medications, including blood thinners (warfarin [Coumadin], aspirin), drugs to treat irregular heart rhythms, drugs to lower blood pressure, immunosuppressants, or herbs and supplements with similar effects, you should not take cat's claw.

- Cat's claw may increase the risk of bleeding and should be discontinued 2 weeks before surgeries or dental procedures.

- **Reminder:** If you have a medical condition, talk to your doctor before taking supplements.

Then, in 1993, an Italian study detected another class of compounds, called quinovic acid glycosides, that have multiple benefits. These may act as antioxidants, ridding the body of cell-damaging molecules called free radicals.

In addition to its antitumor potential, cat's claw may be of value in combating stubborn infections such as sinusitis.

ADDITIONAL BENEFITS

Traditionally, the herb has been relied on to treat pain. Because of its anti-inflammatory properties, it may be effective in relieving joint pain caused by arthritis or gout. Additional studies are needed, however, to define the precise role that cat's claw plays in treating arthritis and other inflammatory complaints.

Some preliminary reports found that cat's claw, in conjunction with conventional AIDS drugs, may benefit people infected with HIV, because it seems to boost the immune response; further studies are necessary, however.

Some experts caution against taking the herb for chronic conditions affecting the immune system, including tuberculosis, multiple sclerosis, and rheumatoid arthritis, because they believe it may overstimulate the immune system and make symptoms worse. Other doctors, however, recommend it for autoimmune disorders, including rheumatoid arthritis and lupus. More research is needed.

▼ HOW TO TAKE IT

DOSAGE

Take 250 mg of a standardized extract in pill form twice a day. Alternatively, consume ⅛ to ⅖ tsp (about 30 drops) of the liquid extract 3 times a day in a glass of water or use as directed by a health-care practitioner.

Pills containing the crude herb (the ground root or inner bark in a nonconcentrated form) are often available in 500- or 1,000-mg capsules. Take these twice daily (up to 2,000 mg a day).

Cat's claw tea is sold in health food stores; use 1 or 2 tsp of dried herb per cup of very hot water (follow package directions). You can drink up to 3 cups a day.

GUIDELINES FOR USE

• You can combine or rotate cat's claw with other immune-stimulating herbs, such as echinacea, goldenseal, reishi and maitake mushrooms, astragalus, or pau d'arco.

• Pregnant or breast-feeding women should avoid cat's claw. In Peru, cat's claw has been long valued as a contraceptive; in animals, it stimulates uterine contractions. This effect suggests that the herb could induce a miscarriage.

Cat's claw tablets are made from the woody inner bark of a South American vine.

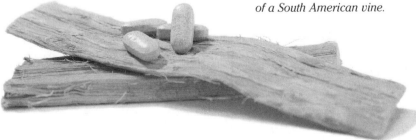

CAYENNE (*Capsicum* species)

This fiery spice, made from dried hot peppers, is said to have originated in Cayenne, French Guiana. Ever since a physician sailing with Columbus first described this pungent fruit, the cayenne pepper's popularity has grown. Today it's valued as a topical painkiller (especially for arthritic joints), digestive aid, and food enhancer.

COMMON USES

- Relieves arthritis pain.
- Reduces nerve pain of shingles (post-herpetic neuralgia), diabetes, surgery, or trigeminal neuralgia (tic douloureux).
- Relieves chronic pain and painful skin.
- May treat cluster headache.

FORMS

- Cream/Ointment
- Tincture/Liquid
- Fresh or dried herb

▼ WHAT IT IS

Derived from several varieties of the *Capsicum* species, cayenne is a hot pepper famous for the fiery taste it brings to Cajun, Mexican, Indian, Asian, and other cuisines. It's a cousin of the bell peppers used in salads and the hot peppers that produce chili powder and hot sauces, but it's unrelated to common black table pepper.

The main active ingredient in cayenne—and what gives the pepper its hotness—is capsaicin (pronounced cap-SAY-sin), an irritating, oily chemical that's also the prime component of pepper sprays sold for self-defense.

▼ WHAT IT DOES

When applied to the skin, capsaicin is an effective painkiller. It causes the depletion of a component in nerve cells called substance P, which transmits pain impulses to the brain.

MAJOR BENEFITS

Regular application of a cream or ointment containing capsaicin can be very effective for relieving the pain of arthritis. It also helps ease lingering post-shingles pain, as well as painful nerve damage from diabetes and from surgery (such as a mastectomy or an amputation).

Preliminary studies indicate that cayenne cream may have other beneficial uses. It may reduce the itching of psoriasis (the itching sensation follows the same nerve pathways as pain). The cream has also shown promise in relieving the aches and pains of fibromyalgia and the coldness in the extremities caused by Raynaud's phenomenon.

Another benefit is the relief of chronic pain.

ADDITIONAL BENEFITS

Cayenne may also relieve severe bladder pain.

  ALERT

SIDE EFFECTS

- Cayenne cream or ointment frequently generates warmth or a mildly unpleasant burning sensation that lasts half an hour or so during the first few days of topical application, but this effect usually disappears after several days of regular use.

- Taken internally, cayenne may cause stomach pain or diarrhea. Capsaicin in the stool can produce a burning sensation during bowel movements.

- Cayenne can sometimes trigger coughing, sneezing, tearing, or an irritated throat. These may be a result of using too much cream or inhaling the powder.

CAUTION

- Never apply cayenne cream to raw or open skin. And avoid touching your eyes and contact lenses; the burning sensation can be intense.

- If you are pregnant or breast feeding, avoid using cayenne. There are insufficient data to recommend its use.

- **Reminder:** If you have a medical condition, talk to your doctor before taking supplements.

Claims that cayenne may reduce heart disease risk (by lowering blood cholesterol and triglyceride levels) or help prevent cancer (by providing vitamin C and other antioxidants) are unfounded.

▼ HOW TO TAKE IT

DOSAGE

Cayenne cream or ointment containing 0.025% to 0.075% capsaicin is most effective with regular daily use; apply a thin layer over the affected areas at least 3 or 4 times a day for pain, rubbing it in well. Pain may take several weeks to subside.

For cluster headache: Apply 0.025% capsaicin cream 2 times a day in nostril on the same side as the headache for 1 week.

GUIDELINES FOR USE

• Because sensitivity to cayenne varies, test it first on a small, particularly painful area. If it works—and this may take a week or more—and causes no lasting discomfort, you can enlarge the coverage area.

• To avoid getting cayenne in the eyes, wash your hands after use with warm, soapy water or wear latex gloves during application and promptly discard them; you can also cover the area with a loose bandage.

• If cayenne does get in your eyes (or other moist mucous membranes) it may cause intense pain and burning but no lasting damage. Flush the affected area with water or milk. To remove cayenne from the skin, wash the area with warm, soapy water. Vinegar may also work, but don't use it in or near your eyes.

• If you're using cayenne cream to relieve pain in your fingers or hands, wait 30 minutes before washing it off to allow the cream to penetrate the skin. In the meantime, avoid touching contact lenses and sensitive areas, such as your eyes and nose.

• Store cayenne cream away from light and extreme heat or cold, and keep it out of the reach of children.

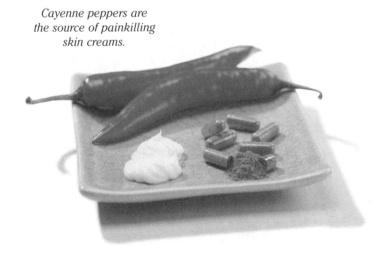

Cayenne peppers are the source of painkilling skin creams.

CHAMOMILE *(Matricaria recutita)*

Sometimes called the world's most soothing plant, chamomile has traditionally been enjoyed as a tea that helps relax the nerves and ease a variety of digestive complaints. In concentrated form, this herb is increasingly found in pills, tinctures, and liquid extracts; it's also included in skin formulas to treat sores and rashes.

COMMON USES

■ Promotes general relaxation and relieves anxiety.

■ May alleviate insomnia.

■ May heal mouth sores and treat diseases of the gums.

■ May soothe skin rashes and burns, including sunburn.

■ May treat bowel inflammation, digestive upset, and heartburn.

FORMS

■ Capsule

■ Dried herb/Tea

■ Liquid extract/Tincture

■ Oil

■ Cream/Ointment

▼ WHAT IT IS

Chamomile is actually two herbs: German chamomile and Roman chamomile. The more popular (and the one discussed in this book) is German—sometimes called Hungarian—chamomile. It comes from the dried flowers of the *Matricaria recutita* plant (its older botanical names are *Matricaria chamomilla* and *Chamomilla recutita*).

The other type of chamomile, known variously as Roman or English chamomile (*Chamaemelum nobile* or *Anthemis nobilis*), has properties similar to those of the German species; it is sold mainly in Europe.

This herb has long been used to prepare a gently soothing tea. Because of its pleasing, applelike aroma and flavor (the name "chamomile" is derived from the Greek *kamai melon,* which means "ground apple"), many people find the ritual of brewing and sipping the tea a relaxing experience.

Concentrated chamomile extracts are also added to creams and lotions or packaged as pills or tinctures. The healing properties of the herb are related in part to its volatile oils, which contain a compound called apigenin, as well as other therapeutic substances.

▼ WHAT IT DOES

Chamomile is a great soother. Its anti-inflammatory, antispasmodic, and infection-fighting effects can benefit the whole body—inside and out. When taken internally, it calms digestive upsets, relieves cramping, and relaxes the nerves. It also works externally on the skin and the mucous membranes of the mouth and eyes, relieving rashes, sores, and inflammation.

MAJOR BENEFITS

When Peter Rabbit's mother put him to bed, she gave him a spoonful of warm chamomile tea. Scientists have confirmed her wisdom. Studies in animals have shown chamomile contains substances that act on the same parts of the brain and nervous system that anti-anxiety drugs affect, promoting relaxation and reducing stress.

Chamomile appears to have a mildly sedating effect, but more important,

 ALERT

SIDE EFFECTS
• Possible side effects include vomiting, increased risk of bleeding, and increased blood pressure.

• Although some red flags have been raised about possible allergic reactions, which cause bronchial tightness or skin rashes, these appear to be so rare that most people don't need to worry about them.

CAUTION
• **Reminder:** If you have a medical condition, are taking medications, are pregnant or breast feeding, or operate heavy machinery, talk to your doctor before taking chamomile.

it also calms the body, making it easier for the person who's taking it to fall asleep naturally.

In addition, the herb has a relaxing, antiinflammatory effect on the smooth muscles that line the digestive tract. It helps ease a wide range of gastrointestinal complaints, including heartburn, diverticular disorders, and inflammatory bowel disease. Women experiencing inflammation of the vagina may also benefit from the effects of chamomile. Chamomile may soothe hemorrhoids and relieve diarrhea in children.

ADDITIONAL BENEFITS

Used externally, chamomile helps soothe skin inflammation. It contains bacteria-fighting compounds that may speed the healing of infections as well. A dressing soaked in chamomile tea, for example, is often beneficial when applied to mild burns. Those suffering from skin conditions such as eczema may also benefit.

For sunburn, chamomile oil can be added to a cool bath or mixed with almond oil and rubbed on sunburned areas. Chamomile creams, available ready-made in health food stores, may relieve sunburn, as well as skin rashes such as eczema.

When used on irritated areas, chamomile may be effective in treating skin

damaged by radiation from cancer treatment.

Some evidence suggests that chamomile may be effective in treating the common cold.

▼ HOW TO TAKE IT

DOSAGE

Tea/infusion: Traditional doses include 10 tbsp or ⅝ cup of boiling water over 2 to 4 g of fresh flower heads, steeped for 10 minutes taken by mouth 3 times daily. One to 4 cups of chamomile tea (from tea bags) taken daily has also been used. *Liquid extract/tincture:* Take ⅛ to ¾ tsp of a liquid extract (1:1 in 45% alcohol), by mouth 3 times daily. Take 1 tbsp of a tincture (1:5 alcohol) 3 to 4 times a day. *Capsules/tablets:* Take 400 to 1,600 mg by mouth daily in divided doses. *Skin use:* Some natural medicine publications have recommended paste, plaster, or ointment containing 3% to 10% chamomile flower heads. *Mouth rinse/gargle:* Use 1% fluid extract or 5% tincture. *Bath:* Use 5 g of chamomile per liter (1 quart) of water.

GUIDELINES FOR USE

• Chamomile is gentle and can be used long term.

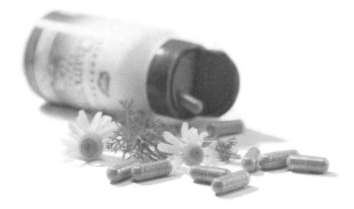

CHASTEBERRY *(Vitex agnus-castus)*

Although chasteberry has been used since ancient times for menstrual complaints, European doctors began prescribing it only in the 1950s. Today, it has become one of the most frequently recommended herbs in Europe for treating bloating, breast tenderness, and other common symptoms of premenstrual syndrome (PMS).

COMMON USES

- Alleviates symptoms of premenstrual syndrome (PMS).
- May regulate menstruation.
- May reduce cyclic breast pain.

FORMS

- Liquid extract/Tincture
- Tablet
- Capsule
- Dried herb/Tea

▼ WHAT IT IS

Also called vitex, chaste tree berry, or monk's pepper, chasteberry is the fruit of the chaste tree. Actually a small shrub with violet flower spikes and long, slender leaves, the chaste tree is native to the Mediterranean region but grows in subtropical climates throughout the world. Its red berries are harvested in the fall and then dried. They resemble peppercorns in shape, and the taste they impart to a therapeutic cup of tea is distinctively peppery.

▼ WHAT IT DOES

The use of chasteberry for "female complaints" dates back to the time of Hippocrates. Although the herb does not actually contain hormones or hormonelike substances, it does spark the pituitary gland (located at the base of the brain) to send a signal to the ovaries to increase production of the female hormone progesterone.

Chasteberry also inhibits the excessive production of prolactin, a hormone that primarily regulates breast milk production but has other less-understood actions as well.

MAJOR BENEFITS

Some scientists believe that women who routinely suffer from premenstrual syndrome (PMS) produce too little progesterone in the last 2 weeks of their menstrual cycle. This deficiency causes an imbalance in the body's natural estrogen-to-progesterone ratio. Chasteberry helps restore hormonal equilibrium, relieving such PMS-related complaints as irritability, bloating, and depression. Studies in Germany indicate that the herb offers at least some relief for PMS symptoms in about 90% of women—and in one-third of them, the symptoms disappear.

Chasteberry's prolactin-lowering action aids in reducing the breast pain and tenderness some women experience prior to menstruation, even if they have no other premenstrual symptoms.

 ALERT

SIDE EFFECTS

- Most people will not have any serious side effects from chasteberry.

- Some people will experience a headache after taking chasteberry.

- In a small percentage of women, studies have shown that stomach irritation or an itchy rash can occur. Discontinue using this herb if you develop any rash.

- Some women may experience an increased menstrual flow or intramenstrual bleeding after taking chasteberry.

CAUTION

- Chasteberry affects hormone production, so it should not be used by women taking hormonal medications, including birth control pills and estrogen, or by those who are pregnant or undergoing in vitro fertilization.

- Chasteberry should be used cautiously when taking medications used to treat certain psychiatric disorders, including schizophrenia and Parkinson's disease.

- **Reminder:** If you have a medical condition, talk to your doctor before taking supplements.

ADDITIONAL BENEFITS

Because high levels of prolactin and low levels of progesterone in the body can inhibit monthly ovulation, chasteberry may be useful for those who are having trouble getting pregnant. The herb works best in women with mild or moderately low progesterone levels. When too much prolactin causes menstruation to stop (a condition called amenorrhea), the herb can help restore a normal monthly cycle.

▼ HOW TO TAKE IT

DOSAGE
Premenstrual syndrome:
Take 1 20–40 mg tablet of standardized chasteberry extract.

Cyclic mastalgia:
For extract, take 60 drops of chasteberry extract daily. For tablet, take 1 tablet daily.

GUIDELINES FOR USE
• Experts recommend taking chasteberry on an empty stomach to increase absorption in the morning for maximum benefits. However, no studies confirm this finding.

• Even after just 10 days, a woman with PMS symptoms will probably notice at least some improvement during her next menstrual cycle. However, it may take 3 months of use to benefit from the full effect of this herb. Six months of treatment with chasteberry may be necessary to correct infertility or amenorrhea.

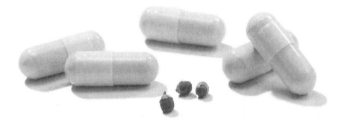

The tiny dark red fruit of the chasteberry tree contains the herb's active ingredients.

CHROMIUM

The second best-selling mineral supplement after calcium in the United States, chromium has been hyped as a fat burner, muscle builder, treatment for diabetes, and weapon against heart disease. Although research has shown that this mineral is essential for growth and health, its more spectacular claims remain controversial.

COMMON USES

■ Essential for the breakdown of protein, fat, and carbohydrates.

■ Helps the body maintain normal blood sugar (glucose) levels.

■ May lower total blood cholesterol, LDL ("bad") cholesterol, as well as triglyceride levels.

■ May enhance weight loss efforts.

■ May lower risk for cardiovascular disease.

■ May protect against Parkinson's disease and treat depression.

FORMS

■ Capsule ■ Softgel

■ Tablet ■ Liquid

▼ WHAT IT IS

Chromium, a trace mineral, comes in several forms. Supplements usually contain chromium picolinate or chromium polynicotinate. Chromium dinicotinic acid glutathione is found in brewer's yeast. Supplements can help people who don't get enough chromium in their diet.

Chromium is found in whole grains, whole-grain breads and cereals, potatoes, prunes, peanut butter, nuts, seafood, and brewer's yeast. Low-fat diets tend to be higher in chromium than high-fat ones.

▼ WHAT IT DOES

Chromium helps the body use insulin, a hormone that transfers blood sugar (glucose) to the cells, where it is burned as fuel. With enough chromium, the body can use insulin efficiently and maintain normal blood sugar levels. Chromium also aids the body as it breaks down protein and fat.

PREVENTION

Getting sufficient chromium may prevent diabetes in people with insulin resistance. This disorder makes the body less sensitive to the effects of insulin, so the pancreas has to produce more and more of it to keep blood sugar levels in check. When the pancreas can no longer keep up with the body's demand for extra insulin, type 2 diabetes develops. Chromium may help avert this progression by aiding the body in using insulin more effectively in the first place.

Chromium also helps break down fats, so it may reduce LDL ("bad") and increase HDL ("good") cholesterol levels, lowering the risk of heart disease.

ADDITIONAL BENEFITS

Chromium may relieve headaches, irritability, and other symptoms of low blood sugar (hypoglycemia) by keeping blood sugar levels from dropping below normal. In people with diabetes, it may help control blood sugar levels.

The mineral's most controversial claims relate to weight loss and muscle building. Although some studies indicate that large doses of chromium picolinate can aid in

  ALERT

SIDE EFFECTS

• Few side effects have been reported from trivalent chromium at recommended doses, but hexavalent chromium may be toxic. The most common complaints include stomach discomfort and nausea or vomiting. It is also possible that chromium may have adverse effects on the heart, kidneys, or liver.

CAUTION

• People with diabetes should consult their physician before taking chromium. This mineral may alter the dosage of insulin or other diabetes medications. Doses of some drugs used to treat conditions such as depression or Parkinson's disease may also need to be changed.

• **Reminder:** If you have a medical condition, talk to your doctor before taking supplements.

weight reduction or increase muscle mass, others have found no benefit. At best, the mineral may give you a slight edge in weight loss when combined with good diet and exercise.

▼ HOW MUCH YOU NEED

No RDA has been established for chromium, but scientists believe that 24 to 45 μg a day can prevent a deficiency. (Even on a healthy, varied diet, getting the maximum of this recommendation would be difficult.)

IF YOU GET TOO LITTLE
A chromium deficiency can lead to inefficient use of glucose. In itself, a lack of chromium is probably not a cause of diabetes, but it can help precipitate the disease in those who are prone to it.

In addition, anxiety, poor metabolism of amino acids, and high blood levels of triglycerides and cholesterol may occur in individuals who don't get enough chromium.

IF YOU GET TOO MUCH
Chromium does not seem to have any adverse effects, although there is some concern that megadoses can impair absorption of iron and zinc. To compensate for reduced absorption, be sure to get plenty of iron and zinc through your diet or supplements.

▼ HOW TO TAKE IT

DOSAGE
Adults (aged 18 or older):
Capsules/tablets: Scientists have studied dosages of 200 to 1,000 μg of chromium per day by mouth, but some believe that adequate dietary intake of chromium is only 24 to 45 μg per day.

Children (younger than 18):
The dosing and safety of chromium have not been studied thoroughly in children, and the use of high doses of chromium is generally not recommended.

GUIDELINES FOR USE
• Take chromium in 200-μg doses with food or a full glass of water to decrease stomach irritation.

• Chromium is better absorbed when combined with foods high in vitamin C (or taken with a vitamin C supplement).

• Both calcium carbonate supplements and antacids can reduce chromium absorption, so don't take them at the same time.

• Don't be confused by labels that suggest that one type of chromium (whether picolinate or polynicotinate) is absorbed better than any other. No reliable research supports these claims.

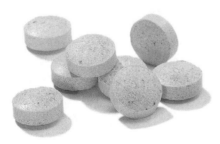
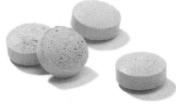

COENZYME Q10

Touted as a wonder supplement, coenzyme Q10 is reputed to enhance stamina, increase weight loss, combat cancer and AIDS, and even stave off aging. Although these claims may be extravagant, this nutrient does show promise for treating a number of conditions ranging from heart disease to weak gums.

COMMON USES

- Treats high blood pressure.
- May improve the symptoms of heart disease, including those from heart failure, cardiomyopathy, angina, and heart attack.
- May protect the heart from injury during surgery or from cardiotoxic chemotherapy.
- May have benefits in breast cancer, HIV/AIDS, Alzheimer's disease, muscular dystrophies, and other degenerative diseases.
- May treat gum disease.

FORMS

- Capsule
- Softgel
- Tablet
- Liquid

▼ WHAT IT IS

Coenzyme Q10, a natural substance produced by the body, belongs to a family of compounds called quinones. When it was first isolated in 1957, scientists called it ubiquinone, because it is ubiquitous in nature. In fact, coenzyme Q10 is found in all living creatures and is also concentrated in many foods, including nuts and oils.

In the past decade, coenzyme Q10 has become one of the most popular dietary supplements around the world. Proponents of the nutrient use it to maintain general good health, as well as to treat heart disease and a number of other serious conditions. Some clinicians believe it is so important for normal body functioning that it should be dubbed "vitamin Q."

▼ WHAT IT DOES

The primary function of coenzyme Q10 is as a catalyst for metabolism—the complex chain of chemical reactions during which food is broken down into packets of energy that the body can use. Acting in conjunction with enzymes (hence the name "coenzyme"), the compound speeds up the vital metabolic process, providing the energy that the cells need to digest food, heal wounds, maintain healthy muscles, and perform countless other bodily functions.

Because of the nutrient's essential role in energy production, it's not surprising that it is found in every cell in the body. It is especially abundant in the energy-intensive cells of the heart, helping this organ beat more than 100,000 times each day.

In addition, coenzyme Q10 acts as an antioxidant, much like vitamins C and E, helping neutralize the cell-damaging molecules known as free radicals.

PREVENTION

Coenzyme Q10 may play a role in preventing cancer, heart attacks, and other diseases linked to free radical damage. It's also used as a general energy enhancer and antiaging

ALERT

SIDE EFFECTS
- Most research suggests that coenzyme Q10 is very safe overall, even in large doses. In rare cases, it may cause stomach discomfort, nausea, vomiting, rash, itching, dizziness, difficult sleeping, irritability, headache, sensitivity to light, fatigue, flulike symptoms, and increased risk of blood clots or bleeding.

CAUTION
- Avoid intense exercise while taking coenzyme Q10; the heart muscle may become unduly strained or fatigued.

- Pregnant or breast-feeding women should be especially vigilant about checking with their doctor before using coenzyme Q10; the nutrient has not been well studied in this group.

- **Reminder:** If you have a medical condition or are taking medications, talk to your doctor before taking supplements.

supplement. Because levels of the compound diminish with age (and with certain diseases), some doctors recommend daily supplementation beginning at about age 40.

MAJOR BENEFITS

Coenzyme Q10 has generated much excitement as a possible therapy for heart disease, especially congestive heart failure or a weakened heart. In some studies, patients with a poorly functioning heart have been found to improve greatly after adding the supplement to their conventional drugs and therapies. Other studies have shown that people with cardiovascular disease have low levels of this substance in their heart.

Further research suggests that coenzyme Q10 may help protect against chemotherapy-induced damage to the heart muscle. In addition, it may be useful in treatment of acute heart attacks and chest pain (angina).

If you have heart disease, talk with your doctor about taking this supplement. Remember, coenzyme Q10 is intended as a complement to—and not as a replacement for—conventional medical treatments. Do not take this nutrient in place of heart drugs or other prescribed medications.

ADDITIONAL BENEFITS

A few small studies suggest that coenzyme Q10 may prolong survival in those with breast cancer, although results remain inconclusive. It also appears to aid healing and reduce pain and bleeding in those with gum disease and to speed recovery after oral surgery. Other benefits may include improving exercise performance and treating gum disease.

The supplement shows some promise against Alzheimer's disease and muscular dystrophies, and it may improve stamina in those with HIV/AIDS.

▼ HOW TO TAKE IT

DOSAGE

Adults (aged 18 or older):
Tablets/capsules/liquid: Most adults can take 75 to 400 mg of coenzyme Q10 or 1 tsp of a 200 mg per ml solution daily.
Topical: Apply topically to the affected area in the mouth in a concentration of 85 mg per ml.
Children (younger than 18): Take 100 mg by mouth twice daily. Safety in children is not well established, so use of this supplement should be discussed with your child's health-care provider.

GUIDELINES FOR USE

• Take this supplement in the morning and evening, preferably with food to enhance absorption.

• Coenzyme Q10 should be continued long term; it may require 8 weeks or longer to notice results.

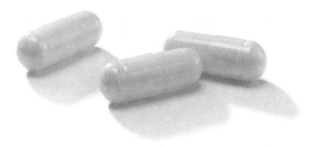

COPPER

Essential in preventing cardiovascular disease, maintaining healthy skin and hair color, and promoting fertility, copper is the least discussed but third most abundant trace mineral in the human body. Even so, some experts now believe that many people may be marginally deficient in this important nutrient.

COMMON USES

- Strengthens blood vessels, bones, tendons, and nerves.
- Helps maintain fertility.
- Ensures healthy pigmentation of hair and skin.
- Promotes blood clotting.

FORMS

- Tablet
- Capsule

▼ WHAT IT IS

Copper, the reddish-brown malleable metal commonly used in cookware and plumbing, is also found in at least 15 proteins in the human body. This mineral is available in nutritional supplement form as copper aspartate, copper citrate, and copper picolinate.

Although it can be obtained from a wide variety of foods, the typical American diet is low in copper, because the foods that are the best sources, such as oysters and liver, are not eaten frequently.

▼ WHAT IT DOES

Copper is essential in the formation of collagen, a fundamental protein in bones, skin, and connective tissue. It also may help the body use its stored iron and play a role in maintaining immunity and fertility.

Involved in the formation of melanin (a dark natural color found in the hair, skin, and eyes), copper promotes consistent pigmentation as well.

PREVENTION

Evidence suggests that copper can be a factor in preventing high blood pressure and heart rhythm disorders (arrhythmias). Some experts believe that it may protect tissues from damage by free radicals, helping prevent cancer, heart disease, and other ailments. Getting enough copper may also help keep cholesterol levels low.

ADDITIONAL BENEFITS

Copper is necessary for the manufacture of many enzymes, especially superoxide dismutase (SOD), which appears to be one of the body's most potent antioxidants. It may also help stave off the bone loss that can lead to osteoporosis.

▼ HOW MUCH YOU NEED

Although there is no daily RDA for copper, adults are advised to obtain 1.5 to 3 mg daily to keep the body functioning normally.

IF YOU GET TOO LITTLE

A true copper deficiency is rare. It usually occurs only in individuals with illnesses such as Crohn's disease or celiac disease or in those with inherited conditions that inhibit copper absorption, such as albinism. Symptoms of deficiency are fatigue; heart

 ALERT

CAUTION

- It's important to take extra copper when using zinc for longer than a month, because zinc interferes with the body's ability to absorb copper.

- **Reminder:** If you have a medical condition, talk to your doctor before taking supplements.

rhythm disorders; brittle, discolored hair; high blood pressure; skeletal defects; and infertility.

Even a mild deficiency may have some adverse health effects. For example, a preliminary study involving 24 men found that a diet low in copper caused a significant increase in LDL ("bad") cholesterol as well as a decrease in HDL ("good") cholesterol. These changes in their cholesterol profiles increased the participants' risk of heart disease.

IF YOU GET TOO MUCH
Just 10 mg of copper taken at one time can produce nausea, muscle pain, and stomachache. Severe copper toxicity from oral copper supplements has not been noted to date. However, some people who work with pesticides containing copper have suffered liver damage, coma, and even death.

▼ HOW TO TAKE IT

DOSAGE
There is no need to consume mega-doses of copper, but it is preferable to get amounts in the upper range of the recommended intake (3 mg a day from food and supplements combined).

Most good multivitamins will contain 1 mg copper, meeting nearly half the daily requirement.

GUIDELINES FOR USE
• It is advisable to take a supplement at the same time every day, preferably with a meal to decrease the chance of stomach irritation.

• If you take zinc supplements for longer than 1 month, add 2 mg of copper to your regimen. People who take antacids regularly may need extra copper as well.

▼ OTHER SOURCES

Shellfish (oysters, lobsters, crabs) and organ meats (liver) are excellent sources of copper. However, if you're concerned about your cholesterol levels, there are many vegetarian foods rich in copper as well. These include legumes; whole grains, such as rye and wheat and products made from them (bread, cereal, pasta); nuts and seeds; vegetables such as peas, artichokes, avocados, radishes, garlic, mushrooms, and potatoes; fruits such as tomatoes, bananas, and prunes; and soy products (tofu, tempeh, soy milk, and soy powder).

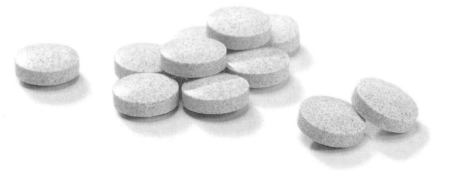

CRANBERRY *(Vaccinium macrocarpon)*

These tangy, ruby-red berries, native to the New World and now such an integral part of the American Thanksgiving tradition, have long been considered nature's cure for the urinary tract infections that frequently plague women of all ages. Modern science has now confirmed that this folk wisdom has real merit.

COMMON USES

- May treat lower urinary tract infections (commonly referred to as bladder infections or cystitis).
- Prevents recurrence of urinary tract infections.
- Helps deodorize urine.
- May acidify urine and prevent kidney stones.

FORMS

- Capsule
- Tablet
- Softgel
- Liquid/Juice
- Fresh or dried fruit
- Tea

▼ WHAT IT IS

The cranberry, an indigenous American plant closely related to the blueberry, has been used for centuries in both healing and cooking. The name is a shortened form of craneberry—the flowers of the low-growing shrub were thought to resemble the heads of the cranes that frequented the bogs where it grew. The berries are now widely cultivated throughout the United States, especially in Massachusetts and Washington State.

In early American medicine, cranberries were crushed and used as poultices for treating wounds and tumors and also as a remedy for scurvy, a gum and bleeding disorder caused by a deficiency of vitamin C. In this century, medicinal interest in cranberry has focused on its important role in preventing and treating urinary tract infections (UTIs), which are caused by *E. coli* and other types of bacteria.

▼ WHAT IT DOES

In the 1920s, it was discovered that people who consumed large amounts of cranberries produced a more acidic urine and that the urine was purified in the process. During this purification process, a powerful substance called hippuric acid was created. It proved to have a strong antibiotic effect on the urinary tract. In fact, it discouraged and sometimes even eliminated the harmful infection-causing bacteria.

More recent studies, however, indicate that cranberry's main infection-fighting capabilities may come from a different property. Cranberry appears to inhibit the adhesion of harmful microorganisms to certain cells lining the urinary tract. This makes the environment a less hospitable place for *E. coli* and other bacteria to replicate, and thus reduces the likelihood of infection.

Scientists have isolated two substances that produce this effect. One is fructose, a sugar that is found in many fruit juices. The other is a poorly under-

 ALERT

SIDE EFFECTS
- There are few known side effects from either the short-term or long-term use of cranberry. Possible side effects are stomach upset, diarrhea, and kidney stones.

CAUTION
- Cranberry is not a substitute for antibiotics during an acute urinary tract infection (UTI). See your doctor if you don't feel better after 24 to 36 hours of using cranberry for a suspected UTI.

- See your doctor right away if symptoms include fever, chills, back pain, or blood in the urine, which may be signs of a kidney infection (upper UTI) requiring medical attention.

- If you are at risk for kidney stones, opt for cranberry juice rather than tablets or capsules, which can be highly concentrated.

- **Reminder:** If you have a medical condition such as diabetes, are taking medications, or are pregnant or breast feeding, talk to your doctor before taking supplements.

stood compound present in cranberry and blueberry juices but absent from grapefruit, orange, guava, mango, and pineapple juices.

MAJOR BENEFITS

Scientists have now confirmed the effectiveness of cranberry in preventing and treating UTIs. Several studies have shown that daily consumption of cranberry, either in juice or capsule form, dramatically reduces the recurrence of UTIs. Women are 10 times more likely to develop these infections than men—in fact, 25% to 35% of women ages 20 to 40 have had at least one. There's no reason, however, why men can't benefit from taking cranberry as well.

Cranberry also appears to shorten the course of urinary tract illness, helping alleviate pain, burning, itching, and other symptoms. It's important to remember, though, that persistent UTIs should be treated promptly with antibiotics to prevent more serious complications. However, cranberry juice can be safely taken along with conventional drugs. It may even help hasten healing.

ADDITIONAL BENEFITS

Because it helps deodorize urine, cranberry should be in the diet of anyone suffering from the embarrassing odors associated with incontinence. Scientific evidence also shows benefits in urostomy care. In addition, cranberry's high vitamin C content makes it a natural vitamin supplement. Evidence also suggests that cranberry may aid absorption of vitamin B_{12} in people using antacids. It also may prevent stomach ulcers.

▼ HOW TO TAKE IT

DOSAGE

To help treat urinary tract infections: Drink 10 oz of cranberry juice cocktail (sweetened) a day, 1 to 2 tbsp a day of 100% cranberry juice (unsweetened), or 1.5 oz of frozen juice concentrate twice daily. For capsules, take 1 to 6 capsules, 300 to 400 mg each, twice daily by mouth with water 1 hour before or 2 hours after meals.

To prevent recurrences: The dose for an infection can be cut in half, to 400 mg of cranberry a day.

GUIDELINES FOR USE

• Cranberry can be taken with or without food. Drinking plenty of water or other fluids along with cranberry and throughout the day should also help speed recovery.

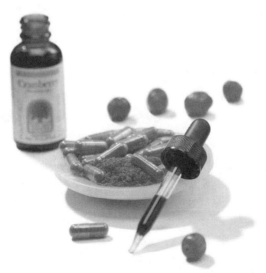

The common cranberry is a source of extracts in liquid and capsule form; both are effective for urinary tract infections.

DANDELION *(Taraxacum officinale)*

Known mostly as a prolific wild weed whose yellow flower dots lawns and roadsides all over the United States, dandelion is grown commercially in Europe. This is because its leaves and roots are a rich source of vitamins and minerals and its active ingredients are particularly useful for treating digestive and liver problems.

COMMON USES

- ■ May improve liver function in people with hepatitis B.
- ■ May have antiinflammatory properties.
- ■ May have a diuretic effect.
- ■ May protect against cancer.
- ■ May have beneficial effects in treating diabetes and colitis.

FORMS

- ■ Capsule
- ■ Tablet
- ■ Liquid/Juice
- ■ Dried or fresh herb/Tea

▼ WHAT IT IS

Dandelion grows wild throughout much of the world and is cultivated in parts of Europe for medicinal uses. Closely related to chicory, this perennial plant can grow up to a foot high; its spatula-shaped leaves are shiny, hairless, and deeply toothed.

The solitary yellow flower blooms for much of the growing season, opening at daybreak and closing at dusk and in wet weather (some cultures have used dandelions to signal the approach of rain). After the flower matures, the plant forms a puffball of seeds that are dispersed by the wind (or by the antics of playful children).

Supplements usually contain the herb's root (which is tapered and sweet to the taste) or leaves, although the whole plant and its flowers are also valued for their healing properties.

▼ WHAT IT DOES

Folk healers have long prescribed dandelion for liver and digestive problems. Because its various active ingredients enhance the performance of the liver, this herb is useful for treating a wide range of disorders.

MAJOR BENEFITS

Studies of dandelion's beneficial effects on the liver have shown that it may improve liver function in people with hepatitis B.

Dandelion is sometimes mixed with other nutritional supplements that bolster liver function, including milk thistle, black radish, celandine, beet leaf, fringe tree bark, inositol, methionine, choline, and others. Such combinations are usually sold as liver or lipotropic ("fat-metabolizing") formulas in health food stores.

ADDITIONAL BENEFITS

Although dandelion leaves have traditionally been used as a diuretic (a unine-producing agent), further studies are needed before dandelion can be recommended for this use.

  ALERT

SIDE EFFECTS

- Dandelion has no serious side effects. In large doses, it may cause a skin rash, stomach upset, or diarrhea. Stop using it if this happens and discuss the reaction with your doctor.

CAUTION

- Dandelion should not be used during acute attacks of gallstones or by people with bile duct problems or a bowel obstruction (often signaled by persistent constipation or lack of bowel movements). Seek professional medical attention.

- If you suffer from plant allergies, be wary of taking dandelion.

- **Reminder:** If you have a medical condition, especially a heart condition, high blood pressure, diabetes, or bowel problems, or are taking medications, talk to your doctor before taking supplements.

One study in humans suggests that an herbal preparation containing dandelion root may help treat chronic pain associated with colitis (inflammation and pain in the large intestine). However, the product tested contained several ingredients, so whether beneficial effects were the result of dandelion is unclear.

Some studies also indicate that dandelion may be of value in treating cancer. The Japanese have patented a freeze-dried extract of dandelion root to use against tumors and the Chinese are using dandelion extracts in fighting breast cancer (a treatment supported by positive effects in animal studies). Additional studies need to be conducted in humans to determine the herb's true effectiveness against specific types of cancer.

As for other medical applications, studies have found that dandelion can lower blood sugar levels in animals, suggesting that it may have some role to play in the treatment of diabetes.

▼ HOW TO TAKE IT

DOSAGE
Dried root: Take 2 to 8 g by creating an infusion (from flowers or leaves) or a decoction (from roots or bark).
Leaf fluid extract: Take ¾ to 1½ tsp of a 1:1 extract in 25% alcohol.
Root tincture: Take 1 or 2 tsp of a 1:5 tincture in 45% alcohol.

GUIDELINES FOR USE
• Drink fresh dandelion juice or liquid extract with water.

• Take pills containing dandelion root extract with or without food.

• Dandelion cannot be recommended for use during pregnancy or breast feeding because of a lack of scientific information.

• Don't use dandelions growing in a lawn or yard medicinally. Instead, get them from health food stores and make sure that they were grown in organic, fertilizer-free soil.

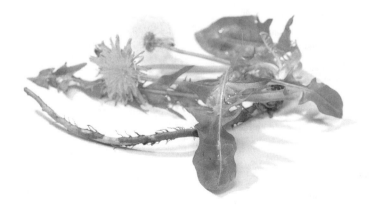

DHEA

Some advocates of the nutritional supplement DHEA call it the fountain of youth. Although the claim may be overblown, this hormone has shown some promise in combating certain age-related diseases. More study is needed, however, to identify the exact effects of DHEA—as well as the people who could benefit most from it.

COMMON USES

- May increase adrenal function.
- May relieve vaginal dryness associated with menopause.
- May increase bone density.
- May increase brain function and well-being in the elderly.
- May stimulate the immune system.

FORMS

- Tablet
- Capsule
- Cream

▼ WHAT IT IS

Nicknamed the "mother of hormones," DHEA, which is scientifically known as dehydroepiandrosterone, is needed by the body to produce many types of hormones, including estrogen and testosterone. DHEA is secreted by the body's two adrenal glands—small organs located on top of the kidneys—as well as by the skin, brain, testicles, and ovaries.

Although women make less DHEA than men, DHEA production in both genders declines dramatically with age; levels are 80% lower at age 70 than at age 30. The significance of these falling DHEA levels, however, has not been determined.

▼ WHAT IT DOES

There has been plenty of hype surrounding DHEA, so it is difficult to separate wishful thinking from sound scientific evidence. DHEA has been said to stimulate weight loss, increase libido, enhance memory, and prevent osteoporosis. All these claims, however, are unsupported.

Studies do indicate that DHEA may improve general well-being in older people (although how isn't clear), reduce the risk of heart disease, ease symptoms of the autoimmune disease lupus, help manage diabetes, and bolster immunity.

MAJOR BENEFITS

DHEA may improve brain function, memory, and overall feelings of well-being in the elderly. DHEA may also improve body mass index, decrease body fat, and increase muscle mass and body density. When DHEA is applied as a cream, it may improve vaginal pain and discomfort associated with menopause. Several studies suggest that DHEA improves well-being, exercise capacity, sex drive, and hormone levels in people with insufficient adrenal function.

Some evidence of DHEA's immune-boosting action was noted in a study of older people who had received flu shots. Their immune response to the weakened flu virus in the injection

---

 ALERT

SIDE EFFECTS

- Few side effects have been reported when DHEA is used at recommended doses. The most common complaints include fatigue, nasal congestion, and headache.

- When used to excess, DHEA supplements can cause acne, extremely oily skin, hair growth in women, breast enlargement in men, deepening of the voice, and mood changes. One animal study demonstrated an association between liver cancer and excessively high doses of DHEA.

CAUTION

- DHEA is a hormone; as such it may be linked to the development of some cancers, such as breast or prostate. Anyone who has these cancers or is at risk for them should not use DHEA.

- **Reminder:** If you have a medical condition, especially adrenal or thyroid disorders; are pregnant or breast feeding; or are taking medications, talk to your doctor before taking DHEA.

was significantly increased after taking DHEA. Researchers are now hopeful that DHEA might improve immune responses in people infected with HIV, the virus that causes AIDS.

ADDITIONAL BENEFITS

Men with high DHEA levels did better on an exercise stress test, a procedure that measures the condition of the heart during physical exertion. These associations weren't seen in women, however. In fact, women who took DHEA seemed to have a slightly higher risk of heart disease.

DHEA has been studied as a treatment for numerous other disorders, including lupus, depression, erectile dysfunction, bacterial infections, severe illnesses in the intensive care unit, ovulation disorders, myotonic dystrophy, chronic fatigue syndrome, clogged arteries, heart failure, and HIV infection. Results to date are inconclusive.

▼ HOW TO TAKE IT

DOSAGE

DHEA supplements should be taken only to raise hormone levels to within a normal range—not to exceed those levels. Start with a low dose (5 to 10 mg a day for women, 25 mg a day for men) and slowly increase the amount to achieve the desired effect. The maximum dose should not exceed 50 mg a day. It's best to take DHEA in the morning. People under age 50 who are healthy don't need the supplement at all.

For vaginal discomfort associated with menopause: Cream: A 10% cream rubbed over a 20-by-20-cm area on both thighs once daily has been used.

GUIDELINES FOR USE

• Although DHEA is readily available in health food stores and vitamin shops, and through the Internet and mail order, it is more potent than many other nutrients or herbs. The long-term effects of DHEA supplementation are simply not known. For this reason, most experts believe that you should take DHEA only under the supervision of a doctor; therefore, try to find a physician who is familiar with the use of this nutritional supplement.

• Before taking DHEA, make sure your doctor checks for prostate cancer (men) or breast cancer (women), because such cancers are influenced by hormone levels in the body.

• Be sure to have a blood test to determine your current DHEA levels, and use this supplement only if your blood level of this hormone is low. After 3 weeks, have another blood test to assess whether your dosage needs adjustment. Once obtained, a satisfactory blood level can often be maintained with as little as 5 to 10 mg of DHEA a week.

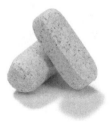

DONG QUAI *(Angelica sinensis, A. acutiloba)*

An ingredient in many herbal "women's supplements," dong quai (also known as angelica) is a traditional tonic used in Asia to aid the female reproductive system. Its popularity is second only to that of ginseng in China and Japan, but Western experts continue to debate the effectiveness of this ancient herb.

COMMON USES
- May help ease menstrual cramps.
- May reduce hot flashes associated with menopause.

FORMS
- Capsule
- Tablet
- Softgel
- Tincture
- Liquid
- Dried herb/Tea

▼ WHAT IT IS

Although dong quai grows wild in Asia, it's also widely cultivated for medicinal purposes in China *(the Angelica sinensis variety)* and in Japan *(A. acutiloba),* where many women take it daily to maintain overall good health.

The most widely available therapeutic form is derived from the root of *A. sinensis,* a plant with hollow stems that grows up to 8 feet tall and has clusters of white flowers. When it's in bloom, angelica resembles Queen Anne's lace, its botanical relative.

Other common names for dong quai include dang gui, tang kuie, and Chinese angelica.

▼ WHAT IT DOES

Generally, dong quai is believed to keep the uterus healthy and to regulate the menstrual cycle. It may also widen blood vessels and increase blood flow to various organs. Even among herbal experts, however, questions linger about its benefits. One reason it has been difficult to assess is that it's often taken along with other herbs.

MAJOR BENEFITS
Traditionally, dong quai has been used for menstrual and menopausal difficulties. Claims for the herb include balancing the menstrual cycle, correcting abnormal bleeding patterns, alleviating symptoms of premenstrual syndrome (PMS), easing menstrual cramps, reducing menopausal hot flashes, and improving the vaginal dryness sometimes associated with menopause.

There are two theories about how dong quai may help relieve these problems. Some herbalists believe it contains plant estrogens (phytoestrogens); these are weaker than estrogens produced by the body, but they do

 ALERT

SIDE EFFECTS
- Dong quai may have a mild laxative effect and may promote heavy menstrual bleeding.

- Dong quai may increase your skin's sensitivity to the sun, resulting in rashes or severe sunburns.

- Components of dong quai may increase the risk of bleeding and should be discontinued 2 weeks prior to major surgical or dental procedures.

CAUTION
- Rarely, other side effects have been reported with dong quai taken alone or in combination with other herbs; these include headache, lightheadedness or dizziness, sedation or drowsiness, insomnia, irritabiliity, fever, sweating, weakness, abnormal heart rhythms, blood pressure abnormalities, wheezing or asthma, hot flashes, worsening premenstrual symptoms, reduced menstrual flow, increased male breast size (gynecomastia), kidney problems (nephrosis), or skin rash.

- Dong quai should not be used by pregnant or breast-feeding women.

- People on anticoagulants (blood thinners) or NSAIDs (nonsteroidal anti-inflammatory drugs) should not take dong quai without consulting a doctor.

- **Reminder:** If you have a medical condition or are taking medications, talk to your doctor before taking supplements.

chemically bind with estrogen receptors in human cells. Because of this, phytoestrogens may minimize the potential negative effects of a woman's own estrogen, which can include an increased risk of breast cancer.

Phytoestrogens also may prevent hot flashes by compensating for the decline in estrogen levels that occurs after menopause.

Other experts attribute the effectiveness of dong quai to its abundance of coumarins. This group of natural chemicals dilates blood vessels, increases blood flow to the uterus and other organs, and stimulates the central nervous system. Coumarins also appear to reduce inflammation and muscle spasms, which may account for dong quai's ability to reduce the severity of menstrual cramps.

ADDITIONAL BENEFITS

Although dong quai is not typically used to lower blood pressure, it does have this effect because it dilates blood vessels, making it easier for the heart to pump blood through the body. The herb is also rich in vitamin B_{12}, and so may help build red blood cells.

Dong quai may aid in treating a variety of other conditions, including arthritis, nerve pain, and pulmonary hypertension. Additional research in these areas is needed bedore treatment recommendations for these claims can be made.

▼ HOW TO TAKE IT

DOSAGE

For PMS, menstrual irregularities, menstrual cramps, or hot flashes: Take 600 mg of dong quai daily. This is also available from 30 drops (1.5 ml) of tincture 3 times a day. In either pill or liquid form, extracts should be standardized to contain 0.8% to 1.1% ligustilide. You can also use a single preparation in which dong quai is combined with menstrual cycle–regulating herbs. Such herbs include chasteberry, licorice, and Siberian ginseng.

GUIDELINES FOR USE

• For symptoms of PMS, use dong quai only on the days that you are not menstruating. For menstrual cramps with PMS, continue using dong quai until menstruation stops. For cramps without PMS, begin taking dong quai

the day before your period is due. For hot flashes, use dong quai daily. Continue the herb for 2 months before deciding if it works.

• Protect yourself from the sun when using dong quai. The plant's root contains compounds called psoralens that can make some people more sensitive to sunlight and cause a rash or severe sunburn.

• Safrole, a volatile oil in dong quai, may be carcinogenic (cancer-causing). Long-term use should be avoided.

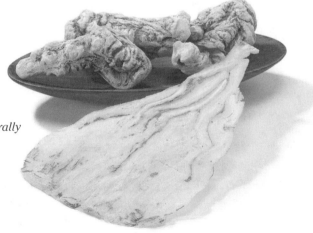

Dong quai's naturally gnarled root is flattened out for medicinal use.

ECHINACEA *(Echinacea angustifolia, E. purpurea, E. pallida)*

Long used by Native Americans, Midwestern settlers, and earlier generations of doctors, this herb, which grows wild on the American prairies, fell out of favor with the advent of modern antibiotics. But echinacea is regaining popularity as a safe and powerful immune system booster to fight colds, the flu, and other infections.

COMMON USES

- Reduces susceptibility to colds and the flu.
- Limits duration and severity of infections.
- Helps treat upper respiratory tract infections.
- May improve white blood cell counts after radiation treatment.
- May help protect against cancer.

FORMS

- Capsule
- Tablet
- Softgel
- Lozenge
- Tincture/Liquid
- Dried herb/Tea

ALERT

SIDE EFFECTS

- Possible side effects include stomach discomfort, nausea, sore throat, rash, drowsiness, headache, dizziness, muscle aches, liver inflammation (hepatitis), and altered blood sugar levels.

CAUTION

- If you're taking antibiotics or other drugs for an infection, use echinacea in addition to, not as a replacement for, those medications.

- Echinacea can overstimulate the immune system and may worsen symptoms of lupus, multiple sclerosis, rheumatoid arthritis, or other autoimmune disorders. It may also be counterproductive in progressive infections such as tuberculosis.

- Because the risks remain unclear, women who are trying to conceive or who are pregnant or breast feeding should avoid using echinacea.

- Severe allergic reactions (anaphylactic shock) have been reported, so if you are allergic to plants in Asteraceae or Compositae family (ragweed, chrysanthemums, marigolds, daisies), you should use caution.

- Echinacea may interact with medications that affect the liver, medications that affect the immune system, antibiotics, econazole nitrate cream (Spectazole), alcohol, and herbs and supplements with similar effects.

- **Reminder:** If you have a medical condition, are a transplant patient, or have a history of liver disease or diabetes, talk to your doctor before taking this supplement.

▼ WHAT IT IS

Also known as the purple, or prairie, coneflower, echinacea (pronounced ek-in-NAY-sha) is a wildflower with daisylike purple blossoms native to the grasslands of the central United States. For centuries, the Plains tribes used the plant to heal wounds and counteract the toxins of snakebites. The herb also became popular with European-American pioneers and their physicians, who considered it an all-purpose infection fighter.

Of the nine echinacea species, three *(Echinacea angustifolia, E. pallida, and E. purpurea)* are used medicinally. They appear in literally hundreds of commercial preparations, which utilize different parts of the plant (flowers, leaves, stems, or roots) and come in a variety of forms. Echinacea contains many active ingredients that are thought to strengthen the immune system and, since the 1990s, has become one of the most popular herbal remedies in the world.

▼ WHAT IT DOES

Echinacea acts by stimulating various immune system cells that are key weapons against infection. In addition, the herb boosts the cells' production of an innate virus-fighting substance called interferon. Because these effects are relatively short-lived, however, the herb is best administered at frequent intervals—as often as every couple of hours during acute infections.

PREVENTION

Echinacea can help prevent the two most common viral ailments—colds and the flu. It is most effective when taken at the first hint of illness. In one study of people who were susceptible to colds, those who used the herb for 8 weeks were 35% less likely to come down with a cold than those given a placebo. Furthermore, they caught colds less often—40 days elapsed between infections versus 25 days for the placebo group. Studies confirm that echinacea is also useful if you're already suffering from the aches, pains, congestion, or fever of colds or the flu. Overall, symptoms are less severe and subside sooner.

ADDITIONAL BENEFITS

Echinacea may prove effective against some types of cancer, particularly in patients whose immune systems are depressed by radiation or chemotherapy. There is good scientific evidence supporting the use of echinacea in the treatment of upper respiratory infections.

Echinacea can be applied to the skin, as well. Its juice promotes the healing of all kinds of wounds, boils, eczema, abscesses, burns, canker or cold sores, and bedsores. To treat a sore throat or tonsillitis, the tincture can be diluted and used as a gargle. Echinacea should not be used to treat genital herpes; there is evidence that it is not effective.

▼ HOW TO TAKE IT

DOSAGE

Because echinacea comes in many different forms, check the product's label for the proper dosage.

For colds and the flu: A high dose is needed—up to 200 mg 5 a times a day. In one major study, patients with the flu who were given 900 mg of echinacea a day did better than those who received either a lower dosage of 450 mg a day or a placebo.

GUIDELINES FOR USE

• Echinacea should be used no longer than 8 weeks, followed by a 1-week interval before you resume taking it. Some studies suggest that with continuous use, the herb's immunity boosting effects diminish. Starting and stopping or rotating it with other herbs may maximize its effectiveness. You can take echinacea with or without food.

• Check the alcohol content of echinacea tinctures; many contain considerable amounts of alcohol, making them unsuitable for children and for people with liver disease or alcoholism.

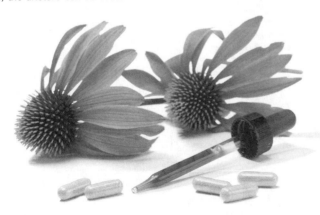

EPHEDRA *(Ephedra sinica, E. intermedia, E. equisetina)*

Sometimes called the world's oldest medicine, this herb has been used in China to treat colds and asthma, probably from as early as 3000 B.C. *Until recently, ephedra was the hottest weight loss drug on the market, but concerns about its abuse and safety caused the FDA to warn against its use and many stores to pull it from their shelves.*

COMMON USES

- Eases congestion and labored breathing caused by allergies or asthma.
- Relieves pressure and congestion in sinus infections (sinusitis).
- Aids in weight loss.

FORMS

- Capsule
- Tablet
- Liquid
- Dried herb/Tea

▼ WHAT IT IS

Also known by its Chinese name *Ma huang*, ephedra is made from the dried stems of *Ephedra sinica*, a shrub native to desert regions of Asia. However, preparations from species such as *E. intermedia* or *E. equisetina* may also be effective. A synthetic version of ephedra's active ingredients is widely used in both prescription and over-the-counter drugs, including hundreds of cold, allergy, asthma, weight loss, and energy-boosting formulas.

Unfortunately, the herb has been abused in recent years; people began taking high doses as a recreational stimulant—leading to heart attacks, strokes, and numerous deaths. Although a ban has not been imposed, the FDA has proposed that all ephedra preparations carry a warning label.

▼ WHAT IT DOES

Ephedra's primary active ingredients, ephedrine and pseudoephedrine, stimulate the central nervous system and open airways.

Ephedra's stimulant effect is stronger than caffeine but less potent than amphetamines or the natural adrenal hormone epinephrine (adrenaline), which causes the "fight-or-flight" response. Ephedra makes the heart beat faster, increases blood pressure,

ALERT

SIDE EFFECTS

- Ephedra can cause rash, dizziness, anxiety, irritability, excitation, headache, increased urination, nausea, vomiting, and constipation.
- Although serious side effects are rare, ephedra can also cause increased blood pressure, rapid heart rate, abnormal heart rhythms, heart attack, stroke, sudden death, seizure, rash, dizziness, anxiety, irritability, excitation, euphoria, headache, paranoia, nervousness, chest tightness, increased urination, tremors, behavior changes, nausea, vomiting, constipation, liver inflammation (hepatitis), decreased blood sugar, and kidney stones. **Note: The FDA has warned against using ephedra, especially when exercising strenuously or taking other stimulants, such as caffeine. Many retailers have taken it off their shelves.**

CAUTION

- **Important:** Check with a qualified health-care professional before taking any product containing ephedra or ephedrine.
- Don't exceed recommended daily dosages. Be sure to factor in amounts from other sources, such as over-the-counter cold remedies.
- People with high blood pressure, abnormal heart rhythm, heart attack, stroke, seizure, eating disorders, anxiety, prostate disease, mental illness, kidney disease, stomach ulcers, heart disease, eye disease, depression, diabetes, thyroid disease, and sleep disorders, and women who are pregnant or breast feeding should not take ephedra.
- People who use caffeine, medications to control blood sugar, alcohol, diuretics ("water pills"), blood pressure medications, certain antidepressants, dexamethasone, anesthesia, oxytocin (Pitosin), medications to treat thyroid disease, amitriptyline, or herbs and supplements should not take ephedra.
- **Reminder:** If you have a medical problem, talk to your doctor before taking supplements.

speeds up the metabolism, and acts as a diuretic.

Ephedra has been used throughout history as a bronchodilator to treat the bronchial and nasal congestion of asthma, allergies, colds, and sinus infections. In the 1920s, U.S. drug companies began extracting active ingredients from the herb and using it in asthma and cold medicines—which they still do today.

MAJOR BENEFITS

Ephedra dilates the small airways in the lungs (the bronchioles), thus relieving congestion and coughing caused by seasonal allergies or mild asthma. Ephedra also helps alleviate symptoms caused by colds, the flu, and sinus infections.

Ephedra may aid in weight loss by making the body burn calories quickly and suppressing the appetite. Serious injuries and deaths associated with the herb, however, have caused the FDA to warn against its use.

ADDITIONAL BENEFITS

Ephedra may be useful in the treatment of low blood pressure. Scientific evidence also suggests that it may enhance sexual arousal. More controversial is the claim that ephedra enhances athletic performance by boosting energy. *Not only is there no scientific basis for this theory, but it has had tragic consequences; a number of athletes have become seriously ill—and several have died—after taking large doses of products containing ephedra.* The herb is currently listed as a banned substance by the U.S. Olympic Committee.

▼ HOW TO TAKE IT

DOSAGE

Check your bottle's label to see how much ephedrine is contained in each dose. Most standardized extracts supply about 5.5% to 6.5% ephedrine (also known as "ephedra alkaloids"). Because of safety concerns, no safe dosing can be recommended. The FDA had suggested a maximum of 8 mg up to every 6 hours (total daily dose of 24 mg) for up to 7 days, but because of current safety concerns, no safe dosing can be recommended.

To make a tea, pour 1 cup of very hot water over 1 tsp of dried ephedra (along with other herbs if desired); steep it for 10 to 15 minutes. Drink 1 or 2 cups a day or take ¼ to 1 tsp ephedra liquid extract (up to 8 mg of ephedrine) in a glass of water up to 3 times daily.

GUIDELINES FOR USE

• You can take this herb long term for certain conditions, such as chronic asthma, but try to use it only as needed—up to 7 days at a time.
• Ephedra interacts with numerous medications, including prescription drugs for heart disease and high blood pressure. Talk to your doctor before using.
• Ephedra may be safely combined with many other herbs, including St. John's wort, but avoid taking ephedra with caffeine or yohimbine, which can cause excessive stimulation.
• If ephedra promotes insomnia, omit your evening dose.

EVENING PRIMROSE OIL (Oenothera biennis)

Native Americans and early settlers in the New World both valued the indigenous evening primrose plant for its healing powers. Today, scientific research is focused largely on the therapeutic effect of the oil derived from the seeds of the plant, which contain a special fat called gamma-linolenic acid (GLA).

COMMON USES

- Eases rheumatoid arthritis pain.
- May minimize symptoms of diabetic nerve damage and may improve diabetes.
- Relieves symptoms of certain skin conditions.
- May improve symptoms of breast cancer, breast cysts, and breast pain.
- May aid weight loss.
- May improve symptoms of chronic fatigue syndrome, multiple sclerosis, and Raynaud's phenomenon.

FORMS

- Capsule
- Softgel
- Oil

▼ WHAT IT IS

Called evening primrose because its light yellow flowers open at dusk, this wildflower grows in North America and Europe. The plant and its root have long been used for medicinal purposes—to treat bruises, hemorrhoids, sore throat, and stomachaches.

The use of its seed oil, which contains gamma-linolenic acid (GLA), is relatively recent. GLA is an essential fatty acid that the body converts to hormonelike compounds called prostaglandins, which regulate a number of bodily functions.

Although the body can make GLA from other types of fat you consume, there is no one food that has appreciable amounts of GLA in it. Evening primrose oil provides a concentrated source: 7% to 10% of its fatty acids are in the form of GLA.

There are, however, other sources of GLA. Both borage seed oil and black currant seed oil actually contain higher amounts of GLA (20% to 26% for borage; 14% to 19% for black currant) than evening primrose oil. They also have a higher percentage of other fatty acids that may interfere with GLA absorption.

Most of the studies investigating the effects of GLA have used evening primrose oil, and for this reason it is the preferred source of GLA. Still, borage oil may be a good substitute: It is less expensive than evening primrose oil and a lower dose is required to produce a therapeutic effect.

▼ WHAT IT DOES

The body produces several types of prostaglandins; some promote inflammation, and others control it. The GLA in evening primrose oil is directly converted to important antiinflammatory prostaglandins, which accounts for most of the supplement's therapeutic effects. In addition, GLA is an important component of cell membranes.

ALERT

SIDE EFFECTS

- In studies, about 2% of the participants using evening primrose oil experienced bloating or abdominal upset. However, consuming it with food may lessen this effect.

- This herb may cause headache, nausea, decreased blood pressure, or loose stools.

CAUTION

- Evening primrose oil may increase the risk of seizures in people taking phenothiazine epileptogenic drugs for conditions such as schizophrenia.

- Avoid using evening primrose oil if you are pregnant or nursing, because the effects on the mother and baby are unknown.

- **Reminder:** If you have a medical condition; are allergic to plants or herbs such as ginger, black cohosh, and oleander; are taking medications; or have surgery scheduled, talk to your doctor before taking supplements.

PREVENTION

In people who have diabetes, the GLA in evening primrose oil has been shown to help prevent nerve damage (neuropathy), a common complication of the disease. In a study of people with mild diabetic neuropathy, 1 year of treatment with evening primrose oil reduced numbness and tingling and other symptoms of the disorder better than a placebo, suggesting that evening primrose may be of value in reversing neuropathy. Evening primrose oil may also improve other nerve conditions.

ADDITIONAL BENEFITS

One of the leading uses for evening primrose oil is to treat eczema, an allergic skin condition that may occur if the body has trouble converting fats from food into GLA. Studies of people with eczema indicate that taking evening primrose oil for 3 to 4 months can help alleviate itching and reduce the need for topical steroid creams and drugs with unpleasant side effects. Evening primrose oil is also effective in treating other skin conditions.

Because of its GLA content, evening primrose oil can help reduce breast pain, breast cysts, and breast cancer.

Research studies have found that symptoms of rheumatoid arthritis, an autoimmune disease characterized by joint pain and swelling, improve when patients take supplements of evening primrose oil or another source of GLA.

▼ HOW TO TAKE IT

DOSAGE

The recommended therapeutic dose of evening primrose oil for adults is generally 3 to 8 g daily in divided doses taken by mouth. The dose for children is 3 g daily in divided doses, not to exceed 0.5 g per kg (2.2 lb) of body weight daily. Standardized capsules of evening primrose oil may contain 320 mg of linotenic acid (LA), 40 mg of GLA, and 10 IU of vitamin E, or may contain 70% LA and 9% GLA.

Evening primrose oil or borage oil can also be applied topically to the fingers to ease the symptoms of poor circulation in Raynaud's phenomenon.

GUIDELINES FOR USE

• Take evening primrose oil or other sources of GLA with meals to enhance the compound's absorption.

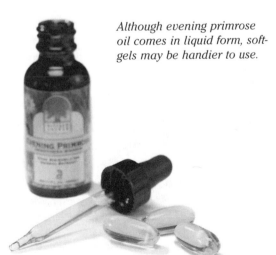

Although evening primrose oil comes in liquid form, softgels may be handier to use.

FEVERFEW *(Tanacetum parthenium)*

Despite its name, feverfew is not a fever reducer but a migraine preventive. For centuries, this herb was relied on to treat headaches, stomach problems, and menstrual irregularities, but feverfew as an herbal remedy virtually disappeared from use until reports calling it a migraine cure began appearing in the late 1970s.

COMMON USES

■ Helps prevent or reduce the intensity of migraines.

■ May relieve pain associated with rheumatoid arthritis.

FORMS

■ Capsule

■ Tablet

■ Liquid

■ Dried herb/Tea

▼ WHAT IT IS

Celebrated for its effect on migraines, feverfew (also known as featherfew or febrifuge) belongs to the flower family that includes daisies and sunflowers. With its clear yellow and white blossoms and feathery yellow-green leaves, this herb resembles chamomile and is often mistaken for it.

The plant's leaves are used medicinally, and although the flowers have no health benefits, they do emit a strong aroma. In the Middle Ages, the plant was believed to purify the air and prevent malaria and other life-threatening diseases. Although feverfew probably can't kill germs in the atmosphere, the odor apparently is quite offensive to bees and bugs, so feverfew planted in your garden can act as a natural insect repellent.

▼ WHAT IT DOES

The active compound in feverfew (a chemical called parthenolide) seems to block substances in the body that widen and constrict blood vessels and cause inflammation.

PREVENTION

Although the exact cause of migraines is unknown, some experts think that they occur when blood vessels in the head constrict and then rapidly dilate. Such a dramatic change can trigger the release of chemicals stored in platelets (the small blood cells involved in blood clotting) that cause pain and inflammation. Researchers speculate that feverfew prevents the sudden dilation of blood vessels and thus inhibits the release of those chemicals. This action makes feverfew a good migraine preventive, but the herb cannot relieve a migraine once it occurs.

Word of mouth among people with chronic migraines led to widespread

---

 ALERT

SIDE EFFECTS

• There have been reports of sores and inflammation of the mucous membranes of the mouth, but this reaction seems to be limited to people who chew the fresh leaves (a common practice before feverfew supplements became available).

• Some people may experience stomach upset, indigestion, gas, constipation, diarrhea, abdominal bloating, or heartburn.

• Skin contact with the plant can cause a rash; anyone who develops a rash after touching feverfew should not use the product internally. People who are allergic to chrysanthemums, daisies, marigolds, ragweed and other members of the Compositae family should not take feverfew.

• Another possible side effect is withdrawal symptoms, including rebound headache, anxiety, fatigue, increased heart rate, muscle stiffness, and joint pain.

CAUTION

• Feverfew should be avoided by people with a history of heart disease, anxiety, or bleeding disorders, or who are taking herbs or dietary supplements with similar effects.

• **Reminder:** If you have a medical condition, are pregnant or breast feeding, or are taking anticoagulant drugs, talk to your doctor before taking this supplement.

use of feverfew, beginning in the 1970s. To determine the herb's effectiveness, British researchers recruited migraine sufferers who had already been using feverfew regularly. The researchers then divided them into two sections. One continued to take feverfew, and the other was given a placebo. Those on the placebo pills soon experienced more frequent—and more intense—headaches. Those in the feverfew group had no increase in migraine occurrences.

Another study showed that feverfew reduced the number of migraines by 24% and that even when the headaches did occur, they were much less severe. The results of these and other research studies have led health authorities in Canada and other countries to approve the use of feverfew for migraine prevention.

ADDITIONAL BENEFITS

The antiinflammatory action of the herb also led to its use as a treatment for the inflamed, sore joints that occur in rheumatoid arthritis (RA). However, a study of RA patients found no additional benefit from taking feverfew in conjunction with medications that are commonly prescribed for this condition. No studies have been done on how the herb might work alone or in combination with other herbal treatments for RA.

▼ HOW TO TAKE IT

DOSAGE

For migraines: You'll want to take 0.5 mg of the active ingredient, parthenolide, daily. To do this, take either 2 to 3 (60 mg) powdered leaves or 70 to 86 (76 mg) dried, chopped leaves, once daily by mouth.

GUIDELINES FOR USE

• The experience of the migraine sufferers in the British study cited above underscores the importance of taking feverfew daily for an extended time, because stopping the herb may lead to a resumption of headaches.

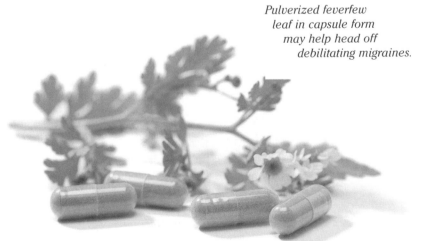

Pulverized feverfew leaf in capsule form may help head off debilitating migraines.

CASE HISTORY

A Migraine Preventive

For a while, Nick L. considered the pricey new migraine medications nothing short of wonder drugs because of their amazing ability to stop the dizzying pain of his headaches. What he really wanted, though, was something that could prevent a migraine from starting. His doctor offered other drugs, but their side effects were troublesome. "Sure, the beta-blockers headed off my migraines," Nick remembers, "but my sex life vanished too."

During a trip to London, he saw a shop sign: "Migraine Sufferers—We have feverfew in stock." Although he was skeptical of herbal therapies, he bought a bottle, and, after affirming the safety and effectiveness of feverfew, he decided to give it a try. "From that point on, it was a migraine-free year," he says. "My first since childhood."

FISH OILS

Several years ago, scientists noticed a curiously low incidence of heart disease among Greenland Inuit despite their high-fat diet. The reason? They were eating cold-water fish rich in omega-3 fatty acids. Later studies confirmed the cardioprotective effect of fish oils and uncovered other benefits as well.

COMMON USES

■ Lowers triglycerides; increases good cholesterol.

■ Helps prevent primary and secondary cardiovascular disease.

■ Reduces blood pressure.

■ Reduces pain and inflammation from rheumatoid arthritis.

FORMS

■ Capsule

■ Softgel

▼ WHAT IT IS

The fat in fish has a form of polyunsaturated fatty acids called omega-3. These differ from the polyunsaturated fatty acids found in vegetable oils (called omega-6), and they have different effects on the body. (Fish don't manufacture such fats but get them from the plankton they eat—the colder the water, the more omega-3 the plankton contains.)

The two most potent forms of omega-3, eicosapentaenoic acid (EPA) and docosahexanoic acid (DHA), are found in abundance in cold-water fish such as salmon, trout, mackerel, and tuna (including the canned variety). The sources of a third type of omega-3, alpha-linolenic acid (ALA), are certain vegetable oils (such as flaxseed oil) and leafy greens (such as purslane). However, ALA doesn't affect the body in the same way that EPA and DHA do.

▼ WHAT IT DOES

Omega-3 fatty acids play a key role in a range of vital body processes, from blood pressure and blood clotting to inflammation and immunity. They may be useful for preventing or treating many diseases and disorders.

PREVENTION

Fish oils appear to reduce the risk of heart disease in several ways. Most important, the presence of omega-3 makes platelets in the blood less likely to clump together and form the clots that lead to heart attacks. Next, omega-3 can reduce triglycerides (blood fats that are related to cholesterol) and may lower blood pressure. In addition, research has shown that omega-3 fatty acids strengthen the heart's electrical system, preventing heart rhythm abnormalities. However, the strongest evidence for the cardiovascular benefits of fish oils comes from studies in which the participants ate fish rather than taking fish oil supplements.

 ALERT

SIDE EFFECTS

• Fish oil capsules may cause belching, flatulence, bloating, nausea, and diarrhea.

• Potential adverse effects include an increase in blood sugar level, increased risk of bleeding, or an increased level of LDL (bad cholesterol).

• Very high doses may result in a slightly fishy body odor.

CAUTION

• Because omega-3 fatty acids inhibit blood clotting, consult a doctor before using fish oil supplements if you have a blood disorder or if you are taking anticoagulants (blood thinners).

• Fish meat may contain methylmercury, and caution is necessary for young children and pregnant or breast-feeding women.

• **Reminder:** If you have a medical condition, especially diabetes or high LDL cholesterol, or are contemplating surgery, talk to your doctor before taking supplements such as fish oil.

Within the artery walls, omega-3 fatty acids inhibit inflammation, which is a factor in plaque buildup. As a result, therapeutic doses of fish oils are one of the few successful ways to prevent the reblockage of arteries that commonly occurs after angioplasty, a procedure in which a small balloon is guided through an artery to a blockage and then is inflated to compress plaque, widen the vessel, and improve blood flow to the heart.

ADDITIONAL BENEFITS

Omega-3 fatty acids are also effective general antiinflammatories, useful for joint problems, lupus, and psoriasis. Studies indicate that people with rheumatoid arthritis experience less joint swelling and stiffness and may even be able to manage on lower doses of antiinflammatory drugs when they take fish oil supplements. Eating fish probably will not supply enough omega-3 to help rheumatoid arthritis and other inflammatory conditions, so fish oil supplements are recommended.

In a year-long study of people with Crohn's disease (a painful type of inflammatory bowel disease), 69% of those taking enteric-coated fish oil supplements (about 3 g of fish oils a day) stayed symptom-free, compared with just 28% of those receiving a placebo. Fish oils may also help ease the inflammation that accompanies menstrual cramps.

In addition, omega-3 fatty acids may play a role in mental health. Some experts believe that there's a correlation between the increasing incidence of depression in the United States and the declining consumption of fish. A preliminary study suggested that omega-3 fatty acids may reduce the severity of schizophrenia by about 25%.

Other preliminary evidence suggests that fish oil has many additional benefits, including prevention of graft failure after heart bypass surgery, cancer prevention, treatment of colon cancer, infant eye and brain development, kidney disease, and cystic fibrosis.

▼ HOW TO TAKE IT

DOSAGE

For hypertriglyceridemia: Take 2,000 mg of fish oils a day.
For heart disease prevention: Take 500 to 3,000 mg of fish oil a day.
For high blood pressure and rheumatoid arthritis: Take 3,000 to 5,000 mg of fish oil a day.

Note: For doses greater than 3,000 mg, you should consult a physician because of an increased risk of bleeding.

GUIDELINES FOR USE

• Fish oil supplements are not necessary for heart disease prevention or treatment if you eat fish at least twice a week.

• Supplements are recommended for rheumatoid arthritis and other inflammatory conditions.

• Take capsules with meals.

• Supplements may be easier to tolerate if you take them in divided doses. Try 1,000 mg 3 times a day instead of 3,000 mg in one sitting.

• Some studies have indicated that high doses of fish oils worsen blood sugar control in people with diabetes; others have shown no effect. To be on the safe side, people with diabetes should not take more than 2,000 mg of fish oil supplements a day without the advice of their doctor.

5-HTP

Americans who are suffering from depression, insomnia, migraines, or obesity may have a new supplement to consider: 5-HTP. Unlike its close chemical cousin, the amino acid tryptophan (which was recalled for safety concerns), 5-HTP appears to be safe—and it may be even more effective than tryptophan.

COMMON USES

- Relieves depression.
- Helps overcome insomnia.
- Aids in weight control.
- Treats migraines.
- May ease pain of fibromyalgia.

FORMS

- Capsule
- Tablet

WHAT IT IS

The nutrient 5-HTP, short for 5-hydroxy-tryptophan, is a derivative of the amino acid tryptophan, which is found in such high-protein foods as beef, chicken, fish, and dairy products. The body makes 5-HTP from the tryptophan present in our diets. It's also in the seeds of an African plant *(Griffonia simplicifolia)*, which is the source of the 5-HTP supplements sold in health food stores.

The focus of much interest, 5-HTP acts on the brain, helping elevate mood, promote sleep and weight loss, and relieve migraines, among other uses. Unlike many other supplements (and drugs) that contain substances with molecules too large to pass from the bloodstream into the brain, 5-HTP is small enough to enter the brain. Once there, it is converted into a vital nervous system chemical, or neurotransmitter, called serotonin. Although it affects many parts of the body, serotonin's most important actions take place in the brain, where it influences everything from mood to appetite to sleep.

Because it is closely related to the amino acid tryptophan, 5-HTP remains somewhat controversial. In 1989, the FDA banned tryptophan supplements—which were often sold as L-tryptophan and used for many of the same purposes as 5-HTP—after reports of a fatal illness among those taking it. The illness was later found to be caused by contamination of the supplement during the manufacturing process, not by the tryptophan itself.

In 1994, 5-HTP began to be sold in the United States as an over-the-counter alternative to tryptophan. Because 5-HTP is not made in the same way as tryptophan, it avoids the contamination problems of its predecessor. Even though safety concerns have been raised, many experts believe the supplement is safe and effective.

 ALERT

SIDE EFFECTS

- The generally mild side effects include nausea, constipation, gas, drowsiness, and reduced sex drive. Nausea usually diminishes within a few days.

- 5-HTP may also have other rare side effects, including lowered cholesterol levels, sodium retention, low blood pressure, pounding heartbeat, slow heart rate, feelings of euphoria and mania, lessened inhibitions, sleepiness, headache, restlessness, rapid speech, anxiety, difficulty sleeping, aggressiveness, and agitation.

CAUTION

- Consult your doctor if you're taking an antidepressant. The combination of 5-HTP with those medications can cause anxiety, confusion, rapid heart rate, sweating, diarrhea, or other adverse reactions.

- Because 5-HTP may alter moods, you should use it with caution if you have a history of mental disorders.

- Do not drive or do hazardous work until you determine how 5-HTP affects you. It can cause drowsiness in some people.

- **Reminder:** If you have a medical or psychiatric condition, are taking drugs that act within the central nervous system, or are pregnant or breast feeding, talk to your doctor before taking 5-HTP.

▼ WHAT IT DOES

5-HTP has been studied as a treatment for such mood disorders as depression, anxiety, and panic attacks because it can boost levels of serotonin in the brain.

Scientists are also investigating whether 5-HTP may work for a diverse array of complaints linked to low serotonin levels, including migraines, fibromyalgia, obesity, eating disorders, PMS, and even violent behavior. Although additional research is needed to determine its effectiveness in treating many of these conditions, preliminary studies suggest that it may be beneficial for some.

MAJOR BENEFITS

For decades, European doctors have been prescribing 5-HTP for the treatment of depression and insomnia. In some cases, it may be more effective, lift depression quicker, and produce fewer side effects than standard anti-depressant drugs. In one study, more than half of the patients who suffered from long-term depression and were resistant to all other antidepressants felt better after taking 5-HTP.

The nutrient has also been shown to promote sleep and improve the quality of sleep by increasing the amount of time people spend in two key sleep stages: deep sleep and REM sleep (the dreaming stage). After dreaming longer, those on 5-HTP awaken feeling more rested and refreshed.

ADDITIONAL BENEFITS

Individuals trying to lose weight or suffering from migraines may benefit from 5-HTP. In one study, overweight women who took the supplement ate fewer calories, lost more weight, and were more likely to feel full while on a diet

than those given a placebo. It may also be useful in relieving severe headaches, including migraines, reducing not only their frequency but also their intensity and duration.

The supplement may also work to increase pain tolerance in those with fibromyalgia, a chronic condition marked by aches and fatigue, in part by helping to relieve any underlying depression. In an Italian study of 200 fibromyalgia sufferers, those who took 5-HTP along with conventional antidepressants had less pain than those receiving either 5-HTP or the drugs alone. If you're taking anti-depressants, don't try 5-HTP without consulting your doctor first. Adverse reactions can occur.

▼ HOW TO TAKE IT

DOSAGE

For depression and most other ailments: Take 50 to 100 mg 3 times a day.
For migraines: Take up to 100 mg 3 times a day if necessary.
For insomnia: Take 100 to 200 mg half an hour before bedtime. When using 5-HTP, it is a good idea to begin with a low dose (such as 50 mg) and gradually increase it if needed.
For fibromyalgia: Take 100 mg 3 times a day.
For appetite control and weight loss: Take 750 to 900 mg a day.

GUIDELINES FOR USE

• To ensure rapid absorption, take 5-HTP on an empty stomach.
• Don't use 5-HTP for more than 3 months without consulting your doctor.
• For weight control, take the supplement 30 minutes before meals.
• Don't use 5-HTP with the mood-enhancing herb St. John's wort or add

it to a St. John's wort/ephedra combination (sometimes recommended for weight control; *see pp. 376 and 377 for warnings against using ephedra*).
• Don't use 5-HTP with a conventional antidepressant.

SHOPPING HINTS

■ Even though a product is billed as 5-HTP, it may include additional herbs or nutrients that you do not need. Carefully check the ingredient list on the label to make sure you know what you're actually getting.

■ Because 5-HTP is typically sold in 50-mg and 100-mg strengths, you can use the smaller dose to increase your dosage more gradually. This will minimize your risk of suffering side effects.

LATEST FINDINGS

■ Although reports of adverse reactions in a few people taking 5-HTP have raised safety concerns, additional study is needed to determine whether these rare reactions are linked to possible contaminants in the supplement. Many experts have found 5-HTP to be safe and effective in large numbers of people.

■ In one study, 20 obese patients took either 5-HTP or a placebo for 12 weeks. During the first 6 weeks, they ate anything they wanted. Over the last 6 weeks, they restricted their daily diet to 1,200 calories. Those on 5-HTP lost 12 lb, compared with barely 2 lb for the placebo group.

FLAVONOIDS

What do citrus fruits, grape seed extract, red wine, pine bark extract, apples, and onions have in common? The answer is that they're all excellent sources of flavonoids, the colorful plant pigments that help us fight a host of disorders—from heart disease and various types of cancer to vision problems and hay fever.

COMMON USES

■ Reduce the risk of heart disease.

■ May prevent breast, prostate, and other types of cancer.

■ Lessen the chance of age-related vision problems, such as cataracts or macular degeneration.

■ Minimize the symptoms of hay fever and asthma.

■ Fight viral infections.

FORMS

■ Capsule

■ Tablet

■ Powder

■ Liquid

▼ WHAT IT IS

More than 4,000 flavonoids (or bioflavonoids, as they are sometimes called on supplement labels) have been identified, and scientists suspect that there may be many more still to be discovered in nature. Flavonoids give color to fruits, vegetables, and herbs and are found in legumes, grains, and nuts.

Flavonoids are also potent antioxidants. Some are even more powerful than vitamin C or vitamin E in neutralizing disease-causing unstable oxygen molecules (free radicals) in the body. So far, however, only a few flavonoids have been studied for their healing potential.

One of these, quercetin (found in onions and apples), also serves as a building block for other flavonoids. Rutin and hesperidin are the most active of the so-called citrus flavonoids,

which, as the name suggests, are present in oranges, grapefruit, tangerines, and other citrus fruits.

Other flavonoids include PCOs (or procyanidolic oligomers, also called proanthocyanidins), anthocyanosides, polyphenols, and genistein. PCOs are plentiful in pine bark and grape seed extracts and in red wine. Anthocyanosides are found in the herb bilberry.

Green tea is the primary source of polyphenols, especially EGCG (epigallocatechin-gallate), which experts believe is possibly the most effective cancer-fighting compound yet discovered. Genistein, found in soy products, has antioxidant properties and can mimic the effects of estrogen. (For more information, see the profiles on these individual supplements.)

▼ WHAT IT DOES

The disease-fighting potential of flavonoids stems from their ability to reduce inflammation, prevent the release of histamine (which causes allergy symptoms such as congestion), fight free radicals, boost immunity, strengthen blood vessels, and increase blood flow, among other actions.

PREVENTION

The flavonoids quercetin and PCOs may protect against heart disease and other circulatory disorders because they inhibit bodily changes that can lead to blocked arteries; they also help strengthen blood vessels in various ways.

Studies from Finland and the Netherlands found that people who get plenty of flavonoids, particularly quercetin, have a reduced risk of developing heart disease or having a stroke. In one study, a diet high in flavonoids appeared to cut the chances of dying from heart disease by 50% in women and 23% in men. Another study reported a 75% drop in stroke risk for men who had the highest intake of flavonoids, compared with those who had the lowest.

Polyphenols and quercetin have shown promise as anticancer compounds. Studies found lower rates of stomach, pancreatic, lung, and possibly breast cancer in people with a high intake of these flavonoids. In addition, soy-based genistein may help fight breast cancer and minimize hot flashes by interacting with estrogen receptors in the body. Quercetin also aids the body in using blood sugar and so may be valuable in preventing diabetes. Furthermore, it inhibits the buildup of sorbitol (a type of sugar) in the lens of the eye, a cause of cataracts.

ADDITIONAL BENEFITS
Quercetin may help relieve hay fever, sinusitis, and asthma because it can block allergic reactions to pollen and reduce inflammation in the airways and lungs. This antiinflammatory action also makes it useful in treating bug bites, eczema, and related skin conditions, as well as inflammatory disorders of the joints and muscles, including rheumatoid arthritis, gout, and fibromyalgia.

Because they strengthen blood vessels, PCOs and citrus flavonoids are helpful in repairing varicose veins and hemorrhoids. Rutin and hesperidin play a role in preventing bruising.

▼ HOW TO TAKE IT

DOSAGE
For general health benefits: Buy a flavonoid mixture that contains several types (such as quercetin, rutin, and hesperidin) and follow the dosage instructions on the label.

For allergies, asthma, gout, and insect bites: Take 500 mg quercetin 2 or 3 times a day.

GUIDELINES FOR USE
• Grape seed extract and green tea are excellent sources of flavonoids and exert an antioxidant effect as well.

• It's usually a good idea to combine flavonoids with vitamin C to enhance their protective properties.

• Quercetin should be taken 20 minutes before meals; other flavonoids can be taken at any time of the day.

SHOPPING HINTS
■ Mixed preparations of citrus flavonoids are the most widely available and the least expensive supplements of this type. They are also the least active, often providing a flavonoid content of only 50%. You'll get more value for your dollar by choosing preparations that contain pure rutin, pure hesperidin, or possibly both.

■ Flavonoids are sometimes mixed with vitamin C, and the combination is labeled and sold as vitamin C complex. It's usually less expensive, however, to buy vitamin C and flavonoids separately, which also allows you to vary your dose as needed.

DID YOU KNOW?
Eating an apple a day has always been associated with good health, and one study has suggested that quercetin may be the magic ingredient. Lung cancer risk fell by 58% in people who ate the most apples (a major source of quercetin) compared with those who ate the fewest apples.

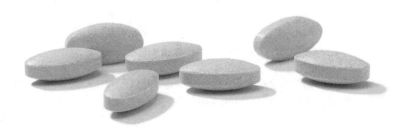

FLAXSEED/FLAXSEED OIL *(Linum usitatissimum)*

A rich source of healing oil, the common flaxseed has been cultivated for more than 7,000 years. The oil prevents and treats cancer, heart disease, and a variety of inflammatory disorders and hormone-related problems. Flaxseed and flaxseed oil have different beneficial effects and are not interchangeable.

COMMON USES

Flaxseed

- Relieves constipation.
- May relieve menstrual breast pain.
- May be useful in the treatment of breast cancer, diabetes, high blood pressure, and kidney disease caused by lupus nephritis.

Flaxseed oil

- May reduce high cholesterol or triglycerides.
- May prevent heart disease.
- May be beneficial in treating HIV/AIDS.

FORMS

- Capsule
- Softgel
- Oil
- Powder

▼ WHAT IT IS

It began as a fiber for weaving—and it remains the basis of natural linen fabric. However, the medicinal properties of flaxseeds quickly became legendary. A slender annual that grows up to 3 feet high and bears blue flowers from February through September, the flax plant was first grown in Europe, then later brought to North America, where it continues to thrive.

Both the oil from the flaxseeds (also known as linseeds) and the seeds are used for therapeutic purposes.

▼ WHAT IT DOES

Flaxseeds are a potent source of essential fatty acids (EFAs)—fats and oils critical for health that the body cannot make on its own. One EFA, alpha-linolenic acid, is known as an omega-3 fatty acid. Found in fish and flaxseeds, omega-3 fatty acids have been acclaimed for protecting against heart disease and for treating many other ailments. Flaxseeds also contain omega-6 fatty acids (in the form of linoleic acid)—the same healthy fats present in many vegetable oils.

In addition, flaxseeds provide substances called lignans, which appear to have beneficial effects on various hormones and may help fight cancer,

ALERT

SIDE EFFECTS

- Possible side effects may include itching, weakness, unstable gait, hives, itching, watering eyes, nasal congestion, sneezing, paralysis, seizures, shortness of breath, lowered blood pressure, nausea, rapid breathing, vomiting, stomach pain, intestinal obstruction, elevated blood sugar levels, menstrual cycle changes, increased risk of bleeding, and prostate cancer.

CAUTION

- Some people are allergic to flaxseed. If you experience any difficulty breathing after taking the supplement, seek immediate medical attention.

- Don't ever take flaxseed oil or ground flaxseeds if you have a bowel obstruction or a history of diarrhea, irritable bowel syndrome, diverticulitis, or inflammatory bowel disease. People with a history of esophageal or gastrointestinal problems should avoid flaxseeds (but not the oil).

- People who have a history of a bleeding disorder, high tryglyceride levels, diabetes, bipolar disorder, thyroid disorder, seizures, or asthma should use caution when taking flaxseed or flaxseed oil.

- **Reminder:** If you have a medical condition, are pregnant or breast feeding, or are taking medications, talk to your doctor before taking supplements.

bacteria, viruses, and fungi. Ounce for ounce, flaxseeds contain up to 800 times the lignans in most other foods.

MAJOR BENEFITS

Essential fatty acids work throughout the body to protect cell membranes— the outer coverings that are gate-keepers for all cells, admitting healthy nutrients and barring damaging sub-stances. That function explains why EFA-rich flaxseed oil has such far-reaching effects.

Flaxseed oil works to lower cholesterol, thereby protecting against heart dis-ease. It may provide benefits as well against angina and high blood pres-sure. A 5-year study at Simmons College in Boston indicated that flaxseed oil may be useful in pre-venting a second heart attack.

Crushed flaxseeds are an excellent natural source of fiber. They add bulk to stools and their oil lubricates the stools, making flaxseeds useful for the relief of constipation.

ADDITIONAL BENEFITS

Flaxseeds seem to have cancer-fighting properties, but further studies are needed. They may reduce the risk of certain cancers, including breast cancer. Studies at the University of Toronto found that the oil may also help treat women with early or advanced breast cancer.

Because flaxseeds contain plant-based estrogens (phytoestrogens) that mimic the female sex hormone estrogen, the oil can have beneficial effects on the menstrual cycle, balancing the ratio of estrogen to progesterone. It may also aid in the treatment of diabetes, high blood pressure, certain kidney diseases, and HIV/AIDS.

▼ HOW TO TAKE IT

DOSAGE

Liquid flaxseed oil is the easiest way to get a therapeutic amount, which ranges from 1 tsp to 1 tbsp once or twice a day. To get 1 tbsp of oil in cap-sule form, you'll need to swallow about 14 capsules, each containing 1,000 mg of oil.

For flaxseed fiber, for constipation, mix 1 to 3 tbsp of ground bulk flaxseeds with a glass of water; drink up to 3 times a day. The treatment may take a day or so to act. For other uses, take 50 g a day of ground, raw flaxseed (or 250 g of flaxseed flour) for up to 4 weeks.

GUIDELINES FOR USE

• Always take flaxseed oil with food, which enhances its absorption by the body. You can also mix it into yogurt, cottage cheese, juice, or other foods and drinks.

• Be sure to take ground flaxseed with plenty of water (a large glass per table-spoon) to prevent it from swelling up and blocking your throat or digestive tract.

• Because flax (both the seeds and the oil) can lessen the absorption of other medications, you should separate doses by at least 2 hours.

FOLIC ACID

Getting enough of this B vitamin could prevent 50,000 deaths each year from cardiovascular disease. It could also reduce by nearly half the number of babies born with common birth defects and possibly prevent many cancers as well. Yet, 9 out of 10 American adults still take far too little folic acid.

COMMON USES
- Protects against birth defects.
- Reduces the risk of heart disease and stroke.
- Lowers risk for several cancers.

FORMS
- Tablet
- Capsule
- Powder
- Liquid

▼ WHAT IT IS

This water-soluble B vitamin, also called folacin or folate, was first identified in the 1940s, when it was extracted from spinach. Because the body can't store folic acid very long, however, you need to replenish your supply daily.

Cooking or even long storage can destroy up to half the folic acid in foods, so supplements may be the best way to get an adequate intake of this vital nutrient.

▼ WHAT IT DOES

In the body, folic acid is used thousands of times a day to make blood cells, heal wounds, build muscle—in fact, it's necessary for every function that requires cell division.

Folic acid is critical to DNA and RNA formation, and it ensures that cells replicate normally. It is especially important in fetal development, helping produce key chemicals for the brain and nervous system.

PREVENTION
Adequate folic acid at conception and for the first 3 months of pregnancy greatly reduces the risk of serious birth defects, including spina bifida.

This B vitamin also appears to regulate the body's production and use of homocysteine, an amino acid–like substance that at high levels may damage the lining of blood vessels, making them more susceptible to plaque buildup. This makes folic acid an important weapon against heart disease.

In addition, folic acid may help the body ward off certain cancers, including those of the lungs, cervix, colon, and rectum.

ADDITIONAL BENEFITS
Folic acid may help depression. Because high levels of homocysteine may contribute to this condition, some experts think folic acid (which is often deficient in people who are depressed) may be of value because this nutrient reduces homocysteine levels. Studies also show that taking folic acid improves the effectiveness of antidepressants in people with low folic acid levels.

 ALERT

CAUTION
- Folic acid supplements, even at normal doses, may mask a type of anemia caused by a vitamin B_{12} deficiency. Unchecked, this anemia can cause irreversible nerve damage and dementia. If you take folic acid supplements, be sure to take extra vitamin B_{12} as well.

- Folic acid may reduce the effectiveness of certain anticonvulsant medications. Consult your doctor before taking folic acid supplements if you take medication for a seizure disorder.

- **Reminder:** If you have a medical or psychiatric condition, talk to your doctor before taking supplements.

Folic acid supplements have been useful in treating gout and irritable bowel syndrome as well. Because high homocysteine levels may be a factor in osteoporosis, folic acid may even help keep bones strong.

▼ HOW MUCH YOU NEED

The current adult RDA for folic acid is 400 µg a day. Supplements are important for older people, who may not get enough of this vitamin in food.

IF YOU GET TOO LITTLE
Although relatively rare, a severe folic acid deficiency can cause a form of anemia (megaloblastic anemia), a sore red tongue, chronic diarrhea, and poor growth (in children). Alcoholics and people who are on certain medications (for cancer or epilepsy) or who have malabsorption diseases (Crohn's, celiac sprue) are susceptible to severe deficiency. Much more common is a low level of folic acid, which causes no symptoms but raises the risk of heart disease or birth defects.

IF YOU GET TOO MUCH
Very large doses—5,000 to 10,000 µg—offer no benefit and may be dangerous for people with hormone-related cancers, such as those of the breast or prostate. High doses may also cause seizures in those with epilepsy or other seizure disorders.

The National Academy of Sciences suggests an upper daily limit of 1,000 µg of folic acid for adults.

▼ HOW TO TAKE IT

DOSAGE
For overall good health and the prevention of heart disease: Take 400 to 800 µg of folic acid a day.
For women who might become pregnant: Take a total of 800 µg a day. (Adequate folic acid stores are important because the vitamin plays a role in a baby's development starting with conception.)
For people with depression: Take 800 to 1,200 µg a day as part of a vitamin B complex supplement.

GUIDELINES FOR USE
• Folic acid can be taken at any time of the day with or without food.

• When taking individual folic acid supplements for any reason, combine them with an additional 1,000 µg of vitamin B_{12} to prevent a B_{12} deficiency.

▼ OTHER SOURCES

Excellent food sources of folic acid include green vegetables, beans, whole grains, and orange juice. Some refined grain products are now fortified with folic acid.

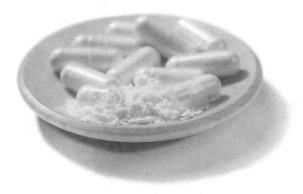

GARLIC *(Allium sativum)*

There was a time when people who wanted to keep their friends wouldn't eat garlic-laced foods and suffer the resulting bad breath. Today, aging baby boomers are more likely to follow the lead of the ancient Egyptians, who worshiped this highly pungent and potent herb for its medicinal and culinary powers.

COMMON USES

- Lowers cholesterol levels.
- Reduces blood clotting.
- May prevent some cancers.
- May produce a slight drop in blood pressure.
- Combats fungal infections.

FORMS

- Tablet
- Capsule
- Softgel
- Fresh herb
- Liquid
- Oil
- Powder

▼ WHAT IT IS

For thousands of years, garlic has been valued for its therapeutic potential. Egyptian pyramid builders took it for strength and endurance, Louis Pasteur investigated its antibacterial properties, and physicians in the two world wars used it to treat battle wounds.

Garlic is related to the onion, scallion, and other plants in the genus *Allium*. The entire plant is odoriferous, but the strongest aroma is concentrated in the bulb, the site of garlic's healing powers and flavor.

Most of garlic's health benefits derive from the more than 100 sulfur compounds it contains. When the bulb is crushed or chewed, alliin, one of the sulfur compounds, becomes allicin, the chemical responsible for garlic's odor and health effects. In turn, some of the allicin is rapidly broken down into other sulfur compounds, such as ajoene, which can also have medicinal properties. Cooking garlic inhibits the formation of allicin and eliminates some of the other therapeutic chemicals.

▼ WHAT IT DOES

Traditionally, garlic has been employed to treat everything from leprosy and parasites to hemorrhoids. Today, researchers are focusing on its potential to reduce the risk of heart disease and cancer.

PREVENTION

The liberal use of garlic in Italy and Spain may partly explain why these countries have such a low incidence of hardening of the arteries (arteriosclerosis). Several studies suggest that garlic can prevent heart disease in various ways. For example, garlic makes platelets (the cells involved in blood clotting) less likely to clump and stick to artery walls, lessening the chance of a heart attack.

There's evidence that the herb dissolves clot-forming proteins, which can affect plaque development. Garlic also lowers blood pressure slightly,

 ALERT

SIDE EFFECTS

- Some people develop heartburn, intestinal gas, diarrhea, bad breath, body odor, burning of the mouth, stomach pain or fullness, poor appetite, vomiting, changes in bacteria of the gut, and constipation when taking garlic, particularly at high doses.

- Other possible side effects include dizziness, sweating, difficulty breathing (asthma), fever, chills, runny nose, decreased blood pressure, change in blood sugar levels, contraction of the uterus, and change in thyroid function.

CAUTION

- People allergic to garlic, hyacinths, tulips, onions, leeks, and chives; who have a history of bleeding disorders, asthma, diabetes, low blood pressure, or thyroid disorders; or who are pregnant or breast feeding should not take garlic supplements.

- **Reminder:** If you have a medical condition; are taking anticoagulants, blood pressure, or cholesterol-lowering medications; or are contemplating surgery, talk to your doctor before taking garlic.

mainly because of its ability to widen blood vessels and help blood circulate more freely. Garlic may also help prevent certain diseases of the eye.

Some studies have examined garlic's effect on cholesterol. Good scientific evidence shows that garlic helps treat high cholesterol, and it may even benefit people with inherited high cholesterol disorders. The herb may interfere with the metabolism of cholesterol in the liver; as a result, less cholesterol is released into the blood.

ADDITIONAL BENEFITS
Garlic may have anticancer properties. It has been found to be particularly effective in preventing digestive cancers and possibly even breast and prostate cancers. Researchers aren't sure how garlic produces these benefits. Several mechanisms may be involved. First, there's the herb's ability to increase the level of enzymes that can detoxify cancer triggers. Then, it blocks the formation of nitrites linked to stomach cancer. Garlic's antioxidant properties are important as well.

Garlic is often effective against infectious organisms—viruses, bacteria, and fungi—because allicin can block the enzymes that give the organisms their ability to invade and damage tissues. It may even treat upper respiratory tract infections. The herb has also been shown to inhibit the fungi responsible for causing athlete's foot and swimmer's ear.

▼ HOW TO TAKE IT

DOSAGE
Adults (aged 18 or older): Raw garlic cloves: Eat ½ to 2 raw garlic cloves (2 to 6 g) up to 4 times a day; ***Garlic pills:*** Take 600 to 900 mg a day in 3 doses; ***Garlic powder:*** Take 0.4 to 1.2 g a day in 3 doses; ***Oil extract of garlic:*** Take 1 or 2 capsules or 0.3 to 0.12 ml 2 times a day; ***Garlic juice:*** Take ½ to 1 tsp 3 times a day; ***Garlic syrup:*** Take ½ to 1½ tsp 3 times a day; ***Tincture:*** Take ½ to 1 tsp of a tincture (1:5; 45% alcohol) 3 times a day.
Children (under 18): There is not enough scientific evidence to recommend garlic supplements for children at this time. The amounts of garlic found in foods are throught to be safe.

GUIDELINES FOR USE
• Garlic can be taken indefinitely.

• If you are using the herb for cholesterol problems, have your blood lipid levels checked in 3 months to see if they have changed; if you haven't derived any benefits, talk to your doctor about other remedies.

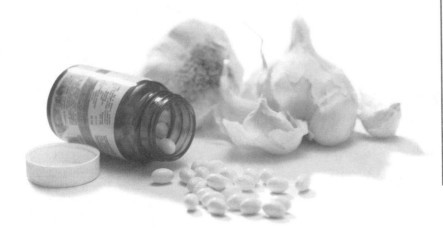

GINGER *(Zingiber officinale)*

From ancient India and China to Greece and Rome, ginger was revered as both a medicinal and culinary spice. Medieval Europeans traced this herb to the Garden of Eden, and it has long been valued by traditional healers. In modern homes and hospitals, it's used to quell nausea and much more.

COMMON USES

■ Alleviates nausea.

■ May relieve pain and inflammation of arthritis.

■ May reduce postoperative nausea and vomiting and motion sickness.

■ May relieve pain associated with rheumatic diseases.

FORMS

■ Capsule
■ Tablet
■ Softgel
■ Oil
■ Liquid
■ Fresh or dried root/Tea
■ Crystallized, candied herb

▼ WHAT IT IS

Renowned for its stomach-settling properties, ginger is native to parts of India and China, as well as to Jamaica and other tropical areas. This warm-climate perennial is related to turmeric and marjoram. Its roots are used for culinary and therapeutic purposes.

As a spice, ginger adds a hot and lemony flavor to foods as disparate as roast pork and gingersnap cookies. Medicinally, it continues to play a major role in traditional healing.

▼ WHAT IT DOES

For thousands of years, all around the globe, this pungent spice has been popular as a treatment for digestive problems, ranging from mild indigestion and flatulence to nausea and vomiting. It's also been helpful for relieving colds and arthritis. Modern research into ginger's active ingredients confirms its effectiveness.

MAJOR BENEFITS

What can you do with a seasick sailor? The answer is, try ginger. In a Danish study, 40 naval cadets took 1 g of powdered ginger a day; they were much less likely to break out in a cold sweat and vomit (classic symptoms of being seasick) than 39 others who took a placebo.

Because ginger works primarily in the digestive tract, boosting digestive fluids and neutralizing acids, it may be a good medical alternative to antinausea drugs that can affect the central nervous system and cause grogginess. Clinical studies of women undergoing exploratory surgery (laparoscopy) or major gynecological surgery show that taking 1 g of ginger before an operation can significantly reduce postoperative nausea and vomiting, a common side effect of anesthetics and other medications given in surgery.

Ginger also appears to counter the nausea created by chemotherapy, although it's best to take it with food.

 ALERT

SIDE EFFECTS

• Ginger is very safe for a broad range of complaints; occasional heartburn is the most common side effect.

CAUTION

• Consult your doctor if unusual or unexpected bleeding develops while taking ginger. Discontinue use 2 weeks prior to surgery and dental procedures because of a risk of bleeding.

• Ginger may relieve morning sickness during the first 2 months of pregnancy (up to 250 mg 4 times a day). Longer use or higher doses should be taken only under a doctor's supervision.

• Chemotherapy patients should not take ginger on an empty stomach because it can irritate the stomach lining.

• People who have a history of irregular heartbeat (arrhythmia) should avoid ginger. Those with a history of ulcers, inflammatory bowel disease, blocked intestines, bleeding disorders, and gallstones should exercise caution using it.

• **Reminder:** If you have a medical condition or are taking medications, talk to your doctor before taking supplements.

Ginger's antinausea effects make it useful for reducing dizziness (common in older patients) as well as for treating morning sickness. For years, ginger has been a staple of folk medicine, serving primarily as a digestive aid.

Ginger supplements (or fresh pulp mixed with lime juice) are also a fine remedy for flatulence.

ADDITIONAL BENEFITS

Ginger's antiinflammatory and pain-relieving properties may help relieve the muscle aches and chronic pain associated with arthritis and other conditions. In a study of 7 women with rheumatoid arthritis (an autoimmune disease characterized by severe inflammation), just 5 to 50 g of fresh ginger or capsules containing up to 1 g of powdered ginger lessened joint pain and inflammation.

▼ HOW TO TAKE IT

DOSAGE

To prevent motion sickness, dizziness, and nausea; reduce flatulence; and relieve chronic pain or rheumatoid arthritis: Take ginger up to 3 times a day or every 4 hours as needed. The usual dose is 100 to 200 mg of the standardized extract in pill form, 1 or 2 g of fresh powdered ginger, or a ½-inch slice of fresh ginger root.

Other preparations, including ginger tea (available in tea bags, or use ½ tsp of grated ginger root per cup of very hot water) or natural ginger ale (containing real ginger), can be used several times a day for similar purposes and for arthritis and pain relief. On trips, try crystallized ginger candy. A 1-inch square, about ¼-inch thick, contains about 500 mg of ginger.

For aching muscles: Rub several drops of ginger oil, mixed with ½ oz almond oil or another neutral oil, on the sore areas.

GUIDELINES FOR USE

• Take ginger capsules with fluid. If you are trying to prevent motion sickness, have ginger 3 to 4 hours before your departure and then take it every 4 hours as needed up to 4 times a day.

• For postoperative nausea, begin taking ginger the day before your operation—but only under a doctor's supervision. Medical oversight is needed because ginger can increase bleeding under certain circumstances.

Whether eaten fresh or taken in capsules, ginger is a potent remedy for nausea and dizziness.

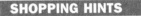

■ Buy ginger supplements standardized to contain "pungent compounds." These consist of gingerols and shogaols—the active ingredients that give ginger its healing properties.

■ Look for natural ginger ales made from real ginger: An 8-oz glass contains about a gram of ginger. Most widely distributed commercial ginger ales have only tiny amounts of ginger or ginger flavoring, which have no therapeutic benefits at all.

FACTS & TIPS

■ The ancient Greeks so prized ginger for digestion that they mixed it into their bread. Thus was born the first gingerbread.

■ American colonists brewed a stomach-soothing remedy called ginger beer—a forerunner of today's ginger ale.

■ For colds or the flu, many folk healers recommend chewing fresh ginger, drinking ginger tea, or squeezing juice from gingerroot into a spoonful of honey. All may help ease the aches and chest tightness associated with these infections.

DID YOU KNOW?

A cup of ginger tea contains the equivalent of about 250 mg of the powdered herb. A heavily spiced Chinese or Indian ginger dish has about twice that amount.

GINKGO BILOBA *(Ginkgo biloba)*

This popular herbal medicine is derived from one of the oldest species of tree on earth, and today it is widely marketed as a general memory booster. Ginkgo biloba does seem to help with age-related memory loss, but whether this high profile herb is a universal "smart pill" that's meant for everyone remains to be seen.

COMMON USES

- Slows progression of Alzheimer's; sharpens memory and concentration.
- May lessen depression and anxiety.
- Alleviates coldness in the extremities and painful leg cramps.
- May help headaches, ringing in the ears (tinnitus), and dizziness.
- May restore impotent men's erections.

FORMS

- Tablet
- Capsule
- Softgel
- Powder
- Liquid

▼ WHAT IT IS

The medicinal form of the herb is extracted from the fan-shaped leaves of the ancient ginkgo biloba tree, a species that has survived in China for more than 200 million years. (The leaves are double- or bi-lobed; hence the name "biloba.")

A concentrated form of the herb called ginkgo biloba extract (GBE) is used to make the dietary supplement that is sold in stores all over the United States today. Commonly called ginkgo, GBE is obtained by drying and milling the plant's leaves and then extracting the active ingredients in a mixture of acetone and water.

▼ WHAT IT DOES

Ginkgo may have beneficial effects on both the circulatory and the central nervous systems. It increases blood flow to the brain and to the arms and legs by regulating the tone and elasticity of blood vessels, from the largest arteries to the tiniest capillaries. It also acts like aspirin by helping reduce the "stickiness" of the blood, thereby lowering the risk of blood clots.

Ginkgo appears to have antioxidant properties as well, mopping up the damaging compounds known as free radicals and aiding in the maintenance of healthy blood cells. Some researchers report that it enhances the nervous system by promoting the delivery of additional oxygen and blood sugar (glucose) to nerve cells.

PREVENTION

Interest now centers on ginkgo's possible role as a preventive for age-related memory loss. Unfortunately, there's little scientific evidence that ginkgo will make most people better able to focus or remember. So far, it is those already suffering from diminished blood flow to the brain—not healthy volunteers—who have benefited most from taking the herb.

Current research is trying to determine whether ginkgo's ability to help prevent blood clots may stave off heart attacks or strokes.

 ALERT

SIDE EFFECTS

- Rarely, ginkgo may cause restlessness, diarrhea, nausea, vomiting, headache, bleeding, muscle weakness, loss of muscle tone, change in blood pressure or blood sugar, and reduced fertility. These effects are usually transient; if they persist, reduce the dosage or stop taking the herb.

CAUTION

- Doses higher than 240 mg a day can cause disorientation and other problems.

- People allergic to members of the Ginkgoaceae family, mango rind, sumac, poison ivy, or cashews should use ginkgo cautiously.

- Do not use ginkgo if you are pregnant.

- **Reminder:** Talk to your doctor before taking ginkgo if you have a medical condition, especially a blood-clotting disorder; are taking medications; are having surgery; or have a psychiatric condition.

MAJOR BENEFITS

The fact that ginkgo aids blood flow to the brain—thus increasing oxygen—is of particular relevance to older people, whose arteries may have narrowed with cholesterol buildup or other conditions. Diminished blood flow has been linked to Alzheimer's and memory loss, as well as to anxiety, headaches, depression, confusion, ringing in the ears, and dizziness. All may be helped by ginkgo.

Ginkgo also promotes blood flow to the arms and legs, making it useful for reducing the pain, cramping, and weakness caused by narrowed arteries in the leg, a disorder called intermittent claudication. There are indications that the herb may improve circulation to the extremities in those with Raynaud's phenomenon, or help victims of scleroderma, an uncommon autoimmune disorder.

ADDITIONAL BENEFITS

In addition, some studies suggest that ginkgo may be of value in treating macular degeneration or diabetes-related eye disease (both leading causes of blindness), as well as some types of hearing loss, by increasing blood flow to the nerve-rich fibers of the eyes and ears.

Ongoing studies are assessing the possible effectiveness of ginkgo in treating conditions that may be related to circulatory or nervous system impairment, including impotence, multiple sclerosis,

and nerve damage that is frequently associated with diabetes. Traditional Chinese healers have long used ginkgo for asthma, because the herb appears to alleviate wheezing and other respiratory complaints.

Gingko can be used to treat some conditions of the eyes. It may also be useful in treating depression and seasonal affective disorder (SAD), multiple sclerosis, and altitude sickness and in reducing side effects associated with chemotherapy.

▼ HOW TO TAKE IT

DOSAGE

Always take supplements that contain ginkgo biloba extract—or GBE—the concentrated form of the herb.

As a general memory booster and for poor circulation: Take 80 to 360 mg of GBE in 2 or 3 divided doses or 3 to 6 ml (about 1 tsp) of 40 mg/ml extract divided into 3 doses. *For Alzheimer's disease, depression, ringing in the ears, dizziness, impotence, or other conditions caused by insufficient blood flow to the brain:* Take up to 240 mg a day.

GUIDELINES FOR USE

• It often takes 4 to 6 weeks, and in some cases up to 12 weeks, to notice the herb's effects.

• You can take ginkgo biloba with or without food.

• Ginkgo biloba is generally considered safe for long-term use when it's taken in recommended dosages.

SHOPPING HINTS

■ Be certain that you buy preparations with ginkgo biloba extract to ensure that you're getting a standardized amount of the active ingredients. GBE supplements should contain at least 24% flavone glycosides (organic substances responsible for the herb's antioxidant and anticlotting properties) and 6% terpene lactones (primarily chemicals called ginkgolides and bilobalides, which improve blood flow and are thought to protect the nerves).

LATEST FINDINGS

■ A yearlong study published in the *Journal of the American Medical Association* evaluated 202 patients with dementia, most of whom also had Alzheimer's disease. Patients who took 120 mg of ginkgo biloba extract a day were more likely to stabilize or improve their mental and social functions, compared with those given a placebo. The effects were modest and of limited duration.

DID YOU KNOW?

Ginkgo trees have two "sexes"— male and female. The nuts from the female tree are still valued in China and Japan as a culinary delicacy with healing properties. Ginkgo seeds are dangerous; however, and should be avoided.

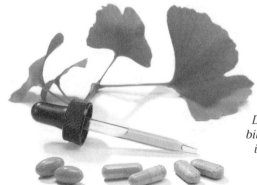

Derived from ginkgo biloba leaves, the herb is effective in either pill or liquid form.

GINSENG (PANAX) *(Panax ginseng)*

A wildly popular herb in the United States and Europe, ginseng is added to everything from fruit juices to vitamin supplements. Most of these products actually contain very little ginseng and are typically ineffective, but supplements made with quality ginseng do indeed exert a variety of protective effects on the body.

COMMON USES

- Boosts mental performance.
- Improves type 2 diabetes.
- May increase exercise performance, improve sense of well-being, and enhance the immune system.
- May treat cardiovascular conditions.
- May decrease menopausal symptoms and restore erectile function.

FORMS

- Tablet
- Capsule
- Softgel
- Powder
- Liquid/Tincture
- Dried herb/Tea

▼ WHAT IT IS

Panax ginseng (also commonly called Asian, Chinese, or Korean ginseng) has been used in Chinese medicine for thousands of years to enhance longevity and the quality of life. *Panax ginseng* is the most widely available and extensively studied form of this herb. Another species, *Panax quinquefolius,* or American ginseng, is grown mainly in the Midwest and exported to China.

The medicinal part of the plant is its slow-growing root, which is harvested after 4 to 6 years, when its overall ginsenoside—the main active ingredient in ginseng—content is at its peak. There are 13 different ginsenosides in all. Panax ginseng also contains panaxans, substances that can lower blood sugar, and polysaccharides, complex sugar molecules that enhance the immune system.

"White" ginseng is simply the dried root; "red" ginseng has been steamed and dried.

Panax ginseng should not be confused with Siberian ginseng *(Eleutherococcus senticosus)*, discussed later.

▼ WHAT IT DOES

The primary health benefits of Panax ginseng derive from its immune-stimulating and antioxidant properties, as well as from its ability to protect the body against the effects of stress.

PREVENTION

Ginseng may help the body combat a variety of illnesses. It stimulates the production of specialized immune cells called "killer T cells," which destroy harmful viruses and bacteria. It may also be useful in treating people with low white blood cell counts.

Studies have also indicated that the herb may inhibit the growth of certain cancer cells. A large Korean study found that the risk of developing cancer in people who took ginseng was half that of those who did not take it.

 ALERT

SIDE EFFECTS

- At the doses recommended here, ginseng is unlikely to cause any noticeable side effects.
- Some women report increased menstrual bleeding or breast tenderness with high doses of ginseng. If this occurs, reduce the dose or stop using it.

CAUTION

- Ginseng may interact with blood thinners or aspirin, medications broken down by the liver, medications used to control blood sugar, some heart medications, blood pressure medications, pseudoephedrine, phenelzine, diuretics, central nervous system stimulants, corticosteroids, hormonal medications, antipsychotics, and herbs and supplements with similar effects.
- **Reminder:** If you have a medical condition or are pregnant or nursing, talk to your doctor before taking ginseng.

Although ginseng powders and tinctures were shown to have cancer-preventive effects, eating fresh ginseng root or drinking ginseng juice or tea did not lower the cancer risk.

ADDITIONAL BENEFITS

Ginseng may benefit people who are feeling fatigued and overstressed and those recovering from a long illness. The herb has been shown to balance the release of stress hormones in the body and support the organs that produce these hormones, namely the pituitary gland and hypothalamus in the brain, and the adrenal glands, located on top of the kidneys. Ginseng may also enhance the production of endorphins, "feel-good" chemicals produced by the brain.

Many long-distance runners and bodybuilders take ginseng to heighten physical endurance. Some nutritionally oriented doctors and herbalists believe that ginseng is able to delay fatigue because it enables the exercising muscles to use energy more efficiently. There is research, however, that contradicts this hypothesis.

Ginseng may be helpful for impotence, but the way it works is not clear. Some of its active ingredients appear to affect smooth muscle tissue and improve erectile function. Men with fertility problems may benefit from ginseng as well, because animal studies indicate that it increases testosterone levels and sperm production.

There is good scientific evidence that ginseng improves mental performance and is useful in treating type 2 diabetes. Other benefits may include treating cardiovascular conditions, including high blood pressure, congestive heart failure, and cardiovascular disease.

▼ HOW TO TAKE IT

DOSAGE

Select a product that is standardized to contain at least 4% to 7% ginsenosides.

Ginseng tablets/capsules: Take 100 mg of ginseng extract (4% ginsenosides) once or twice daily.
Ginseng liquid/fluid: Take a decoction of 1 to 2 g in ⅓ cup of water, a 1:1 (g per ml) fluid extract as 1 to 2 ml daily, or 1 to 2 tsp of a 1:5 tincture (g per ml).

GUIDELINES FOR USE

• Start at the lower end of the dosage range and increase your intake gradually until you begin to feel better.
• Some experts recommend that you stop taking ginseng for a week every 2 or 3 weeks and then resume your regular dose. In some cases, ginseng may be rotated with other immune-stimulating herbs, such as astragalus or Siberian ginseng.
• The combination of ginseng and caffeine may intensify any side effects, so cut back on (or avoid) caffeine.

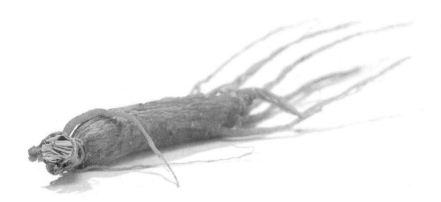

GLUCOSAMINE

This promising and popular arthritis fighter helps build cartilage, which provides cushioning at the tips of the bones. It also protects and strengthens the joints as it relieves the pain and stiffness that often accompany this degenerative condition. Although your body produces some glucosamine, a supplement is more effective.

COMMON USES

■ Relieves pain, stiffness, and swelling caused by osteoarthritis or rheumatoid arthritis, which affect the knees, fingers, and other joints.

■ Helps reduce arthritic back and neck pain.

■ May have beneficial effects in blood circulation problems, temporomandibular joint (TMJ) disorders, and inflammatory bowel disease.

FORMS

■ Capsule
■ Tablet
■ Powder

▼ WHAT IT IS

Scientists have long known that the body manufactures a small amount of glucosamine (pronounced glue-KOSE-a-mean), a fairly simple molecule that contains the sugar glucose. It's found in relatively high concentrations in the joints and connective tissues, where the body uses it to form the larger molecules necessary for cartilage repair and maintenance.

In recent years, glucosamine has become available as a nutritional supplement. Various forms are sold, including glucosamine sulfate and N-acetyl-glucosamine (NAG). Glucosamine sulfate is the preferred form

for arthritis: It is readily used by the body (90% to 98% is absorbed through the intestine) and appears to be very effective for this condition.

▼ WHAT IT DOES

Although some experts hail glucosamine as an arthritis cure, no one supplement can claim that title. It does, however, provide significant relief from pain and inflammation for about half of arthritis sufferers—especially those with the common age-related form known as osteoarthritis. It can also help people with rheumatoid arthritis and other types of joint injuries, and it offers additional benefits as well.

MAJOR BENEFITS

Approved for the treatment of arthritis in at least 70 countries around the world, glucosamine has been shown to ease pain and inflammation, increase range of motion, and help repair aging and damaged joints in the knees, hips, spine, and hands.

Studies have shown that glucosamine may be even more effective for relieving pain and inflammation than aspirin, ibuprofen, and other nonsteroidal anti-inflammatory drugs (NSAIDs)—and without the side effects of NSAIDs. NSAIDs, commonly taken by arthritis sufferers, mask arthritis pain, but they do little to combat the progression of the disease—and may even make it worse by impairing the body's ability to build cartilage.

 ALERT

SIDE EFFECTS
• Glucosamine is virtually free of severe side effects, but drowsiness, insomnia, headache, increased nail growth, rash, sun sensitivity, heart palpitations, elevated blood pressure, water retention, stomach upset, heartburn, diarrhea, nausea, vomiting, constipation, decreased appetite, abdominal pain, flatulence, or eye cataract formation may occur in some people.

CAUTION
• Glucosamine may interact with certain diuretic drugs, necessitating higher doses of the diuretic. It may also interact with medications used to alter blood sugar levels and herbs and supplements with similar effects. Consult your doctor for guidance.

• People who have a history of diabetes mellitus, shellfish allergy, iodine sensitivity, kidney disease, cataracts, or active peptic ulcer disease should exercise caution when using glucosamine.

• **Reminder:** If you have a medical condition or are or wish to become pregnant, talk to your doctor before taking supplements.

In contrast, glucosamine helps make cartilage and may repair damaged joints. Although it can't do much for people with advanced arthritis, when cartilage has completely worn away, it may benefit the millions of people with mild to moderately severe symptoms.

ADDITIONAL BENEFITS

As a joint strengthener, glucosamine may be useful for the prevention of arthritis and many forms of age-related degenerative joint disease. It may also improve symptoms of temporo-mandibular joint (TMJ) disorder.

In addition to aiding joints and connective tissues, glucosamine promotes a healthy lining in the digestive tract and may be beneficial in treating ailments such as inflammatory bowel disease. It is included in various "intestinal health" preparations sold in health food stores, usually in the form of NAG (N-acetyl-glucosamine), which tends to act specifically on the intestinal lining.

There is some scientific evidence to suggest that glucosamine may have beneficial effects in patients suffering from blood circulation problems.

▼ HOW TO TAKE IT

DOSAGE

The standard dosage for arthritis and other conditions is 500 mg glucosamine sulfate 3 times a day. For convenience, the entire dose of 1,500 mg can be taken once daily in either pill or powder form. (Packets containing a daily dose of powdered glucosamine are convenient; mix it into a glass of water.)

This amount (1,500 mg) has been shown to be safe for all individuals and effective for most. People weighing more than 200 lb or taking diuretics may need higher daily doses (about 900 mg per 100 lb of body weight); talk to your doctor about determining an appropriate dosage.

GUIDELINES FOR USE

• Glucosamine is typically taken long term and appears to be very safe. It may not bring relief as quickly as pain relievers or antiinflammatories (it usually works in 2 to 8 weeks), but its benefits are far greater and longer lasting when it's used over an extended period of time.
• Take glucosamine with meals. Food will help minimize the chance of digestive upset.
• Glucosamine's antiarthritis effects may be enhanced by using it along with another supplement, such as chondroitin sulfate (a related cartilage-building compound), niacinamide (a form of the B vitamin niacin), or S-adenosylmethionine (SAMe), a form of the amino acid methionine. Other supplements that are sometimes taken along with glucosamine for the relief of arthritis include boswellia, a tree extract from India; sea cucumber, an ancient Chinese remedy; and the topical pain reliever cayenne cream.

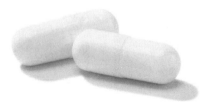

GOLDENSEAL *(Hydrastis canadensis)*

For centuries, the Cherokee, Iroquois, and other Native American tribes have valued the root of the goldenseal plant as a remedy for everything from insect bites and bloating to eye infections and stomachaches. Today, this versatile herb is officially recognized as a medicine in 11 countries—though not yet in the United States.

COMMON USES

- May bolster the immune system.
- May treat eye infection.
- May help treat the common cold and upper respiratory tract infections.
- May fight malaria and infectious diarrhea.

FORMS

- Capsule
- Softgel
- Liquid
- Dried herb/Tea
- Ointment/Cream

▼ WHAT IT IS

The dried root of this perennial herb has long been used to soothe inflamed or infected mucous membranes. Today, it is appreciated for its ability to help the body fight infection.

The plant was first called goldenseal in the nineteenth century, deriving its name from the rich yellow of the root and the small cuplike scars found there. These scars, which appear on the previous year's root growth, resemble the wax seals that were once used to close envelopes—hence the name "goldenseal."

Related to the buttercup, goldenseal is native to North America and once grew wild from Vermont to Arkansas. As interest in the herb's medicinal properties grew, however, the plant was extensively harvested. Currently, most of the goldenseal on the market is commercially cultivated in Oregon and Washington.

The key medicinal compounds in goldenseal are the alkaloids berberine and hydrastine. Berberine is also responsible for the root's rich yellow color—so vibrant, in fact, that Native Americans and early settlers utilized goldenseal as a dye as well as a medicinal herb. Because the alkaloids have a bitter taste, goldenseal tea often includes other herbs. It can be mixed with a sweetener such as honey.

▼ WHAT IT DOES

The primary benefit of goldenseal is its overall effect on immunity. Not only does it increase the immune system's production of germ-fighting compounds, this herb can combat both bacteria and viruses directly.

PREVENTION

Taking goldenseal at the first sign of a cold or the flu may prevent the illness from developing fully—or at least greatly minimize the symptoms—by enhancing the activity of virus-fighting white blood cells.

ADDITIONAL BENEFITS

Goldenseal may fight bacteria and may be useful in fighting upper respiratory tract infections, malaria, and infectious diarrhea.

As one of several herbs that stimulate the immune system—others include echinacea, pau d'arco, and astragalus—goldenseal may play a role in relieving the symptoms of chronic fatigue syndrome, a disabling disorder that may be partially caused by a weakened immune system.

Once cooled and strained, goldenseal tea can be used as an eyewash to relieve certain eye infections. Be sure to prepare a fresh batch daily and store it in a sterile container, so the tea won't get contaminated.

▼ HOW TO TAKE IT

DOSAGE

Tablets/capsules: Take 500 to 1,000 mg of goldenseal 3 times daily.
Liquid: Take 0.3 to 1 ml of liquid or fluid extract (1:1 in 60% ethanol) 3 times daily, 0.5 to 1 g as a decoction (boiling the bark or roots) 3 times daily, or ⅔ to ⅘ tsp as a tincture (1:10 in 60% ethanol) 3 times daily.

For eye infections: Use 1 tsp dried herb per pint of hot water. Steep, finely strain, cool, and apply as an eyewash 3 times a day; make a new solution every day.

GUIDELINES FOR USE

• Take goldenseal with meals.

• Use goldenseal only when you feel as if you're coming down with a cold, the flu, or some other illness, and use it only for the duration of the illness.

• As a general rule, don't use goldenseal for more than 3 weeks at a time. And wait 2 weeks, at least, before taking it again.

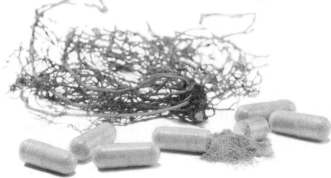

The root of the goldenseal plant is dried and then ground to a fine powder for use in supplements.

CASE HISTORY

Go for the Gold

Alexa K. always reacted badly to antibiotics. Although she knew she needed them for her sinus infections, the side effects (dizziness, nausea, diarrhea) often made the drugs worse than the illness.

When an herbalist told her to try goldenseal extract, her doctor was skeptical. "Look," he said, "try the goldenseal, but keep my prescription handy. If you don't feel better, you can always get it filled."

Alexa took the goldenseal, and in a few days her sinus infection was gone—without a single side effect. Now goldenseal is a part of her sinus first-aid kit. At the first sign of an infection, she starts taking it, along with the immune stimulator echinacea.

Although antibiotics are sometimes necessary, in the last few years Alexa has often been able to avoid them. "Those miserable side effects are history!" she happily reports.

GOTU KOLA *(Centella asiatica)*

Because this herb from India has long been a favorite food of elephants, notoriously long-lived animals, many people associate its use with longevity. Even though scientific research hasn't shown that this plant can extend your life, studies have found that gotu kola does provide many other important health benefits.

COMMON USES

■ Improves blood circulation problems and varicose veins.

■ May improve diabetes-related cardiovascular disease.

■ May reduce anxiety.

■ May speed healing.

FORMS

■ Capsule

■ Tablet

■ Liquid

■ Powder

■ Dried herb/Tea

▼ WHAT IT IS

The medicinal use of gotu kola has its roots in India, where the herb continues to be part of the ancient healing tradition called ayurveda. Word of its therapeutic benefits for skin disorders gradually spread throughout Asia and Europe. In fact, gotu kola has been prescribed in France to treat burns and other wounds since the 1880s.

A red-flowered plant that thrives in hot, swampy areas, gotu kola grows naturally in India, Sri Lanka, Madagascar, middle and southern Africa, Australia, China, and the southern United States.

The appearance of this slender, creeping perennial changes depending on whether it's growing in water (broad, fan-shaped leaves) or on dry land (small, thin leaves). The plant's leaf is most commonly used medicinally.

▼ WHAT IT DOES

Whether taken internally or applied externally as a compress, gotu kola has many beneficial effects. The herb's workhorse substances are chemicals called triterpenes (especially asiaticoside), which appear to enhance the formation of collagen in bones, cartilage, and connective tissue. In addition, they promote healthy blood vessels and help produce neurotransmitters, the chemical messengers in the brain.

MAJOR BENEFITS

Gotu kola's singular effect on connective tissue—promoting its healthy development and inhibiting the formation of hardened areas—makes this herb potentially important for treating many skin conditions. It can be therapeutic for burns, keloids (overgrown scar tissue), and wounds (including surgical incisions and skin ulcers).

Gotu kola also seems to strengthen cells in the walls of blood vessels, improving blood flow and making it valuable for the treatment of varicose veins. Research results have been

 ALERT

SIDE EFFECTS
• Possible side effects include skin rash, nausea, sedation, increased cholesterol, fatigue, increased blood sugar, decreased fertility, cancer, and allergic reactions. If you experience these symptoms, reduce the dosage or stop using the herb.

CAUTION
• Women who are pregnant, trying to conceive, or are breast feeding; people who are allergic to gotu kola, asiaticoside, asiatic acid, or madecassic; and people who have a history of high cholesterol, cancer, or diabetes should not take gotu kola.

• Possible drug interactions include medications that cause drowsiness, cholesterol-lowering medications, medications used to control blood sugar levels, steroids, phenylbutazone, and herbs and supplements with similar effects.

• **Reminder:** If you have a medical condition, talk to your doctor before taking supplements.

impressive. In more than a dozen studies observing gotu kola's effect on veins (which are surrounded by supportive connective tissue sheaths), about 80% of patients with varicose veins and similar problems showed substantial improvement. There is also evidence to suggest that it may improve diabetes-related cardiovascular disease.

ADDITIONAL BENEFITS

Gotu kola has been used to increase mental acuity for thousands of years. Most current research does not support its use for improving memory; however, it may play a role in reducing anxiety.

▼ HOW TO TAKE IT

DOSAGE

To treat varicose veins: Take 40 to 60 mg of the standardized extract or 400 to 600 mg of the dried whole herb 3 times a day.
For burns: Apply gotu kola liquid extract or a strong (cooled) gotu kola tea (see below) to the burn twice a day.

GUIDELINES FOR USE

• You can use both the oral and topical preparations of the herb over the same period of time.

• Internally, gotu kola is usually taken in the form of a tablet or capsule with or without meals.

• Topically, a gotu kola tea or a liquid extract can be applied to the skin for burns, wounds, incisions, or scars. To apply gotu kola topically, soak a compress in tea or in 1 to 2 tsp of liquid extract and apply it directly to problem areas. Start with a relatively weak solution and increase the strength as needed.

• To brew gotu kola tea, steep 1 or 2 tsp of dried leaf in a cup of very hot water for 10 to 15 minutes.

SHOPPING HINTS

■ When buying gotu kola supplements, look for those products that are standardized to contain 10% asiaticoside, an active ingredient in the herb. If you cannot find the standardized extract, you may substitute 400 to 500 mg of the crude herb for each 200 mg dose of the standardized extract.

FACTS & TIPS

■ Gotu kola is also known as *Centella asiatica*, talepetrako, Indian pennywort, Indian water navelwort, or hydrocotyle. A plant native to Europe, marsh pennywort *(Hydrocotyle vulgaris)*, is a related species, but it has no known therapeutic properties.

■ Although the names sound similar, there's no relationship between gotu kola and the kola (or cola) nut, which is used in cola soft drinks. The kola nut is a stimulant containing caffeine; gotu kola is a very mild sedative and caffeine-free.

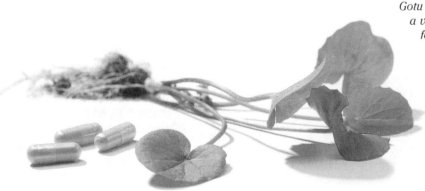

Gotu kola leaf is sold in a variety of supplement forms, including capsules.

GRAPE SEED EXTRACT

With antioxidant properties many times more powerful than those found in better-known nutrients (including vitamin C and vitamin E), grape seed extract is a heart-smart and cancer-smart botanical. It also has the power to improve vascular health, protect brain cells, and increase your overall well-being in many ways.

COMMON USES

- Treats blood vessel disorders.
- Protects against vision damage.
- Lessens the risk of heart disease and cancer.
- May reduce skin damage and redness from sunlight and ultraviolet light.
- Reduces swelling after surgery or injury.

FORMS

- Capsule
- Tablet
- Liquid

▼ WHAT IT IS

This extract made from the tiny seeds of red grapes is a flavonoid and one of Europe's leading natural treatments. Plant substances with potent antioxidant potential, flavonoids protect the cells from damage by unstable oxygen molecules called free radicals.

Grape seed extract contains procyanidolic oligomers (PCOs), also called proanthocyanidins. Once called pycnogenols (pik-NODGE-en-alls), PCOs are believed to play an important role in preventing heart disease and cancer.

"Pycnogenol" with a capital P is the trademark for a specific PCO derived from maritime pine bark; it can be used in place of grape seed extract, but it is more expensive and many practitioners don't believe it's worth the extra cost.

▼ WHAT IT DOES

Grape seed extract exerts a powerful, positive influence on blood vessels. Not coincidentally, the active substances in this extract, PCOs, are key ingredients in one of the drugs most frequently prescribed for blood vessel (vascular) disorders in Western Europe.

Because grape seed extract is both oil- and water-soluble, it can penetrate all types of cell membranes, delivering antioxidant protection throughout the body. Moreover, it is one of the few substances that can cross the blood-brain barrier, which means it has the potential to protect brain cells from free radical damage.

MAJOR BENEFITS

With its powerful ability to enhance the health of blood vessels, grape seed extract may reduce the risk of heart attack and stroke and also strengthen fragile or weak capillaries and increase blood flow, particularly to the extremities. For this reason, many experts find it a beneficial supplement for almost any type of vascular insufficiency as well as for conditions that are associated with poor vascular function,

---

 ALERT

SIDE EFFECTS
- Few side effects from grape seed extract have been reported, and no toxic reactions have been noted.

- In theory, grape seed may increase the risk of bleeding.

CAUTION
- You may need to stop taking grape seed before some surgeries; discuss this with your doctor.

- Grape seed use during pregnancy and breast feeding has not been studied and cannot be recommended.

- Grape seed oil interacts with medications that increase the risk of bleeding, certain enzyme inhibitors, cholesterol-lowering drugs, medications broken down by the liver, and herbs and supplements with similar effects.

- **Reminder:** If you have a medical condition, talk to your doctor before taking supplements.

including diabetes, varicose veins, some cases of impotence, numbness and tingling in the arms and legs, and even painful leg cramps.

Because it can have an impact on even the tiniest blood vessels, grape seed extract also benefits circulation in the eye. It is frequently recommended as a supplement to combat macular degeneration and cataracts, two of the most common causes of blindness in older people. If you use computers on a regular basis, grape seed extract may also be for you. At least one study showed that 300 mg daily for just 60 days reduced eye strain associated with computer monitor work and improved contrast vision.

Many experts now endorse grape seed extract for its cancer-fighting properties. Working as antioxidants, PCOs correct damage to the genetic material of cells that could possibly cause tumors to form.

ADDITIONAL BENEFITS

Helping preserve and reinforce the collagen in the skin, grape seed extract is often used in the treatment of connective tissue disorders, such as rheuma-

toid arthritis. In Europe, it is often included in cosmetic creams to improve skin elasticity.

Grape seed oil may also decrease injury to the liver and inflammation of the pancreas (pancreatitis). It may thin the blood, relieve the symptoms of premenstrual syndrome (PMS), and treat attention deficit and hyperactivity disorder (ADHD).

▼ HOW TO TAKE IT

DOSAGE

Choose supplements that are standardized to contain 92% to 95% proanthocyanidins, or PCOs.

For antioxidant protection: Take 100 mg daily.
For therapeutic benefits: Dose is usually 200 mg daily.

GUIDELINES FOR USE

• After 24 hours, only about 28% of grape seed extract's active components remain in the body. It's important to take supplements at the same time every day, particularly when they are used to combat disease.

• Grape seed extract is best used with other antioxidants such as vitamins C and E; money-saving combination products are available.

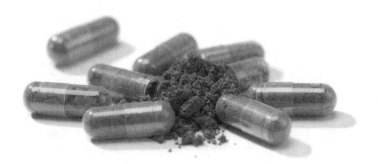

GREEN TEA *(Camellia sinensis)*

According to legend, around 2700 B.C. a Chinese emperor sat under a tea shrub, and a few leaves fell into his cup of hot water. Presto! Green tea was born. Now, modern research has found that this type of tea—a staple of the Asian diet—contains one of the most promising anticancer compounds ever discovered.

COMMON USES

- May help prevent cancer.
- May protect against heart disease, reduce cholesterol, and aid in weight loss.
- May inhibit tooth decay.
- Promotes longevity.
- May enhance mental performance, alertness, and memory.
- May offer protection against the damaging effects of the sun.
- May treat asthma.

FORMS

- Capsule
- Tablet
- Liquid
- Powder
- Tea

▼ WHAT IT IS

Green tea is made from the dried leaves of *Camellia sinensis*, a perennial evergreen shrub.

The traditional process that yields green tea is simple. The leaves from the tea plant are first steamed and then rolled and dried. The steaming kills enzymes that would otherwise ferment the leaves.

With other types of tea, the leaves are allowed to ferment either partially (for oolong tea) or fully (for black tea). The lack of fermentation, however, gives green tea its unique flavor and, more important, preserves virtually all of the naturally present polyphenols (strong antioxidants that can protect against cell damage).

Other substances in green tea that also appear to have medicinal properties are fluoride, catechins, and tannins.

▼ WHAT IT DOES

Green tea contains compounds that may provide powerful protection against several cancers and, possibly, against heart disease. It also fights infection and promotes longevity.

PREVENTION

The rate of certain types of cancer is lower among people who drink green tea. In one large-scale study, researchers found that Chinese men and women who drank green tea as seldom as once a week for 6 months had lower rates of rectal, pancreatic, and possibly colon cancer than those who rarely or never drank it. In women, the risk of rectal and pancreatic cancer was nearly cut in half. Preliminary research suggests that green tea may also fight breast, stomach, and skin cancers.

Studies investigating how green tea might guard against cancer have pointed to the potency of its main antioxidant, a polyphenol dubbed EGCG (for epigallocatechin-gallate). Some scientists believe that EGCG may be one of the most effective anticancer compounds ever discovered, protecting cells from damage and strengthening the body's own production of antioxidant enzymes.

ALERT

SIDE EFFECTS

- Green tea is very safe as both a supplement and as a beverage. People who are sensitive to caffeine, however, may not want to drink too much green tea, because each cup contains about 40 mg of caffeine.

- Because of its caffeine content, pregnant women and those who are breast feeding should limit their green tea consumption to 2 cups a day.

- Caffeine may be habit forming, resulting in tolerance and physiological dependence. Abrubt discontinuation may result in withdrawal symptoms such as headache, irritation, nervousness, anxiety, tremor, or dizziness.

CAUTION

- **Reminder:** If you have a medical condition or are taking medications or other supplements, talk to your doctor before taking supplements.

According to a study from Ohio's Case Western Reserve University, EGCG seems to signal cancer cells to stop reproducing by stimulating a natural process of programmed cell death called apoptosis. Remarkably, EGCG does not harm healthy cells. In addition, research at the Medical College of Ohio indicates that EGCG inhibits the production of urokinase, an enzyme that cancer cells need in order to grow. In animals, blocking urokinase shrinks tumors and sometimes causes cancer to go into complete remission.

ADDITIONAL BENEFITS

The antioxidant effect of green tea's polyphenols may also help protect the heart. In laboratory studies, these compounds appeared to suppress the blood vessel damage caused by LDL cholesterol, thought to be an initial step in the buildup of plaque in the arteries. A Japanese study of 1,371 men linked daily green tea consumption to the prevention of heart disease.

In addition, green tea contains fluoride, which may help protect against tooth decay and provides an overall antibacterial effect.

Green tea can be taken in supplement form or enjoyed as a soothing beverage.

▼ HOW TO TAKE IT

DOSAGE

You can get the benefits of green tea by taking either green tea capsules or tablets or by drinking several cups of the brew each day. Your aim should be to get 240 to 320 mg of polyphenols.

When using supplements, buy those standardized to contain at least 50% polyphenols. At this concentration, two 250-mg supplements would provide 250 mg of polyphenols. Studies show that 4 cups of freshly brewed green tea supplies the recommended amount of polyphenols.

Green tea supplements have very little caffeine. The recommended dose of green tea supplements provides the same amount of polyphenols as 4 cups of green tea, but generally contains only 5 to 6 mg of caffeine.

GUIDELINES FOR USE

• Take green tea supplements at meals with a full glass of water.

• Drink freshly brewed green tea on its own or with meals. To make the tea, use 1 tsp of green tea leaves per cup of very hot (but not boiling) water. Let the brew steep for 3 to 5 minutes; then strain and drink it.

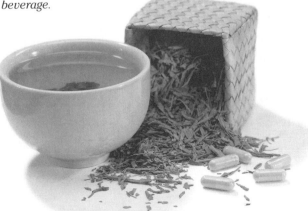

GUGULIPID *(Commiphora mukul)*

Since antiquity, practitioners of ayurvedic medicine in India have used the gum resin of the mukul myrrh tree to treat obesity and arthritis. Now a modern purified extract called gugulipid has been found to be as effective as some prescription drugs for lowering cholesterol and triglyceride levels in the blood.

COMMON USES

- Helps lower high blood cholesterol and high blood triglycerides.
- Treats arthritis inflammation.
- May aid weight loss.
- May treat acne.

FORMS

- Capsule
- Tablet
- Powder

WHAT IT IS

Gugulipid comes from the gummy resin of the small thorny mukul myrrh tree native to India. The tree's resin is closely related to the richly perfumed Biblical myrrh, traditionally used for purification purposes.

Called gum guggul ("guggulu"), the resin itself has been part of ayurveda, the traditional medicine of India, for thousands of years. Guggulu, however, has toxic compounds. Fortunately, modern Indian pharmacologists have devised a way to extract the active components in the resins and leave the toxic substances behind. The result is the standardized extract called gugulipid.

WHAT IT DOES

The active ingredients in gugulipid, known as guggulsterones, appear to affect the way the body metabolizes fat and cholesterol. These compounds also have antiinflammatory and antioxidant properties.

PREVENTION

If you have high blood cholesterol levels, you are at increased risk for developing coronary heart disease. Studies suggest that gugulipid can lower these levels; it is the guggulsterones, in particular, that seem to stimulate the liver to break down the most harmful form of cholesterol, LDL.

In addition, gugulipid sometimes elevates the levels of protective HDL cholesterol. A study of 205 people in India found that gugulipid, in combination with a low-fat diet, reduced total cholesterol by an average of 24% in more than 75% of the participants.

In another study comparing the efficacy of gugulipid with that of clofibrate, a prescription cholesterol-lowering medication, total cholesterol dropped by 11% in the gugulipid group and by 10% in the clofibrate group. In addi-

---

 ALERT

SIDE EFFECTS

- Rarely, taking gugulipid may cause stomach upset, headache, restlessness, apprehension, nervousness, diarrhea, vomiting, belching, hiccups, increased bleeding, increased thyroid function, decreased cholesterol, increased risk of bleeding, weight reduction, or allergic reaction (rash).

CAUTION

- Never use the crude gum guggul, or guggulu, which can cause rashes, diarrhea, stomach pain, and loss of appetite. Opt for the standardized gugulipid products instead.

- Be sure to consult your doctor before trying gugulipid if you suffer from liver disease, diarrhea, thyroid disorders, anorexia, bulimia, or a bleeding disorder.

- Pregnant or breast-feeding women should not take gugulipid.

- People taking medications that lower blood pressure, thyroid medications, cholesterol-lowering medications, blood thinners, and herbs and supplements with similar effects should not take gugulipid.

- **Reminder:** If you have a medical condition, talk to your doctor before taking supplements.

tion, nearly two-thirds of those taking gugulipid experienced increases in HDL cholesterol levels on average; however, no change in HDL was seen in those using clofibrate.

In animal studies, gugulipid has been shown to prevent the formation of artery-blocking plaque and even to help reverse existing plaque. In addition, it inhibits blood platelets from sticking together, and thus may protect against blood clots, which often trigger heart attacks.

ADDITIONAL BENEFITS
Studies lend support to two of the traditional uses for guggul: treating arthritis and obesity.

Results from animal studies indicate that the antiinflammatory action of guggulsterones may be as powerful as that of over-the-counter pain medications, such as ibuprofen, making this herb useful in treating arthritis. Its anti-inflammatory action also suggests that gugulipid may be effective for acne; in fact, one study showed it had a beneficial effect on this condition.

There is some evidence that gugulipid stimulates the production of thyroid hormones, increasing the rate at which the body burns calories. In one small study, Indian researchers reported that in overweight patients, gugulipid supplements sparked significant weight loss. Much of the weight loss came from a reduction in fat around the abdomen, which is associated with an increased risk of heart disease and diabetes. Any effective long-term weight control program, of course, must begin with a low-fat, high-fiber diet and a regular exercise program.

▼ HOW TO TAKE IT

DOSAGE
To lower cholesterol: Take 500 to 1,000 mg of gugulipid by mouth daily or take a product that contains 25 mg of guggulsterone 1 to 3 times daily or 50 mg twice daily.

GUIDELINES FOR USE
• You can take gugulipid with or without meals.

• Don't stop seeing your doctor for a cholesterol problem and never substitute a gugulipid product for a cholesterol-lowering medication without getting your doctor's approval first.

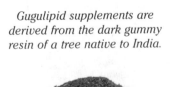

Gugulipid supplements are derived from the dark gummy resin of a tree native to India.

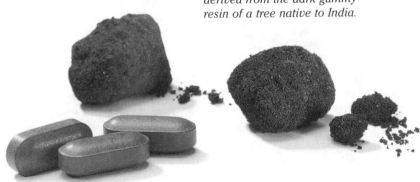

411

GYMNEMA *(Gymnema sylvestre)*

This woody plant has been used in India to treat diabetes for more than 2,000 years. Other names for gymnema include gurmar, meshasringi, periploca of the woods, and chi geng teng.

COMMON USES

- Aids treatment of diabetes

FORMS

- Extract
- Capsules

▼ WHAT IT IS

Gymnema sylvestre is a woody, climbing plant native to India. The leaves are the part used most often medicinally, but the stem is believed also to possess some therapeutic value. The leaves have been used in India for more than 2,000 years to treat *madhu meha*, or "honey urine" (diabetes). It has been used alone and as a component of the ayurvedic medicinal compound *Tribang shila*, a mixture of tin, lead, zinc, *Gymnema*

sylvestre leaves, neem *(Melia azadirachta)* leaves, mamijava *(Enicostemma littorale)*, and jambul *(Eugenia jambolana)* seeds. Traditional healers observed that chewing the leaves of gymnema resulted in a reversible loss of sweet taste perception.

Chewing the leaves has been noted to diminish the ability to discriminate sweet tastes. This, together with the herb's ability to decrease blood sugar levels, may have prompted the Hindi name *gurmar*, or "sugar destroyer." Gymnema has a long history of use in individuals with diabetes.

Gymnema has become a popular natural product used in the management of blood sugar levels in individuals with diabetes and is believed by some to play a role in reducing serum lipids.

▼ WHAT IT DOES

MAJOR BENEFITS

Several studies suggest that gymnema can lower blood sugar levels in people with certain types of diabetes. Gymnema appears to do this by greatly increasing the number of insulin-secreting beta cells in the pancreas while returning blood sugar levels to near normal. It may increase the activity of enzymes responsible for glucose uptake and utilization. These studies were small

 ALERT

SIDE EFFECTS
- Gymnema may lower blood sugar levels and may alter the ability to taste sweet foods.

CAUTION
- People allergic to plants in the Asclepiadaceae (milkweed) family should avoid gymnema.

- If you also taking prescription drugs, herbs, or supplements that may lower blood sugar levels, you should exercise caution when using gymnema. If you are taking oral drugs for diabetes or are using insulin, you should be monitored closely by your doctor while using gymnema. You may need to adjust your dosage.

- Gymnema may decrease the body's absorption of oleic acid (a fatty acid). It may also affect the absorption of other nutritionally important lipids or fat-soluble vitamins, such as A, D, E, or K, but research is inconclusive.

- Do not use gymnema if you are pregnant or breast feeding; there is insufficient information on its safety and effectiveness.

Reminder: If you have a medical condition, talk to your doctor before taking supplements.

and of poor quality; better research is needed to determine safety and dosing.

Researchers at Georgetown University compared the effects of chromium, vanadium, and gymnema in rats with sugar-induced hypertension. They found that gymnema, unlike the trace minerals chromium and vanadium, reduced blood cholesterol but did not reduce the high blood pressure caused by dietary sugar.

ADDITIONAL BENEFITS

The following uses for gymnema are possible but are *as yet unproven:* as an aphrodisiac, a laxative, or a snake venom antidote; to treat cardiovascular disease, constipation, cough, diuresis (increased urination), gout, high cholesterol, high blood pressure, hyperglycemia, liver disease, malaria, obesity, rheumatoid arthritis, or stomach ailments; or to stimulate the uterus or digestion.

▼ HOW TO TAKE IT

DOSAGE

Extract/Capsules: Take 200 mg of the gymnema extract called GS4 twice a day by mouth. This dosage has been studied for the treatment of diabetes in adults. No dosage for capsules can be recommended at this time. The dosage on the bottle for capsules sold in health food stores, however, is typically 1 capsule (260 mg dried extract and 50 mg leaf) 3 times daily, preferably with food.

GUIDELINES FOR USE

• The dosing and safety of the use of gymnema by children have not been studied thoroughly. You should discuss doses with your child's doctor before giving gymnema to your child.

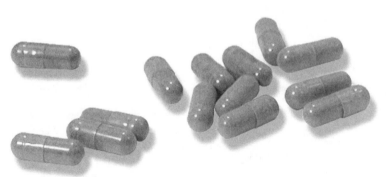

Gymnema capsules are made from a woody, climbing plant (Gymnema sylvestre) *native to India.*

SHOPPING HINTS

■ Note that products containing gymnema that are advertised as appetite suppressants (and part of a diet control plan) may not be useful for diabetes control. Check the label.

■ Alternately, nonstandardized extracts, or those with lower gymnemic acid content, may also be helpful in blocking sugar absorption.

LATEST FINDINGS

■ Further research being done at Creighton University, in Omaha, Nebraska, will use a standardized formula and will be conducted on people with type 2 diabetes.

■ In the early 1990s, researchers at India's University of Madras found that high doses (40 g of dried herb daily) of gymnema extracts may help repair or regenerate the pancreas's beta cells. Beta cells are important in the production and secretion of insulin, so taking gymnema may result in the reversal of beta cell damage and may reduce a diabetic's need for insulin and other medications.

DID YOU KNOW?

Gymnema has also been used in African healing traditions, by Tanzanian healers as an aphrodisiac, for example. Other traditional applications include use as an antimalarial agent, a digestive stimulant, a laxative, a diuretic, and a snake venom antidote.

HAWTHORN *(Crataegus oxyacantha)*

If your doctor confirms that you have any form of heart disease, you'll want to know all about hawthorn. Historically used as a diuretic and as a treatment for kidney and bladder stones, this herb today is widely prescribed in Europe as a natural heart remedy for conditions ranging from mild hypertension to angina.

COMMON USES

- Relieves chest pain from angina.
- Helps the heart pump more efficiently in people with congestive heart failure.
- May improve cardiovascular disorders.

FORMS

- Tablet
- Capsule
- Liquid
- Powder
- Dried herb/Tea

▼ WHAT IT IS

For centuries, hawthorn, a shrub that grows to 30 feet, has been trimmed to hedge height and planted along the edges of fields or property lines. As a divider, it looks attractive and discourages trespassers. It produces pretty white flowers and vibrant red berries, but it also sports large thorns, and the flowers on some varieties smell like rotting meat.

The plant has long been associated with bad luck and death, because the crown of thorns that Christ wore at the Crucifixion is widely believed to have been woven from haw-thorn twigs.

Given this reputation, it's surprising that anyone got close enough to dis-cover hawthorn's cardioprotective benefits, but obviously a number of people in different eras and locations—from the ancient Greeks to the Native Americans—did consider the herb a potent tonic for the heart.

The modern use of hawthorn origi-nated with a nineteenth-century Irish physician who treated heart disease quite successfully. Because he closely guarded his heart formula, his secret remedy was not revealed to be tincture of hawthorn berry until after his death in the 1890s.

▼ WHAT IT DOES

Hawthorn is an herb that directly benefits the workings of the heart. It can help dilate blood vessels, increase the heart's energy supply, and improve its pumping ability. These powerful cardiac effects can probably be traced to hawthorn's abundant supply of plant compounds called flavonoids—and especially pro-cyanidolic oligomers (PCOs), which are potent antioxidants.

ALERT

SIDE EFFECTS

- There have been reports of nausea, sweating, fatigue, and skin rash, but these side effects are uncommon. Other possible side effects may include palpitations, irregular or fast heart rhythm, sleeplessness, agitation, diffi-culty breathing, and headache. Stop taking the herb and consult your doc-tor if any of these reactions occur.

- In people who don't have heart disease, large doses of hawthorn can cause very low blood pressure, which can lead to dizziness and fainting.

CAUTION

- Hawthorn may interact with heart medications, blood pressure medica-tions, phenylephrine, ephedrine or ephedra, cholesterol-lowering medica-tions, and herbs and supplements with similar effects. Talk with your doctor before trying hawthorn, and never stop taking a drug that's been prescribed for you (or reduce the dose) without your doctor's consent.

- Chest pain (angina) is a very serious symptom of heart trouble; don't expect hawthorn to stop an acute angina attack. See your doctor.

- People who have a history of low blood pressure, irregular heartbeat, asthma, or insomnia or women who are pregnant or breast feeding should not take hawthorn.

- **Reminder:** If you have a medical condition, talk to your doctor before taking supplements.

MAJOR BENEFITS

Strong scientific evidence confirms the usefulness of hawthorn in the treatment of congestive heart failure. It seems to block enzymes that weaken the heart muscle, thereby strengthening its pumping power. This property is especially useful for individuals with mild congestive heart failure who don't require strong heart medications, such as digitalis. Moreover, the antioxidant properties of hawthorn may help protect against damage associated with the buildup of plaque in the coronary arteries.

▼ HOW TO TAKE IT

DOSAGE

The recommended dose of hawthorn extract ranges from 300 to 450 mg a day in pill form, and from 1 to 3 tsp (5 to 15 ml) of the liquid extract, depending on the type of heart condition.

People at risk for heart disease may wish to take a 100 to 150 mg supplement or 1 tsp of the liquid extract daily as a heart disease preventive.

GUIDELINES FOR USE

• Hawthorn should be used only under the supervision of a qualified healthcare provider.

• If you're on large doses, hawthorn works best when the daily amount is divided and taken at 3 different times during the day.

• Hawthorn may take 1 to 2 months to build up in your system before it produces noticeable results.

SHOPPING HINTS

■ When buying hawthorn, look for standardized extracts that contain at least 1.8% vitexin, sometimes called vitexin-2-rhamnoside. This is the main heart-protecting substance in the herb.

LATEST FINDINGS

■ In an 8-week German study of 136 people with mild to moderate congestive heart failure, those who took hawthorn extract reported less shortness of breath, less ankle swelling, and better exercise performance than those given a placebo. Physical exams and laboratory tests confirmed that the condition of the hawthorn group improved and the condition of the placebo group worsened.

DID YOU KNOW?

Hawthorn varieties grow in Europe, eastern Asia, northern Africa, and the United States. It is also known as whitethorn and mayflower—in fact, the Pilgrim ship *Mayflower* was named after the hawthorn blossom.

Hawthorn supplements may contain the plant's leaves and flowers, its red berries, or a combination of all three.

HORSE CHESTNUT *(Aesculus hippocastanum)*

Horse chestnut seeds have been used medicinally in Europe and Asia for centuries. The horse chestnut tree is native to Asia and northern Greece, but it is now cultivated in many areas. Scientists have found evidence that horse chestnut can help in the treatment of certain blood circulation problems.

COMMON USES

■ May help treat chronic venous insufficiency (a condition in which blood pools in the veins of the lower legs, causing swelling and possibly causing leg ulcers).

ALERT

SIDE EFFECTS

• If you have known allergies to horse chestnut or any of the chemicals found in horse chestnut (such as esculin, flavonoids, biosides, triosides of quercetins, and oligosaccharides, including 1-ketose or 2-ketose), you should avoid using horse chestnut seed extract products. Allergic skin rashes (contact dermatitis) have been reported after the use of a skin cream containing horse chestnut seed extract.

• Few side effects have been reported from horse chestnut seed extract when taken by mouth at recommended doses. The most common problems are stomach upset and muscle spasms. Less common side effects are headache, skin rash, dizziness, liver problems, and kidney problems.

CAUTION

• Intravenous or injected horse chestnut seed extract may cause anaphylactic shock (a severe allergic reaction) or other serious reactions and should be avoided.

• Some animal studies found that horse chestnut seed extract may lower blood sugar levels.

• In theory, horse chestnut seed extract may increase the risk of bleeding. You may need to stop taking horse chestnut seed extract before some surgeries; discuss this with your doctor.

• *Warning:* Eating the flower, branch bark, leaf, or raw seeds of horse chestnut can cause serious side effects or death.

• Do not take horse chestnut seed extract if you are pregnant or breast feeding; research on its effects is inconclusive.

• No adverse drug interactions have been reported, but if you are taking anticoagulants (blood thinners) or antiplatelets, agents that may lower blood sugar levels, oral drugs for diabetes, insulin, or herbs or supplements with the same effects, talk to your doctor before taking horse chestnut seed extract. Dosing adjustments may be necessary.

Reminder: If you have a medical condition, talk to your doctor before taking supplements.

FORMS

■ Horse chestnut seed extract (HCSE)

■ Seeds   ■ Capsules

■ Fruit

▼ WHAT IT IS

Horse chestnut is a member of the genus *Aesculus* and the family Hippocastanaceae. The fruit has a thick husk and contains from 1 to 6 seeds. The plant has pink and white flowers. Indigenous to the mountains of Greece, Bulgaria, the Caucasus, northern Iran, and the Himalayas, horse chestnut is now cultivated internationally, particularly in Europe and Russia.

Horse chestnuts have been used medicinally for centuries. People in India have roasted, peeled, and mashed chestnut seeds and then leached them in lime in order to render them less toxic. Extracts of the bark have been used as a yellow dye.

▼ WHAT IT DOES

MAJOR BENEFITS

Scientific evidence best supports the use of horse chestnut seed extract for a condition called chronic venous insufficiency. This term is more common in Europe than the United States. It describes several different problems that may be caused by the failure of veins in the lower legs to work correctly. These problems include leg swelling (edema), pain, itching, varicose veins, breakdown of skin, and skin ulcers. A number of studies have suggested that horse chestnut seed extract, together with other treatments, such as compression stockings, may help these problems. These studies were small, of low quality, and not fully convincing, however. Better research is necessary to provide a clear answer. If you experience sudden leg swelling, consult your doctor immediately.

ADDITIONAL BENEFITS

Although such claims are *unproven*, horse chestnut seed extract may also help in the treatment of benign prostatic hypertrophy (BPH), fluid in the lungs (pulmonary edema), gallbladder pain (colic), gallbladder infection (cholecystitis), gallbladder stones (cholelithiasis), bladder disorders (incontinence, cystitis), bruising, cough, vein clots (deep venous thrombosis), diarrhea, dizziness, fever, hemorrhoids, kidney diseases, leg cramps, liver congestion, lung blood clots (pulmonary embolism), menstrual pain, nerve pain, osteoarthritis, pancreatitis, rectal complaints, "rheumatism," rheumatoid arthritis, skin conditions, postoperative or posttraumatic soft tissue swelling, ringing in the ears (tinnitus), ulcers, and whooping cough.

▼ HOW TO TAKE IT

DOSAGE

Horse chestnut seed extract:
Take 300 mg by mouth every 12 hours for up to 12 weeks.

Horse chestnut seed extract capsules: No dosage can be recommended at this time. The dosage on the bottle for capsules sold in health food stores, however, is typically one 150-mg capsule daily.

GUIDELINES FOR USE

• Because little research has been done on its effects on children, horse chestnut seed extract should not be given to children. Death has occurred when children have eaten raw horse chestnut seeds or have drunk tea made from horse chestnut leaves and twigs.

• Horse chestnut seed extract should be used only at recommended doses for up to 12 weeks. Consult your doctor immediately if you experience side effects.

• Scientists have not been able to prove that horse chestnut is safe for women who are pregnant or breast feeding, but one study of 52 women taking horse chestnut reported no ill effects after 2 weeks of its use.

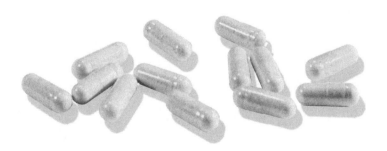

IODINE

Many people associate iodine with the orange-brown topical antiseptic their mothers swabbed on their childhood scrapes and bruises. The real value of this potent trace mineral is its role in the health of the thyroid gland, where it is involved in numerous biological functions that we couldn't live without.

COMMON USES
- Corrects an iodine deficiency.
- Ensures proper functioning of the thyroid gland.
- May help treat fibrocystic breasts.

FORMS
- Tablet
- Capsule
- Liquid

▼ WHAT IT IS

Although the body needs just tiny amounts of iodine, this mineral is so crucial to an individual's overall health that in the 1920s government officials decided that it should be added to a foodstuff common to nearly everyone: table salt. The introduction of iodized salt into the American diet virtually eliminated one severe form of mental retardation called cretinism.

Despite the recognized importance of this vital mineral, however, about 1.6 billion people in the world, mostly in underdeveloped countries, still suffer from iodine deficiency.

▼ WHAT IT DOES

Unique among minerals, iodine has only one known function in the body— it is essential to the thyroid gland for manufacturing thyroxine, a hormone that regulates metabolism in all the body's cells.

PREVENTION
By getting enough iodine, pregnant women can prevent certain types of mental retardation in the fetus.

ADDITIONAL BENEFITS
Unlike many other minerals, iodine does not seem to help in the treatment of specific diseases; however, it does play a fundamental role in ensuring the health of the thyroid, the butterfly-shaped gland that surrounds the windpipe (trachea).

When your iodine intake is adequate, your body contains about an ounce of it. About 75% of that amount is stored in the thyroid. This organ controls the body's overall metabolism, which determines how quickly and efficiently calories are burned. It also regulates growth and development in children, reproduction, nerve and muscle function, the breakdown of proteins and fats, the growth of nails and hair, and the use of oxygen by every cell in the body.

There is some evidence that iodine derived from an organic source may be effective in reducing the pain of fibrocystic breasts, but patients should discuss this type of supplementation with their doctor first.

▼ HOW MUCH YOU NEED

The RDA for iodine is 150 µg daily for adult men and women. Most

ALERT

CAUTION
- Because iodine deficiency is rarely seen in people in developed countries, take iodine supplements only if prescribed by your physician.

- **Reminder:** If you have a medical or psychiatric condition, talk to your doctor before taking supplements.

people meet or exceed this amount by using iodized salt (1 tsp of iodized salt contains more than 300 µg of iodine).

IF YOU GET TOO LITTLE
Thanks to the widespread use of iodized salt, not a single case of iodine deficiency has been reported in the United States since the 1970s.

Among the first signs of iodine deficiency, now rarely seen, is an enlarged thyroid gland, known as a goiter. Lack of iodine can cause the gland to expand in an attempt to increase its surface area and trap as much of the iodine in the bloodstream as possible.

If your iodine intake is low, your thyroid hormone level may well be low too. This condition can lead to fatigue, dry skin, an increase in blood fats, a hoarse voice, delayed reflexes, and reduced mental clarity. See your doctor if you have these symptoms.

IF YOU GET TOO MUCH
There is very little risk of iodine overdose, even at levels 10 to 20 times the RDA. However, if you ingest 30 times the RDA, you are likely to experience a metallic taste, mouth sores, swollen salivary glands, diarrhea, vomiting, headache, a rash, and difficulty breathing. Ironically, a goiter can also develop if you consistently take extremely large amounts of iodine.

▼ HOW TO TAKE IT

DOSAGE
You probably get all the iodine you need from iodized salt or from regular servings of seafood. Iodine is also a standard ingredient in many multivitamin and mineral supplements.

Even if you are on a strict, very low-salt diet for high blood pressure, you probably don't require extra iodine, although you can safely take 150 µg a day.

People taking a thyroid hormone should always discuss their condition with a doctor before taking individual iodine supplements.

GUIDELINES FOR USE
• When prescribed, iodine supplements can be taken at any time of day with or without food.

▼ OTHER SOURCES

Although the most abundant source of iodine is iodized table salt, the mineral can also be found in saltwater fish and in sea vegetation such as kelp. Soil in coastal areas also tends to be iodine-rich, as are the dairy products produced by cows grazing there. The same is true for fruits and vegetables grown in soil with a high iodine content.

Commercial baked goods—such as breads and cakes—are other good sources of iodine. Although iodized salt is not used in commercial baking, these products are often made with dough conditioners that contain iodine.

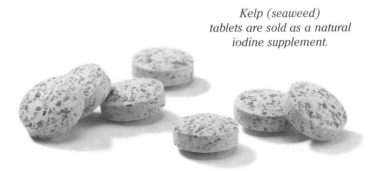

Kelp (seaweed) tablets are sold as a natural iodine supplement.

IRON

A surprising number of Americans get too little iron—and few realize that a lack of this vital mineral can make them weak, unable to concentrate, and more susceptible to infection. Too much iron, however, can be dangerous. A blood test can show whether you would benefit from an iron supplement.

COMMON USES

■ Treats iron deficiency anemia.

■ Often needed during pregnancy, by women with heavy menstrual periods, or in other situations determined by your doctor.

FORMS

■ Tablet

■ Capsule

■ Softgel

■ Liquid

▼ WHAT IT IS

Needed throughout the body, iron is an essential part of hemoglobin, the oxygen-carrying component of red blood cells. The mineral is also found in myoglobin, which supplies oxygen to the muscles of the body, and is it part of many important enzymes and immune system compounds.

The body, which gets most of the iron it requires from food, carefully monitors its iron status, absorbing more of the mineral when demand is high (during periods of rapid growth such as pregnancy or childhood) and less when stores of it are adequate.

Because the body loses iron when bleeding, many menstruating women have low iron levels. Dieters, vegetarians, and endurance athletes may experience iron deficiencies as well.

▼ WHAT IT DOES

By helping the blood and muscles deliver oxygen, iron supplies energy to every cell in the body. Yet, iron deficiency is surprisingly common in the United States. According to federal statistics, 9% of adolescent girls and 11% of women under age 50 are deficient in this mineral.

Although it is very difficult to develop an iron deficiency from poor nutrition (iron is found in many foods), women with heavy menstrual periods and people with certain medical conditions may need supplements to prevent or correct the severe condition known as iron deficiency anemia.

MAJOR BENEFITS
Keeping your body well supplied with iron provides energy, helps your immune system function at its best, and gives your mind an edge. Studies show that even mild iron deficiency—well short of the levels commonly associated with anemia—can cause adults to have a short attention span and teens to do poorly in school.

▼ HOW MUCH YOU NEED

The RDA for iron in men of all ages and women over age 50 is 8 mg a day. For younger women, it's 18 mg daily (during pregnancy, 27 mg a day). To combat anemia, additional iron—either

ALERT

CAUTION

• Never take an iron supplement unless you are following your doctor's recommendation. More than 1 million Americans have an inherited disease called hemochromatosis, which causes them to absorb too much iron—and most don't even know it. (Early symptoms include fatigue and aching joints.)

• Taking iron on your own could mask a cause of anemia, such as a bleeding ulcer, and prevent a doctor from making an early, lifesaving diagnosis.

• **Reminder:** If you have a medical condition, talk to your doctor before taking supplements.

through diet or supplements—is typically needed for a period of weeks or months.

IF YOU GET TOO LITTLE

If you get too little iron in your diet or lose too much through heavy menstrual periods, stomach bleeding (commonly caused by arthritis drugs), or cancer, your body draws on its iron reserve. Initially, there are no symptoms, but as your iron supply dwindles, so does your body's ability to produce healthy red blood cells. The result is iron deficiency anemia, marked by weakness, fatigue, paleness, breathlessness, palpitations, and increased susceptibility to infection.

IF YOU GET TOO MUCH

Some studies link too much iron to an increased risk of chronic diseases, including heart disease and colon cancer. Excess iron can be particularly dangerous for adults with a genetic tendency to overabsorb it (hemochromatosis) and for children, who are especially susceptible to iron overdose.

▼ HOW TO TAKE IT

DOSAGE

Iron supplements should be taken only under your doctor's supervision; self-treatment can be dangerous. Anemia requires a careful diagnosis and treatment to correct the underlying cause.

When a doctor recommends it, iron is typically taken in a form called ferrous salts—usually ferrous sulfate, ferrous fumarate, or ferrous gluconate. A typical prescribed dose provides about 30 mg of iron 1 to 3 times daily.

Most men and postmenopausal women do not need iron supplements and should make sure iron is not included in their daily multivitamin.

GUIDELINES FOR USE

• Iron is best absorbed when taken on an empty stomach. If iron upsets your stomach, have it with meals, preferably with a small amount of meat and a food or drink rich in vitamin C, such as broccoli or orange juice, to help boost the amount of iron your body absorbs.

• Never take iron for more than 6 months without having your blood iron levels rechecked by your doctor.

▼ OTHER SOURCES

Iron-rich foods include liver, beef, and lamb. Clams, oysters, and mussels also contain iron.

Vegetarians can get plenty of iron from beans and peas, leafy greens, dried fruits (apricots, raisins), seeds (pumpkin, squash, sunflower), and fortified breakfast cereals. Brewer's yeast, kelp, blackstrap molasses, and wheat bran are also exceptionally good sources.

Cooking tomatoes or other acidic foods in a cast iron pot adds iron to meals as well; a healthful amount leaches out of the cookware into the food.

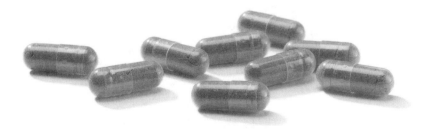

KAVA *(Piper methysticum)*

When English explorer Captain James Cook sailed the South Pacific in the 1700s, the kava-laced drink his crew sampled on tropical islands along the way may have eased the stress of the long journey. The herb has long been appreciated for its calming effects, and it continues to attract new enthusiasts.

COMMON USES
- Combats anxiety.
- Eases panic attacks.

FORMS
- Capsule
- Tablet
- Softgel
- Liquid
- Dried herb/Tea

▼ WHAT IT IS

A member of the pepper family, kava (also known as kava-kava) is a shrub that thrives on many South Pacific islands. The name "kava" refers not only to the herb but also to a traditional beverage made by crushing the plant's root into a pulp, adding water or coconut milk, and straining it into coconut shells.

For thousands of years, kava has played a major role in social events and religious rituals among Pacific islanders. In fact, island ceremonies—whether those welcoming royalty or simply hosting a neighborhood get-together—wouldn't be complete without kava, which serves a purpose similar to that of alcohol in other societies—namely, inducing a sense of well-being and fostering social discourse.

The kava plant, with its heart-shaped leaves, bears sterile flowers and can be propagated only by dividing the roots, which are thick and gnarled. These can weigh up to 22 lb. Today, in many parts of the South Pacific, kava is widely cultivated for the medicinal properties of its roots and is exported to herb shops throughout the world.

▼ WHAT IT DOES

Kava root contains a number of compounds (the most prominent are known as kavalactones), which have a wide range of therapeutic effects. In many European countries, doctors currently prescribe kava for the treatment of anxiety, stress, restlessness, and insomnia. Kava recently has been withdrawn from several European markets, however, because of safety concerns and numerous reports of severe liver damage. Scientists aren't sure how it works but believe that kava targets the limbic system, a primitive part of

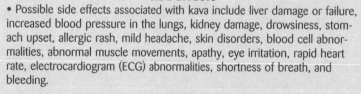

ALERT

SIDE EFFECTS
- Possible side effects associated with kava include liver damage or failure, increased blood pressure in the lungs, kidney damage, drowsiness, stomach upset, allergic rash, mild headache, skin disorders, blood cell abnormalities, abnormal muscle movements, apathy, eye irritation, rapid heart rate, electrocardiogram (ECG) abnormalities, shortness of breath, and bleeding.

CAUTION
- Don't take more than the recommended dose. Higher doses can cause disorientation or intoxication, and even recommended doses taken for more than 3 months can increase the risk of adverse reactions.

- Pregnant or breast-feeding women should not use kava.

- Avoid taking kava if you have a history of liver disease, Parkinson's disease, heart disease, lung disease, eye disease, or blood cell disorders or are taking medications to treat those disorders.

- Avoid alcohol while taking kava. Also avoid driving or operating heavy machinery, because kava may cause drowsiness.

- **Reminder:** If you have a medical or psychiatric condition, talk to your doctor before taking supplements.

the brain that (among other things) regulates emotions.

MAJOR BENEFITS

Kava is known primarily for its anxiety-relieving benefits. It can be useful for reducing general stress and nervousness, as well as for warding off the intense bouts of anxiety known as panic attacks. Kava may also have a calming, sedative effect on individuals who are trying to stop smoking or wean themselves off alcohol. Its relaxing properties may help insomniacs fall asleep. Those with mild to moderate depression, who often suffer from anxiety, may likewise benefit from the herb's properties.

Unlike conventional tranquilizers, kava doesn't appear to dull the mind. Some studies even show that it improves mental reaction time. People taking kava rarely seem to develop a tolerance to the herb. Also, kava generally doesn't seem to be addictive.

▼ HOW TO TAKE IT

DOSAGE

Because of safety concerns, no safe dosage can be recommended. Taking 300 mg of standardized kava extract by mouth in 3 divided doses a day has been found to be beneficial in human studies. Consult your doctor if you have been taking kava for more than 3 months, because prolonged use increases the chance of side effects.

GUIDELINES FOR USE

• Do not exceed the recommended dose. Higher dosages can lead to intoxication or disorientation. One man in Utah was convicted of driving under the influence after spending the evening consuming 16 cups of kava tea, which caused him to stagger, slur his speech, and drive as if drunk on alcohol.

• Look for extracts standardized to contain at least 30% of the herb's active ingredients, which are called kavalactones. Most U.S. standardized kava brands have 50 to 110 mg kavalactones per tablet or capsule. You can also look for products containing kavapyrones—another name for the active ingredient—which varies with preparation. Most human studies used 70 to 240 mg kavapyrones daily.

• Kava is sometimes combined with herbal supplements that affect the brain, such as the antidepressant St. John's wort.

• Kava usually acts within minutes, but for some people with severe anxiety, the full benefits may not be apparent until up to 8 weeks after first taking the herb.

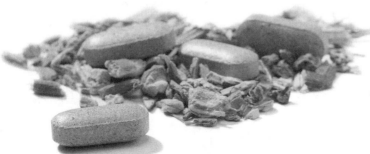

The dried root of the tropical kava plant can be made into stress-relieving pills or a soothing tea.

LAVENDER

The name lavender is derived from the Latin *lavare*, meaning to wash. In ancient Greece, Persia, and Rome, it was used as a perfume in baths and laundry and as an antiseptic. Today, lavender aromatherapy provides relief from the stress of everyday life.

COMMON USES

- Relieves anxiety and induces sleep.
- May relieve rheumatoid arthritis pain.
- May help in the treatment of cancer.

FORMS

- Aromatherapy
- Oil
- Fresh and dried flowers
- Tea

▼ WHAT IT IS

Lavender is native to the Mediterranean, the Arabian Peninsula, Russia, and Africa. It has been used in cosmetics and medicine throughout history. In modern times, lavender is cultivated around the world, and the fragrant oils of its flowers are used in aromatherapy, baked goods, candles, cosmetics, detergents, jellies, massage oils, perfumes, powders, shampoo, soaps, and tea.

English lavender (*Lavandula angustifolia*) is the most common species of lavender used, although other species, including *L. burnamii, L. dentata, L. dhofarensis, L. latifolia,* and *L. stoechas,* are also in use.

MAJOR BENEFITS

Many people find lavender aromatherapy to be relaxing, and several studies have reported it to relieve anxiety in those who have used it. These trials have been small and methodologically flawed, however. Overall, the weight of the evidence suggests that lavender has a small positive effect, although additional data from well-designed studies are required before the evidence can be considered strong.

Small phase 1 human trials of the lavender component perillyl alcohol for cancer treatment have suggested safety and tolerability, although its effects have not been proven.

Lavender aromatherapy is also used as a hypnotic, although there is insufficient evidence to support this use.

ADDITIONAL BENEFITS

Although the results are unproven, lavender has also been used to treat many conditions, including acne, anxiety, asthma, bronchitis, carpal tunnel syndrome, circulation problems, colic, the common cold, depression, diabetes, discomfort after childbirth, dizziness, fatigue, fever, gas, general pain,

  ALERT

SIDE EFFECTS

- People with allergies to lavender may have skin irritation after contact.

- Lavender may cause nausea, vomiting, headache, and chills after inhaling it or absorbing it through the skin. You may experience those effects, as well as constipation, appetite loss, confusion, and drowsiness, if you ingest large doses of lavender or perillyl alcohol, an ingredient in lavender.

CAUTION

- The essential oil of lavender may be poisonous if taken internally.

- Lavender may cause skin rashes and sun sensitivity.

- Some cancer patients have experienced low blood cell counts (neutropenia) after high doses of perillyl alcohol (a constituent of lavender).

- Do not take lavender if you are pregnant or breast feeding. Lavender may cause women to start menstruating if they ingest it in large doses.

- Lavender may increase the amount of drowsiness caused by some drugs, supplements, and alcohol. Exercise caution when driving or operating machinery while using lavender and taking these drugs. In theory, taking lavender by mouth may increase the risk of bleeding when used with some drugs or supplements. In theory, lavender may also add to the cholesterol-lowering effects of other drugs and supplements.

Reminder: If you have a medical condition, talk to your doctor before taking supplements.

hangover, heartburn, HIV infection, indigestion, infertility, lice, low blood pressure, migraine and tension headaches, minor burns, motion sickness, nausea and vomiting, parasites and worms, psychosis, seizures and epilepsy, sores, sprains, toothache, and varicose veins. It has also been used as an antibacterial, antifungal, and antiinflammatory agent; an antioxidant; an aphrodisiac; an appetite stimulant; a diuretic; a douche; an insect repellent; and as an aid in wound healing and recovery from exercise. It has been used to relieve menstrual period problems and the symptoms of menopause.

▼WHAT IT DOES

Lavender aromatherapy is traditionally believed to be relaxing. It is thought to produce circulatory, electrical, central nervous system, and brain reactions similar to those induced by tranquilizers.

A small study of people with rheumatoid arthritis reported no pain relief after massage with lavender aromatherapy. However, patients in this study used fewer painkillers after the massage, which suggests that they may have felt less pain. It is not clear if this benefit was because of the massage or the aromatherapy.

Animal studies suggest that an ingredient in lavender called perillyl alcohol may help treat cancer when taken by mouth. Research has focused on cancers of the breast, pancreas, and intestine. Small studies have been done in humans, but there is not enough evidence to recommend lavender for any type of cancer. There is not enough scientific evidence to recommend lavender aromatherapy for rheumatoid arthritis pain.

▼ HOW TO TAKE IT

DOSAGE (ADULTS)

Aromatherapy: Add 2 to 4 drops of lavender oil to 2 to 3 cups of boiling water and inhale the steam once a day.

Bath: Add 6 drops of lavender oil or ¼ to ½ cup of dried lavender flowers to bath water.

Massage: Add 1 to 4 drops of lavender to a base oil and use for massage.

GUIDELINES FOR USE

There is not enough scientific evidence to recommend lavender for children younger than 18 years of age.

Although lavender aromatherapy may help relieve anxiety and restlessness, scientific evidence does not support the use of lavender for any other health problems. Oral forms of lavender are not recommended because of their possible side effects, especially for women who are pregnant or breast feeding, people at high risk of bleeding, and for children. People taking anticoagulants or drugs that cause drowsiness should use lavender with caution. Call your doctor immediately if you have any side effects.

LECITHIN AND CHOLINE

These closely related nutrients are members of the B-vitamin family, and although you may never have heard of them, they are essential for every cell in your body. Because they are particularly important for the liver and nerves, it's not surprising that so many nutritionists urge Americans to get more of them.

COMMON USES

■ Help prevent gallstones.

■ May strengthen the liver, making them useful in the treatment of hepatitis and cirrhosis.

■ May boost memory and enhance brain function.

■ May diminish the symptoms of Parkinson's disease.

FORMS

■ Capsule   ■ Powder/Grains

■ Tablet   ■ Liquid

■ Softgel

▼ WHAT IT IS

Lecithin (pronounced LESS-a-thin) is a fatty substance found in many animal- and plant-based foods, including liver, eggs, soybeans, peanuts, and wheat germ. It is often added to processed foods—including ice cream, chocolate, margarine, and salad dressings—to help blend, or emulsify, the fats with water. The body manufactures its own supply as well.

Lecithin is considered an excellent source of the B-vitamin choline, primarily in the form called phosphatidylcholine. Once in the body, phosphatidylcholine breaks down into choline, so that when you take lecithin or absorb it from foods your body gets choline.

Only 10% to 20% of the lecithin found in plants and other natural sources consists of phosphatidylcholine. You can buy lecithin supplements that contain higher concentrations of phosphatidylcholine, but they can be very expensive. For most situations, just taking plain lecithin, rather than the more costly phosphatidylcholine, works fine.

Dietary lecithin is a primary source of choline, but choline is also found in liver, soybeans, egg yolks, grape juice, peanuts, cabbage, cauliflower, and other foods. You can also buy choline supplements, and choline is often included as an ingredient in B-complex vitamins or other combination formulas.

▼ WHAT IT DOES

Lecithin and choline are needed for a range of body functions. They help build cell membranes and facilitate the movement of fats and nutrients into and out of cells. They aid in reproduction and in fetal and infant development, they're essential to liver and gallbladder health, and they may help the heart. Choline is also a key component of the brain chemical acetylcholine, which plays a major role in memory and muscle control.

ALERT

SIDE EFFECTS

• Choline supplements may cause rash, insomnia, headaches, cold symptoms, or worsening depression.

• In high doses, lecithin and choline may cause sweating, nausea, vomiting, bloating, and diarrhea. Taking very high dosages of choline (10 g a day) may produce a fishy body odor or a heart rhythm disorder.

CAUTION

• Because individual lecithin, choline, or phosphatidylcholine supplements can increase levels of acetylcholine, they should not be used by people who have a history of depression. Symptoms of worsening depression and mood destabilization have been reported.

• People with kidney or liver problems or who are taking certain medications or stimulants should exercise caution when taking lecithin and choline.

• **Reminder:** If you have a medical or psychiatric condition, talk to your doctor before taking supplements.

As a result of these far-flung effects, lecithin and choline have been touted for almost everything—from curing cancer and AIDS to lowering cholesterol. Even though the evidence for some of these claims is weak, these nutrients should not be dismissed out of hand.

MAJOR BENEFITS
Lecithin and choline may be especially helpful in the treatment of gallbladder and liver diseases. Lecithin is a key component of bile, the fat-digesting substance, and low levels of this nutrient are known to precipitate gallstones. Taking supplements with lecithin or its purified extract, phosphatidylcholine, may treat or prevent this disorder.

Lecithin may also be beneficial for the liver. The results of a 10-year study on baboons showed that it prevented severe liver scarring and cirrhosis caused by alcohol abuse; other studies have indicated that it helps liver problems associated with hepatitis.

Choline is often included in liver complex formulas along with other liver-strengthening supplements, such as the B-vitamin inositol, the amino acid methionine, and the herbs milk thistle and dandelion. These preparations, often called lipotropic combinations or factors, can protect against the buildup of fats in the liver, improve the flow of fats and cholesterol through the liver and gallbladder, and help the liver rid the body of dangerous toxins.

Lecithin and choline may be especially helpful in treating liver or gallbladder diseases, such as hepatitis, cirrhosis, or gallstones.

ADDITIONAL BENEFITS
These two nerve-building nutrients may be useful for improving memory in those with Alzheimer's disease, preventing neural tube birth defects (spina bifida), boosting performance in endurance sports, and treating twitches and tics (tardive dyskinesia) caused by antipsychotic drugs. Preliminary research shows that choline may have a role in treating disorders of the brain, spinal cord, or blood vessels, coma, and postsurgical recovery.

▼ HOW TO TAKE IT

DOSAGE
Lecithin is usually given in a dosage of two 1,200-mg capsules twice a day. It can also be taken in a granular form: 1 tsp contains 19 grains or 1,200 mg of lecithin.

Choline can be obtained from lecithin, although phosphatidylcholine (500 mg 3 times a day) or plain choline (500 mg 3 times a day) may be a better source. Choline can also be taken as part of a lipotropic combination product.

Lecithin and choline have no RDAs, although the scientific group that sets nutritional standards has established what's called an adequate intake (AI) for choline: 550 mg for men and 425 mg for women.

GUIDELINES FOR USE
• Lecithin and choline should be taken with meals to enhance absorption.

• Granular lecithin has a nutty taste and can be easily incorporated into your diet by sprinkling it on foods or mixing it into drinks.

LICORICE *(Glycyrrhiza glabra)*

In ancient Greece, licorice calmed coughs and soothed stomachs. In China, it's still thought to lengthen life. In fact, modern research has found that this versatile herb boosts immunity, fights viruses, treats ulcers, reduces inflammation, protects the liver, eases menopause and, applied topically, even relieves eczema.

COMMON USES

- Helps treat eczema.
- Promotes hepatitis recovery.
- May aid healing canker sores.
- May inhibit the spread of the herpes simplex virus, which causes cold sores and sores on the genitals and buttocks.

FORMS

- Capsule/Tablet
- Liquid
- Wafer
- Lozenge
- Cream
- Dried herb/Tea

▼ WHAT IT IS

One of the most extensively used and thoroughly studied herbal remedies, licorice has a long medicinal history. It was one of the first foods investigated by the National Cancer Institute's experimental food program.

Cultivated in Turkey and Greece, the licorice plant—a member of the pea family—is a tall shrub with bluish flowers. Its medicinal properties are in the root, or rhizome, which contains glycyrrhizin. Licorice is also a source of hundreds of other potentially beneficial substances, including plant estrogens and flavonoids.

Licorice root is made into capsules, tablets, liquids, and cream for therapeutic use. Because it has a sweet, musty taste, licorice root is frequently combined with other herbs to mask their bitterness.

Another form, DGL, or deglycyrrhizinated licorice, has had the glycyrrhizin removed; it is available in capsules and chewable wafers. The two types of licorice have different uses and effects on the body.

▼ WHAT IT DOES

The glycyrrhizin in licorice stimulates the adrenal glands to produce certain hormones, reduces inflammation, and increases the levels of interferon, a virus-fighting substance manufactured by the immune system. Other compounds in licorice are potent antioxidants and may also mimic the effects of estrogen in the body. DGL has a beneficial effect on the digestive tract.

MAJOR BENEFITS

The licorice extracts DGL and carbenoxolone have been proposed as possible therapies for viral hepatitis. They also have been studied for treating peptic ulcers. DGL (but not car-

ALERT

SIDE EFFECTS

- Licorice contains a chemical called glycyrrhizic acid, which causes many side effects. Deglycyrrhizinated licorice (DGL), available in capsule or wafer form, has had this acid removed and is considered safer for use than the other forms. Licorice may affect hormone systems in the body, causing sodium and fluid retention and low potassium levels.
- It may cause high blood pressure and have negative effects on the brain, with symptoms of serious headache, nausea, vomiting, and one-sided weakness. It may also cause abnormally low testosterone levels in men or high prolactin levels in women. These adverse effects may make it difficult to become pregnant and may cause menstrual abnormalities.
- High doses of licorice may cause temporary vision problems or loss.

CAUTION

- Do not exceed recommended dosages. Have your blood pressure monitored if you take licorice root longer than 1 month.
- Avoid licorice if you are pregnant or if you have heart, kidney, or liver disease or high blood pressure.
- Don't take licorice if you are on blood pressure medications, diuretics, hormone replacement therapy, or oral corticosteroids (i.e., prednisone).
- **Reminder:** If you have a medical condition, especially relative to the heart, kidney, or liver, or are taking medications or supplements, talk to your doctor before taking licorice.

benoxolone) may offer some benefits. Some research also suggests that licorice extracts DGL and carbenoxolone may provide benefits for treating canker sores. Studies in these areas have been small and inconclusive.

The DGL form does not work in the same way as licorice root. DGL enhances the body's production of substances that coat the esophagus and stomach, protecting them from the corrosive effects of stomach acid.

In fact, in several studies, DGL was more effective than standard prescription antiulcer medications. It works only when mixed with saliva, however, which is why the chewable wafer form of DGL is preferred for digestive problems. These wafers can also speed the healing of canker sores.

ADDITIONAL BENEFITS

There may be some benefits of licorice for high potassium levels caused by a condition called hypoaldosteronism. There is early evidence in humans that supports this use. However, a qualified health-care provider should supervise treatment.

Available studies have not found any benefit from carbenoxolone cream when applied topically to treat genetal herpes infections.

▼ HOW TO TAKE IT

DOSAGE

Licorice powdered root (4% to 9% glycyrrhizin): Take 1 to 4 g in 3 or 4 doses daily by mouth.
Licorice fluid extract (10% to 20% glycyrrhizin): Take ⅖ to ⅕ tsp per day.
DGL extract tablets: Take 380 to 1,140 mg 3 times daily, 20 minutes before meals.
Carbenoxolone gel or cream: Apply 2% cream or gel 5 times a day for 7 to 14 days to treat herpes simplex virus skin lesions.

GUIDELINES FOR USE

• Licorice should be used for only 4 to 6 weeks unless under direct medical supervision. This is based on the use of relatively large daily doses, 5 to 15 g per day. Many experts believe that extended treatments may be safe if lower doses are used.

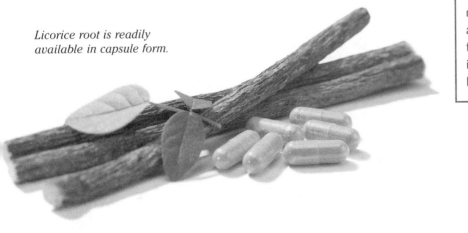

Licorice root is readily available in capsule form.

MAGNESIUM

Although little heralded, magnesium seems to be one of the most important health-promoting minerals. Studies suggest that besides enhancing approximately 300 enzyme-related processes in the body, magnesium may help prevent or combat many chronic diseases ranging from asthma and fibromyalgia to heart disease.

COMMON USES

■ Helps protect against heart disease and irregular heartbeat (arrhythmia).

■ Eases fibromyalgia symptoms.

■ Lowers high blood pressure.

■ May help reduce the severity of asthma attacks.

■ Improves symptoms of premenstrual syndrome (PMS).

■ Aids in preventing the complications of diabetes.

FORMS

■ Capsule

■ Tablet

■ Powder

▼ WHAT IT IS

The average person's body contains just an ounce of magnesium, but this small amount is vital to a number of bodily functions. Many people do not have adequate stores of magnesium, often because they rely too heavily on processed foods, which contain very little of this mineral. In addition, magnesium levels are easily depleted by stress, certain diseases or medications, and intense physical activity.

For this reason, nutritional supplements may be necessary for optimal health. They are available in several forms, including magnesium aspartate, magnesium carbonate, magnesium gluconate, magnesium oxide, and magnesium sulfate.

▼ WHAT IT DOES

One of the most versatile minerals, magnesium is involved in energy production, nerve function, muscle relaxation, and bone and tooth formation. In conjunction with potassium and calcium, magnesium regulates heart rhythm and clots blood; it also aids in the production and use of insulin.

PREVENTION

Research indicates that magnesium is beneficial for the prevention and treatment of heart disease. Studies have shown that the risk of dying of a heart attack is lower in areas with "hard" water, which contains high levels of magnesium. Some researchers speculated that if everyone drank hard water, the number of deaths from heart attacks might decline by 19%. Magnesium appears to lower blood pressure and has also been found to aid recovery after a heart attack by inhibiting blood clots, widening arteries, and normalizing dangerous arrhythmias.

Preliminary studies suggest that an adequate intake of magnesium may prevent type 2 (non-insulin-dependent) diabetes. Researchers at Johns Hopkins University measured magnesium levels in more than 12,000 people who did not have diabetes and tracked them for 6 years to see who developed the disease. Individuals with the lowest magnesium levels had a 94% greater chance of developing the disease than

ALERT

SIDE EFFECTS

• Some people develop nausea and diarrhea with magnesium supplements. If this happens to you, try reducing the dose or taking magnesium gluconate or magnesium sulfate, which are easier on the digestive tract.

CAUTION

• People with kidney disease should consult their physician before taking magnesium supplements.

• Magnesium can make tetracycline antibiotics less effective. Consult your doctor before combining them.

• **Reminder:** If you have a medical condition, talk to your doctor before taking supplements.

those with the highest levels. (These study results, however, apply only to Caucasians; magnesium levels don't seem to affect diabetes in African Americans.) Future studies are needed to see if magnesium supplements can prevent the disease.

ADDITIONAL BENEFITS

Because magnesium relaxes muscles, it's useful for sports injuries and fibromyalgia. It also seems to ease PMS and menstrual cramps and may increase bone density in post-menopausal women, helping stem the onset of osteoporosis.

In addition, magnesium expands airways, which aids in the treatment of asthma and bronchitis. Studies are inconclusive about magnesium's role in preventing or treating migraines, but one study said it may improve the effect of sumatriptan, a prescription drug used for migraines.

▼ HOW MUCH YOU NEED

The RDA for magnesium is 400 mg a day for men ages 19 to 30, 310 mg for women, 420 mg a day for men ages 31 to 70, and 320 mg for women. Higher doses of magnesium are required for disease prevention or treatment, as well as for women who take oral contraceptives.

IF YOU GET TOO LITTLE

Even moderate deficiencies can raise the risk of heart disease and diabetes. Severe deficiencies can result in irregular heartbeat, fatigue, muscle spasms, irritability, nervousness, and confusion.

IF YOU GET TOO MUCH

Magnesium can cause serious side effects—including muscle weakness,

lethargy, confusion, and difficulty breathing—if the body can't process high doses properly. Overdosing on magnesium, however, is rare, because the kidneys are usually efficient at eliminating excess amounts.

▼ HOW TO TAKE IT

DOSAGE

For heart disease prevention: Take 400 mg a day.
For arrythmias, congestive heart failure, and asthma: Take 400 mg twice a day.
For fibromyalgia: Take 150 mg magnesium with 600 mg malic acid twice a day.
For high blood pressure: Take 400 to 800 mg a day.
For diabetes: Take 500 mg a day.

GUIDELINES FOR USE

• Magnesium is best absorbed when taken with each meal.

• Because magnesium can reduce the effectiveness of tetracycline antibiotics, take magnesium supplements 1 to 3 hours before or after the antibiotic medication.

▼ OTHER SOURCES

Good food sources of magnesium are whole grains, nuts, legumes, dark green leafy vegetables, and shellfish.

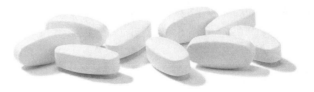

MELATONIN

Hailed by some proponents as a potent antiaging hormone, melatonin has been credited with almost miraculous effects on a wide variety of ailments, including cancer, heart disease, and cataracts. It is probably most effective, however, as a natural sleep aid to ease insomnia and overcome jet lag.

COMMON USES

- Relieves insomnia.
- Promotes restful sleep, even during nighttime pain or stress-related disturbances in sleep.
- Diminishes the effects and shortens the course of jet lag.

FORMS

- Capsule
- Softgel
- Tablet
- Liquid
- Lozenge

▼ WHAT IT IS

First identified in 1958, this naturally occurring hormone is manufactured by the pineal gland, a pea-sized organ deep in the brain. All humans and most animals secrete melatonin throughout their lives, with the highest levels occurring during childhood. As we age, however, the production of melatonin declines, leading some researchers to theorize that melatonin supplementation might benefit all older people.

Natural melatonin levels vary widely. About 1% of the population has very low levels, and another 1% has levels 500 times above normal. There's no correlation, however, between these amounts and specific health concerns or sleep patterns.

▼ WHAT IT DOES

One of the main functions of melatonin is to regulate cycles of sleep and wakefulness. It does so by helping set the brain's internal clock, creating what are known as circadian rhythms—the body's daily biorhythms that govern everything from sleeping and waking times to digestive functions and the release of a variety of hormones linked to reproduction and other body processes.

In order to produce melatonin, the body responds to light cues, making more melatonin when it's dark outside (production begins around dusk and peaks between 2 A.M. and 4 A.M.) and less during the day. This daily cyclical melatonin secretion is what tells the body when to sleep and when to waken.

MAJOR BENEFITS

Melatonin may be most effective as a sleep aid. Various studies of both young and elderly adults indicate that in some people, melatonin shortens the time needed to fall asleep and improves sleep quality by decreasing the number of times they waken

▲ ALERT ▲

SIDE EFFECTS

- No serious risks have been associated with 3 mg or less of melatonin, but long-term studies of 6 months or more have yet to be done.

- Melatonin can cause drowsiness within 30 minutes; its effect may last for several hours. Don't drive or handle heavy machinery during this time.

- Side effects can include headache, stomach upset, itchy skin, depression (transient), fast heartbeat, lethargy, or disorientation. Fuzzy thinking; vivid, unpleasant dreams; and even a worsening of insomnia may occur.

CAUTION

- Let your doctor know if you're taking melatonin. It may interact with certain medications as well as with alcohol and caffeine.

- Don't take melatonin if you are pregnant, breast feeding, or trying to get pregnant (investigators are examining its effect on the menstrual cycle).

- Melatonin may affect hormone levels in the body.

- Melatonin should not be taken by people with liver problems, depression, heart disease, or a neurological disorder.

- **Reminder:** If you have a medical or psychiatric condition, talk to your doctor before taking supplements.

during the night. It may be beneficial when chronic pain or stress causes sleep disturbances.

Melatonin can also help restore normal sleep patterns in people who do night shift work or in those suffering from jet lag as a result of crossing time zones. Melatonin may also relieve sleep disturbances with a wide variety of causes, including schizophrenia, Alzheimer's, bipolar disorder, neuropsychiatric disorders in children, and depression. Moreover, it works without producing the addictive effects of conventional sleep medications.

ADDITIONAL BENEFITS

Some studies suggest that when combined with certain cancer drugs, melatonin may help destroy malignant cells. Another study conducted in Holland in 1995 found that when taken in conjunction with birth control pills, melatonin has an estrogen-countering effect that may offer protection against some forms of breast cancer.

Melatonin may help treat several types of cancers, including melanoma and gastrointestinal, breast, and brain tumors. Although melatonin's antioxidant activity may improve the effectiveness of conventional treatments and reduce side effects, there is a lack of controlled human research at this time to recommend for or against the use of melatonin as a treatment for any cancer.

Additional conditions melatonin may benefit include AIDS, headache (migraine, cluster, and tension type), high blood pressure, childhood epilepsy, Parkinson's disease, and seasonal affective disorder.

▼ HOW TO TAKE IT

DOSAGE

For improving normal sleep: Take 0.3 to 3 mg 30 to 60 minutes before bedtime.
For other sleep disturbances or disorders: Take up to 5 to 10 mg before bedtime. Lower doses, 0.5 to 2 mg, should be used by the elderly.
For headache: Take 10 mg every evening.
For high blood pressure: Take 1 mg every evening.
For cancer: Take up to 20 to 40 mg as an additional therapy for limited periods of time.

GUIDELINES FOR USE

• To combat insomnia, stick to a precise schedule, taking supplements at the same time every evening.

• Begin with the lowest dose and increase it as needed.

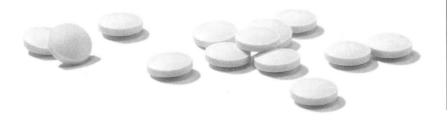

MILK THISTLE *(Silybum marianum)*

The medicinal use of milk thistle (widely called silymarin after its active ingredient) can be traced back thousands of years to the time of the ancient Greeks and the Romans. Today, researchers have completed more than 300 scientific studies that attest to the benefits of this herb, particularly for treating liver-related ailments.

COMMON USES

- May protect the liver from all kinds of toxins, including drugs, poisons, and chemicals.
- May improve liver disorders such as cirrhosis and hepatitis.
- Reduces liver damage from drinking excessive alcohol.
- Aids in the treatment and prevention of gallstones.

FORMS

- Tablet
- Capsule
- Softgel
- Liquid

▼ WHAT IT IS

Known by its botanical name, *Silybum marianum,* as well as by its principal active ingredient, silymarin, milk thistle is a member of the aster family. The purple flowers and milky white leaf veins of this herb, which early settlers brought from Europe to North America, are a common sight along the East Coast and in California; the plant also grows as a weed in other parts of the United States and around the world. It blooms from June through August, and the shiny black seeds used for medicinal purposes are collected at the end of summer.

▼ WHAT IT DOES

Milk thistle is one of the most extensively studied and documented herbs in use today. Scientific research continues to validate its healing powers, particularly for the treatment of liver-related disorders.

Most of its effectiveness stems from a flavonoid complex of three liver-protecting compounds collectively known as silymarin, which constitutes 4% to 6% of the ripe seeds.

MAJOR BENEFITS

Among the most important benefits of milk thistle is its ability to fortify the liver, which is one of the body's most important organs, second in size only to the skin. The liver processes nutrients, including fats and other foods. In addition, it breaks down and neutralizes, or detoxifies, many drugs, chemical pollutants, and alcohol.

Milk thistle helps enhance and even strengthen this vital organ by preventing the depletion of glutathione, an amino acid–like compound that is essential to the detoxifying process. What's more, studies show that milk thistle can increase glutathione concentration by up to 35%. This herb is also an effective gatekeeper, limiting the number of toxins that the liver processes at any given time.

Milk thistle is a powerful antioxidant as well. Even more potent than vitamins C

ALERT

SIDE EFFECTS

- Possible side effects include stomach upset, headache, itching, appetite loss, gas, heartburn, joint pain, impotence, decreased blood sugar, and anaphylactic shock.

- In some people, it may have a slight laxative effect for a day or two.

CAUTION

- Milk thistle may interact with medications broken down by the liver, medications used to control blood suugar, phenytoin (Dilantin), and herbs and supplements with similar effects.

- Any liver disease requires careful medical evaluation and treatment under the supervision of a physician.

- **Reminder:** If you have a medical condition, are pregnant or nursing, are allergic to plants in the aster family, or are taking prescription medications, talk to your doctor before taking milk thistle.

and E, it helps prevent damage from highly reactive free radical molecules. Furthermore, it promotes the regeneration of new, healthy liver cells, which replace old, damaged ones. Milk thistle eases a range of serious liver ailments, including viral infections (hepatitis) and scarring of the liver (cirrhosis).

This herb is so potent that it's sometimes given in an injectable form in the emergency room to combat the life-threatening, liver-destroying effects of poisonous mushrooms. In addition, because excessive alcohol depletes glutathione, milk thistle can aid in protecting the livers of alcoholics or those recovering from alcohol abuse.

ADDITIONAL BENEFITS
In cancer patients, milk thistle limits the potential for drug-induced damage to the liver after chemotherapy treatments, and it hastens recovery by speeding removal of toxic substances that can accumulate in the body.

Scientific evidence also has shown that it may be beneficial in treating high cholesterol.

▼ HOW TO TAKE IT

DOSAGE
The recommended dose for milk thistle is 230 to 420 mg of standardized extract a day divided into 2 or 3 doses (up to 8,000 mg daily has been used, but safety is not known). Doses for Silipide, a special milk thistle product designed to be better absorbed by the body, are 160 to 480 mg a day.

Milk thistle is often combined with other herbs and nutrients, such as dandelion, choline, methionine, and inositol. This combination may be labeled "liver complex" or "lipotropic factors" ("lipotropic" refers to the formula's fat-metabolizing properties; it prevents the buildup of fatty substances in the liver). For proper dosage, follow package directions.

GUIDELINES FOR USE
• Milk thistle seems most effective when taken between meals.

• The benefits of milk thistle may be noticeable within a week or two, although long-term treatment is often needed for chronic conditions.

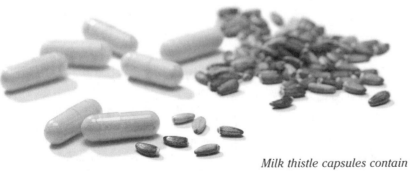

Milk thistle capsules contain powdered extracts derived from the seeds of the plant.

MUSHROOMS *(Shiitake, maitake, reishi, and PSK)*

Shiitake, reishi, and maitake are more than just exotic-sounding ingredients on a Japanese menu. In fact, they (along with an extract called PSK) are members of a special group of medicinal mushrooms that Asians have heralded for centuries as longevity tonics, immune-system boosters, and cancer fighters.

COMMON USES

- May build immunity.
- Help prevent cancer.
- May enhance cancer treatments.
- Help prevent heart disease.
- May lower blood pressure.
- May lower blood sugar.

FORMS

- Capsule
- Tablet
- Liquid
- Powder
- Tea
- Dried mushrooms
- Fresh mushrooms

▼ WHAT IT IS

For millennia, traditional Asian medicine has cherished certain mushrooms for their health-promoting effects. These include maitake *(Grifola frondosa)*, reishi *(Ganoderma lucidum)*, and shiitake *(Lentinus edodes)*. More recently, an extract from the mushroom *Coriolus versicolor*, called PSK, has also been found to be a potent cancer fighter.

Although other mushrooms—tree ear and oyster mushrooms, for example—may also provide some health benefits, most of the attention and research have concentrated on the four types mentioned above.

These mushrooms are available as powders (in loose form for tea or in capsules or tablets) or as liquid extracts, which concentrate their potency. Dried reishi mushrooms and fresh and dried shiitake and maitake may be found in Asian groceries and some gourmet stores, but for therapeutic purposes, supplements are preferred. Maitake, reishi, and shiitake mushroom powders are sometimes combined in one capsule.

▼ WHAT IT DOES

Medicinal mushrooms have varied effects, including boosting the body's immune system, lowering cholesterol, acting as an anticoagulant, and playing a supporting role for other agents in the treatment of cancer.

ALERT

SIDE EFFECTS

- Shiitake, maitake, and reishi, as well as *Coriolus versicolor*, are all safe when used in appropriate doses. Allergies to all varieties have been reported; these cause rashes and respiratory problems.

- Other side effects may include an increased risk of bleeding, gastric bleeding, low blood pressure, low blood sugar, dizziness, dry mouth, nosebleed, breast tenderness, and bone pain.

CAUTION

- Pregnant or breast-feeding women should consult a physician before trying any of the mushrooms medicinally.

- People taking anticoagulant drugs (including a daily aspirin) should avoid reishi supplements because the mushrooms contain compounds that also "thin" the blood. Because of this effect, mushrooms should be discontinued 2 weeks before surgery or dental procedures. People who have bleeding or blood disorders or a history of hypotension, hypoglycemia, gastric ulcers, active gastrointestinal bleeding, or hemophilia should avoid medicinal use of mushrooms.

- Mushrooms may interact with certain medications, including medications that lower the blood pressure, antiviral drugs, immunosuppressive agents, antibiotics, certain pain-relieving medications, medications that lower cholesterol, drugs to treat diabetes, amphetamines, and herbs and supplements with similar effects.

- **Reminder:** If you have a medical condition, talk to your doctor before taking supplements.

MAJOR BENEFITS

Maitake and *Coriolus versicolor* are commonly used in Japan to strengthen the immune systems of people undergoing chemotherapy treatment for cancer. Studies have shown that maitake extracts increase the effectiveness of lower chemotherapy doses while protecting healthy cells from the damage such drugs can cause.

The Japanese have been employing the PSK extract from *Coriolus versicolor* as an adjunct to chemotherapy for many years. (In the United States, a similar product is labeled simply *Coriolus versicolor* extract.) Several studies have suggested that PSK can improve survival rates in people who have stomach, colon, or lung cancer, but more research is needed.

For example, shiitake mushrooms contain a carbohydrate compound called lentinan, which promotes the body's production of T cells and other immune system components. Laboratory studies show that *Coriolus versicolor* might be able to overpower HIV in the test tube; more research is needed, however, to see if it can do the same in the human body.

Other people with compromised immune systems—such as those with chronic fatigue syndrome—may benefit from medicinal mushrooms too.

ADDITIONAL BENEFITS

Shiitake, maitake, and reishi may help fight heart disease by reducing the tendency of blood to clot, lowering blood pressure, and possibly reducing cholesterol levels.

▼ HOW TO TAKE IT

DOSAGE

For immune system support for cancer: Take 500 mg of reishi, 400 mg of shiitake, and 200 mg of maitake mushrooms 3 times a day or 3,000 mg of *Coriolus versicolor* divided into 2 doses a day.
For heart disease or HIV/AIDS: Take 1,500 mg of reishi and 600 mg of maitake daily.

GUIDELINES FOR USE

• The effects of medicinal mushrooms aren't dramatic and may need several months to appear.

• For best results, divide the supplements into 2 or 3 daily doses and take them with or without food.

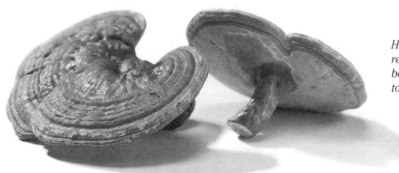

Helpful for stress, dried reishi mushrooms can be simmered in water to make a calming tea.

NETTLE *(Urtica dioica)*

The healing powers of this herb date to the third century B.C., when it was used to remove venom from snakebites. Today, scientists are confirming that nettle, with its stinging leaves, has a valuable role to play in treating hay fever and prostate symptoms as well as in alleviating the pain and inflammation of gout.

COMMON USES

■ May reduce pain and inflammation from arthritis.

■ Relieves allergy symptoms, particularly hay fever.

■ May ease prostate symptoms.

FORMS

■ Capsule

■ Tincture

■ Liquid

■ Dried herb/Tea

▼ WHAT IT IS

Strange as it may sound, the original interest in using nettle for medicinal purposes probably was inspired by the plant's ability to irritate exposed skin. Nettle leaves are covered with tiny hairs—hollow needles actually—that sting and burn on contact. This effect was believed to be beneficial for joint pain (stinging oneself with nettle is an old folk remedy for arthritis), and for centuries nettle leaf poultices were applied to draw toxins from the skin.

Also considered a nutritious food, nettle leaves taste like spinach. They are particularly high in iron and other minerals and are rich in carotenoids and vitamin C as well. (Opt for young shoots, which have no stingers.) The plant often grows up to 5 feet tall in parts of the United States and Canada as well as in Europe.

▼ WHAT IT DOES

Stinging yourself with nettle leaves probably won't help your joint pain, but nettle tea or fresh nettle juice applied as a compress or nettle supplements taken orally may relieve inflamed joints, especially in people with certain forms of arthritis.

MAJOR BENEFITS

Nettle (specifically the root) may be suitable for men with an enlarged prostate not caused by cancer. This condition, called benign prostatic hyperplasia (BPH), occurs when the prostate enlarges and narrows the urethra (the tube that transports urine out of the bladder), making urination difficult. Nettle may aid in slowing prostate growth.

ADDITIONAL BENEFITS

Nasal congestion and watery eyes result when the body produces an inflammatory compound called histamine in response to pollen and other allergens. Nettle is a good source of quercetin, a flavonoid that has been shown to inhibit the release of hista-

---

 ALERT

SIDE EFFECTS
• Nettle is considered safe, with only a minimal risk of causing an allergic reaction. There have been some reports, however, that nettle root in particular may irritate the stomach, causing indigestion and diarrhea.

• Handling the fresh nettle plant itself can cause skin redness and irritation.

CAUTION
• Don't ever substitute nettle for a prescription medication for prostate problems without consulting your doctor.

• Nettle leaf preparations can cause complications in people with swelling (edema) related to heart or kidney problems.

• People with diabetes or a body fluid imbalance, or women who are pregnant or breast feeding, should exercise caution when using nettle.

• Nettle may interact with medications that lower blood pressure, medications used to treat prostate conditions, diuretics, antiinflammatory agents, blood thinners, and herbs and supplements with similar effects.

Reminder: If you have a medical condition, talk to your doctor before taking supplements.

mine. In one study of allergy sufferers, more than half the participants rated nettle moderately to highly effective in reducing allergy symptoms when compared with a placebo.

▼ HOW TO TAKE IT

DOSAGE

For allergies: Take 250 mg of nettle leaf standardized extract 3 times a day, as needed. Alternatively, take 600 mg of freeze-dried leaves daily for 1 week at the onset of symptoms.

For BPH: Use 250 mg of nettle root standardized extract twice a day in combination with the herb saw palmetto (160 mg twice a day) or *Pygeum africanum* (100 mg twice a day).

For arthritis: Take 50 mg of stewed nettle leaves in combination with 50 mg of diclofenac tablets (see p. 93) daily for 14 days.

For topical use: Apply the underside of a leaf cut from a fresh nettle plant to the painful area with gentle pressure for 30 seconds, moving the leaf twice; do this twice daily for 1 week.

GUIDELINES FOR USE

• In any of its forms, take nettle with food to minimize stomach upset.

• If you want to try the fresh leaves as a vegetable, keep in mind that the young shoots can be eaten raw, but older leaves (with mature, stinging hairs) must be cooked before eating to inactivate the stingers.

Supplements are a convenient way to get the diuretic and antihistamine effects of nettle leaves.

PAU D'ARCO *(Tabebuia impetiginosa)*

Rumored to have been prescribed by the ancient Incas to treat serious ailments, the herb pau d'arco, found in South American rain forests, has been investigated as a remedy for infectious diseases and cancer. Although its anticancer properties are debatable, pau d'arco may indeed combat a variety of infections.

COMMON USES

- Treats vaginal yeast infections.
- Helps get rid of warts.
- Reduces inflammation of the airways in bronchitis.
- May be useful in treating immune-related disorders such as asthma, eczema, psoriasis, and bacterial and viral infections.

FORMS

- Capsule
- Tablet
- Softgel
- Powder
- Liquid
- Dried herb/Tea

▼ WHAT IT IS

Pau d'arco is obtained from the inner bark of a tree—*Tabebuia impetiginosa*—indigenous to the rain forests of South America. Native tribes have taken advantage of its healing powers for centuries. Pau d'arco is also known as *lapacho, taheebo,* or *ipe roxo*. In the United States, however, it's always sold as pau d'arco.

The therapeutic ingredients in pau d'arco include a host of potent plant chemicals called naphthoquinones. Of these, a particular one called lapachol has been the most intensely studied by research investigators.

▼ WHAT IT DOES

Lapachol and other compounds in pau d'arco help destroy the microorganisms that can cause diseases and infections ranging from malaria and the flu to yeast infections. Most people, however, are interested in the potential cancer-fighting properties of this herb.

MAJOR BENEFITS

Pau d'arco appears to combat bacteria, viruses, and fungi; reduce inflammation; and support the immune system. One of its best-documented uses is for vaginal yeast infections. Herbalists often recommend a pau d'arco tea douche to restore the normal chemical environment of the vagina.

In capsule, tablet, tincture, or tea form, pau d'arco may be effective in strengthening immunity in people with chronic fatigue syndrome, HIV or AIDS, or chronic bronchitis. The herb's antiinflammatory properties likewise benefit acute bronchitis, which involves inflammation of the respiratory passages, as well as muscle pain. A tincture of pau d'arco applied directly to warts is useful in eradicating them.

ADDITIONAL BENEFITS

Pau d'arco's anticancer activity is subject to continuing debate. Because of the herb's traditional reputation as a cancer fighter, the National Cancer Institute (NCI) investigated it, identifying lapachol as its most active ingredient.

 ALERT

SIDE EFFECTS

- Whole-bark products are generally safe; they do not produce the side effects of high doses of lapachol. If pau d'arco tea or supplements cause stomach upset, take them with food.

- Unusual bruising or bleeding, pink urine, or severe nausea or vomiting are signs of an adverse reaction to pau d'arco. Stop taking the herb and call your doctor if they develop.

CAUTION

- Pregnant or breast-feeding women should avoid pau d'arco.

- Be careful if using pau d'arco with anticoagulant medications. The herb can amplify the drugs' blood-thinning actions, posing the risk of excessive bleeding and other problems. Consult your doctor for guidance.

- **Reminder:** If you have a medical condition, talk to your doctor before taking supplements.

In animal studies, pau d'arco showed promise in shrinking tumors, so the NCI began human trials using high doses of lapachol in the 1970s. Again, there was some evidence that lapachol was active in destroying cancer cells, but participants taking a therapeutic dose suffered serious side effects, including nausea, vomiting, and blood-clotting problems. As a result, research on lapachol and its source, pau d'arco, to treat cancer was abandoned.

Critics of this investigation believe that using therapeutic doses of pau d'arco—and not simply the isolated compound lapachol—would have produced similar benefits without the potentially danger-ous blood-thinning effects. It's likely that lapachol interferes with the action of vitamin K, needed for the blood to clot properly. Some researchers sug-gest that other compounds in pau d'arco supply some vitamin K, so use of the whole herb would not interfere with blood clotting. Others think that combining lapachol with vitamin K sup-plements might make it possible for people to take doses of lapachol high enough to permit its potential anti-tumor action to be further studied without provoking a reaction.

Despite the controversy, many practi-tioners rely on the historical evidence of pau d'arco's anticancer action and often recommend it as a complement to conventional cancer treatment.

▼ HOW TO TAKE IT

DOSAGE
The typical daily dosage when using pau d'arco in capsule or tablet form is 250 mg twice a day; in liquid extract form it is 1 tsp twice a day.

This dose of pau d'arco is often recommended for chronic fatigue syndrome or HIV and AIDS, alternating with other immune-boosting herbs such as echinacea or goldenseal.

Pau d'arco is also commonly con-sumed as a tea in dried herb form. To make it, steep 2 or 3 tsp of pau d'arco in 2 cups of very hot water; drink the tea over the course of a day.

GUIDELINES FOR USE
• Many herbalists recommend using whole-bark products (not those that contain just lapachol). They suspect that the herb's healing properties come from the interaction of the full range of plant chemicals in the bark.

• **For vaginal yeast infections:** Let pau d'arco tea cool to lukewarm before using it as a douche.

• **For warts:** Apply a compress soaked in pau d'arco liquid extract to the affected area at bedtime and leave it on all night. Repeat the treatment until the wart disappears.

Pau d'arco can be taken as a supplement or brewed as a tea.

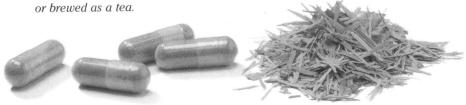

PEPPERMINT *(Mentha piperita)*

For centuries this powerfully aromatic herb has provided relief for indigestion, colds, and headache. Today, medicinal peppermint is most prized for its ability to soothe the digestive tract, easing indigestion, irritable bowel syndrome, and other complaints. It's also useful for relieving muscle aches and freshening stale breath.

COMMON USES

- May relieve nausea and indigestion.
- Eases symptoms of diverticulosis and irritable bowel syndrome.
- Sweetens breath.
- May relieve tension headaches and nasal congestion.
- May treat urinary tract infections.

FORMS

- Capsule
- Tincture/Liquid
- Oil
- Dried or fresh herb/Tea
- Ointment/Cream

▼ WHAT IT IS

Peppermint is cultivated worldwide for use as a flavoring agent and an herbal medicine. A natural hybrid of spearmint and water mint, peppermint has square stems and oval, pointed dark green or purple leaves and lilac flowers. For medicinal purposes, the plant's leaves and stems are harvested just before the flowers bloom in summer.

The major active ingredient of peppermint is its volatile oil, which is made up of more than 40 different compounds. The oil's therapeutic effect comes mainly from menthol (35% to 55% of the oil), menthone (15% to 30%), and menthyl acetate (3% to 10%). Medicinal peppermint oil is made by steam-distilling the parts of the plant that grow above the ground.

▼ WHAT IT DOES

Particularly effective in treating digestive disorders, peppermint relieves cramps and relaxes intestinal muscles. It freshens the breath and may clear up nasal congestion as well.

MAJOR BENEFITS

Peppermint oil relaxes the muscles of the digestive tract, helping relieve intestinal cramping and gas. Its antispasmodic effect also makes it useful for alleviating the symptoms of irritable bowel syndrome, a common disorder characterized by abdominal pain, alternating bouts of constipation and diarrhea, and indigestion.

The menthol in peppermint aids digestion because it stimulates the flow of natural digestive juices and bile. This explains why peppermint oil is often included in over-the-counter antacids.

You can put the oil directly on your tongue; it provides a minty antidote to bad breath.

As a tea or oil, peppermint serves as a mild anesthetic to the stomach's

---

 ALERT

SIDE EFFECTS

- Peppermint leaves in recommended doses generally produce no side effects. However, peppermint oil taken by mouth may cause headache; dizziness; heartburn and burning, slow heart rate; or muscle tremor.

- Topical peppermint oil can cause allergic skin rashes (especially if you're applying heat as well), mouth sores, and eye irritation. If side effects occur, stop using the herb.

CAUTION

- Because peppermint oil relaxes gastrointestinal muscles, it may aggravate the symptoms of a hiatal hernia or gallbladder disease.

- Avoid large doses of peppermint oil during pregnancy.

- Peppermint oil should not be applied to the nostrils or chest of infants and children under age 5 years because it can cause a choking sensation.

- Never ingest pure menthol, a major ingredient in peppermint oil; as little as 1 tsp (2 g) can cause a severe reaction.

- **Reminder:** If you have a medical condition or are taking medications, talk to your doctor before taking peppermint.

mucous lining, which helps reduce nausea and motion sickness. The tea may ease symptoms of diverticulosis, including gas and bloating.

ADDITIONAL BENEFITS

When rubbed on the skin, peppermint oil relieves pain by stimulating the nerves that perceive cold while muting those that sense pain, making it a welcome remedy for aching muscles.

The jury is out on whether peppermint helps treat coughs or colds. Some tests show that the aromatic plant has no effect. Commission E, a German health board recognized as an authority on the scientific investigation of herbs, however, found that peppermint was an effective decongestant that reduced inflammation of the nasal passageways. In addition, many people with colds report that inhaling peppermint's menthol enables them to breathe more easily. Drinking warm peppermint tea also may offer relief from the bronchial constriction of asthma.

▼ HOW TO TAKE IT

DOSAGE

For the treatment of irritable bowel syndrome and nausea: Try enteric-coated capsules containing peppermint oil, because they release peppermint oil where it's needed most—in the small and large intestines rather than in the stomach. Take 1 or 2 cap-

The oil from peppermint leaves helps relieve many digestive complaints.

sules (containing 0.2 ml of oil per capsule) 2 or 3 times a day between meals.
To freshen the breath: Place a few drops of peppermint oil on the tongue.
To relieve gas and calm the stomach: Make a tea by steeping 1 or 2 tsp of dried peppermint leaves in a cup of very hot water for between 5 and 10 minutes; be sure to cover the cup to keep the volatile oil from escaping.
For congestion: Drink up to 4 cups of peppermint tea a day. For inhalation, inhale 3 to 4 drops of oil added to about ⅔ cup of hot water up to 3 times per day or use 1% to 5% essential oil as a nasal ointment to relieve congestion.
For pain relief: Add a few drops of peppermint oil to ½ oz of a neutral oil. Apply to the affected areas up to 4 times daily.
For headache relief: Apply 10% peppermint oil (in methanol) to the skin of the forehead and temples multiple times per day.

GUIDELINES FOR USE

• Take enteric-coated capsules between meals.
• Drink a cup of peppermint tea 3 or 4 times a day, right after or between meals.
• Apply peppermint oil or ointments containing menthol no more than 3 or 4 times a day.
• To use peppermint tincture, put 10 to 20 drops of the tincture in a glass of water and drink; to take the liquid extract, put ½ to 1 tsp of the extract in a glass of water and drink.

PHOSPHORUS

If you compiled a list of nutrients the body could not live without, phosphorus would be near the top. Although the main function of phosphorus is building strong bones and teeth (in conjunction with calcium), this mineral is needed by virtually every cell. Fortunately, the chance of developing a phosphorus deficiency is very small.

COMMON USES
- Builds strong bones and maintains skeletal integrity.
- Helps form tooth enamel and strengthens teeth.

FORMS
- Capsule
- Tablet
- Powder
- Liquid

▼ WHAT IT IS

Phosphorus is the second most abundant mineral in the body (after calcium), and up to 1½ lb of it are found in the average person. Although 85% of this mineral is concentrated in the bones and teeth, the rest is distributed in the blood and in various organs, including the heart, kidneys, brain, and muscles.

Phosphorus interacts with a variety of other nutrients, but its most constant companion is calcium. In the bones, the ratio of calcium to phosphorus is about 2:1. In other tissues, however, the amount of phosphorus is higher.

▼ WHAT IT DOES

There is hardly a biological or cellular process that does not, directly or indirectly, involve phosphorus. In some instances, the mineral works to protect cells, strengthening the membranes that surround them. In other cases, it acts as a kind of biological escort, assisting a variety of nutrients, hormones, and chemicals in doing their jobs. There's also evidence that phosphorus helps activate the B vitamins, enabling them to provide all their benefits.

MAJOR BENEFITS
One of phosphorus's most important functions is to team up with calcium to build bones and aid in maintaining a strong, healthy skeleton. The calcium-phosphorus partnership is also crucial for strengthening the teeth and helping keep them strong.

In addition, phosphorus joins with fats in the blood to make compounds called phospholipids, which, in turn, play structural and metabolic roles in cell membranes throughout the body. Furthermore, without phosphorus, the body could not convert the proteins, carbohydrates, and fats it absorbs from food into energy.

The mineral is needed to create the molecule known as adenosine triphosphate, or ATP, which acts like a tiny battery charger, supplying vital energy to every cell in the body.

ADDITIONAL BENEFITS
Phosphorus serves as a cell-to-cell messenger. In this capacity, it helps the coordination of such body pro-

ALERT

CAUTION
- The greatest risk associated with phosphorus may be getting too much, which some experts caution may lead to a calcium deficiency. Never take phosphorus supplements without discussing it with your doctor first.

- In the rare instance of a phosphorus deficiency—such as from kidney or digestive disease or a severe burn—phosphorus supplementation must be medically supervised.

- **Reminder:** If you have a medical condition, talk to your doctor before taking supplements.

cesses as muscle contraction, the transmission of nerve impulses from the brain to the body, and the secretion of hormones. An adequate phosphorus supply may therefore enhance your physical performance and be effective in fighting fatigue.

In addition, the mineral is necessary for maintaining the pH (the acid-base balance) of the blood and for manufacturing DNA and RNA, the basic components of our genetic makeup.

▼ HOW MUCH YOU NEED

Because phosphorus is found in so many foods, the need for supplements is virtually nonexistent. The RDA for phosphorus in men and women is the same, 700 mg daily. In the past, many nutritionists recommended that phosphorus and calcium be taken in a 1:1 ratio, but more recently experts have advised that this ratio has little practical benefit. Most people today consume more phosphorus than calcium in their diet.

IF YOU GET TOO LITTLE

Although rare, a deficiency of phosphorus can lead to fragile bones and teeth, fatigue, weakness, a loss of appetite, joint pain and stiffness, and an increased susceptibility to infection. A mild deficiency may produce a modest decrease in energy.

IF YOU GET TOO MUCH

There are no immediate adverse effects from getting too much phosphorus.

However, some experts caution that over the long term, excessive phosphorus intake may inhibit calcium absorption, but it's uncertain whether this can result in a calcium deficiency that threatens bone health.

▼ HOW TO TAKE IT

DOSAGE

Most people get all the phosphorus they require through their daily diet. In addition, a small amount of phosphorus may be included in daily multivitamin and mineral supplements.

If you have a medical condition that depletes this mineral, such as a bowel ailment or failing kidneys, your doctor will prescribe an appropriate dosage.

GUIDELINES FOR USE

• Never take individual phosphorus supplements without being under a doctor's supervision.

▼ OTHER SOURCES

High-protein foods, such as meat, fish, poultry, and dairy products, contain a lot of phosphorus. It is also used as an additive in many processed foods. Soft drinks, particularly colas, often have large amounts.

Phosphorus is present in grain products as well, although whole-grain breads and cereals may include ingredients that partially reduce the absorption of this mineral.

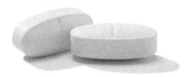

POTASSIUM

You're probably careful not to eat too much sodium (salt), especially if you're watching your blood pressure. You might also want to focus your efforts, however, on getting more potassium. For some people, stocking up on this mineral may be as important to blood pressure control as limiting the sodium they eat.

COMMON USES
- Helps lower blood pressure.
- May prevent high blood pressure, heart disease, and stroke.

FORMS
- Tablet
- Liquid
- Powder

▼ WHAT IT IS

The third most abundant mineral in the body after calcium and phosphorus, potassium is an electrolyte—a substance that takes on a positive or negative charge when dissolved in the watery medium of the bloodstream. Sodium and chloride are electrolytes, too, and the body needs a balance of these minerals to perform a host of essential functions. Almost all of the potassium in the body is found inside the cells.

▼ WHAT IT DOES

Along with the other electrolytes, potassium is used to conduct nerve impulses, initiate muscle contractions, and regulate heartbeat and blood pressure. It controls the amount of fluid inside the cells, and sodium regulates the amount outside, so the two minerals work together to balance fluid levels in the body.

Potassium also enables the body to convert blood sugar (glucose)—its primary fuel—into a stored form of energy (glycogen) that's held in reserve by the muscles and liver.

PREVENTION
Study after study has shown that people who get plenty of potassium in their diet have lower blood pressure than those who get very little. This effect holds true even when sodium intake remains high (although reducing sodium produces better results).

In one study, 54 people on medication for high blood pressure were divided into two groups. Half followed their regular diet; the other half added 3 to 6 servings of potassium-rich foods a day. After a year, 81% of those getting extra potassium were able to reduce their drug dosages significantly compared with only 29% of the individuals following their regular diets.

ADDITIONAL BENEFITS
Through its effects on blood pressure, potassium may also decrease the risk of heart disease and stroke. In one study, a group of people with hypertension who ate 1 serving of a food high in potassium every day reduced their risk of fatal stroke by 40%. A 12-year investigation found that men who got the least amount of potassium were 2½ times more likely to die from a stroke than men who consumed the most; for women with a low potassium

 ALERT

CAUTION
- Do not take potassium supplements without consulting your doctor if you have kidney disease, are taking corticosteroids, or are using any medication for high blood pressure or heart disease.

- **Reminder:** If you have a medical condition, talk to your doctor before taking supplements.

intake, the risk of fatal stroke was nearly 5 times greater.

▼ HOW MUCH YOU NEED

There is no RDA for potassium, but most experts recommend 2,000 to 3,000 mg a day. More may be needed to control blood pressure.

IF YOU GET TOO LITTLE
Potassium is found in a wide variety of foods, so it is practically impossible not to get enough of this mineral to perform the basic body functions. A serious deficiency can occur if an individual is taking a potent diuretic (a drug that reduces fluid levels in the body) or is suffering from an extreme case of diarrhea or vomiting. The first sign of deficiency is muscle weakness and nausea. If potassium is not replaced, low levels could lead to heart failure.

IF YOU GET TOO MUCH
Potassium toxicity is highly unlikely because most people can safely consume up to 18 g a day. Toxicity usually occurs only if an individual has a kidney disorder or takes too many potassium supplements. Signs of potassium overload include muscle fatigue and an irregular heartbeat. Even in small doses, potassium supplements may cause stomach irritation and nausea.

▼ HOW TO TAKE IT

DOSAGE
Most people don't need potassium supplements unless they are taking certain diuretic medications. Try to get sufficient potassium in your daily diet; if you want extra insurance, take no more than 500 mg of potassium in supplement form a day.

People who use ACE inhibitors (such as captopril or enalapril) for high blood pressure or angina and those who have kidney disease should not take potassium supplements at all.

GUIDELINES FOR USE
• If you use potassium supplements, take them with food to decrease stomach irritation.

• Many nutrition-conscious doctors believe that you really don't need to take potassium supplements unless specifically advised to do so by your health-care practitioner. Potassium-rich foods are a better option for those who wish to maintain good health.

▼ OTHER SOURCES

Fresh fruits and vegetables—such as bananas, oranges and orange juice, and potatoes—are very high in potassium. Meats, poultry, milk, and yogurt are also good sources.

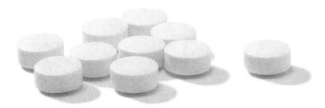

PSYLLIUM *(Plantago psyllium, P. ovata)*

These tiny plant seeds are so rich in fiber that they've been prescribed for constipation and a wide range of other digestive ailments for more than 500 years. Now, new research is finding that psyllium offers an added benefit as well: The seeds appear to lower blood cholesterol levels both safely and effectively.

COMMON USES
- Relieves constipation and diarrhea.
- May treat diverticular disease and irritable bowel syndrome.
- May lower cholesterol.
- May treat high blood sugar.

FORMS
- Powder
- Capsule
- Wafer

▼ WHAT IT IS

Odorless and nearly tasteless, psyllium comes from the small, reddish-brown to black seeds of the *Plantago psyllium* plant. Also known as the plantain, it should not be confused with the edible banana-like fruit of the same name *(Musa paradisiaca)* or with the herb plantain *(Plantago lanceolata)* sometimes recommended for coughs.

Plantago psyllium grows as a weed in numerous places around the world, and it is commercially cultivated in Spain, France, India, Pakistan, and other countries.

Various species of the plant, most commonly the seeds of *Plantago psyllium* and *P. ovata*, are used in herbal medicine. These seeds, so tiny that they are sometimes called "flea seeds," are generally dried, ground, and sold in powder, capsule, or chewable tablet (wafer) form. Psyllium is sometimes added to breakfast cereals.

▼ WHAT IT DOES

When mixed with water, the fibrous, mucilage-covered husks of psyllium seeds form a gellike mass that absorbs excess water from the intestines and creates larger, softer stools. Psyllium helps lower cholesterol by binding to cholesterol-rich bile in the digestive tract, causing the body to draw cholesterol from the bloodstream.

As an inexpensive source of soluble fiber (the kind of fiber that blends with water), it's particularly suitable for those people who don't eat enough fiber-rich foods, such as whole grains (oats are particularly rich in soluble fiber), beans, fruits, and vegetables.

MAJOR BENEFITS
Psyllium can help normalize bowel function in a wide variety of disorders, including constipation, diarrhea, diverticulosis, hemorrhoids, and irritable bowel syndrome. It does so by a single mechanism: water absorption, which lends bulk to stools. In the case of

 ALERT

SIDE EFFECTS
- Psyllium can cause temporary bloating and increased flatulence because it supplies fiber. Avoid these problems by slowly increasing psyllium intake over several days.

- Other side effects such as rash, cold symptoms, or difficulty breathing may be caused by psyllium allergies.

- Don't exceed recommended doses; taking larger quantities of psyllium can reduce your body's ability to absorb certain minerals.

CAUTION
- Always take psyllium with plenty of liquid. Without lots of fluid, it is possible to develop an intestinal blockage, which can cause severe, painful constipation.

- Some people are allergic to psyllium. Reactions are often quick, marked by a rash, itching, and in severe cases, difficulty breathing or swallowing. Get immediate medical help.

- **Reminder:** If you have a medical condition, or are taking medications, especially those that lower blood sugar level, or laxatives, talk to your doctor before taking psyllium.

constipation, the added water and bulk help soften stools, making them easier to pass.

Although psyllium doesn't cure hemorrhoids, passing softer stools reduces irritation in the tender area. In one study, 84% of hemorrhoid sufferers receiving a supplement containing psyllium reported less bleeding and pain. Psyllium has also been reported to have a soothing effect on those with irritable bowel syndrome.

In people with diverticular disease—in which small pockets in the intestine's lining trap fecal particles and become susceptible to infection—psyllium bulks the stools and speeds their passage through the intestine, helping alleviate the problem. Psyllium's ability to absorb large amounts of excess water from loose stools is an effective treatment for diarrhea.

ADDITIONAL BENEFITS
Although psyllium has been used for constipation for centuries, only in the 1980s did scientists discover another benefit: This herb reliably lowers levels of blood cholesterol, especially the "bad" LDL cholesterol that can stick to artery walls and lead to heart disease. In several studies of men and women with high cholesterol levels, taking in 10 g or more of psyllium daily for 6 weeks or longer lowered LDL from 6% to 20% more than consuming a low-fat diet did. Sometimes, simply adding psyllium to your diet is enough to eliminate the need for cholesterol-lowering medications.

This fiber source may also play a role in weight-loss programs. By absorbing water, psyllium fills the stomach, providing a sense of fullness. It also delays the emptying of food from the stomach, thus extending the length of time you feel full.

In a small British study, women who took psyllium with water 3 hours before they ate consumed less fat and fewer calories during the meal itself. Whether this effect persists and leads to long-term weight loss, however, is unknown. Psyllium can also help stabilize levels of glucose (sugar) in the blood, which may control food cravings.

▼ HOW TO TAKE IT

DOSAGE
The dose of a psyllium product depends on the concentration of soluble fiber in the product and can range from 1 tsp 3 times a day to 3 tbsp 3 times a day. Read the package carefully to determine the correct dose of your psyllium product.

GUIDELINES FOR USE
• Relief of constipation usually occurs in 12 to 24 hours, although it can take as long as 3 days.

• Because psyllium absorbs water, always consume it with large amounts of fluid. Dissolve psyllium powder in water (or juice), drink it, and then drink another glass of water or juice. In addition to this fluid, drink 6 to 8 glasses of water a day.

• Take psyllium 2 hours or more after taking medications or other supplements so it doesn't inhibit the absorption of the drugs.

• If you are pregnant, have diabetes, or have an obstructed bowel (possibly signaled by persistent constipation or abdominal pain), check with a doctor before using psyllium.

PYGEUM *(Pygeum africanum)*

Pygeum has been used in Africa for many generations to treat the symptoms of what is now known as benign prostatic hyperplasia, or BPH, a condition often affecting older men. Only since the 1960s and 1970s have medical practitioners and herbalists in the West begun to catch up to their African counterparts.

COMMON USES

■ Treats benign prostatic hyperplasia (BPH), commonly called "enlarged prostate."

FORMS

■ Capsule

▼ WHAT IT IS

The *Pygeum africanum* extract tree is a tall evergreen of the family Rosaceae found in central and southern Africa. Its bark has been used medicinally for thousands of years and was historically powdered and used to make a tea drunk to relieve urinary disorders. The African plum tree has become endangered because of the demand for its bark to process *P. africanum* extract.

Phytosterols, including beta-sitosterol; pentacyclic triterpenoids, including ursolic and oleaic acids; and ferulic esters of long-chain fatty alcohols, including ferulic esters of docosanol and tetracosanol, have been suggested as active constituents of *P. africanum*.

▼ WHAT IT DOES

Pygeum has been observed to improve urinary symptoms associated with enlargement of the prostate gland or prostate inflammation. It is thought that the pentacyclic triterpenoids present in pygeum help rid the body of substances that bind to prostate walls and thus maintain sound prostrate and reproductive system health.

MAJOR BENEFITS

A lipophilic extract of the bark of *Pygeum africanum* is used in the treatment of a mildly to moderately enlarged prostate (BPH) in several European countries, especially France and Italy. Numerous studies have suggested the effectiveness of *P. africanum* extract in improving symptoms of BPH, including International Prostate Symptom Score, quality of life, residual urine volume, urine flow rate, urinary hesitancy or frequency, pain associated with urination, and frequency of nocturia (nighttime urination) in men with mild to moderate symptoms. The majority of trials conducted since the 1970s show improvement in BPH symptoms,

 ALERT

SIDE EFFECTS
• Pygeum has been well tolerated in studies and is generally well tolerated in the recommended dose of 100 to 200 mg a day. Some people may experience stomach discomfort, including diarrhea, constipation, stomach pain, or nausea. Stomach upset is usually mild and does not typically cause people to stop using pygeum.

CAUTION
• People with known allergies to pygeum should avoid this herb. Signs of allergy include rash, itching, and shortness of breath.

• Pygeum cannot be recommended for use during pregnancy or breast feeding because of a lack of scientific information and possible effects on a women's hormones. The herb could cause birth defects or spontaneous abortion.

• Children should not use pygeum.

• Always have urinary problems or symptoms of prostate problems checked by a doctor before beginning treatment with pygeum.

Reminder: If you have a medical condition, talk to your doctor before taking supplements.

including frequency of nocturia, urine flow rate, and residual urine volume, with the administration of *P. africanum* extract, lending some credibility to its popular use in Europe.

Although pygeum improves bothersome symptoms associated with prostate enlargement or irritation, it does not seem to reverse the condition. It is unclear whether pygeum is more effective or better tolerated than are other common medical therapies, including surgery. Scientists are conducting ongoing clinical trials comparing the effects of pygeum with conventional medical therapies for BPH.

ADDITIONAL BENEFITS

Although effectiveness is unproven, pygeum is sometimes used as an aphrodisiac and as an aid to sexual performance. It has also been used to treat fever, impotence, inflammation, kidney disease, malaria, male baldness, psychosis, and stomach upset, although effectiveness in these areas is also unproven.

Pygeum may help in the treatment of prostate problems if used with the herbs saw palmetto (*Serenoa repens*) or stinging nettle (*Urtica dioica*).

Products containing both stinging nettle and pygeum are available.

▼ HOW TO TAKE IT

DOSAGE

There are no standard or well-studied doses of pygeum, and many different doses are used traditionally. Safety of use beyond 12 months has not been studied.

To treat benign prostatic hypertrophy: Take 100 to 200 mg of pygeum extract in capsule form by mouth in 1 or 2 equal doses.

There are not enough scientific data to recommend pygeum for use in children, and pygeum is not recommended because of potential side effects.

GUIDELINES FOR USE

• Always have symptoms of prostate problems checked by a doctor.

• Studies have found pygeum to be well tolerated at recommended doses.

• Safety of use beyond 12 months has not been studied.

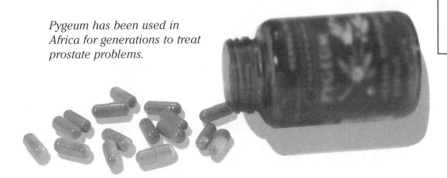

Pygeum has been used in Africa for generations to treat prostate problems.

SAW PALMETTO *(Serenoa repens)*

Native Americans regularly consumed this herb as a food and used it as a tonic, so they were probably not plagued by prostate problems. Long a favorite in Europe, saw palmetto is now one of the 10 best-selling supplements in the United States as well. This is definitely an herb with a man's troubles in mind.

COMMON USES

■ Eases frequent nighttime urination, weak urine flow, and other symptoms of an enlarged prostate.

■ Relieves prostate inflammation.

■ May prevent male pattern hair loss.

FORMS

■ Capsule   ■ Liquid

■ Tablet   ■ Dried herb/Tea

■ Softgel   ■ Suppositories

▼ WHAT IT IS

The saw palmetto, a small palm tree that grows wild from Texas to South Carolina, gets its name from the spiny saw-toothed stems that lie at the base of each leaf. With a life span of nearly 700 years, the plant seems almost indestructible, resisting drought, insect infestation, and fire.

Its medicinal properties are derived from the blue-black berries, which are usually harvested in August and September. This process is sometimes hazardous; harvesters can easily be cut by the razor-sharp leaf stems, and they risk being bitten by the diamondback rattlesnakes that make their home in the shade of this scrubby palm.

▼ WHAT IT DOES

Saw palmetto has a long history of folk use. Native Americans valued it for treating disorders of the urinary tract. Early colonists, noting the vitality of animals who fed on the berries, gave the fruits to frail individuals as a general tonic. Through the years, it's also been employed to relieve persistent coughs and improve digestion. Today, saw palmetto's main claim to fame rests on its ability to relieve the symptoms of an enlarged prostate gland—a use verified by a number of reputable scientific studies.

MAJOR BENEFITS

In Italy, Germany, France, and other countries, doctors routinely prescribe saw palmetto for the benign (non-cancerous) enlargement of the prostate gland known medically as BPH, which stands for "benign prostatic hyperplasia," or "hypertrophy."

When the walnut-sized prostate gland becomes enlarged, a common condition that affects more than half of men over age 50, it can press on the

 ALERT

SIDE EFFECTS

• Although relatively uncommon, possible side effects include bleeding, stomach pain, nausea, vomiting, bad breath, constipation, diarrhea, ulcers, yellowing of the skin from liver or gallbladder disorders (jaundice), headache, dizziness, insomnia, depression, breathing difficulties, muscle pain, high blood pressure, chest pain, and abnormal heart rhythm.

• Men may experience difficulty with erections, testicular discomfort, breast tenderness, and changes in sexual desire.

• Very rarely, men develop breast enlargement. If side effects occur, lower the dose or stop taking the herb altogether.

CAUTION

• Anyone finding blood in the urine or having trouble urinating should see a doctor before taking saw palmetto. These symptoms could be related to prostate cancer.

• People with health conditions involving the stomach, liver, heart, or lungs; people taking medications that thin the blood, hormonal medications, or birth control pills; or people with a hormone-sensitive condition should exercise caution when saw palmetto.

• Women who are pregnant or breast feeding should not take the herb.

• **Reminder:** If you have a medical condition, talk to your doctor before taking supplements.

urethra, the tube that carries urine from the bladder through the prostate and out the penis. The resulting symptoms typically include frequent urination (especially at night), weak urine flow, painful urination, and difficulty emptying the bladder completely. Researchers believe that saw palmetto relieves the symptoms of BPH in various ways. Most important, it appears to alter levels of various hormones that cause prostate cells to multiply. In addition, the herb may act to curb inflammation and reduce tissue swelling.

Studies have found that saw palmetto produces fewer side effects (such as impotence) and quicker results than the conventional prostate drug finasteride (Proscar). Saw palmetto took only about 30 days to become effective, compared with at least 6 months for the prescription medication.

▼ HOW TO TAKE IT

DOSAGE
The usual dosage is 160 to 320 mg of standardized extract in pill or capsule form daily in 1 or 2 divided doses.

You can also take saw palmetto as 1 or 2 g of ground, dried, or whole berries, ½ to ¾ tsp of 4:1 tincture 3 times daily, or ⅛ to ⅖ tsp of fluid extract of berry pulp (1:1) 3 times daily. A tea can be made by slowly simmering 2 tsp of dried berry with 24 oz of water; drink 4 oz of the tea 3 times daily. Rectal suppositories should be taken as 640 mg once daily.

Be careful if you're thinking about taking higher amounts. Scientific studies have not examined the effects of daily doses of more than 320 mg.

Choose saw palmetto supplements made from extracts standardized to contain 85% to 95% fatty acids and sterols—the active ingredients in the berries that are responsible for the herb's therapeutic effects.

GUIDELINES FOR USE
• Because saw palmetto has a bitter taste, those using the liquid form may want to dilute the extract in a small amount of water.

• The herb can be taken with or without food, although taking it with breakfast or dinner will minimize the risk of stomach upset.

• Although some herbal healers recommend sipping a tea made from saw palmetto, such a brew may not contain therapeutic amounts of the active ingredients, so it will provide few real benefits for the treatment of BPH.

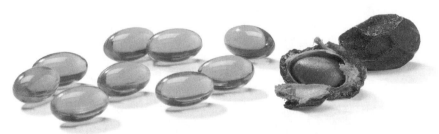

The dried fruit of the saw palmetto tree, often processed into softgels, provides a potent remedy for prostate complaints.

SELENIUM

Although researchers didn't discover the importance of this trace mineral until 1979, selenium quickly gained prominence as a potentially powerful cancer fighter. Today, many experts believe selenium to be such a potent antioxidant that it could prove to be a key disease-fighting nutrient for a host of other ailments as well.

COMMON USES

- Helps in the prevention of cancer and heart disease.
- Protects against cataracts and macular degeneration.
- Fights viral infections; reduces the severity of cold sores and shingles; may slow the progression of HIV/AIDS.
- Helps relieve rheumatoid arthritis and lupus symptoms.

FORMS

- Capsule
- Tablet

▼ WHAT IT IS

A trace mineral essential for many body processes, selenium is found in soil. In the body, selenium is present in virtually every cell but is most abundant in the kidneys, liver, spleen, pancreas, and testes.

▼ WHAT IT DOES

Selenium acts as an antioxidant, blocking the rogue molecules known as free radicals that damage DNA. It's part of an antioxidant enzyme (called glutathione peroxidase) that protects cells against environmental and dietary toxins, and is often included in antioxidant "cocktails" with vitamins C and E. This combination may help guard against a wide range of disorders—from cancer, heart disease, cataracts, and macular degeneration to strokes and even aging—thought to be caused by free radical damage.

MAJOR BENEFITS

Selenium has received a lot of attention for its role in combating cancer. A dramatic 5-year study conducted at Cornell University and the University of Arizona showed that 200 micrograms (µg) of selenium daily resulted in 63% fewer prostate tumors, 58% fewer colorectal cancers, 46% fewer lung malignancies, and a 39% overall decrease in cancer deaths. In other studies, selenium showed promise in preventing cancers of the ovaries, cervix, rectum, bladder, esophagus, pancreas, and liver, as well as leukemia.

Studies of cancer patients indicate that people with the lowest selenium levels developed more tumors, had a higher rate of disease recurrence, a greater risk of cancer spreading, and a shorter overall survival rate than those with high blood levels of selenium.

Selenium can also protect the heart, primarily by reducing the "stickiness" of the blood and decreasing the risk of clotting—which, in turn, lowers the risk of heart attack and stroke. Also, selenium increases the ratio of HDL ("good") cholesterol to LDL ("bad") cholesterol, critical for a healthy heart.

Smokers or those who've already had a heart attack or stroke may gain the greatest cardiovascular benefits from selenium supplements, but everyone can profit from taking selenium in a daily high-potency multivitamin.

 ALERT

CAUTION

- Don't exceed recommended doses. In some people, taking selenium long term—at doses of 900 µg a day—can cause serious side effects, such as skin rashes, nausea, fatigue, hair loss, fingernail abnormalities, and depression.

- **Reminder:** If you have a medical condition, talk to your doctor before taking supplements.

ADDITIONAL BENEFITS

Selenium may be useful in preventing cataracts and macular degeneration, the leading causes of impaired vision or blindness in older Americans. It is also vital for converting thyroid hormone, which is needed for the proper functioning of every cell in the body, from a less active form (called T4) to its active form (known as T3).

In addition, selenium is essential for a healthy immune system, assisting the body in defending itself against harmful bacteria and viruses as well as cancer cells. Its immune-boosting effects may play a role in fighting the herpes viruses that are responsible for cold sores and shingles, and it is also being studied for possible effectiveness against HIV, the virus that causes AIDS.

When combined with vitamin E, selenium appears to have some anti-inflammatory benefits. These two nutrients may relieve chronic conditions such as rheumatoid arthritis, psoriasis, lupus, and eczema.

▼ HOW MUCH YOU NEED

The RDA for selenium is 55 μg for men and women daily. To produce major benefits, up to 600 μg a day may be needed.

IF YOU GET TOO LITTLE

Most Americans consume enough selenium in their daily diet, so deficiencies of this mineral are rare. Falling below the RDA, however, may lead to higher incidences of cancer, heart disease, immune problems, and inflammatory conditions of all kinds, particularly those affecting the skin. Insufficient amounts of selenium during pregnancy could increase the risk of birth defects (especially those involving the heart) or, possibly, sudden infant death syndrome (SIDS). Early symptoms of selenium deficiency include muscular weakness and fatigue.

IF YOU GET TOO MUCH

It's hard to get too much selenium from your diet, but if you're taking this mineral in supplement form, remember that the margin of safety between a therapeutic dose of selenium (up to 600 μg a day) and a toxic dose (as little as 900 μg) is quite small compared with other nutrients. Specific symptoms of selenium toxicity include nervousness, depression, nausea and vomiting, a garlicky odor to the breath and perspiration, and a loss of hair and fingernails.

▼ HOW TO TAKE IT

DOSAGE

Most experts agree that the optimum dose for long-term use of selenium should fall between 100 μg and 400 μg daily. Up to 600 μg daily may be taken for a limited time as a treatment for viral infections or as part of a cancer treatment program.

GUIDELINES FOR USE

• Vitamin E greatly enhances selenium's effectiveness; be sure to get 400 IU of it daily.

▼ OTHER SOURCES

The most abundant sources of selenium include Brazil nuts, seafood, poultry, and meats. Grains, particularly oats and brown rice, may also have significant amounts of the mineral, depending on the selenium content of the soil in which they were grown.

SHARK CARTILAGE

Not usually friends to humans, sharks are finally getting a warmer welcome, largely thanks to a tough, rubbery material in their skeletons. Although many claims are made for shark cartilage—the most spectacular being that it cures cancer—its actual role in the treatment of disease remains uncertain.

COMMON USES

- May help fight cancer.
- May relieve pain from inflammatory joint diseases such as rheumatoid arthritis or osteoarthritis.
- May temper the lesions of the skin disease psoriasis.
- May improve vision loss caused by macular degeneration.

FORMS

- Tablet
- Capsule
- Powder

▼ WHAT IT IS

Bone forms the framework of the human body. Cartilage does the same for sharks. This elastic substance, which is softer than bone but tough and fibrous, is found in people as well: in the nose, for example, and around the joints. Shark cartilage products have become popular worldwide as a much hyped remedy for a variety of ills. Harvested from the head and fins, the cartilage is cleaned, dried, and ground into a fine white powder.

There is much debate, however, about whether the supplement is effective. Solid evidence proving its health benefits lags significantly behind the glowing testimonials. What's more, ecological concern is mounting because shark populations around the globe appear to be declining rapidly because of overfishing.

▼ WHAT IT DOES

Most researchers greet the claims made for shark cartilage—from curing cancer and AIDS to healing arthritis and herpes—with skepticism. Some believe that stomach acids digest shark cartilage, rendering oral supplements ineffective; others say that even if the body does absorb the cartilage, it has no demonstrable therapeutic benefits.

If shark cartilage does contain healing ingredients, they are present only in very small amounts at best. Although a few promising studies have been conducted, additional research is needed to confirm—or disprove—the effectiveness of this controversial supplement.

MAJOR BENEFITS

Research dating back to the 1980s sparked interest in this supplement's greatest claim to fame—its supposed ability to battle cancer. Observing that sharks rarely get cancer, investigators began studying various substances from sharks. In their research, they noted that shark cartilage blocks the growth of new blood vessels.

Because blood vessel growth is essential for tumors—providing them with an oxygen-rich blood supply that allows

ALERT

SIDE EFFECTS
- Possible side effects associated with shark cartilage may include gastrointestinal distress, slow healing of wounds, decreased strength and sensation, fatigue, weakness, dizziness, low blood pressure, heartbeat irregularities, liver inflammation (hepatitis), and altered blood sugar levels.

CAUTION
- People who have a history of heart attack, vascular disease, heart rhythm abnormalities (arrhythmias), or heart disease, or are pregnant or breast feeding, should not take shark cartilage. People with a history of liver or kidney disorders; a tendency to form kidney stones; or breast cancer, prostate cancer, multiple myeloma, squamous cell lung cancer, or diabetes should exercise caution when taking this supplement.

- **Reminder:** If you have a medical condition or are taking diuretics, diabetes medication, or supplements with similar effects, talk to your doctor before taking this supplement.

them to survive and grow—the researchers speculated that the cartilage might fight cancer. (Cancer therapies that inhibit blood vessel growth became headline news when two drugs that shrink tumors—called angiostatin and endostatin—were isolated in the laboratory.)

Other theories have been advanced for shark cartilage's supposed anticancer effects, and studies in laboratories and with animals suggest that it may have some cancer-fighting benefits. Studies have generally failed to show any significant benefits to people with cancer, however, even when shark cartilage was given in very high doses. In fact, a leading maker of shark cartilage supplements has admitted that they are "probably not effective" against cancer.

ADDITIONAL BENEFITS
Shark cartilage may have antiinflammatory properties that make it useful for treating diseases such as rheumatoid arthritis and the skin ailment psoriasis. In one study, animals given a shark cartilage extract experienced less pain and inflammation from substances that irritate the skin.

Shark cartilage may also ease symptoms of osteoarthritis by facilitating the delivery of cartilage-building nutrients to the joints, thereby stimulating cartilage repair while reducing cartilage breakdown. (Most doctors, however, believe that there are more effective remedies for this purpose, such as the nutritional supplement glucosamine.)

Scientific evidence also shows that shark cartilage may be of benefit in treating macular degeneration.

▼ HOW TO TAKE IT

DOSAGE
For disorders such as arthritis: Dosages of about 2,000 mg of shark cartilage 3 times a day are sometimes recommended.
For cancer: Practitioners sometimes recommend doses as high as 200 to 2,000 mg per 2.2 lb (1 kg) of body weight a day divided into 2 to 4 doses, which could mean up to 136,000 mg for someone weighing 150 lb—a substantial expense for a supplement with unproven value.

GUIDELINES FOR USE
• Some researchers suggest taking the supplement on an empty stomach to minimize exposure to stomach acids that could destroy its active ingredients. Acidic fruit juices should be avoided for 15 to 30 minutes before and after taking it.
• Because of the large amounts recommended to treat cancer (in some cases the equivalent of more than 100 capsules a day), the powder form may be more convenient and less expensive.
• Those concerned about fishy taste may prefer tablets or capsules.

LATEST FINDINGS
■ According to one Canadian study, shark cartilage helps treat psoriasis, a condition marked by excessive inflammation and growth of new blood vessels in the skin. To mimic the disease, investigators applied a chemical irritant to the arms of nine healthy volunteers. When spread on the skin prior to the application of the irritant, an extract of shark cartilage effectively curtailed inflammation. In a follow-up study, the extract also soothed the rashes of those who actually had psoriasis.

■ Although shark cartilage is often promoted for its cancer-fighting properties, the supplement appeared to have no effect in a study conducted by the Cancer Treatment Research Foundation. Sixty patients with breast, colon, lung, prostate, and other advanced cancers took many spoonfuls of shark cartilage 3 times a day. Over 10 months, the supplement had no discernible effect on their tumors.

DID YOU KNOW?
In Japan, shark fin soup is thought to be a longevity booster.

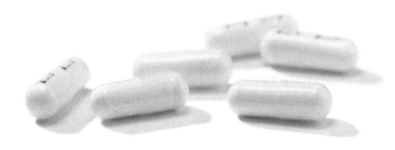

SIBERIAN GINSENG *(Eleutherococcus senticosus)*

This ancient Chinese tonic, rediscovered by the Russians after World War II, helps an individual withstand stress more effectively. A series of studies has now shown that this herb appears to benefit the whole body, sharpening physical and mental performance and restoring vitality during times of overwork or illness.

COMMON USES

- Combats stress-related illness.
- Fights fatigue; restores energy.
- Enhances immunity and helps relieve symptoms of chronic fatigue syndrome and fibromyalgia.
- Supports sexual function; may improve fertility in both sexes.
- Eases symptoms of menopause.
- May boost mental alertness in people with Alzheimer's disease.

FORMS

- Tablet
- Capsule
- Softgel
- Tincture/Liquid
- Powder
- Dried herb/Tea

▼ WHAT IT IS

Also called eleuthero, Siberian ginseng is a distant botanical cousin of *Panax ginseng*, which is the better known of the two. Although not as revered (or as expensive) as the *Panax* species, Siberian ginseng has been used in China for thousands of years to enhance the body's vital energy *(qi)*, restore memory, and prevent colds and the flu. It is derived from *Eleutherococcus senticosus,* a plant native to eastern Russia, China, Korea, and Japan; supplements are usually made from the dried roots.

Siberian ginseng gained prominence among Western doctors in the 1950s, after a Russian health researcher, I. I. Brekhman, completed experiments examining its effects on thousands of men and women. His studies demonstrated that Siberian ginseng could help healthy people withstand physical stress, improve their immune systems, and increase their mental and physical performance. Subsequent research revealed the herb's potential for treating specific ailments.

▼ WHAT IT DOES

Siberian ginseng contains substances that exert beneficial effects on the adrenals (the small glands on top of the kidneys that secrete stress-fighting hormones). It also raises energy levels and enhances immunity. Studies show that the herb is effective in protecting against all kinds of physical stresses: heat, cold, and even radiation. It heightens mental alertness and allows the mind to focus in adverse situations. By reducing the effects of stress and supporting the immune system, Siberian ginseng may also be of value in decreasing the risk of many chronic illnesses.

MAJOR BENEFITS

Siberian ginseng is often recommended as a general revitalizer for people who are fatigued (including those recovering from illness and those who are overworked). It's also suggested for people whose ability to work is impaired or for those whose concentration is weak.

Studies in Russia involving 2,100 healthy men and women ages 19 to 72 who were given extracts of the herb found that Siberian ginseng improved the

ALERT

SIDE EFFECTS

- The herb appears to be very safe at recommended doses. In rare cases, it may cause mild diarrhea, menstrual irregularities, or agitation.

- Some report feeling restless after taking Siberian ginseng, so don't use it too close to bedtime.

CAUTION

- Siberian ginseng may interfere in hazardous ways with heart medications, including digoxin and antihypertensives. Consult your doctor.

- Don't take it while menstruating, and stop taking it if you become pregnant.

- **Reminder:** If you have a medical condition, talk to your doctor before taking supplements.

following: physical labor performance; accuracy at proofreading; the ability to adapt to hot temperatures, as well as to a high-altitude, low-oxygen environment; and the ability to withstand the nausea of motion sickness.

Because it also enhances immunity, Siberian ginseng is frequently included in nutritional support programs for people with chronic fatigue syndrome or fibromyalgia. In addition, it may benefit people in the early stages of Alzheimer's disease by increasing mental alertness.

ADDITIONAL BENEFITS
By altering hormone levels and toning the uterus, Siberian ginseng may play a role in treating menstrual irregularities and menopausal symptoms. Taken between menstrual periods, it may also be useful in preventing female infertility.

The herb may be suitable as a fertility aid for men as well. When alternated with *Panax ginseng*, it may be of value for some cases of impotence.

Traditionally, the Chinese have utilized Siberian ginseng to suppress colds and the flu; the herb's efficacy may partly be related to its ability to improve the immune system. Russian studies have supported this use. In a very large study, more than 13,000 auto workers who took the herb one winter reported suffering 40% fewer respiratory tract infections during that period than in previous winters.

Siberian ginseng has also been employed to treat certain heart conditions and to lower blood sugar; laboratory studies suggest that Siberian ginseng may help protect against some types of cancer or boost the effects of conventional chemotherapy drugs. More studies are needed to verify these and other potential benefits.

▼ HOW TO TAKE IT

DOSAGE
For stress, fatigue, and other complaints: Take 100 to 300 mg of a standardized extract 2 or 3 times a day or 1 tsp of liquid extract once or twice a day.
For menstrual disorders: Use Siberian ginseng along with herbs such as chasteberry, dong quai, and licorice. Commercial combinations are available.

GUIDELINES FOR USE
• Siberian ginseng can be taken on a long-term basis. However, some authorities suggest using it for 3 months and then stopping for a week or two.

• German health authorities do not recommend Siberian ginseng for people who have high blood pressure. There are few studies, however, that indicate any adverse reactions in this group.

LATEST FINDINGS
■ In Germany, Siberian ginseng is approved for use as an invigorating tonic for fatigue, weakness, an inability to work, impaired concentration, and convalescence from illness. It may not be effective, however, at enabling a fit and well-nourished American athlete to run any faster or longer. When 20 highly trained distance runners were given Siberian ginseng, they didn't perform any better on treadmill tests than their peers on placebos.

DID YOU KNOW?
After the Chernobyl nuclear accident, many Russians were offered Siberian ginseng to help minimize the effects of the radiation.

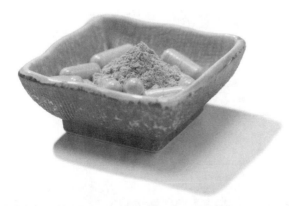

SOY ISOFLAVONES

Soy has shown great promise in reducing the uncomfortable hot flashes associated with menopause. Used as a phytoestrogen in Asia for hundreds of years, it has been the subject of new research indicating that it may help protect against certain chronic diseases, including osteoporosis, heart disease, and some cancers.

COMMON USES

- Reduces menopausal hot flashes.
- Reduces cholesterol and may decrease risk for cardiovascular disease.
- Reduces diarrhea in children.
- Excellent source of protein.
- May forestall certain cancers.
- May help prevent osteoporosis.

FORMS

- Capsule
- Tablet
- Soy protein powder

▼ WHAT IT IS

Found in soybean products such as tofu and soy milk and also sold in supplement form, isoflavones are powerful compounds known as phytoestrogens. These plant-based substances are chemically similar to the hormone estrogen (produced in the body) but are much weaker. Phytoestrogens, however, can bind to estrogen receptors in the cells and produce various important health benefits.

Most research on soy isoflavones has been done with people who regularly ate soy products. Therefore, even though most supplements contain the major isoflavones in soybeans (genistein and daidzein), it's not clear whether isoflavones are the only beneficial compounds in soy.

▼ WHAT IT DOES

As phytoestrogens, soy isoflavones have two important effects. First, when estrogen levels are high, phytoestrogens can block the more potent forms of estrogen produced by the body and may help prevent hormone-driven diseases, such as breast cancer. Second, when estrogen levels are low, as they are after menopause, phytoestrogens can substitute for the body's own estrogen, possibly reducing hot flashes and preserving bones. Soy isoflavones may also have antioxidant and anticoagulant effects.

PREVENTION
Research indicates that soybean products help protect against heart disease by lowering LDL ("bad") cholesterol and significantly increasing HDL ("good") cholesterol. Soy seems most effective in people with high cholesterol levels. In those with near-normal cholesterol levels, its effects are less powerful and larger amounts are needed to produce the same benefits. Soy products may also inhibit the oxidation of LDL cholesterol, the first step in the accumulation of artery-clogging plaque. In addition, laboratory studies have

shown that the genistein in soy helps prevent blood clots from forming.

In Asian countries where soy is a dietary staple, rates of certain cancers are much lower than they are in the United States. Studies have indicated that regular consumption of soy foods may protect against cancers of the breast, prostate, and endometrium. In animal studies, adding soy protein to the diet significantly reduced tumor formation and the likelihood that cancer, once developed, will spread.

The phytoestrogens in the soy are most likely responsible for this effect. Researchers speculate that the iso-flavone genistein may block a protein called tyrosine kinase, which promotes the growth and proliferation of tumor cells. This effect may be why soy is also associated with a lower risk of prostate cancer in men. Genistein has potent antioxidant properties as well, and for these reasons, it may one day prove useful against cancer–but more research is clearly needed.

ADDITIONAL BENEFITS

Studies show that hot flashes and other symptoms of menopause are relatively rare in Asia, where women generally eat a lot of soy products. In addition, in one Western study, women who added 45 g of soy flour to their daily diet experienced a notable 40% reduction in the occurrence of menopause-related hot flashes.

Soy isoflavones may also help women maintain bone density. One study of postmenopausal women found that consuming 40 g of soy protein a day resulted in a significant increase in bone mineral density in the spine, an area often weakened by osteoporosis (brittle bone disease).

Soy may also benefit a variety of other conditions, including gallstones, Crohn's disease, diarrhea, cyclical breast pain, type 2 diabetes, high blood pressure, kidney disease, and obesity; however, more research needs to be conducted before strong recommendations about these claims can be made.

▼ HOW TO TAKE IT

DOSAGE

Experts don't know the amount of soy isoflavones needed to produce a thera-peutic effect. In Asian countries, the isoflavone consumption ranges from 25 to 200 mg a day. Some researchers now believe that an intake of 50 to 120 mg a day might be the minimum amount necessary.

The supplements on the market vary in the types of isoflavones they contain and the total amount of isoflavones per pill. Choose a product that supplies a mixture of isoflavones–it should include both genistein and daidzein–and take enough pills to obtain 50 to 100 mg isoflavones a day.

Feed infants and children soy formula to treat diarrhea. Because of potential safety concerns, a qualified health-care provider should be consulted regarding the choice of infant formula.

GUIDELINES FOR USE

• Most experts recommend that you try to get your soy isoflavones from soy foods. In addition to their isoflavone content, these foods are good sources of protein, so they can replace red meat and other foods high in saturated fat.
• The amount of isoflavones in soy-beans–and therefore any product made from them–varies. Eating 1 to 2 serv-ings of soy products a day is probably

sufficient. (A serving equals 3½ oz tofu or miso, 1 cup soy milk, or ½ cup soy flour, cooked soybeans, or texturized vegetable protein.) Or, you might want to get your isoflavones from a combina-tion of foods and supplements.
• Another alternative is soy powder, which contains both soy protein and isoflavones; mix it into juice, milk, or shakes. Take soy supplements with a large glass of warm water right before eating breakfast and dinner.

SPIRULINA AND KELP

Health enthusiasts are looking to the lakes and seas for algae and plant proteins that are powerful food supplements. Although spirulina and kelp have inspired hype as well as hope, these aquatic plants actually do contain various helpful substances, with benefits ranging from sweetening the breath to helping the thyroid.

ALERT

SIDE EFFECTS

- Nausea or diarrhea may develop in those taking spirulina or kelp.

- Up to 3% of the population is sensitive to iodine and may experience adverse reactions to long-term ingestion of kelp—including a painful enlargement of the thyroid gland that disappears once kelp consumption is discontinued.

- Spirulina may cause headache, muscle pain, flushing of the face, sweating, and difficulty concentrating.

- Kelp may cause worsening of acne; increased salivation; stomach irritation; brassy taste; abnormal bleeding; nerve toxicity; increased blood levels of calcium, magnesium, potassium, and sodium; lowered blood sugar; diarrhea; and increased thyroid activity (hyperthyroidism).

CAUTION

- Kelp may aggravate the condition of people taking medication for an overactive thyroid. Consult your doctor before taking this supplement with any thyroid medication.

- People with a history of thyroid disease, bleeding, acne, kidney disease, blood clots, nerve disorders, high blood pressure, stroke, or diabetes should avoid using kelp.

- **Reminder:** If you have phenylketonuria (PKU) or another medical condition or are taking medications or other supplements, talk to your doctor before taking kelp or spirulina. If you are pregnant or breast feeding, do not use spirulina.

▼ WHAT IT IS

Spirulina and kelp are two very different types of aquatic algae. The smaller of the two, spirulina (also known as blue-green algae), is actually a single-celled microorganism, or microalga, that closely resembles a bacterium. Because its spiral-shaped filaments are rich in the plant pigment chlorophyll, spirulina turns the lakes and ponds where it grows a dark blue-green.

Kelp (also known as bladderwrack) is another beneficial protector—one that comes from the sea. Derived from various species of brown algae known as *Fucus* or *Laminaria,* this long-stemmed seaweed is a prime source of iodine, crucial in preventing thyroid problems.

▼ WHAT IT DOES

Spirulina and kelp have been used medicinally for thousands of years in China. Their devotees make many claims—ranging from increased libido to reduced hair loss—but most of these benefits remain highly speculative. The algae do, however, have some confirmed powers.

MAJOR BENEFITS

Because it is a prime source of chlorophyll, spirulina is ideal for combating one of life's most bothersome complaints—bad breath. It can be an extremely effective remedy, provided the condition is not caused by gum disease or chronic sinusitis. Many commercial chlorophyll breath fresheners contain spirulina as a key ingredient.

The high iodine content of kelp makes it useful for treating an underactive thyroid caused by a shortage of iodine. Scientific evidence shows that it can even treat goiter. This remedy is rarely necessary, however, because iodized salt supplies plenty of this mineral.

Kelp is also marketed as a weight loss aid, but it's probably effective only in the rare cases when weight gain is caused by an iodine-deficient, underactive thyroid. Kelp should be taken for the treatment of thyroid disorders only with a doctor's supervision.

ADDITIONAL BENEFITS
Sometimes spirulina and kelp are included in vegetarian and macrobiotic diets. Spirulina contains protein, vitamins (including B_{12} and folic acid), carotenoids, and other nutrients. In addition to iodine, kelp provides carotenoids, as well as fairly low concentrations of fatty acids, potassium, magnesium, calcium, iron, and other nutrients. There are many less expensive—and better tasting—sources of vitamins and minerals than spirulina and kelp, including many common garden vegetables.

Some scientific evidence suggests that spirulina may be effective in treating diabetes and high cholesterol, aiding in weight loss, and fighting precancerous mouth lesions. Kelp may also help lower blood sugar, which helps treat diabetes. It has antioxidant properties, which help fight cancer.

Kelp and spirulina may also boost energy, relieve arthritis, enhance liver function, prevent heart disease and

certain cancers, boost immunity, suppress HIV and AIDS, and protect cells against damage from X rays or heavy metals, but more research is needed.

▼ HOW TO TAKE IT

DOSAGE
As a concentrated nutritional source: Use a commercial, chlorophyll-rich "green" drink (the label will often say if the chlorophyll is derived in part from spirulina) and follow package directions regarding preparation.

To freshen the breath with spirulina: Mix 1 tsp of spirulina powder in half a glass of water. Swish around in your mouth, then swallow. Or, chew a tablet thoroughly, then ingest it. Repeat 3 or 4 times a day or as needed.

To use kelp for an underactive thyroid: Use only when recommended by your doctor; if iodine is needed, your doctor can prescribe an appropriate dose. Take 200 to 600 mg of soft capsules (alcohol extract) daily, or take tablets 3 times a day and gradually increase to 24 tablets a day. Kelp (bladderwrack) and seaweed patches are sold commercially as weight loss products, although their effectiveness is not proven.

For high cholesterol: Take 1.4 g of spirulina 3 times daily with meals for 8 weeks.

For diabetes mellitus (type 2): Take 1 g of spirulina twice daily with meals.

Weight loss: Take 200 mg of spirulina tablets 3 times daily just before eating.

Oral leukoplakia (precancerous mouth lesions): Take 1 g of *Spirulina fusiformis* daily for up to a year.

GUIDELINES FOR USE
• Take it with food to minimize the chances of digestive upset.
• Pregnant or breast-feeding women should avoid kelp because of its high

iodine content (spirulina seems to be very safe).
• Note that blue-green algae, especially types that are usually harvested in uncontrolled settings (*Anabaena* spp., *Aphanizomenon* spp., and *Microcystis* spp.), may contain heavy metals.

ST. JOHN'S WORT *(Hypericum perforatum)*

Ancient Greeks and Romans believed that this herb could deter evil spirits. Today, St. John's wort has found new and widespread popularity as a natural antidepressant, a gentle alternative to conventional medications with far fewer side effects.

COMMON USES

- Treats depression.
- May help relieve symptoms of premenstrual syndrome (PMS) and menopause.
- May have beneficial effects in treating anxiety disorders, obsessive-compulsive disorder, and seasonal affective disorder.

FORMS

- Tablet
- Capsule
- Softgel
- Liquid
- Cream/Ointment

▼ WHAT IT IS

A shrubby perennial bearing bright yellow flowers, St. John's wort is cultivated worldwide. It was named for Saint John the Baptist because it blooms around June 24, the day celebrated as his birthday; "wort" is an old English word for plant.

For centuries, St. John's wort was used to soothe nerves and to help the healing of wounds, burns, and snakebites. Herbal supplements are made from the plant's dried flowers, which contain a number of therapeutic substances, including a healing pigment called hypericin.

▼ WHAT IT DOES

St. John's wort is most often used to treat mild depression. Scientists aren't sure exactly how the herb works, but it's believed to boost levels of the brain chemical serotonin, which is key to mood and emotions.

MAJOR BENEFITS

A careful analysis of 23 different studies of St. John's wort concluded that the herb is as effective as antidepressant drugs—and more effective than a placebo—in the treatment of mild to moderate depression. Another study, however, showed that St. John's wort was not effective for treating major serious clinical depression. In such cases, conventional antidepressant therapy is appropriate.

ALERT

SIDE EFFECTS

- Possible side effects include stomach upset, skin reactions, fatigue, drowsiness, restlessness, anxiety, sexual dysfunction, dizziness, headache, dry mouth, weight loss, and increased thyroid levels.

- Avoid prolonged exposure to sunlight while taking St. John's wort; it may increase sensitivity to the sun, especially with high doses or prolonged use.

CAUTION

- If you're taking conventional antidepressant drugs, consult your doctor before switching to St. John's wort. Never alter a drug dose on your own.

- St. John's wort affects the metabolism of many medications broken down in the liver, including birth control pills, warfarin (Coumadin), cyclosporine, digoxin, antidepressants, antibiotics, loperamide (Imodium), migraine medications, irinotecan (CPT-11), HIV/AIDS drugs, theophylline, herbs and supplements with similar effects, and foods containing tyramine or tryptophan (such as cheese, wine, yogurt, caffeine, soy sauce, and chocolate).

- If you develop hives or have difficulty breathing (rarely, people have allergic reactions), get immediate medical help.

- People with a history of thyroid disorders should use St. John's wort cautiously.

- Pregnant or breast-feeding women should not take St. John's wort.

- **Reminder:** If you have a medical or psychiatric condition or are taking medications, talk to your doctor before taking supplements.

Some people are leery of conventional antidepressants because of their potential for causing undesirable side effects, especially reduced sexual function. St. John's wort has fewer bothersome side effects than these drugs.

St. John's wort seems so promising that the National Institutes of Health (NIH) has been conducting a major study of its effectiveness that involves more than 330 patients who are suffering from depression.

ADDITIONAL BENEFITS

St. John's wort may also be helpful for many conditions associated with depression, such as anxiety, obsessive-compulsive disorder, premenstrual syndrome (PMS), and menopause.

This herb promotes sound sleep and may be especially valuable when depression is marked by fatigue, sleepiness, and low energy levels. It may also aid in treating "wintertime blues" (seasonal affective disorder), a type of depression that develops in the fall and winter and dissipates in the bright sunlight of spring and summer.

▼ HOW TO TAKE IT

DOSAGE

The recommended dose is 300 mg of an extract standardized to contain 0.3% hypericin 3 times a day. Supplements containing 450 mg are also available and can be taken twice a day. Opt for standardized extracts whenever possible; they tend to be of higher quality than nonstandardized formulations.

GUIDELINES FOR USE

• Take St. John's wort with food in order to prevent the fairly common side effect of mild stomach irritation.

• Women taking birth control pills should avoid taking St. John's wort; it causes an increase in the rate at which estrogens are broken down, which decreases their effectiveness. Several pregnancies resulting from women taking both St. John's wort and birth control pills have been reported in Germany.

• Like a prescription antidepressant, the herb must build up in your blood before it becomes effective, so be sure to allow at least 4 weeks to determine whether it works for you. It can be used long term as needed.

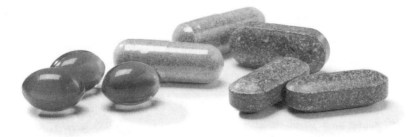

In softgels, capsules, or tablets,
St. John's wort can be very effective
for mild depression.

TEA TREE OIL *(Melaleuca alternifolia)*

For centuries, Australian aborigines relied on the leaves of a native tree to fight infections. Dubbed the "tea tree" by English explorer Captain Cook, its leaves produce an oil that is valued throughout the world as a potent antiseptic. Studies have also confirmed its powerful ability to combat bacteria and fungal infections.

COMMON USES

■ Disinfects and promotes the healing of cuts and scrapes.

■ May treat acne, certain bacteria infections, genital herpes, and vaginal infections.

■ May fight athlete's foot, fungal nail infections, and thrush (caused by *Candida albicans*).

FORMS

■ Oil   ■ Cream

■ Gel   ■ Vaginal suppository

▼ WHAT IT IS

A champion infection fighter, tea tree oil has a pleasant nutmeglike scent. The oil comes from the leaves of the *Melaleuca alternifolia,* or tea tree, a species that grows only in Australia (and is completely different from the *Camellia* species used to make black, oolong, and green teas for drinking).

Extracted through a steam distillation process, quality tea tree oil contains at least 40% terpinen-4-ol (the active ingredient that is responsible for its healing effects) and less than 5% cineol, a substance believed to counteract the medicinal properties of the oil. With the rise of antibiotics after World War II, tea tree oil fell out of favor. Interest in its use has revived, and today more than 700 tons of tea tree oil are produced annually.

▼ WHAT IT DOES

Tea tree oil is used topically to treat a variety of common infections. Once applied to the skin, the oil makes it impossible for many disease-causing fungi to survive. Several studies have shown that it fights various bacteria as well, including some that are resistant to powerful antibiotics. Experts think that one reason tea tree oil is so effective is that it readily mixes with skin oils, allowing it to attack the infective agent quickly and actively.

MAJOR BENEFITS

Tea tree oil's antiseptic properties are especially useful for treating cuts and scrapes as well as insect bites and stings. The oil promotes healing of minor wounds, helps prevent infection, and minimizes any future scarring.

As an antifungal agent, tea tree oil fights the fungus *Trichophyton*, the culprit in athlete's foot, jock itch, and some nail infections. It may also be effective against *Candida albicans* and *Tri-*

ALERT

SIDE EFFECTS

• Although tea tree oil can irritate sensitive skin, it otherwise appears to be safe for topical use.

• Possible but rare side effects of tea tree oil include rash, reduced immune system function, abdominal pain, diarrhea, drowsiness, confusion, coma, muscle tremor, poor coordination, and reduced hearing.

CAUTION

• Keep tea tree oil away from eyes and mucous membranes.

• If you accidentally ingest the oil, call a doctor or poison control center immediately.

• People using tretinoin (Retin-A), benzoyl peroxide, salicylic acid, isotretinoin (Accutane), or herbs and supplements with drying effects or that make skin sensitive to the sun (for example, St. John's wort or capsaicin) should avoid using tea tree oil.

• People who are allergic to tea tree oil or to plants of the myrtle (Myrtaceae) family, have a history of eczema, or are pregnant or breast feeding should not use tea tree oil.

• Consult your doctor before applying tea tree oil to deep, open wounds.

• **Reminder:** If you have a medical condition, talk to your doctor before using supplements.

chomonas vaginalis, two of the organisms that cause vaginal infections.

ADDITIONAL BENEFITS

Tea tree oil may help treat acne. In one study, a gel containing 5% tea tree oil was shown to be as effective against acne as a lotion with 5% benzoyl peroxide, the active ingredient in most over-the-counter acne medications. There were fewer side effects with tea tree oil; specifically, it caused less scaling, dryness, and itching than the benzoyl peroxide formula.

Another study found that a solution containing 0.5% tea tree oil offered protection against *Pityrosporum ovale,* a common dandruff-causing fungus. Sometimes tea tree oil is suggested as a treatment for genital herpes, which is caused by a virus, but studies have not confirmed this use.

▼ HOW TO TAKE IT

DOSAGE

To treat athlete's foot, skin wounds, acne, or nail infections: Apply a drop or two of pure, undiluted tea tree oil to the affected areas of the skin. For athlete's foot (tinea pedis),

apply 10% tea tree oil cream to the feet twice daily after they have been thoroughly washed and dried. For acne, apply tea tree oil 5% gel to acne-prone areas of the skin daily. For fungal nail infections, apply 100% tea tree oil to the affected area twice daily for 6 months.

To treat vaginal yeast infections: Insert a commercially available tea tree oil vaginal suppository every 12 hours for up to 5 days. If symptoms of the yeast infection persist, be sure to contact your doctor.

GUIDELINES FOR USE

• Tea tree oil is for topical use only. Never take tea tree oil orally. If you or a child ingests it, call your doctor or a poison control center right away.

• Rarely, tea tree oil can cause an allergic skin rash in some people. Before using the oil for the first time, be sure to dab a small amount onto your inner arm with a cotton swab. If you are allergic, your arm will quickly become red or inflamed. If this response occurs, dilute the tea tree oil by adding a few drops to a tablespoon of bland oil, such as vegetable oil or almond oil, and try the arm test again. If you have no skin reaction, it's safe to apply the diluted tea tree oil elsewhere on the body.

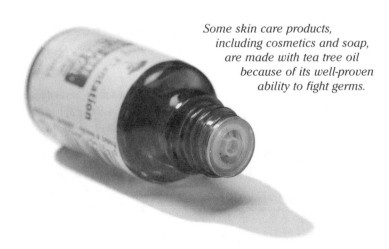

Some skin care products, including cosmetics and soap, are made with tea tree oil because of its well-proven ability to fight germs.

TRACE MINERALS

The old adage that good things come in small packages certainly is true for a group of nutrients known as trace minerals. Some of these tiny nutritional powerhouses are poorly understood, but others are known to be essential for everything from strong bones (silicon and boron) to a healthy heart (manganese).

COMMON USES

Boron, silicon, and fluoride
- Aid in building strong bones, teeth, and nails.

Manganese
- Treats heart arrhythmias, osteoporosis, epileptic seizures, sprains, and back pain.

Vanadium
- May aid people with diabetes.

Molybdenum
- Helps the body use iron.

FORMS
- Tablet
- Capsule
- Powder
- Liquid

▼ WHAT IT IS

Trace minerals are those the body needs in only minuscule amounts. For example, although the average-sized person carries around approximately 3 lb of calcium, the trace mineral manganese weighs in at only .0004 of an ounce.

Some trace minerals, such as copper, iron, magnesium, selenium, and zinc, have been studied extensively and are included elsewhere in this book. Others discussed here include boron, fluoride, manganese, molybdenum, silicon, and vanadium.

▼ WHAT IT DOES

The vast majority of trace minerals act as coenzymes, which—in partnership with the proteins known as enzymes—facilitate chemical reactions throughout the body. They aid in forming bones and other tissues, assist in growth and development, make up part of the genetic material DNA, and help the body burn fats and carbohydrates.

PREVENTION
Preliminary evidence suggests that some trace minerals (like their big brother calcium) are good for bones and may be effective against osteoporosis. Along with silicon, manganese helps build strong bones and connective tissue, the durable substance that holds much of the body together.

Boron may enhance bone health by preventing calcium loss and activating the bone-maintaining hormone estrogen, whereas vanadium seems to stimulate bone-building enzymes. Fluoride is known mainly for its ability to prevent cavities, but some studies suggest that it may also aid in protecting against bone fractures.

ADDITIONAL BENEFITS
In addition to strengthening bones, manganese is part of the enzyme superoxide dismutase, a potent antioxidant that plays a role in protecting cells throughout the body. Furthermore, some evidence suggests that manganese may benefit people with epilepsy by reducing the likelihood of seizures.

Researchers are investigating the possibility that silicon may be useful in guarding against heart disease. Blood

 ALERT

CAUTION
- Molybdenum may aggravate symptoms of gout.

- Boron can affect hormone levels and should be used cautiously by those at risk for breast or prostate cancer.

- Manganese may be toxic for anyone with liver or gallbladder disease.

- **Reminder:** If you have a medical condition, talk to your doctor before taking supplements.

vessel walls concentrate this mineral, and people who get more silicon in their diet may have a decreased risk of this disease. Because silicon also strengthens connective tissue, it is sometimes used to nourish hair, skin, and nails. Molybdenum helps the body use its stores of iron and assists in the burning of fat for energy. Vanadium may be beneficial for people with diabetes because of its ability to enhance or mimic the effects of the hormone insulin, which regulates blood sugar (glucose) levels.

▼ HOW MUCH YOU NEED

There is no RDA for many trace minerals, because scientific evidence is too scanty to provide a firm requirement. Instead, an adequate intake (AI) has been established for some. For manganese, it's 2.3 mg for men and 1.8 mg for women; for fluoride, 4.0 mg for men and 3.0 mg for women; for molybdenum, 45 micrograms (μg) for both men and women. For boron and vanadium there is no AI; however, a safe upper limit has been set at 20 mg for boron and 1.8 mg for vanadium for both men and women. No RDA or AI has been set for silicon.

IF YOU GET TOO LITTLE
A fluoride deficiency makes people more prone to cavities, and a low boron intake may weaken bones. Deficiencies of manganese, vanadium, and silicon (determined mostly from animal studies) can result in poor growth and development, imbalances in cholesterol levels, and problems making insulin.

IF YOU GET TOO MUCH
In most cases, there is no reason to take high doses of these trace minerals. However, the majority do not cause serious adverse reactions when ingested in large amounts. Manganese toxicity, which has been noted in people inhaling the metal in mines, can cause severe psychiatric disorders, violent rages, poor coordination, and stiff muscles. Very high doses of boron may produce diarrhea, vomiting, nausea, and fatigue. Too much vanadium can cause cramping, diarrhea, and a green tongue.

▼ HOW TO TAKE IT

DOSAGE
Many bone-building formulas and multivitamin and mineral supplements contain varying doses of trace minerals, including up to 3 mg of boron, 10 mg of manganese, 25 mg of silicon, and 10 μg of vanadium.

You probably don't need to take individual trace minerals, although single supplements such as manganese (up to 100 mg a day) are available. For most people, a balanced diet plus a high-quality multivitamin or mineral will supply all the needed trace minerals.

GUIDELINES FOR USE
• Boron is probably best taken as part of a bone-building supplement that also contains calcium, manganese, magnesium, and other minerals. Manganese absorption may be impaired by a high iron intake.

▼ OTHER SOURCES

Manganese is present in whole grains, pineapple, nuts, and leafy greens. Nuts and leafy greens also supply boron, as do broccoli, apples, and raisins. Vanadium is found in whole grains, shellfish, mushrooms, soy products, and oats. Silicon is available in whole grains, turnips, beets, and soy products.

VALERIAN *(Valeriana officinalis)*

It's 3 o'clock in the morning, and you're wide awake—again. You wish there was something that you could safely take to help you fall asleep. Valerian may be just the natural remedy that you're looking for, because this herb gently induces slumber without the unpleasant side effects of conventional drugs.

COMMON USES

■ Promotes restful sleep.

■ Soothes stress and anxiety.

■ Reduces the amount of time it takes to fall asleep.

■ Helps in the treatment of insomnia.

FORMS

■ Capsule

■ Tablet

■ Softgel

■ Liquid

■ Dried herb/Tea

▼ WHAT IT IS

In Germany, Great Britain, and other European countries, valerian is officially approved as a sleep aid by medical authorities. A perennial plant native to North America and Europe, valerian has pinkish-colored flowers that grow from a tuberous rootstock, or rhizome.

Harvested when the plant is 2 years old, the rootstock contains a number of important compounds—valepotriates, valeric acid, and volatile oils among

them—that at one time or another were each thought to be responsible for the herb's sedative powers. Many experts believe that valerian's effectiveness may be the result of synergy among the various compounds.

▼ WHAT IT DOES

Taken for centuries as an aid to sleep, valerian can also act as a calming agent in stressful daytime situations. It is used in treating anxiety disorders and conditions worsened by stress, such as diverticulosis and irritable bowel syndrome.

MAJOR BENEFITS

Compounds in valerian seem to affect brain receptors for a nerve chemical (neurotransmitter) called gamma-aminobutyric acid, or GABA. Valerian promotes sleep and eases anxiety through this interaction.

Unlike benzodiazepines—drugs such as diazepam (Valium) or alprazolam (Xanax), commonly prescribed for these disorders—valerian is not addictive and does not make you feel drugged. Rather than inducing sleep directly, valerian calms the brain and body so sleep can occur naturally.

According to various studies, valerian works as well as prescription drugs for many individuals, and when compared

ALERT

SIDE EFFECTS

• Possible side effects include headache, excitability, stomach upset, uneasiness, dizziness, unsteadiness, low body temperature (hypothermia), reduced concentration, and morning drowsiness. Insomnia may occur with use longer than 2 to 4 months.

• Valerian withdrawal may occur with abrupt discontinuation, causing confusion and rapid heartbeat.

CAUTION

• For about 2 or 3 hours after you take valerian, avoid driving or performing hazardous tasks that require you to be alert and focused.

• Avoid alcohol while taking valerian.

• People taking benzodiazepines, barbiturates, narcotics, antidepressants, beta-blockers, loperamide (Imodium), St. John's wort, antiseizure medication, or herbs and supplements with similar effects should not take valerian.

• People with liver disease should avoid using valerian.

• If you are pregnant or breast feeding, do not use valerian.

• **Reminder:** If you have a medical or psychiatric condition, talk to your doctor before taking supplements.

with a placebo, it appears to lull a person to sleep. In one study, 128 people were given one of two valerian preparations or a placebo. It was found that the herb improved sleep quality. Those taking valerian fell asleep more quickly and woke up less often than those receiving a placebo. In another study involving insomniacs, nearly all participants reported improved sleep when taking valerian, and 44% classified their sleep quality as perfect.

Although modern interest in valerian as an antianxiety aid is relatively recent, the herb is increasingly recommended by herbalists and nutritionally oriented physicians for this purpose.

▼ HOW TO TAKE IT

DOSAGE
For mild insomnia in adults (aged 18 or older): Aqueous or aqueous ethanol extract: Take 1.5 to 3 g of herb by mouth 30 to 60 minutes before going to bed. Tea: Steep 1.5 to 3 g of valerian root in 5 oz or ⅔ cup of boiling water for 5 to 10 minutes, then drink it 30 to 60 minutes before going to bed.
For mild insomnia in children (younger than 18): The dosage and safety of valerian have not been studied thoroughly in children; therefore, valerian is not recommended.
For sedation or stress reduction: Aqueous or aqueous ethanol extract: Take 100 to 600 mg by mouth before or after stressful events. Tea: Steep 1.5 to 3 g of valerian root in 5 oz or ⅔ cup of boiling water; drink it 5 to 10 minutes before or after stressful events.

Valerian has only been recommended for 4 to 6 weeks of use. It should not be used for longer periods without the supervision of a health-care provider.

GUIDELINES FOR USE
• If you opt for the liquid extract, try blending it with a little honey or sugar to make this herb, which is a bit unpleasant tasting, more palatable.

• It is not a good idea to rely on any substance, herbal or not, to fall asleep every night. Therefore, don't take valerian nightly for more than 2 weeks in a row.

The root of the valerian plant contains compounds that relax the mind and promote sleep.

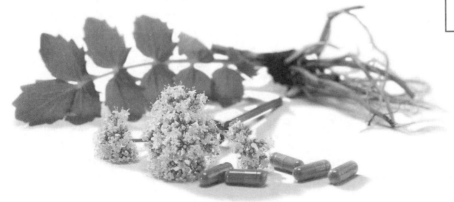

VITAMIN A

One of the first vitamins to be discovered, this essential nutrient keeps your eyesight keen, your skin healthy, and your immune system strong. It follows that an extra dose of vitamin A may help treat various eye problems, a number of skin disorders, and a wide range of infections.

COMMON USES

- Treats skin disorders.
- May enhance immunity.
- Necessary for growth and differentiation of the body's tissues.
- Helps prevent cancer and certain malignancies.
- May reduce the effects of the sun and aging on the skin.
- Vital for good vision.
- Maintains eye health.

FORMS

- Tablet
- Capsule
- Softgel
- Liquid

▼ WHAT IT IS

Vitamin A, a fat-soluble nutrient, is stored in the liver. The body gets part of its vitamin A from animal fats and makes part in the intestine from beta-carotene and other carotenoids in fruits and vegetables. Vitamin A is present in the body in various chemical forms called retinoids—so named because the vitamin is essential to the health of the retina of the eye.

▼ WHAT IT DOES

This vitamin prevents night blindness, maintains the skin and cells that line the respiratory and gastrointestinal tracts, and helps build healthy teeth and bones. It is vital for normal reproduction, growth, and development, too. In addition, vitamin A is crucial to the immune system, including the plentiful supply of immune cells that line the airways and digestive tract and form an important line of defense against infectious disease.

MAJOR BENEFITS
Vitamin A is perhaps best known for its ability to maintain vision, especially night vision, assisting the eye in adjusting from bright light to darkness. It can also alleviate such specific eye complaints as "dry eye."

By boosting immunity, vitamin A greatly strengthens resistance to infections, including sore throat, colds, the flu, and bronchitis. It may also combat cold sores and shingles (caused by a herpesvirus), warts (a viral skin infection), eye infections, and vaginal yeast infections—and perhaps even control bothersome allergies.

The vitamin may help the immune system battle against breast and lung cancers and improve survival rates in those with leukemia; in addition, animal studies suggest that it inhibits melanoma, an often deadly form of skin cancer. Another benefit for cancer patients is that vitamin A may possibly enhance the effectiveness of chemotherapy.

ADDITIONAL BENEFITS
Vitamin A was first used in the 1940s to treat skin disorders, including acne and psoriasis, but the doses were high and toxic. Scientists later developed

 ALERT

CAUTION

- Like vitamin D (another fat-soluble vitamin), vitamin A can build up to toxic levels, so be careful not to get too much.

- If you're pregnant or plan to become pregnant, don't take more than 5,000 IU of vitamin A daily; higher doses may cause birth defects. Practice effective birth control when taking doses of more than 5,000 IU and for at least a month afterward.

- **Reminder:** If you have a medical condition, talk to your doctor before taking supplements.

safer vitamin A derivatives (notably retinoic acid); now sold as prescription drugs, these include the acne and anti-wrinkle cream Retin-A. Lower doses of vitamin A (25,000 IU a day) can be used to treat a range of skin conditions, including acne, dry skin, eczema, rosacea, and psoriasis. Vitamin A also promotes healing of skin wounds and can be applied to cuts, scrapes, and burns; it may hasten recovery from sprains and strains.

Women with heavy or prolonged menstrual periods are sometimes deficient in this vitamin, so supplements may be of value in treating this condition as well.

▼ HOW MUCH YOU NEED

The RDA for vitamin A is 2,300 IU a day for adult women (over age 19) and 3,000 IU a day for adult men (over age 19).

IF YOU GET TOO LITTLE
Although quite rare in the United States, a vitamin A deficiency can cause night blindness (or even total blindness) and a greatly lowered resistance to infection. Milder cases of deficiency do occur, especially in the elderly, who often have vitamin-poor diets. Infections such as pneumonia can deplete vitamin A stores.

IF YOU GET TOO MUCH
An overabundance of vitamin A can be a real problem. A single dose of 500,000 IU may induce weakness and

vomiting, and 25,000 IU a day for 6 years has been reported to cause serious liver disease (cirrhosis). Signs of toxicity include dry, cracking skin and brittle nails; hair that falls out easily; bleeding gums; weight loss; irritability; fatigue; and nausea.

▼ HOW TO TAKE IT

DOSAGE
Multivitamins supply vitamin A, often in the form of beta-carotene. The recommended amount is 4,000 IU for women and 5,000 IU for men. Children should take vitamin A supplements beyond what is contained in children's multivitamins because of an increased risk of toxicity.

GUIDELINES FOR USE
• Take vitamin A supplements with food; a little fat in the diet aids absorption.

• Vitamin E and zinc help the body use vitamin A, which in turn boosts absorption of iron from foods.

▼ OTHER SOURCES

Vitamin A is richly represented in fish, egg yolks, butter, organ meats such as liver (3 oz provide more than 9,000 IU), and fortified milk (check the label to be sure). Dark green, yellow, orange, and red fruits and vegetables have large amounts of beta-carotene and many other carotenoids, which the body makes into vitamin A on an as-needed basis.

VITAMIN B₁ (THIAMINE)

Concerns about getting enough thiamine disappeared in the 1940s, when a law was passed requiring that the B vitamins removed during the milling of refined grains be added back into commercial bread and cereal products. Severe thiamine deficiency is a thing of the past, but even a moderate deficit has health consequences.

COMMON USES

- Aids energy production.
- Promotes healthy nerves.
- May improve mood.
- Strengthens the heart.
- Soothes heartburn.

FORMS

- Tablet
- Capsule

▼ WHAT IT IS

An often overlooked but key member of the B-complex vitamin family, thiamine is known as vitamin B₁ because it was the first B vitamin discovered. Most people get enough thiamine in their diet to meet their basic needs; however, experts believe some people, especially older adults, are mildly deficient in this nutrient.

Thiamine is available as an individual supplement, but it's best to get it from a B-complex supplement, because it works closely with the other B vitamins.

▼ WHAT IT DOES

Thiamine is essential for converting the carbohydrates in foods into energy. It also plays a role in promoting healthy nerves and may be useful in treating certain types of heart disease.

MAJOR BENEFITS

In people with congestive heart failure (CHF), thiamine can help improve the pumping power of the heart. Thiamine levels in the body are depleted by long-term treatment with diuretic drugs, which are often prescribed for CHF patients to reduce the fluid buildup associated with the disease. In one study, CHF patients who took furosemide (a diuretic) were given either 200 mg a day of thiamine or a placebo. After 6 weeks, the thiamine group showed a 22% improvement.

By helping maintain healthy nerves, thiamine may minimize numbness and tingling in the hands and feet. This problem frequently plagues people with diabetes or other diseases that cause nerve damage.

ADDITIONAL BENEFITS

In combination with choline and pantothenic acid (also B vitamins), thiamine can enhance the digestive process and provide relief from heartburn. Some researchers think that a thiamine deficiency is linked to mental illnesses, including depression, and that high-dose thiamine supplementation may be beneficial.

Thiamine may also boost memory in people with Alzheimer's disease, but evidence is far from conclusive. However, the confusion that is common in older adults after surgery may be prevented by additional doses of thiamine in the weeks before an operation. Doctors also use thiamine to treat the psychosis related to alcohol withdrawal.

 ALERT

SIDE EFFECTS

- There are no adverse side effects associated with thiamine.

CAUTION

- **Reminder:** If you have a medical or psychiatric condition, talk to your doctor before taking supplements.

Antiseizure medications interfere with the vitamin's absorption, so people taking them may need extra thiamine; this may also reduce the fuzzy thinking that such drugs can cause.

▼ HOW MUCH YOU NEED

To maintain good health and to prevent a thiamine deficiency, the RDA of 1.2 mg a day for men and 1.1 mg a day for women is sufficient. Higher doses are recommended for therapeutic use.

IF YOU GET TOO LITTLE
A mild thiamine deficiency may go unnoticed. Its symptoms are irritability, weight loss, depression, and muscle weakness. A severe thiamine deficiency causes beriberi, a disease that leads to mental impairment, the wasting away of muscle, paralysis, nerve damage, and eventually death. Once rampant in many countries, beriberi is rare today. It is seen only in parts of Asia where the diet consists mainly of white rice, which is stripped of thiamine and other nutrients during milling. In the United States, thiamine is added to white bread, cereals, pasta, and white rice.

IF YOU GET TOO MUCH
There are no adverse effects associated with high doses of thiamine, because the body is efficient at eliminating excess amounts through the urine.

▼ HOW TO TAKE IT

DOSAGE
Specific disorders can benefit from supplemental thiamine.

For congestive heart failure: Take 200 mg of thiamine daily.
For numbness and tingling: Take 100 mg of thiamine a day (50 mg as part of a B-complex supplement and 50 mg of extra thiamine).
For depression: Take 50 mg daily as part of a B complex.
For heartburn: Take 500 mg a day in the morning.
For alcoholism: Take 150 mg daily (50 mg as part of a B complex and an extra 100 mg).

GUIDELINES FOR USE
• Thiamine is best absorbed in an acid environment. Try to take it with meals, when stomach acid is produced to digest the food you're eating.

• Divide your dose and have it twice a day, because high doses are readily flushed out of the body through urine.

▼ OTHER SOURCES

Lean pork is probably the best dietary source of thiamine, followed by whole grains, dried beans, and nuts and seeds. Enriched grain products also contain thiamine.

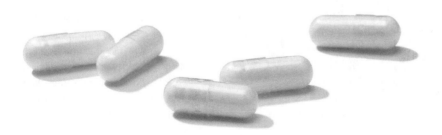

VITAMIN B₂ (RIBOFLAVIN)

For decades, riboflavin, also known as vitamin B₂, was largely overlooked. Thanks to exciting new research, this vitamin has been praised for its potential healing powers, including battling painful migraines, preventing sight-robbing cataracts, treating nerve-related conditions, healing skin blemishes—and much more.

COMMON USES

- Prevents or delays the onset of cataracts.
- Reduces the frequency and severity of migraines.
- Improves skin blemishes caused by rosacea.

FORMS

- Tablet
- Capsule
- Liquid
- Powder

▼ WHAT IT IS

Looking through a microscope in 1879, scientists discovered a fluorescent yellow-green substance in milk, but not until 1933 was the substance identified as riboflavin. This water-soluble vitamin is part of the B-complex family, which is involved in transforming protein, fats, and carbohydrates into fuel for the body.

Found naturally in many foods, riboflavin is also added to fortified breads and cereals. It is easily destroyed when exposed to light. Inadequate riboflavin intake often accompanies B-vitamin deficiencies, which are a common problem in the elderly and alcoholics. Riboflavin is available as a single supplement, in combination with other B vitamins (vitamin B complex), or as part of a multivitamin.

▼ WHAT IT DOES

The body depends on riboflavin for a wide range of functions. It plays a vital role in the production of thyroid hormone, which speeds up metabolism and helps ensure a steady supply of energy. Riboflavin also aids the body in producing infection-fighting immune cells; it works in conjunction with iron to manufacture red blood cells, which transport oxygen to all the cells in the body. In addition, it converts vitamins B₆ and B₃ (niacin) into active forms so that they can do their work.

Riboflavin produces substances that assist powerful antioxidants, such as vitamin E, in protecting cells against damage from the naturally occurring, highly reactive molecules known as free radicals.

Riboflavin is essential for tissue maintenance and repair—the body uses extra amounts to speed the healing of wounds after surgery, burns, and other injuries. The vitamin is also necessary to maintain the function of the eye, and it may be important for healthy nerves, too.

PREVENTION

By boosting antioxidant activity, riboflavin protects many body tissues—particularly the lens of the eye. It therefore may help prevent the formation of cataracts, the milky opacities in the lens that impair the vision of many older people. Ophthalmologists urge everyone, especially those with a family history of this eye disorder, to get an adequate and steady supply of riboflavin throughout life.

  ALERT

CAUTION

- Consult your doctor if you are taking oral contraceptives, antibiotics, or psychiatric drugs, which can affect riboflavin needs.

- **Reminder:** If you have a medical or psychiatric condition, talk to your doctor before taking supplements.

The vitamin has also been proven highly effective in reducing the frequency and severity of migraine headaches. Migraine sufferers are believed to have reduced energy reserves in the brain, and riboflavin may prevent attacks by increasing the energy supply to brain cells.

ADDITIONAL BENEFITS

Riboflavin has proven valuable in treating skin disorders, including rosacea, which causes facial flushing and skin pustules in many adults.

In combination with other B vitamins, including vitamin B_6 and niacin, riboflavin may help protect against a broad range of nerve and other ailments, including Alzheimer's disease, epilepsy, numbness and tingling, and multiple sclerosis, as well as anxiety, stress, and even fatigue. Some doctors will prescribe extra riboflavin supplementation to treat sickle cell anemia, because many patients with this condition have a riboflavin deficiency.

▼ HOW MUCH YOU NEED

The daily RDA for riboflavin is 1.3 mg for men and 1.1 mg for women. These amounts prevent general deficiencies; larger doses are usually prescribed for specific conditions.

IF YOU GET TOO LITTLE

Classic deficiency symptoms include cracking and sores in the corner of the mouth and increased sensitivity to light, with tearing, burning, and itchy eyes. The skin around the nose, eyebrows, and earlobes may peel, and there may be a skin rash in the groin area. A low red blood cell count (or anemia), resulting in fatigue, can also occur.

IF YOU GET TOO MUCH

Excess riboflavin isn't dangerous because the body excretes any extra in the urine. However, high intakes of this vitamin can turn the urine bright yellow—which is a harmless but somewhat unsettling side effect.

▼ HOW TO TAKE IT

DOSAGE

For cataract prevention: The usual dosage is 25 mg a day.
For rosacea: Dosages of 50 mg a day are recommended.
For migraines: Even higher amounts may be needed—up to 400 mg a day.

Many one-a-day vitamins meet the RDA for riboflavin; high-potency multivitamins may contain much higher amounts—30 mg or more. Mixed vitamin B formulas typically contain 50 or 100 mg of riboflavin along with other B vitamins, including niacin, thiamine, vitamins B_6 and B_{12}, and folic acid.

GUIDELINES FOR USE

• Don't take riboflavin with alcohol, which reduces its absorption in the digestive tract.

▼ OTHER SOURCES

Good sources of riboflavin include milk, cheese, yogurt, liver, beef, fish, fortified breads and cereals, avocados, mushrooms, and eggs.

FACTS & TIPS

■ Americans get about half their riboflavin from milk and other dairy products.

■ Milk stored in a clear glass bottle loses 75% of its riboflavin after just a few hours because the vitamin is extremely sensitive to light. That's one reason milk comes in opaque bottles or cardboard cartons.

■ Eating a well-balanced diet is especially important for elderly people because many of them are deficient in riboflavin.

LATEST FINDINGS

■ In one European study, 55 patients who suffered 2 to 8 migraines per month were given 400 mg of riboflavin a day. After 3 months, patients experienced, on average, 37% fewer headaches—a rate commonly achieved only with prescription migraine drugs. Riboflavin has far fewer side effects than those drugs, and it's much cheaper.

DID YOU KNOW?

You'd have to drink approximately 72 8-oz glasses of milk to get 30 mg of riboflavin, the amount found in many high-potency multivitamins.

VITAMIN B₃ (NIACIN)

This B vitamin has been in the limelight as a potent cholesterol-lowering agent because it rivals some prescription drugs in its effectiveness for this common condition. Niacin in its various forms also shows promise in the prevention and treatment of arthritis and a host of other ailments.

COMMON USES

- Lowers cholesterol.
- May improve circulation.
- May ease symptoms of arthritis.
- Useful in the prevention of hardening of the arteries (atheroclerosis) and heart attack recurrence.
- May prevent progression of type 1 diabetes.

FORMS

- Capsule
- Tablet

▼ WHAT IT IS

Also known as vitamin B₃, niacin is available as a supplement in three forms: nicotinic acid (or nicotinate), niacinamide, and inositol hexaniacinate (niacin bound to inositol, a member of the B-vitamin family). The body can also make niacin by converting the amino acid tryptophan—found in eggs, milk, and poultry—into the vitamin. About half of the niacin supplied by the average diet comes from the body's processing of tryptophan.

In supplement form, both nicotinic acid and niacinamide can satisfy your nutritional requirement for this B vitamin, but each of the three forms has its own specific role in treating disease.

▼ WHAT IT DOES

Niacin is needed to release energy from carbohydrates. It is also involved in controlling blood sugar, keeping the skin healthy, and maintaining the nervous and digestive systems.

PREVENTION
High doses of niacin raise HDL ("good") cholesterol while lowering LDL ("bad") cholesterol and triglyceride levels. In fact, studies show that niacin may be more effective than prescription cholesterol-lowering drugs in reducing the risk of heart disease, mainly because it's one of the few agents that is known to boost HDL. There is good scientific evidence supporting the use of niacin in preventing atherosclerosis and heart attack reoccurrence.

The cholesterol-lowering forms of niacin are nicotinic acid and inositol hexaniacinate. Although both are effective, inositol hexaniacinate is a safer form to use because it doesn't cause skin flushing and is less likely to cause liver damage.

ADDITIONAL BENEFITS
Niacinamide seems to have an anti-inflammatory effect and may help

 ALERT

CAUTION

- Stick to recommended doses. Excessive amounts of niacin can cause serious health problems.

- Consult your doctor before using any form of niacin if you have diabetes, low blood pressure, bleeding problems, glaucoma, gout, liver disease, abnormal heart rhythm (arrhythmia), heart disease, asthma, anxiety, panic attacks, thyroid disorders, or ulcers. All can be aggravated by niacin.

- Because of drug interactions, people taking other medications and supplements should not take niacin.

- Pregnant or breast-feeding women should avoid therapeutic doses of niacin.

- If you take a daily therapeutic dose of 1,000 mg or more of any form of niacin, be sure to see a doctor every 3 months to have your liver enzymes measured.

- **Reminder:** If you have a medical or psychiatric condition, talk to your doctor before taking supplements.

repair cartilage. Some scientific evidence supports its use in treating osteoarthritis.

High doses of niacinamide may reverse the development of type 1 diabetes—the form that typically appears before age 30—if this vitamin is given early enough. This therapy should be tried only with medical supervision.

▼ HOW MUCH YOU NEED

The RDA for niacin is 14 mg for women and 16 mg for men daily. Far higher doses are required to lower cholesterol and treat other disorders.

IF YOU GET TOO LITTLE
A slight niacin deficiency will cause patches of irritated skin, appetite loss, indigestion, and weakness. Severe deficiencies (practically nonexistent in industrialized countries) result in pellagra, a debilitating disease. Symptoms include a rash in areas exposed to sunlight, vomiting, a bright red tongue, fatigue, and memory loss.

IF YOU GET TOO MUCH
Therapeutic doses of nicotinic acid may cause stomach upset, flushing and itching of the skin, and liver damage (at high doses, niacinamide may also harm the liver). To prevent these side effects, substitute inositol hexaniacinate whenever possible; it eliminates skin flushing and greatly reduces the risk of liver damage. If you're taking any form of niacin for long periods, have your doctor do periodic blood tests to monitor your liver. Doses of inositol hexaniacinate higher than

2,000 mg a day may have a blood-thinning effect.

▼ HOW TO TAKE IT

DOSAGE
For lowering cholesterol or preventing atherosclerosis or heart attack recurrence: Take 500 to 1,000 mg of inositol hexaniacinate 3 times a day. Doses are usually started lower and increased gradually. When trying to reduce cholesterol, use the vitamin for 2 months; if your cholesterol levels continue unchanged, stop taking the supplement.
For arthritis: Take 1,000 mg niacinamide 3 times a day, but only under a doctor's supervision.

GUIDELINES FOR USE
• Take any form of niacin with meals or milk to decrease the likelihood of stomach upset.

• Therapeutic doses of niacin often cause a flushing of the skin in the face, which is bothersome but harmless. This may be lessened by taking a dose of aspirin or ibuprofen before each dose of niacin.

▼ OTHER SOURCES

Niacin is found in foods high in protein, such as chicken, beef, fish, and nuts. Breads, cereals, and pasta are also enriched with niacin. Although they're low in niacin, milk and other dairy products, as well as eggs, are good sources of the vitamin because they're high in tryptophan.

FACTS & TIPS
■ Don't use over-the-counter timed-release niacin. It was developed to stop the skin flushing that high doses of nicotinic acid can cause, but studies show that it can damage the liver.

LATEST FINDINGS
■ In a study of niacin's effect on high cholesterol, participants who took niacin supplements had a 17% drop in LDL ("bad") cholesterol levels, a 16% rise in HDL ("good") cholesterol levels, and an 18% reduction in triglyceride levels.

■ The results of a study of niacinamide's effect on osteoarthritis showed that people who took the supplement for 12 weeks experienced more joint flexibility, less inflammation, and less need for antiinflammatory drugs than those who were given a placebo.

DID YOU KNOW?
Pasta is often enriched with niacin, but you'd have to eat 7 cups of cooked pasta to meet the RDA for this vitamin.

VITAMIN B$_6$

This remarkable nutrient is probably involved in more bodily processes than any other vitamin or mineral. Government surveys have indicated, however, that one-third of all adults—and half of all women—are not getting enough B$_6$ in their diet. In addition, this vitamin seems to play a role in treating PMS, asthma, and carpal tunnel syndrome.

COMMON USES

- Helps prevent cardiovascular disease and strokes.
- Helps lift depression.
- Eases insomnia.
- Treats carpal tunnel syndrome.
- May lessen PMS symptoms.
- Helps relieve asthma attacks.

FORMS

- Tablet
- Capsule
- Liquid
- Powder

▼ WHAT IT IS

Vitamin B$_6$, unequivocally the "work-horse" of nutrients, performs more than 100 jobs innumerable times a day. It functions primarily as a coenzyme, a substance that acts in concert with enzymes to speed up chemical reactions in the cells.

Another name for vitamin B$_6$ is pyridoxine. In supplement form, it is available as pyridoxine hydrochloride or pyridoxal-5-phosphate (P-5-P). Either form satisfies most needs, but some nutrition-conscious physicians prefer P-5-P because it may be better absorbed.

▼ WHAT IT DOES

Forming red blood cells, helping cells make proteins, manufacturing brain chemicals (neurotransmitters) such as serotonin, and releasing stored forms of energy are just a few of the functions of vitamin B$_6$. There is also evidence that vitamin B$_6$ plays a role in preventing and treating many diseases.

PREVENTION

Getting enough B$_6$ through the diet or supplements may help prevent heart disease. Working with folic acid and vitamin B$_{12}$, this vitamin assists the body in processing homocysteine, an amino acid–like compound that has been linked to an increased risk of heart disease and other vascular disorders when large amounts are present in the blood.

ADDITIONAL BENEFITS

Some women suffering from premenstrual syndrome (PMS) report that vitamin B$_6$ provides relief from many of the symptoms. This beneficial effect probably occurs because of the vitamin's involvement in clearing excess estrogen from the body.

In its role as a building block for neurotransmitters, vitamin B$_6$ may be useful in reducing the likelihood of having epileptic seizures, as well as relieving depression. In fact, up to 25% of people with depression may be deficient in vitamin B$_6$.

In addition, this vitamin maintains nerve health. People with diabetes, who are at risk for nerve damage, can also benefit from B$_6$. Furthermore, it is effective in easing the symptoms of

---

 ALERT

CAUTION

• Long-term use of high doses of vitamin B$_6$ may cause nerve damage. Stop taking the supplement and call your doctor if you develop any new numbness or tingling.

• Because of the risk of unwanted reactions, consult your doctor before taking a vitamin B$_6$ supplement if you also take an anticonvulsant medication or the prescription drug levodopa for Parkinson's disease.

• **Reminder:** If you have a medical or psychiatric condition, talk to your doctor before taking supplements.

carpal tunnel syndrome, which involves nerve inflammation in the wrist. For people with asthma, vitamin B$_6$ may reduce the intensity and frequency of attacks; it is especially important for those people who are taking the asthma drug theophylline.

▼ HOW MUCH YOU NEED

The RDA for vitamin B$_6$ is 1.3 mg a day for women and men younger than age 50, 1.5 mg a day for women older than age 50, and 1.7 mg a day for men older than age 50. Therapeutic doses are usually higher.

IF YOU GET TOO LITTLE
One survey found that half of all American women fail to meet the RDA for vitamin B$_6$. Women taking oral contraceptives may have especially low levels of this vitamin. Mild deficiencies of vitamin B$_6$ can raise homocysteine levels, increasing the risk of heart and vascular diseases.

Symptoms of severe deficiency, which is rare, are skin disorders such as dermatitis, sores around the mouth, and acne. Neurological signs include insomnia, depression, and, in really extreme cases, seizures and brain wave abnormalities.

IF YOU GET TOO MUCH
High doses of vitamin B$_6$ (more than 2,000 mg a day) can cause nerve damage when taken for long periods. In rare cases, prolonged use at lower doses (200 to 300 mg a day) can have the same consequence. Fortunately, nerve damage is completely reversible once you discontinue the vitamin. If you're using B$_6$ for nerve pain and you experience any new numbness or tingling, stop taking the vitamin and call your doctor. Doses up to 100 mg a day are safe, even for long-term use.

▼ HOW TO TAKE IT

DOSAGE
You can keep homocysteine levels in check with just 3 mg of B$_6$ a day, but a daily dose of 50 mg is often recommended. Higher doses are needed for therapeutic uses.

For PMS: Take 100 mg of B$_6$ a day.
For acute carpal tunnel syndrome: Take 50 mg of B$_6$ or P-5-P 3 times a day.
For asthma: Take 50 mg of B$_6$ twice a day.

GUIDELINES FOR USE
• Vitamin B$_6$ is best absorbed in doses of no more than 100 mg at a time. When taking higher doses, this more gradual intake will also decrease your chances of nerve damage.

▼ OTHER SOURCES

Fish, poultry, meats, chickpeas, potatoes, avocados, and bananas are all good sources of vitamin B$_6$.

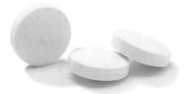

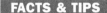

VITAMIN B$_{12}$

This vitamin is plentiful in most people's diets, but after age 50 some individuals have only a limited ability to absorb B$_{12}$ from food. Supplements are usually recommended, because mild deficiencies may increase the risk of heart disease, depression, and possibly Alzheimer's disease.

COMMON USES

- Prevents a form of anemia.
- Helps reduce depression.
- Thwarts nerve pain, numbness, and tingling.
- Lowers the risk of heart disease.
- May improve multiple sclerosis and tinnitus (ringing in the ears).

FORMS

- Tablet
- Capsule
- Lozenge

▼ WHAT IT IS

Also known as cobalamin, vitamin B$_{12}$ was the last vitamin to be discovered. In the late 1940s, it was identified as the substance in calf's liver that cured pernicious anemia, a potentially fatal disease primarily affecting older adults.

Vitamin B$_{12}$ is the only B vitamin the body stores in large amounts, mostly in the liver. The body absorbs B$_{12}$ through a very complicated process. Digestive enzymes in the presence of enough stomach acid separate B$_{12}$ from the protein in foods. The vitamin then binds with a substance called intrinsic factor (a protein produced by cells in the stomach lining) before being carried to the small intestine, where it is absorbed.

Low levels of stomach acid or an inadequate amount of intrinsic factor—both of which occur with age—can lead to deficiencies. However, because the body has good reserves of B$_{12}$, it can take several years for a shortfall to develop.

▼ WHAT IT DOES

Vitamin B$_{12}$ is essential for cell replication and is particularly important for red blood cell production. It maintains the protective sheath around nerves (myelin), assists in converting food to energy, and plays a critical role in the production of DNA and RNA, the genetic material in cells.

PREVENTION

Moderately high blood levels of homocysteine, an amino acid–like substance, have been linked to an increased risk of heart disease. Working with folic acid, vitamin B$_{12}$ helps the body process homocysteine and so may lower that risk.

Because of its beneficial effects on the nerves, vitamin B$_{12}$ may help prevent a number of neurological disorders, as well as the numbness and tingling often associated with diabetes. It may also play a part in treating depression.

ADDITIONAL BENEFITS

Research shows that low levels of B$_{12}$ are common in people with Alzheimer's disease. Whether this deficiency is a contributing factor to the disease or simply a result of it is unknown.

The nutrient does, however, keep the immune system healthy. Some studies suggest that it lengthens the amount of time between infection with the HIV virus and the development of AIDS.

 ALERT

CAUTION

- If you take a vitamin B$_{12}$ supplement, you must also have a folic acid supplement. A high intake of one can mask a deficiency of the other.

- Excessive alcohol hinders absorption of vitamin B$_{12}$.

- **Reminder:** If you have a medical or psychiatric condition, talk to your doctor before taking supplements.

Other research indicates that adequate B_{12} intake improves immune responses in older people.

With its beneficial effect on nerves, vitamin B_{12} may lessen ringing in the ears (tinnitus). As a component of myelin, it is valuable in treating multiple sclerosis, a disease that involves the destruction of this nerve covering. Through its role in cell replication, B_{12} may relieve symptoms of rosacea.

▼ HOW MUCH YOU NEED

The RDA for vitamin B_{12} is 2.4 micrograms (μg) a day for adults, but many experts recommend that you get 100 to 400 μg. Supplements of vitamin B_{12} are very important for older people and vegans (who eat no meat products).

IF YOU GET TOO LITTLE
Symptoms of a vitamin B_{12} deficiency include fatigue; depression; numbness and tingling in the extremities, caused by nerve damage; muscle weakness; confusion; and memory loss. Dementia and pernicious anemia can develop; both are reversible if caught early.

The level of vitamin B_{12} in the blood decreases with age. Individuals with ulcers, Crohn's disease, or other gastrointestinal disorders are at risk for B_{12} deficiencies, as are those taking prescription medication for epilepsy (seizures), chronic heartburn, or gout.

IF YOU GET TOO MUCH
Excess vitamin B_{12} is readily excreted in urine; there are no known adverse effects from a high intake of B_{12}.

▼ HOW TO TAKE IT

DOSAGE
A typical multiple vitamin usually contains between 50 and 100 μg of vitamin B_{12}, which is sufficient to prevent a B_{12} deficiency. However, a general dose of 1,000 μg of vitamin B_{12} a day is useful for heart disease prevention, pernicious anemia, numbness and tingling, tinnitus, multiple sclerosis, and rosacea.

If blood tests show that you're deficient in B_{12}, it may be that you are not producing enough intrinsic factor, and B_{12} shots or a prescription nasal spray may be necessary. Ask your doctor.

GUIDELINES FOR USE
• Take vitamin B_{12} once a day, preferably in the morning, along with at least 400 μg of folic acid.

• Most multivitamins contain at least the RDA of vitamin B_{12} and folic acid; B-complex supplements have higher amounts. For larger, therapeutic amounts, look for a supplement with just vitamin B_{12} or B_{12} with folic acid.

• Using a sublingual (under the tongue) form enhances absorption.

▼ OTHER SOURCES

Animal foods are the primary source of B_{12}. These include organ meats, oysters, sardines and other fish, eggs, meat, and cheese. Brewer's yeast is another source. Some breakfast cereals are fortified with this vitamin.

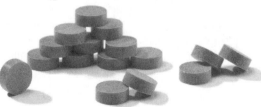

VITAMIN C

This vitamin is probably better known and more widely used than any other nutritional supplement sold in the United States today, but even if you think you're familiar with vitamin C, read on. You may be quite surprised to discover exactly how versatile and health-enhancing this popular nutrient truly is.

COMMON USES

■ Helps prevent cataracts and macular degeneration.

■ Protects against some forms of cancer and heart disease.

■ May treat some diseases of the blood.

■ Has powerful antioxidant properties.

FORMS

■ Tablet

■ Capsule

■ Liquid

■ Powder

▼ WHAT IT IS

As early as 1742, lemon juice was known to prevent scurvy, a disease that plagued long-distance sailors. Not until 1928, however, was the healthful component in lemon juice identified as vitamin C. Its antiscurvy, or anti-scorbutic, effect is the root of vitamin C's scientific name: ascorbic acid.

Today, interest in vitamin C is based less on its ability to cure scurvy than on its potential to protect cells. As the body's primary water-soluble antioxidant, vitamin C helps fight damage caused by unstable oxygen molecules called free radicals—especially in those areas that are mostly water, such as the interior of cells.

▼ WHAT IT DOES

Vitamin C is active throughout the body. It helps strengthen the capillaries (the tiniest blood vessels) and cell walls and is crucial for the formation of collagen (a protein found in connective tissue). In these ways, vitamin C prevents bruising, promotes healing, and keeps ligaments (which connect muscle to bone), tendons (which connect bone to bone), and gums strong and healthy. It also aids in producing hemoglobin in red blood cells and assists the body in absorbing iron from foods.

PREVENTION

As an antioxidant, vitamin C offers protection against cancer and heart disease; several studies have shown that low levels of this vitamin are linked to heart attacks.

In addition, vitamin C may lengthen life. In one study, men who consumed more than 300 mg of vitamin C a day (from food and supplements) lived longer than men who consumed less than 50 mg a day.

Another study found that over the long term, vitamin C supplements protect against cataracts, a clouding of the eye's lens that interferes with vision. Women who took vitamin C for 10 years or more had a 77% lower rate of early "lens opacities," the beginning stage of cataracts, than women who didn't take vitamin C.

 ALERT

SIDE EFFECTS

• Large amounts of vitamin C (more than 2,000 mg a day) can cause loose stools, diarrhea, and gas; if such reactions occur, lower your dose.

• Megadoses can increase the risk of kidney stones and can result in rebound scurvy if you stop taking it suddenly.

CAUTION

• There is some evidence that megadoses of vitamin C can actually increase cell damage rather than help prevent it. Lower your dose to recommended levels and consult your doctor if you have any concerns.

• Don't take more than 500 mg a day if you have kidney disease or hemochromatosis, a genetic tendency to store excess iron (vitamin C enhances iron absorption).

• Vitamin C can distort the accuracy of medical tests for diabetes, colon cancer, and hemoglobin levels. Let your doctor know if you're taking it.

Regular use of vitamin C has also been shown to prevent another type of age-related degeneration of the eye, macular degeneration.

ADDITIONAL BENEFITS

For people with type 1 diabetes, which interferes with the transport of vitamin C into cells, supplements of 1,000 to 3,000 mg a day may prevent complications of the disease, such as eye problems and high cholesterol levels.

The antioxidant properties of vitamin C may also help control some diseases of the blood; however, it is not as effective as the standard treatment.

▼ HOW MUCH YOU NEED

The RDA for vitamin C for men is 90 mg a day, and it is 75 mg for women (smokers need an additional 35 mg). But even conservative experts think an optimal intake is at least 200 mg a day, and they recommend higher doses for the treatment of specific diseases.

IF YOU GET TOO LITTLE

You'd have to consume less than 10 mg a day to get scurvy, but getting less than 50 mg of vitamin C a day has been linked with an increased risk of heart attack, cataracts, and a shorter life.

IF YOU GET TOO MUCH

Large doses of vitamin C—more than 2,000 mg a day—can cause loose stools, diarrhea, gas, and bloating; all can be corrected by reducing your daily dose. At this level, the vitamin may interfere with the absorption of copper and selenium, so be sure you consume enough of these minerals in foods or supplements.

▼ HOW TO TAKE IT

DOSAGE

For general health: Get 500 mg of vitamin C a day through food and supplements.
For the treatment of various diseases: Depending on the condition, about 1,000 mg a day may be appropriate for lessening symptoms.

GUIDELINES FOR USE

• Vitamin C is best taken with meals.

• Experts recommend taking the vitamin in combination with other antioxidants, such as vitamin E and flavonoids. This helps with absorption and enables the body to recycle its antioxidants, minimizing risks associated with taking high doses of a single antioxidant.

▼ OTHER SOURCES

Citrus fruits and juices, broccoli, red peppers, dark greens, strawberries, and kiwifruit are all good sources of vitamin C.

VITAMIN D

Commonly called the sunshine vitamin (because your body makes all it needs when you're exposed to enough sunlight), vitamin D is essential for bone health and may slow the progression of arthritis. It is also believed to strengthen the immune system and possibly prevent some cancers.

COMMON USES

- Aids the body's absorption of calcium.
- Promotes healthy bones.
- Strengthens teeth.
- May protect against some types of cancer.

FORMS

- Tablet
- Capsule
- Softgel
- Liquid

▼ WHAT IT IS

Technically a hormone, vitamin D is produced in the body when the skin is exposed to the ultraviolet B (UVB) rays in sunlight. Theoretically, spending a few minutes in the sun each day supplies all the vitamin D your body needs, but many people don't get enough sun to generate adequate vitamin D, especially in the winter.

What's more, the body's ability to manufacture vitamin D declines with age. Vitamin D deficiencies thus are common in older people, but even young adults may not have sufficient vitamin D stores.

One study of nearly 300 patients (of all ages) hospitalized for a variety of causes found that 57% of them did not have high enough levels of vitamin D. Of particular concern was the observation that a vitamin D deficiency was present in a third of the people who obtained the recommended amount of vitamin D through diet or supplements.

This finding suggests that current recommendations for vitamin D may not be high enough.

▼ WHAT IT DOES

The basic function of vitamin D is to regulate blood levels of calcium and phosphorus, helping build strong bones and healthy teeth.

PREVENTION

Studies have shown that vitamin D is important in the prevention of osteoporosis, a disease that causes porous bones and thus an increased risk of fractures. Without sufficient vitamin D, the body cannot absorb calcium from food or supplements—no matter how much calcium you consume. When blood calcium levels are low, the body will move calcium from the bones to the blood to supply the muscles—especially the heart—and the nerves with the amount they need. Over time, this reallocation of calcium leads to a loss of bone mass.

ADDITIONAL BENEFITS

Scientists continue to discover more about the functions of vitamin D in the body. Some studies suggest that it is important for a healthy immune system. Others indicate that it may help prevent prostate, colon, and breast cancers.

The results of one study showed that adequate vitamin D slowed the

 ALERT

CAUTION

- Overuse of vitamin D supplements can result in elevated blood levels of calcium, leading to weight loss, nausea, and heart and kidney damage.

- Avoid taking vitamin D supplements with antacids containing magnesium or with thiazide diuretics (indapamide, hydrochlorothiazide, and others).

- **Reminder:** If you have a medical condition, talk to your doctor before taking supplements.

progression of osteoarthritis in the knees, although it did not prevent the disease from developing initially.

▼ HOW MUCH YOU NEED

The government-established level of intake (called AI, or adequate intake) sufficient to maintain healthy blood levels of vitamin D is 200 IU a day for people 50 or under, 400 IU for those ages 51 to 70, and 600 IU for those over age 70. Many experts, however, think the recommendations for people over age 50 are too low.

IF YOU GET TOO LITTLE
A vitamin D deficiency can harm the bones, causing a bone-weakening disease in children (rickets) and increasing the risk of osteoporosis in adults. A deficiency can also cause diarrhea, insomnia, nervousness, and muscle twitches. The likelihood of a child developing rickets today is remote, however, because vitamin D is added to milk. In addition, children typically spend enough time in the sunshine to generate ample vitamin D.

IF YOU GET TOO MUCH
Although your body effectively rids itself of any extra vitamin D it makes from sunlight, overloading on supplements may create problems. Daily doses of 1,000 to 2,000 IU over 6 months can cause constipation or diarrhea, headache, loss of appetite, nausea and vomiting, heartbeat irregularities, and extreme fatigue. Continued high doses weaken the bones and allow calcium to accumulate in soft tissues, such as the muscles.

▼ HOW TO TAKE IT

DOSAGE
As little as 10 to 15 minutes of midday sunlight on your face, hands, and arms 2 or 3 times a week can supply all the vitamin D you need.

If you are over age 50, if you don't drink milk (which is fortified with vitamin D), if you don't get outdoors much between the hours of 8 A.M. and 3 P.M., or if you always wear sunscreen, you might want to consider taking vitamin D supplements.

Many experts recommend 400 to 600 IU a day for people over age 50 and 800 IU for those over age 70; 200 to 400 IU a day is probably sufficient for younger adults.

GUIDELINES FOR USE
• Supplements can be taken at any time of day with or without food.

• Most daily multivitamins contain up to 400 IU of vitamin D. It is also often found in calcium supplements.

▼ OTHER SOURCES

Vitamin D is added to milk; 1 cup contains 100 IU. Some breakfast cereals are fortified with 40 to 100 IU of vitamin D in each serving. Fatty fish, such as herring, salmon, and tuna, are naturally rich in the vitamin.

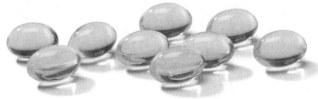

VITAMIN E

A superstar nutrient with much touted antioxidant capabilities, vitamin E offers a multitude of preventive benefits, including protection against heart disease, cancer, eye problems, and a broad range of other disorders. Working at the body's cellular level, vitamin E may even slow the aging process.

COMMON USES

■ Helps protect against heart disease, certain cancers, and various other chronic ailments.

■ May delay or prevent cataracts.

■ Enhances the immune system.

■ Protects against secondhand smoke and other pollutants.

■ Aids in skin healing.

FORMS

■ Capsule

■ Tablet

■ Softgel

■ Cream

■ Oil

■ Liquid

▼ WHAT IT IS

Vitamin E is a generic term for a group of related compounds called toco-pherols, which occur in four major forms: alpha-, beta-, delta-, and gamma-tocopherols. Alpha-tocopherol is the most common and most potent form of the vitamin. Because it is fat-soluble, vitamin E is stored for relatively long periods in the body, mainly in fat tissue and the liver.

Vitamin E is found in only a few foods, and many of these are high in fat, which makes it difficult to get the amount of vitamin E you require while on a healthy low-fat diet. Therefore, supplements can be very useful in supplying optimal amounts of this nutrient.

▼ WHAT IT DOES

One of vitamin E's basic functions is to protect cell membranes. It also helps the body use selenium and vitamin K. Vitamin E's current reputation comes from its disease-fighting potential as an antioxidant—meaning it assists in destroying or neutralizing free radicals, the unstable oxygen molecules that cause damage to cells.

PREVENTION

By safeguarding cell membranes and acting as an antioxidant, vitamin E may play a role in preventing cancer. Some of the most compelling research to date suggests that vitamin E can help protect against cardiovascular disease, including heart attack and stroke, by reducing the harmful effects of LDL ("bad") cholesterol and by preventing blood clots.

In addition, vitamin E may offer protection because it works to reduce inflammatory processes that have been linked to heart disease. Findings from two large studies suggested that vitamin E may reduce the risk of heart disease by 25% to 50%—and it may prevent chest pain (angina) as well. Other findings suggest that taking vitamin E with vitamin C may help block some of the harmful effects of a fatty meal.

ADDITIONAL BENEFITS

Because it protects cells from free radical damage, some experts think that vitamin E may slow the aging process. There is also evidence to suggest that it improves immune function in the elderly, combats toxins from

ALERT

CAUTION

• Always tell your doctor that you are taking vitamin E supplements.

• People on prescription blood-thinning drugs (anticoagulants) or daily aspirin should consult their doctor before using vitamin E.

• Because of the risk of abnormal bleeding, do not take vitamin E 2 days before or after elective surgery.

• **Reminder:** If you have a medical condition, talk to your doctor before taking supplements.

cigarette smoke and other pollutants, treats Parkinson's disease, postpones the development of cataracts, and slows the progression of Alzheimer's disease.

Other research found that vitamin E can relieve the severe leg pain caused by a circulatory problem called intermittent claudication. It may alleviate premenstrual breast pain and tenderness as well. In addition, many people report that applying creams or oils containing vitamin E to skin wounds helps promote healing.

▼ HOW MUCH YOU NEED

The RDA for vitamin E is 15 mg (in the form of alpha-tocopherol) for all adults over age 19—which is equal to 22 IU of *d*-alpha tocopherol (natural E) or 33 IU of *dl*-alpha tocopherol (the synthetic form found in supplements and some fortified foods). Although this amount may be enough to prevent deficiency, higher doses are needed to provide the full antioxidant effect.

IF YOU GET TOO LITTLE
Intakes of vitamin E below the RDA can lead to neurological damage and can shorten the life of red blood cells. If you are eating a balanced diet, however, you are probably not at risk.

IF YOU GET TOO MUCH
No toxic effects from large doses of vitamin E have been discovered, although too much can raise the risk of bleeding. Minor side effects, such as headaches and diarrhea, have rarely been reported. Large doses of vitamin E can interfere with the absorption of vitamin A.

The maximum amount considered safe by government standards (the tolerable

upper limit) is 1,000 mg (equal to 1,500 IU of natural vitamin E or 1,200 IU of *dl*-alpha-tocopherol, synthetic vitamin E).

▼ HOW TO TAKE IT

DOSAGE
To obtain the disease-fighting potential of vitamin E, many experts recommend 400 to 800 IU daily in capsule or tablet form. (This total includes amounts you get in a multivitamin.) Vitamin E may be particularly effective when taken with vitamin C.

GUIDELINES FOR USE
• Try to take vitamin E supplements at the same time every day. Combining it with a meal decreases stomach irritation and increases the absorption of this fat-soluble vitamin.

• Experts recommend taking the vitamin in combination with other antioxidants, such as vitamin C. This helps with absorption and enables the body to recycle its antioxidants, minimizing risks associated with taking high doses of a single antioxidant.

• For topical use, break open a capsule and apply the oil directly to your skin or use a commercial cream containing vitamin E as needed.

▼ OTHER SOURCES

Wheat germ is an outstanding dietary source of vitamin E; 1 oz (about 2 tbsp) contains the equivalent of 54 IU. Beneficial amounts of vitamin E are also found in vegetable oils, nuts and seeds (hazelnuts, almonds, sunflower seeds), green leafy vegetables, and whole grains.

SHOPPING HINTS
■ Although alpha-tocopherol is the most clinically studied form of vitamin E, there's evidence that the natural form ("*d*") may be even better. This is because the natural form contains a mixture of tocopherols whereas the synthetic ("*dl*") only contains alpha. The only way to get the mixture is to take the natural vitamin E.

LATEST FINDINGS
■ In one study of thousands of smokers, vitamin E supplements reduced the risk of prostate cancer by 33% and the death rate from the disease by 41%. The dosage was 50 IU a day, indicating that even low doses of vitamin E may offer protective benefits.

■ Taking vitamin E supplements may strengthen the immune systems of older people. In a study of 88 healthy subjects age 65 and older, those taking 200 IU of vitamin E each day showed the greatest increase in immune system responses (such as a buildup of antibodies to fight disease).

DID YOU KNOW?
You'd have to eat 4 lb of hazelnuts or 245 tbsp of mayonnaise to get the vitamin E supplied by one 400-IU capsule.

VITAMIN K

Doctors have long used vitamin K, which promotes blood clotting, to help heal incisions in surgical patients and to prevent bleeding problems in newborns. This vitamin also aids in building strong bones and may be useful for combating the threat of osteoporosis in older women.

COMMON USES

■ Reduces the risk of internal hemorrhaging.

■ Protects against bleeding problems after surgery.

■ Helps build strong bones and ward off or treat osteoporosis.

FORMS

■ Tablet

■ Liquid

▼ WHAT IT IS

In the 1930s, Danish researchers noted that baby chickens fed a fat-free diet developed bleeding problems. They eventually solved the problem with an alfalfa-based compound that they named vitamin K, for Koagulation.

Scientists now know that most of the body's vitamin K needs are met by bacteria in the intestines that produce this vitamin, and only about 20% comes from foods. Deficiencies are rare in healthy people, even though the body doesn't store vitamin K in high amounts.

Natural forms of vitamin K come from chlorophyll—the same substance that gives plants such as alfalfa their green color. Synthetic vitamin K supplements are also available by prescription. Other names for vitamin K are phytonadione and menadiol.

▼ WHAT IT DOES

This single nutrient sets in motion the entire blood-clotting process as soon as a wound occurs. Without it, we might bleed to death. Researchers have discovered that vitamin K plays a protective role in bone health as well.

PREVENTION

Doctors often recommend preventive doses of vitamin K if bleeding or hemorrhaging is a concern. Even when no deficiency exists, surgeons frequently order vitamin K before an operation to reduce the risk of postoperative bleeding. Under medical supervision, vitamin K can also be prescribed for excessive menstrual bleeding.

Although not yet a widely accepted treatment, vitamin K may provide great benefits for those suffering from osteoporosis. Some studies have shown that it helps the body make use of calcium and decreases the risk of fractures. Vitamin K may be especially important for bone health in older women. Because of this, it is included among the ingredients in many bone-building formulas.

Consult your doctor before taking vitamin K prior to an operation, because certain types of surgery and prolonged bed rest may increase risk for unwanted blood clots.

ADDITIONAL BENEFITS

Vitamin K may play a role in cancer prevention and may help those undergoing radiation therapy. Some findings also put vitamin K in the arsenal of heart-smart nutrients, and some evidence suggests that it may halt the

ALERT

CAUTION

• Supplemental vitamin K (more than is found in a multivitamin) should be taken only with your doctor's consent.

• High doses of vitamin E may counteract the blood coagulation properties of vitamin K, increasing the risk of bleeding.

• People taking blood-thinning medications (anticoagulants) or who are at high risk for blood clots should avoid vitamin K because it may counteract the medication's effects and cause an increased risk for blood clots.

• **Reminder:** If you have a medical condition, talk to your doctor before taking supplements.

buildup of disease-causing plaque in arteries and reduce the blood level of LDL ("bad") cholesterol. More research is needed to define the role of vitamin K in these and other disorders.

▼ HOW MUCH YOU NEED

An adequate intake (AI) has been established for vitamin K. Because vitamin K needs are met by the body, the daily AI is low: 120 µg for men and 90 µg for women age 19 and older.

IF YOU GET TOO LITTLE
In healthy people, a vitamin K deficiency is rare, because the body manufactures most of what it requires. In fact, deficiencies are found only in those with liver disease or intestinal illnesses that interfere with fat absorption. However, vitamin K levels can decrease as a result of using antibiotics long term.

One of the first signs of a deficiency is a tendency to bruise easily. Those at risk need careful medical monitoring because they could bleed to death in the event of a serious injury.

IF YOU GET TOO MUCH
It's hard to get too much vitamin K because it's not abundant in any one food (except leafy greens). Although even megadoses are not toxic, high

doses can be dangerous if you're taking anticoagulants. Large doses may also cause flushing and sweating.

▼ HOW TO TAKE IT

DOSAGE
Multivitamins often contain between 25 and 60 µg of vitamin K. Bone-building formulas provide about 300 µg a day, the equivalent of adding a large leafy salad to your daily diet. Higher doses (such as those in prenatal multivitamins) may be prescribed under medical supervision for those with specific medical needs.

GUIDELINES FOR USE
• When prescribed, vitamin K should be taken with meals. Food enhances its absorption.

▼ OTHER SOURCES

Leafy green vegetables, including (per cup of vegetable) kale (547 µg), Swiss chard (299 µg), and turnip greens (138 µg), are richest in vitamin K. Broccoli, spring onions, and brussels sprouts are also good sources. Other foods with some vitamin K are pistachios, vegetable oils, meats, and dairy products.

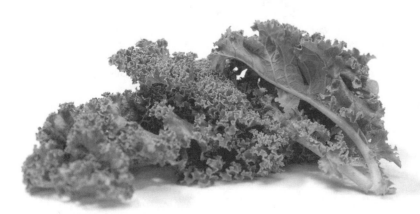

A cup of kale provides the equivalent of more than 5 100-µg tablets of vitamin K.

WHITE WILLOW BARK *(Salix alba)*

Used for thousands of years to treat fevers and headaches, white willow bark contains a chemical forerunner of today's most popular painkiller, aspirin. Effective for pain, inflammation, and fever, the herb is sometimes called "herbal aspirin"; fortunately, it causes few of that drug's side effects or complications.

COMMON USES

- Relieves acute and chronic pain.
- May reduce arthritis inflammation.
- May lower fevers.

FORMS

- Capsule
- Tablet
- Liquid
- Powder
- Dried herb/Tea

▼ WHAT IT IS

White willow bark comes from the stately white willow tree, which can grow up to 75 feet tall. In China, its medicinal properties have been appreciated for centuries. Not until the eighteenth century, however, was the herb recognized as a pain reliever and fever reducer in the West. European settlers brought the white willow tree to North America, where they discovered that local tribes were using native willow species to alleviate pain and fight fevers.

In 1828, the plant's active ingredient, salicin, was isolated by German and French scientists, and 10 years later, European chemists manufactured salicylic acid, a chemical cousin to aspirin, from it. Regular aspirin, or acetylsalicylic acid, was later created from meadowsweet, another herb containing salicin.

By the end of the nineteenth century, the Bayer Company had begun commercially producing aspirin, which was marketed as a new and safer pain reliever than wintergreen and black birch oil, the herbs commonly employed for reducing pain at that time.

All parts of the white willow contain salicin, but concentrations of this chemical are highest in the bark, which is collected in early spring from trees that are 2 to 5 years old. *Salix alba,* or white willow, is the most popular species for medicinal use, but other types of willow including *Salix fragilis* (crack willow), *Salix purpurea* (purple willow), and *Salix daphnoides* (violet willow), are also rich in salicin. These species are often sold simply as willow bark in health food stores.

▼ WHAT IT DOES

In the body, the salicin from white willow bark is metabolized to form sali-

ALERT

SIDE EFFECTS

- This herb rarely causes side effects at recommended doses.

- White willow bark may prolong the bleeding time and induce allergic reactions in people allergic to salicylates (made in plants to fend off soil bacteria and pests).

- Higher doses can lead to stomach upset, nausea, or tinnitus (ringing in the ears). If any of these reactions occur, lower the dosage or stop taking the herb. See your doctor if side effects persist.

CAUTION

- Do not consume white willow bark with aspirin; it can amplify the side effects of the drug. Anyone who has been told to avoid aspirin or other salicylates should refrain from using white willow bark. This advice applies to people who are allergic to aspirin and to those with ulcers or other gastrointestinal disorders.

- Never give white willow bark to a child or teenager under age 16 who has a cold, the flu, or chicken pox.

- Avoid white willow bark if you also take an anticoagulant medication; there is an increased risk of bleeding.

- Other possible drug interactions include alcohol, medications to treat high blood pressure, beta-blockers, certain antiseizure medications, diuretics, certain pain medications, probenicid, sulfonylureas, sulfinpyrazone, valproic acid, and herbs and supplements with similar effects.

- **Reminder:** If you have a medical condition or are pregnant or breast feeding, talk to your doctor before taking this supplement.

cylic acid, which reduces pain, fever, and inflammation. Although the herb is slower acting than aspirin, its beneficial effects last longer and it causes fewer adverse reactions. Most notable, it does not promote stomach bleeding—one of aspirin's potentially serious side effects.

MAJOR BENEFITS

White willow bark can be very effective for relieving headaches as well as acute muscle aches and pains. It can also alleviate all sorts of chronic pain, including back and neck pain. When recommended for arthritis, especially if there is pain in the back, knees, and hips, it can reduce swelling and inflammation and increase joint mobility.

In addition, white willow bark may help ease the pain of menstrual cramps—the salicin interferes with the action of hormonelike chemicals called prostaglandins, which can contribute to inflammation and cause pain.

ADDITIONAL BENEFITS

White willow bark, like aspirin, may be useful for bringing down fevers.

▼ HOW TO TAKE IT

DOSAGE

Take 1 or 2 pills 3 times a day, or as needed to relieve pain, lower a fever, or reduce inflammation (follow package instructions). Note that no scientific studies have been conducted to test its ability to reduce fever.

Look for preparations that are standardized to contain 15% salicin. This dosage provides between 60 and 120 mg of salicin a day. Standardized extracts can also be taken in liquid or powder form.

White willow bark teas are likely to be less effective than standardized extracts, because they supply only a small amount of pain-relieving salicin.

GUIDELINES FOR USE

• White willow bark is safe to use long term. It has a bitter, astringent taste, so pill form is probably the most convenient way to take it.

• Taking aspirin puts youngsters with a fever at risk for a potentially fatal brain and liver condition called Reye's syndrome. Salicin, the therapeutic ingredient in white willow bark, is not likely to cause this problem because it is metabolized differently than aspirin. However, the herb's similarities to the painkiller warrant extra caution. For children and teenagers, acetaminophen is a better choice than white willow bark or aspirin.

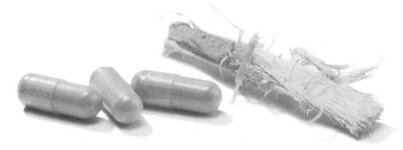

Bark from the white willow tree (dried, concentrated, and packaged into pills) is the source of a potent natural pain reliever.

SHOPPING HINTS

■ Buy white willow bark extract standardized to contain 15% salicin—the aspirin-like active ingredient in the herb.

■ Although white willow bark tea is sometimes recommended as a pain reliever, you should take only standardized extracts in pill, powder, or liquid form. Because the bark contains 1% or less salicin, you'd probably have to drink at least several quarts of tea to get an effective dose.

■ If white willow bark doesn't help pain, try other pain-relieving herbs, such as meadowsweet, feverfew, cat's claw, or pau d'arco.

LATEST FINDINGS

■ One study has confirmed earlier reports that white willow bark appears to be quite safe. Among 41 patients with long-standing arthritis who were treated for 2 months with white willow bark (as well as other herbs), only three people taking the herbs had mild adverse reactions, including headache and digestive upset—all of which also occurred in those who were given a placebo.

DID YOU KNOW?

Native Americans and early settlers chewed willow twigs "until the ears ring" to relieve headache pain. Today, ringing in the ears is recognized as a sign that you've taken too much of the herb or its drug counterpart, aspirin.

WILD YAM

Misconceptions about the active ingredients in wild yam have led to much marketing hype. The herb has been hailed as a natural alternative to hormone replacement therapy for menopause and has been suggested to treat other conditions. Research is still needed to prove its effectiveness.

COMMON USES

- May relieve menopauseal symptoms.
- May lower cholesterol.
- May have hormonal properties.

FORMS

- Capsule
- Tablet
- Softgel
- Tincture
- Cream
- Dried herb/Tea

 ## WHAT IT IS

Wild yam is not related, even distantly, to the familiar vegetable most commonly served at Thanksgiving. (In fact, those orange tubers aren't true yams at all but rather sweet potatoes.) A native plant of North and Central America, the wild yam was first used medicinally by the Aztecs and Mayans because of its pain-relieving qualities.

Later, European settlers took advantage of the wild yam's therapeutic properties and utilized it for treating joint pain and colic. The root is the part of the plant that has medicinal value.

WHAT IT DOES

Wild yam has been extolled for its ability to mimic certain hormones—especially progesterone—and is said to relieve menopausal or PMS symptoms. Most of these claims, however, remain scientifically unproven. This belief is likely based on the historical fact that Mexico's wild yam was used in laboratories to manufacture steroid hormones in the 1960s. It is true that wild yam contains a substance called diosgenin, which can be converted to progesterone in the laboratory, but the human body is unable to make this conversion. Laboratory studies and small studies in humans have not found reliable evidence of wild yam having hormonal effects.

Some holistic practitioners, however, have reported that patients suffering from premenstrual syndrome (PMS) and menopausal symptoms experienced good results with wild yam cream—which is applied to the soft areas of the body (belly and thighs). How the cream helps is unclear. Sometimes manufacturers of the creams add laboratory-synthesized progesterone, which could account

 ## ALERT

SIDE EFFECTS

- Wild yam has been well tolerated in studies, although some people may experience stomach discomfort. A rash may be caused by wild yam allergy.

- In extremely large amounts, wild yam supplements and tinctures can cause nausea and diarrhea.

- Avoid wild yam if you have a known allergy to wild yam or any member of the Dioscoreaceae plant family. Signs of allergy include rash, itching, and shortness of breath.

- Wild yam may interact with various medications, including antiinflammatory drugs, so consult your doctor and pharmacist before using wild yam products.

- Wild yam cannot be recommended during pregnancy or breast feeding because of the risk of birth defects or spontaneous abortion. Pregnant women whould especially avoid tinctures because of the high alcohol content (15% to 90%).

CAUTION

- Wild yam may alter blood sugar and cholesterol levels. Use wild yam carefully if you take drugs to control your blood sugar or cholesterol levels. Consult your health-care provider immediately if you have any side effects.

- People who have had blood clots or strokes and women who take hormone replacement therapy or birth control pills should use wild yam products cautiously. In addition, women with fibroids, endometriosis, or cancer of the breast, uterus, or ovary should be aware that these are hormone-sensitive conditions that may be affected by agents with hormonal properties, such as wild yam.

- Children and pregnant or breast-feeding women should not use wild yam.

- **Reminder:** If you have a medical condition, talk to your doctor before taking supplements.

for some of the therapeutic effects. (This progesterone is not always listed on the product label.) At this time, despite the positive patient reports, the value of pure wild yam creams has yet to be scientifically proven.

When taken in capsule, tincture, or tea form, however, wild yam does have other medicinal effects. Some herbalists believe that crude forms of this herb may help hormonal imbalances associated with PMS and menopause because it contains estrogen-like substances. Studies suggesting that wild yam may help treat menstrual cramps and hot flashes and headaches associated with menopause have been small and have had flaws in their designs, however.

Wild yam has been observed to have cholesterol-lowering effects in animal research and in a few low-quality reports in humans. It has been used hisorically to treat heart disease, but there is not enough research in this area to make a recommendation.

MAJOR BENEFITS
Research on wild yam therapy is inconclusive, so no major benefits can be identified at this time.

▼ HOW TO TAKE IT

DOSAGE
Products containing wild yam may be standardized to 10% diosgenin per dose. There are no standard or well-studied doses of wild yam, and many different doses are used traditionally. The following dosages are for adults 18 years or older.

Dried root: Take 2 to 4 g or 1 to 2 tsp by mouth daily in 2 or 3 divided doses.
Capsules: Take 250 mg by mouth 1 to 3 times daily or 450 to 900 mg of *Dioscorea* extract daily.
Liquid: Take ⅖ to ⅕ tsp of tincture (1:1 in 45% alcohol) by mouth in 3 divided doses daily.
Topical cream: Vaginal creams containing wild yam are available, but there is no widely accepted dose. Effects from absorption into the blood stream have not been shown.

GUIDELINES FOR USE
• There are not enough scientific data to recommend wild yam for use by children, and wild yam is also not recommended because of potential side effects. It should only be used for children under close supervision of a qualified health-care provider.

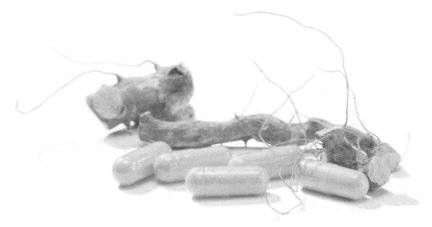

ZINC

Everyone needs zinc. This mineral fuels enzymes that do everything from manufacturing DNA to healing wounds and keeping the body's hormones in balance. Zinc is a crucial component of a strong immune system, and it fights the common cold. Still, many Americans don't get enough of this vital nutrient.

COMMON USES

- May boost immunity and help fight a variety of infections.
- Boosts fertility.
- Treats childhood malnutrition.
- Treats leg ulcers and sores caused by herpes.
- Treats taste and smell disorders and some dental complaints.
- Heals skin ailments and relieves digestive complaints.

FORMS

- Tablet
- Capsule
- Lozenge
- Liquid

▼ WHAT IT IS

An essential mineral required by every cell in the body, zinc is concentrated in the muscles, bones, skin, kidneys, liver, pancreas, eyes, and, in men, the prostate. It is plentiful in drinking water and in some foods, including meat. Your body does not produce zinc, so it depends on external sources for its supply.

▼ WHAT IT DOES

Zinc plays a critical role in hundreds of body processes—from cell growth and sexual maturation and immunity to the development of taste and smell. Consequently, everyone who takes a daily multivitamin and mineral supplement should be certain that it contains zinc.

Individual supplements are also available for specific problems.

MAJOR BENEFITS

Scientific evidence has shown that zinc effectively treats a wide variety of diseases and conditions, including acne, childhood malnutrition, gastrointestinal disease, and leg ulcers. Scientific evidence also supports its use for dental problems, herpes, taste and smell disorders, and Wilson's disease.

Zinc has beneficial effects on various hormones, including the sex and thyroid hormones. It shows promise for enhancing fertility in both women and men.

ADDITIONAL BENEFITS

Necessary for the proper functioning of the immune system, zinc may also help protect the body against colds, the flu, conjunctivitis, and other infections. In a study of 100 people in the initial stages of a cold, those who sucked on zinc lozenges every 2 or 3 hours recovered from the illness about 3 days sooner than those who sucked on placebo lozenges. Zinc lozenges may also speed the healing of canker sores and sore throat.

Because zinc affects so many body systems, it has many other uses. It stimulates the healing of wounds and skin irritations, making it useful for acne, burns, psoriasis, and rosacea, and it promotes the health of the hair and scalp. Zinc may also help treat diaper rash and other skin conditions.

▼▼▼ ALERT ▼▼▼

SIDE EFFECTS
- Possible side effects of higher doses may include nausea, vomiting, abdominal cramping, hepatitis, liver failure, intestinal bleeding, kidney problems, various types of anemia, and increased respiratory infections in children.

CAUTION
- Don't take too much zinc. More than 100 mg daily can, over the long term, impair immunity. It can also interfere with copper absorption, leading to anemia.

- Zinc supplements may alter the absorption and effectiveness of medications such as tetracycline, captropril, pancreatic enzymes, thiazide diuretics, and supplements such as vitamin A and niacin. Consult your doctor before taking them together.

- **Reminder:** If you have a medical condition, talk to your doctor before taking supplements.

Zinc has been shown to slow vision loss in people with macular degeneration, a common cause of blindness in those over age 50. In one Japanese study, tinnitus (ringing in the ears) improved after participants took zinc. Zinc may also be useful for osteoporosis, hemorrhoids, inflammatory bowel disease, and ulcers.

Preliminary research has shown that zinc may help treat cancer, diseases of the central nervous system, diabetes, human papilloma virus, kidney disease, leprosy, menopause, rheumatoid arthritis, and sickle cell anemia in adults. Zinc may also stimulate metabolism and promote health in the elderly, healthy pregnancy, and pregnancy outcome.

▼ HOW MUCH YOU NEED

The RDA for zinc is 8 mg for women and 11 mg for men daily. Higher doses are reserved for specific complaints.

IF YOU GET TOO LITTLE

Severe zinc deficiency is rare in the United States, but a mild zinc deficiency can lead to poor wound healing, more colds and the flu, a muted sense of taste and smell, and skin problems such as acne, eczema, and psoriasis. It can result in impaired blood sugar tolerance (and an increased diabetes risk) and a low sperm count.

IF YOU GET TOO MUCH

Long-term use of more than 100 mg of zinc a day has been shown to impair immunity and lower levels of HDL ("good") cholesterol. One study reported a connection between excess zinc and Alzheimer's, but evidence is scant. Larger doses (more than 200 mg a day) can cause nausea, vomiting, and diarrhea.

▼ HOW TO TAKE IT

DOSAGE

As a general supplement: Take 30 mg daily. *For acne:* Take 135 mg daily or apply 1.2% zinc topically. *For gastrointestinal disease:* Take 300 mg zinc acexamate daily. *For infertility:* Take 50 mg daily. *For leg ulcers:* Take 660 mg of zinc sulfate daily. *For taste disorders:* Take 100 mg daily. *For Wilson's disease:* Take 150 mg daily. *For the common cold:* Take 10 to 23 mg of zinc per lozenge every 2 waking hours, not to exceed 150 mg a day. Children should take 10 mg a day or 1 mg per 2.2 lb (1 kg) of body weight. *For childhood malnutrition:* Take 10 mg a day or 1 mg per 2.2 lb (1 kg) of body weight. *For topical use:* Acne: 1.2% zinc. Dental application: 0.5% zinc citrate. Herpes: 0.3% zinc.

GUIDELINES FOR USE

• Take zinc 1 hour before or 2 hours after a meal; if it causes stomach upset, have it with a low-fiber food.
• If you also use iron supplements, do not take them at the same time as zinc.
• Take zinc at least 2 hours after taking antibiotics.
• Taking zinc for longer than 1 month may interfere with copper absorption, so add 2 mg of copper for every 30 mg of zinc.
• Phosphorus-, calcium-, or fiber-rich foods, such as milk, cheese, poultry, and bran, may interfere with the absorption of zinc.

▼ OTHER SOURCES

When looking for foods rich in zinc, think protein. Zinc is abundant in beef, pork, liver, poultry (especially dark meat), eggs, and seafood (especially oysters). Cheese, beans, nuts, and wheat germ are other good sources, but the zinc in these foods is less easily absorbed than the zinc in meat.

DRUG INTERACTIONS

▼

Many people believe that herbs and other "natural" supplements are so gentle that they're safe to use under any circumstances. Actually, a number of them interact in unwanted ways with prescription and over-the-counter (OTC) drugs, intensifying or blunting the action of the medications or even producing dangerous side effects.

Although research in the area of herb-drug interactions has increased, there is still much to be learned about the potential for problems.

To be safe, if you regularly take a prescription or OTC medication—or even another dietary supplement—consult your doctor before adding an herbal remedy to your regimen. After all, part of the reason that herbs can be so helpful is that they contain active (which can mean potentially interactive) ingredients.

In the same vein, if you have a medical or psychiatric condition or are getting prepared for elective surgery, be sure to consult your doctor or pharmacist before trying any dietary supplement.

This section lists common drug classes and highlights interactions with popular dietary supplements that have been documented. Although far from comprehensive, the list illustrates how real the risk for unwanted side effects and adverse reactions can be when combining drugs and herbs.

Even if you don't see the name of your particular drug listed, the interactions may apply to all the drugs in that class. Always check the individual supplement profile in this book for specific information on any substance you are considering taking; current data on known interactions with common medications will be listed there.

ANTACIDS

The effectiveness and safety of *antacid medications* may be altered by the use of the following dietary supplements:
- **Iron** (take 2 hours before or after the antacid)
- **Vitamin D**

ANTIBIOTICS

A number of supplements may lessen the effectiveness of **oral antibiotics** (*doxycycline, minocycline, tetracycline,* and others). To reduce the risk of problems, take the supplement at least 2 hours before or after the antibiotic. Supplements that may interact adversely with common oral antibiotics include the following:
- **Calcium**
- **Iron**
- **Magnesium**
- **Psyllium**
- **Zinc**

ANTICOAGULANTS

Certain supplements may interact dangerously with anticoagulants (blood thinners) such as **warfarin** and daily **aspirin,** intensifying the effect of the medication and possibly leading to excessive bleeding. These supplements include the following:
- **Feverfew**
- **Fish oils**
- **Garlic**
- **Ginger**
- **Ginkgo biloba**
- **Pau d'arco**
- **Reishi mushrooms**
- **Vitamin E**
- **Vitamin K** (counteracts rather than intensifies the effects of the anticoagulant medication)
- **White willow bark**

ANTIDEPRESSANTS

There are a number of supplements that should not be taken with **antidepressants** of any type without consulting your doctor. Common medications in this category are **fluoxetine (Prozac), paroxetine (Paxil),** and **sertraline (Zoloft).** When these are used with the following supplements there is a risk of serious adverse interactions:
- **Melatonin**
- **St. John's wort**

Medications in the class of antidepressants known as **monoamine oxidase (MAO) inhibitors,** such as **phenelzine (Nardil)** and **tranylcypromine (Parnate),** should not be taken within 14 days of certain dietary supplements because of a risk of anxiety, confusion, excessive sedation, and other potentially serious reactions. These supplements include the following:
- **Ephedra**
- **5-HTP**
- **Ginseng (Panax)**
- **St. John's wort**

ANTIHISTAMINES

Certain supplements may cause excessive drowsiness when taken with *sedating antihistamines.* These supplements include the following:

- **5-HTP**
- **Kava**
- **Melatonin**
- **Valerian**

CHOLESTEROL DRUGS

Cholesterol-lowering agents classified as *"statins"* (*lovastatin* and *simvastatin,* for example) should not be taken with certain supplements because of a risk of serious interactions. These supplements include the following:

- **Iron**
- **Niacin**
- **St. John's wort**

COLD REMEDIES

Prescription and over-the counter (OTC) remedies containing *ephedrine* or *pseudoephedrine* should not be combined with the following supplements:

- **Ephedra**
- **5-HTP**

DIABETES DRUGS

Medications taken for diabetes, such as *insulin* and *oral diabetes drugs,* should be taken cautiously with certain supplements. There may be a risk of adverse side effects (such as enhanced blood sugar–lowering actions) or changes in the effectiveness of the medications. These supplements include the following:

- **Alpha-lipoic acid**
- **Cat's claw**
- **Chromium**
- **Dandelion**
- **Ephedra**
- **Ginseng (Panax)**
- **Siberian ginseng**

DIURETICS

Medications that reduce the amount of fluid in the body through increased urination are known as *diuretics.* There are three basic types: potassium-sparing, loop, and thiazide.

Potassium-sparing diuretics (for example, the drugs *amiloride, spironolactone,* and *triamterene*) should not be taken with certain supplements without consulting your doctor because of a risk of hyperkalemia (too much potassium in the blood) and associated problems. These supplements include the following:

- **Phosphorus**
- **Potassium**

Agents classified as *loop diuretics* (for example, the drugs *bumetanide, ethacrynic acid, furosemide,* and *torsemide*) should not be used with certain supplements because of the risk of increasing or decreasing the drug's diuretic effect. These supplements include the following:

- **Dandelion**
- **Ephedra**
- **Ginseng (Panax)**
- **Glucosamine**

Agents classified as *thiazide diuretics* (for example, the drugs *chlorothiazide, indapamide, hydrochlorothiazide,* and *metolazone*) should not be used with certain supplements because of the risk of increasing or decreasing the drug's diuretic effect or, in some cases, of causing serious side effects. These supplements include the following:

- **Aloe vera**
- **Calcium**
- **Dandelion**
- **Ephedra**
- **Glucosamine**
- **Hawthorn**
- **Licorice**
- **Potassium**

HEART AND BLOOD PRESSURE DRUGS

Many herbs and dietary supplements pose serious risks when taken with prescription cardiac and antihypertensive (blood pressure–lowering) medications. Consult your doctor before combining any such medication with a dietary supplement. This precaution applies to any type of *calcium channel blocker, beta-blocker, angiotensin-converting enzyme (ACE) inhibitor, nitrate medication, digitalis drug,* or *cardiac glycoside* (*digitoxin* or *digoxin*). Notable and potentially serious interactions or side effects have been documented with the following supplements:

- **Aloe vera** (juice form)
- **Ephedra**
- **Flavonoids** (specifically, a citrus bioflavonoid preparation containing naringin, a flavonoid present in grapefruit but not in oranges)
- **Garlic** (supplement form)
- **Ginseng (Panax** or **Siberian)**
- **Hawthorn**
- **Licorice**
- **Potassium**
- **Phosphorus**
- **St. John's wort**

MUSCLE RELAXANTS

Some supplements should not be combined with certain muscle relaxants (for example, the medications *carisoprodol, cyclobenzaprine,* and *metaxalone*) because there is a risk of causing excessive drowsiness, loss of alertness, and other unwanted reactions. These supplements include the following:

- **5-HTP**
- **Kava**
- **Melatonin**
- **Valerian**

NARCOTIC PAIN RELIEVERS

Certain supplements should not be taken with **codeine, hydrocodone/ acetaminophen,** or any other **narcotic analgesics** because excessive drowsiness and other dangerous complications may result. These supplements include the following:

- **5-HTP**
- **Goldenseal**
- **Kava**
- **Melatonin**
- **Valerian**

NEUROLOGY DRUGS

Risk of overstimulation, stomach upset, and other problems can occur when certain **nervous system stimulants,** such as **methylphenidate (Ritalin),** are combined with the following supplements:

- **Ephedra**
- **Ginseng (Panax)**

NSAIDS

Some supplements pose the risk of hyperkalemia (excessive amounts of potassium in the blood) if taken with **NSAIDs (nonsteroidal anti-inflammatory drugs)** such as **ibuprofen, ketoprofen,** and **naproxen,** for example. These supplements include the following:

- **Phosphorus**
- **Potassium**

Taken long-term, the NSAID **aspirin** carries the risk of excessive blood-thinning and bleeding when combined with certain supplements. These supplements include the following:

- **Feverfew**
- **Fish oils**
- **Garlic**
- **Ginkgo biloba**
- **Reishi mushrooms**
- **White willow bark**

OB-GYN DRUGS

Many supplements affect hormone levels and should be combined with **oral contraceptives**, **hormone replacement therapy medications**, and **other gynecological drugs** only after discussion with a doctor. Interactions could lessen the potency of the drug or even cause harm. These supplements include the following:

- **Black cohosh**
- **Cat's claw**
- **Chasteberry**
- **Soy isoflavones**
- **St. John's wort**

PARKINSON'S DRUGS

Two supplements in particular pose a risk of interactions when taken with the anti-Parkinson medication **levodopa**. Consult your doctor before combining Parkinson's medication with the following:

- **5-HTP**
- **Vitamin B$_6$**

PSYCHIATRIC DRUGS

Certain supplements can interfere with the action of a wide range of psychiatric medications such as **antipsychotic, antianxiety,** and **antimanic drugs.** These supplements include the following:

- **Ginseng (Panax)**
- **Iodine**
- **Kava**
- **5-HTP**

SEDATIVES/TRANQUILIZERS

Excessive drowsiness and other side effects associated with alertness and concentration have occurred when **sleep aids** and other **sedatives** and **tranquilizers** have been taken with the following supplements:

- **Black cohosh**
- **5-HTP**
- **Goldenseal**
- **Kava**
- **Melatonin**
- **Valerian**

SEIZURE/EPILEPSY DRUGS

The effect of some anticonvulsants (the drugs **phenytoin, carbamazepine,** and **gabapentin,** for example) may be compromised if you are using the following B-vitamin supplements:

- **Folic acid**
- **Vitamin B$_6$**

Corticosteroids taken orally (the drugs **beclomethasone** and **prednisone,** for example) should not be combined with certain supplements because of the risk of adverse interactions. These supplements include the following:

- **Aloe vera** (juice form)
- **Ginseng (Panax)**
- **Melatonin**
- **Phosphorus**

THYROID DRUGS

Common thyroid medications (the drugs **methimazole** and **propylthiouracil,** for example) should not be used with certain supplements because of the risk of adverse interactions or reduced effectiveness of the prescription medication. These supplements include the following:

- **Iodine**
- **Kelp**

A poison control center can provide valuable instruction in the event of a potential drug overdose or other emergency involving an ingested substance. The places below, listed by state, are all certified by the American Association of Poison Control Centers. Each is staffed 24 hours a day by trained personnel who can answer questions about what to do in the event of a possible drug overdose or poisoning with a toxic substance. Calling the national toll-free number (800) 222-1222 will connect you directly to a regional poison center for your area. In addition, many hospitals and medical centers provide emergency services within a local area. Keep your area numbers handy in the event of an emergency. In addition, keep a bottle of ipecac syrup on hand, in case you are told to "induce vomiting," as well as a supply of activated charcoal. (TTY = teletypewriter; TDD = telecommunications device for the deaf)

Alabama
Alabama Poison Center, Tuscaloosa
(800) 222-1222
(800) 462-0800 (AL only; also TDD)
(205) 345-0609

Regional Poison Control Center,
Birmingham
(800) 222-1222
(205) 939-9720

Alaska
Oregon Poison Control Center,
Portland, OR
(800) 222-1222
(503) 494-8600

Arkansas
Arkansas Poison and Drug Information
Center, Little Rock
(800) 222-1222
(800) 641-3805 (TTY/TDD)
(501) 686-5540

Arizona
Arizona Poison and Drug Information
Center, Tucson
(800) 222-1222
(520) 626-7899

Banner Regional Poison Control Center,
Phoenix
(800) 222-1222
(602) 495-4884

California
California Poison Control System,
Fresno/Madera Division
(800) 876-4766 (CA only)
(800) 972-3323 (TTY/TDD)
(559) 622-2300

California Poison Control System, San
Diego Division
(800) 876-4766 (CA only)
(800) 972-3323 (TTY/TDD)
(858) 715-6300

California Poison Control System, San
Francisco Division
(800) 876-4766 (CA only)
(800) 972-3323 (TTY/TDD)
(415) 502-6000

California Poison Control System,
Sacramento Division
(800) 876-4766 (CA only)
(800) 972-3323 (TTY/TDD)
(916) 227-1400

Colorado
Rocky Mountain Poison and Drug
Center, Denver
(800) 332-3073 (CO only)
(800) 222-1222
(303) 739-1127 (TTY/TDD)
(303) 739-1100

Connecticut
Connecticut Poison Center, Farmington
(800) 222-1222
(866) 218-5372 (TTY/TDD)
(860) 679-4540

Delaware
The Poison Control Center,
Philadelphia, PA
(800) 222-1222
(215) 590-8789 (TTY/TDD)
(215) 590-2003

District of Columbia
National Capital Poison Center,
Washington, D.C.
(800) 222-1222 (also TTY)
(202) 362-8563 (TTY/TDD)
(202) 362-3867

Florida
Florida Poison Information Center–
Jacksonville
(800) 222-1222 (also TTY)
(800) 282-3171 (TTY/TDD)
(904) 244-4465

Florida Poison Information Center–
Miami
(800) 222-1222 (also TTY)
(305) 585-5250

Florida Poison Information Center–
Tampa
(800) 222-1222 (also TTY)
(813) 844-7044

Georgia
Georgia Poison Center, Atlanta
(800) 222-1222
(404) 616-9287 (TTY/TDD)
(404) 616-9237

Hawaii
Rocky Mountain Poison and Drug
Center, Denver, CO
(800) 222-1222
(800) 362-3585 (Neighbor Islands only)
(808) 941-4411 (Oahu only)
(303) 739-1127 (TTY/TDD)
(303) 739-1100

Idaho
Rocky Mountain Poison and Drug
Center, Denver, CO
(800) 222-1222
(800) 860-0620 (ID only)
(303) 739-1127 (TTY/TDD)
(303) 739-1100

Illinois
Illinois Poison Center, Chicago
(800) 222-1222
(312) 906-6185 (TTY/TDD)
(312) 906-6136

Indiana
Indiana Poison Center, Indianapolis
(800) 222-1222
(800) 382-9097
(317) 962-2323 (IN only)
(317) 962-2336 (TTY)
(317) 962-2335

Iowa
Iowa Statewide Poison Control Center,
Sioux City
(800) 222-1222
(712) 279-3710

Kansas
Mid-America Poison Control Center,
Kansas City
(800) 222-1222
(913) 588-6639 (TTY/TDD)
(913) 588-6638

Kentucky
Kentucky Regional Poison Center,
Louisville
(800) 222-1222
(502) 589-8222 (Metro Louisville)
(502) 629-7264

Louisiana
Louisiana Drug and Poison Information
Center, Monroe
(800) 222-1222
(800) 256-9822 (LA only)
(318) 342-3648

Maine
Northern New England Poison Control
Center, Portland
(800) 222-1222
(877) 299-4447 (TTY/TDD)
(207) 842-7222

Maryland
Maryland Poison Center, Baltimore
(800) 222-1222
(410) 706-1858 (TTY/TDD)
(410) 706-7604

National Capital Poison Center,
Washington, DC
(800) 222-1222 (also TTY)
(202) 362-8563 (TTY/TDD)

Massachusetts
Regional Center for Poison Control and
Prevention, Boston
(800) 222-1222
(888) 244-5313 (TTY/TDD)
(617) 355-6609

Michigan
Children's Hospital of Michigan Regional
Poison Control Center, Detroit
(800) 222-1222
(800) 356-3232 (TTY/TDD)
(313) 745-5335

DeVos Children's Hospital Regional
Poison Center, Grand Rapids
(800) 222-1222 (also TTY)
(616) 391-9099

Minnesota
Hennepin Regional Poison Center,
Minneapolis
(800) 222-1222 (also TTY)
(612) 347-3144

Mississippi
Mississippi Regional Poison Control
Center, Jackson
(800) 222-1222
(601) 984-1675

Missouri
Missouri Regional Poison Center,
St. Louis
(800) 222-1222
(314) 612-5705 (TTY/TDD)
(314) 772-8300

Montana
Rocky Mountain Poison and Drug
Center, Denver, CO
(800) 222-1222
(800) 525-5042 (MT only)
(303) 739-1127 (TTY/TDD)
(303) 739-1100

Nebraska
The Poison Center, Omaha
(800) 222-1222
(402) 955-5555 (NE only)

Nevada
Oregon Poison Center, Portland, OR
(northern Nevada)
(800) 222-1222 (also TTY/TDD)
(503) 494-8600

Rocky Mountain Poison and Drug
Center, Denver, CO (southern Nevada)
(800) 222-1222
(800) 446-6179 (NV only)
(303) 739-1127 (TTY/TDD)
(303) 739-1100

New Hampshire
New Hampshire Poison Center,
Lebanon
(800) 222-1222
(603) 650-6318

New Jersey
New Jersey Poison Information and
Education System, Newark
(800) 222-1222
(973) 926-8008 (TTY/TDD)
(973) 926-9280

New Mexico
New Mexico Poison and Drug
Information Center, Albuquerque
(800) 222-1222 (also TTY)
(505) 272-4261

New York
Central New York Poison Center, Syracuse
(800) 222-1222
(313) 464-7078

Finger Lakes Regional Poison and Drug Center, Rochester
(800) 222-1222
(585) 273-3854 (TTY/TDD)
(585) 273-4155

Long Island Regional Poison and Drug Information Center, Mineola
(800) 222-1222
(516) 747-3323 (TTY/TDD Nassau)
(516) 924-8811 (TTY/TDD Suffolk)
(516) 663-4574

New York City Poison Control Center
(800) 222-1222
(212) 689-9014 (TTY/TDD)
(212) 447-8152
(212) 447-2666

Western New York Poison Center, Buffalo
(800) 222-1222
(800) 888-7655 (NY only)
(716) 878-7871

North Carolina
Carolinas Poison Center, Charlotte
(800) 222-1222
(704) 395-3795

North Dakota
Hennepin Regional Medical Center, Minneapolis, MN
(800) 222-1222 (also TTY)
(612) 347-3144

Ohio
Central Ohio Poison Center, Columbus
(800) 222-1222
(614) 228-2272 (TTY/TDD)
(614) 722-2635

Cincinnati Drug and Poison Information Center
(800) 222-1222
(800) 253-7955 (TTY/TDD)
(513) 636-5063

Greater Cleveland Poison Control Center, Cleveland
(800) 222-1222
(216) 844-1573

Oklahoma
Oklahoma Poison Control Center, Oklahoma City
(800) 222-1222 (also TTY/TDD)
(405) 271-1122 (TTY/TDD)

Oregon
Oregon Poison Center, Portland
(800) 222-1222 (also TTY/TDD)
(503) 494-8600

Pennsylvania
Pittsburgh Poison Center
(800) 222-1222
(412) 390-3300

Central Pennsylvania Poison Center, Hershey
(800) 222-1222
(717) 531-8335 (TTY)
(717) 531-7057

The Poison Control Center, Philadelphia
(800) 222-1222
(215) 590-8789 (TTY/TDD)
(215) 590-2003

Rhode Island
Regional Center for Poison Control and Prevention, Boston, MA
(800) 222-1222
(888) 244-5313 (TTY/TDD)
(617) 355-6609

South Carolina
Palmetto Poison Center, Columbia
(800) 222-1222
(800) 922-1117 (SC only)
(803) 777-7909

South Dakota
Hennepin Regional Medical Center, Minneapolis, MN
(800) 222-1222 (also TTY)
(612) 347-3144

Tennessee
Middle Tennessee Poison Center, Nashville
(800) 222-1222
(615) 936-2047 (TTY/TDD)
(615) 936-0760

Southern Poison Center, Memphis
(800) 222-1222 (also TTY/TDD)
(901) 448-6800

Texas
Central Texas Poison Center, Temple
(800) 222-1222
(254) 724-7405

North Texas Poison Center, Dallas
(800) 222-1222 (TX only)
(214) 589-0911

South Texas Poison Center, San Antonio
(800) 222-1222
(210) 567-5762

Texas Panhandle Poison Center, Amarillo
(800) 222-1222
(806) 354-1630

Southeast Texas Poison Center, Galveston
(800) 222-1222 (also TTY/TDD)
(409) 766-4403

West Texas Regional Poison Center, El Paso
(800) 222-1222
(915) 534-3800

Utah
Utah Poison Control Center, Salt Lake City
(800) 222-1222
(801) 581-7504

Vermont
Northern New England Poison Center,
Portland, ME
(800) 222-1222
(877) 299-4447
(207) 842-7222

Virginia
Blue Ridge Poison Center, Charlottesville
(800) 222-1222
(804) 924-0347

National Capital Poison Center,
Washington, DC
(800) 222-1222 (also TTY)
(202) 362-8563 (TTY/TDD)
(202) 362-3867

Virginia Poison Center, Richmond
(800) 222-1222
(804) 828-4780

Washington
Washington Poison Center, Seattle
(800) 222-1222
(800) 572-0638 (TTY/TDD, WA only)
(206) 517-2394 (TTY/TDD)
(206) 517-2350

West Virginia
West Virginia Poison Center, Charleston
(800) 222-1222
(304) 388-9698 (TTY/TDD)
(304) 347-1212

Wisconsin
Children's Hospital of Wisconsin Poison
Center, Milwaukee
(800) 222-1222
(414) 266-2542 (TTY/TDD)
(414) 266-2952

Wyoming
The Poison Center, Omaha, NE
(800) 222-1222
(402) 955-5555

▼

There are hundreds of health information organizations in the United States. They offer a range of services, from sending literature on a specific disorder or providing updates on the latest drugs and treatments to making referrals to physicians, hospitals, or local support groups. Some focus on a single disease or area of health; others operate on a national level and offer general advice on a wide range of health issues.

Which type of group or organization is right for you depends on your particular needs. When looking for additional informa-tion or support, a good place to start is with your doctor, who may be able to recommend specific groups for you to contact. You can also refer to the list of major national health informa-tion organizations below. Many have toll-free phone numbers or fax lines. Others can be contacted via the Internet or e-mail. This is a limited listing. There are many more associations that offer valuable patient support. If one organization doesn't have the information you need, a staff member may be able to refer you to another one that does.

Agency for Healthcare Research and Quality (AHRQ)
540 Gaither Road
Rockville, MD 20850
(301) 427-1364
Internet site: http://www.ahrq.gov
An information clearinghouse sponsored by the U.S. Department of Health and Human Services. Offers publications on back pain, HIV infection, living with heart disease, and many other topics.

American Academy of Pediatrics
141 Northwest Point Boulevard
Elk Grove Village, IL 60007-1098
(847) 434-4000
Internet site: http://www.aap.org
Offers child-related publications on antibiotics, safety, first aid, and more.

American Cancer Society (ACS)
1599 Clifton Road, NE
Atlanta, GA 30329-4251
(800) ACS-2345 (227-2345)
Internet site: http://www.cancer.org
A national organization offering information on the management of all types of cancer. Makes referrals to local self-help organizations.

American Cancer Society
Response Line
(800) ACS-2345 (227-2345)
Provides publications and information about cancer and its treatment.

American Diabetes Association
ATTN: National Call Center
1701 North Beauregard Street
Alexandria, VA 22311
(800) DIABETES (342-2383)
Internet site: http://www.diabetes.org
Provides information and public education programs on diabetes.

American Dietetic Association
120 South Riverside Plaza, Suite 2000
Chicago, IL 60606-6995
(800) 877-1600
Internet site: http://www.eatright.org
The organization also answers food and nutrition questions and makes referrals to registered dietitians.

American Heart Association
7272 Greenville Avenue
Dallas, TX 75231
(800) 242-8721
Internet site: http://www.americanheart.org
A national organization with many local branches, offering pamphlets and public education programs on all aspects of car-diovascular health. Check your telephone book for a branch near you.

American Self-Help Clearinghouse
St. Clare's Riverside Medical Center
25 Pocono Road
Denville, NJ 07834
(973) 625-7101
A not-for-profit agency that makes referrals to more than 700 national self-help groups. Also provides information on how to start your own local self-help group.

Arthritis Foundation
P.O. Box 7669
Atlanta, GA 30357-0669
(800) 283-7800
Internet site: http://www.arthritis.org
Makes referrals to local chapters and pro-vides information on the causes and treat-ment of rheumatoid arthritis, osteoarthritis, and other musculoskeletal disorders. Also provides services to improve quality of life for people with arthritis.

Cancer Information Service
Office of Cancer Communications
National Cancer Institute
(800) 4-CANCER (422-6237)
Internet: http://cis.nci.nih.gov/
A hotline of the National Cancer Institute, offering information on cancer, smoking cessation, and other topics.

Centers for Disease Control and Prevention (CDC)
Office of Public Affairs
1600 Clifton Road, NE
Atlanta, GA 30333
(800) 311-3435
(404) 639-3534
Internet site: http://www.cdc.gov
A U.S. government agency dealing with issues of public health, including AIDS and other infectious diseases, environmental concerns, and occupational safety.

CDC National AIDS Hotline
(800) 342-AIDS (342-2437)
Sponsored by the Centers for Disease Control and Prevention. Offers publications and referrals to thousands of community-based organizations that deal with AIDS and HIV infection.

CDC National STD Hotline
(800) 227-8922
Sponsored by the Centers for Disease Control and Prevention. Provides anony-mous, detailed information on sexually transmitted diseases.

CDC Travel Health Line
(877) FYI-TRIP (394-8747)
Fax-on-command: (888) 232-3299
Internet site: http://www.cdc.gov/travel/
Sponsored by the Centers for Disease Control and Prevention. Detailed health advice tailored to specific international travel destinations.

Food and Drug Administration (FDA)
5600 Fishers Lane
Rockville, MD 20857-0001
(888) INFO-FDA (463-6332)
Internet site: http://www.fda.gov
The U.S. government agency that aims to protect consumers against impure and unsafe foods, drugs, and cosmetics. Answers questions, listens to complaints, and makes referrals to other appropriate agencies. Offers FDA publications on drug labeling, safe use of medications, food and nutrition, and other topics.

National Cancer Institute
National Institutes of Health
NCI Public Inquiries Office, Suite 3036A
6116 Executive Boulevard, MSC 8322
Bethesda, MD 20892-8322
800-4-CANCER (422-6237)
(301) 435-3848
CancerFax: (800) 624-2511
(301) 402-5874
Internet site: http://www.nci.nih.gov
A branch of the National Institutes of Health that provides information on dozens of types of cancers.

National Eye Institute
2020 Vision Place
Bethesda, MD 20892-3655
(301) 496-5248
Internet site: http://www.nei.nih.gov
A branch of the National Institutes of Health that provides information on various eye ailments.

National Heart, Lung, and Blood Institute
NHLBI Health Information Center
Attention: Web site
P.O. Box 3015
Bethesda, MD 20824-0105
(301) 592-8573
(301) 496-0554
Internet site: http://www.nhlbi.nih.gov
A branch of the National Institutes of Health that provides written material on cardiovascular and respiratory health.

National Institute of Allergy and Infectious Diseases (NIAID)
NIAID Office of Communications and Public Liaison
31 Center Drive MSC 2520
Bethesda, MD 20892-2520
(301) 496-5717
Internet site: http://www.niaid.nih.gov

Provides information on pollen allergies, dust allergies, sexually transmitted diseases, and other topics.

National Institute of Arthritis and Musculoskeletal and Skin Diseases (NIAMS)
Information Clearinghouse
1 AMS Circle
Bethesda, MD 20892-3675
(877) 22-NIAMS (226-4267)
(301) 495-4484
Internet site: http:/www.nih.gov/niams/
A branch of the National Institutes of Health offering information on arthritis, osteoporosis, various skin diseases, and other topics.

National Institute of Child Health and Human Development
P.O. Box 3006
Rockville, MD 20847
(800) 370-2943
Internet site: http://www.nichd.nih.gov/
A branch of the National Institutes of Health that provides information on issues of child health and development.

National Institute of Diabetes and Digestive and Kidney Disorders (NIDDK)
Office of Communications and Public Liaison
31 Center Drive MASC 2560
Bethesda, MD 20892-2560
(301) 496-3583
Internet site: http://www.niddk.nih.gov/
A branch of the National Institutes of Health that offers information on diabetes, digestive disorders, endocrine and metabolic disorders, kidney disease, nutrition and obesity, and urologic disease.

National Institute on Aging
31 Center Drive, MSC 2292
Bethesda, MD 20892
(800) 222-2225
(301) 496-1752
Internet site: http://www.nih.gov/nia/
A branch of the National Institutes of Health that provides information and publications on arthritis, accident prevention, incontinence, cancer, menopause, osteoporosis, nutrition, heart disease, and other topics of interest to older adults.

National Institutes of Health
9000 Rockville Pike
Bethesda, MD 20892
(301) 496-4000
Internet site: http://www.nih.gov
The principal medical research arm of the U.S. government. Makes referrals to appropriate federal agencies.

National Institute of Mental Health (NIMH)
Office of Communications
6001 Executive Boulevard, Rm. 8184, MSC 9663
Bethesda, MD 20892-9663
(866) 615-NIMH (615-6464)
(301) 443-4513
Internet site: http://www.nimh.nih.gov/
Makes referrals to local mental health associations and offers publications on depression, bipolar disorder, anxiety, phobias, panic disorder, Alzheimer's disease, and other conditions.

National Library of Medicine
Public Health Service
National Institutes of Health
8600 Rockville Pike
Bethesda, MD 20894
(888) FIND-NLM (346-3656)
(301) 594-5983
Internet site: http://www.nlm.nih.gov/
One of the world's largest health science libraries. Open to the public. Offers reference services to general consumers.

National Self-Help Clearinghouse (NSHC)
365 Fifth Avenue
Suite 3300
New York, NY 10016
(212) 817-1822
Internet site: http://www.selfhelpweb.org/
Provides referral services to local self-help groups and organizations.

National Women's Health Information Center
8550 Arlington Boulevard, Suite 300
Fairfax, VA 22031
(800) 994-WOMAN (994-9662)
http://www.4woman.gov
A branch of the Department of Health and Human Services. Provides general fact sheets on various issues in women's health.

GLOSSARY

▼

ACE inhibitor: An abbreviation for angiotensin-converting enzyme inhibitor, a type of *antihypertensive* drug. ACE inhibitors prevent the formation of angiotensin II, a naturally occurring substance that constricts blood vessels, causing blood pressure to rise.

active ingredient: The chemical component of a drug preparation that exerts the desired therapeutic effects. The active ingredient is commonly what we think of as the "drug." Drugs contain *inactive ingredients* as well, such as the binders and colorings added to a pill to hold it together and give it its characteristic color.

acute: Short, severe, nonchronic; designates an illness or condition that typically lasts no more than a week or two.

addiction: A term used to describe physical dependence on a drug; psychological factors may also play a role in addiction.

adverse reaction: A harmful and unintended response to a drug.

agonist: A drug or other compound that stimulates activity in specific cells, setting into motion particular chemical reactions and bodily processes.

allergic drug reaction: An exaggerated immune response to a drug, which can result in hives, itching, or, in serious cases, shock and breathing difficulty. People who are allergic to one drug, such as penicillin, may also be allergic to chemically related drugs in the same drug class.

alternative medicine: Any of various approaches to healing, such as herbal therapies and acupuncture, that fall outside the domain of conventional mainstream medicine.

amino acids: Chemical substances, found in foods and produced in the body that are used to build protein.

aminoglycoside: One of a group of chemically related *antibiotics* that is used to treat a variety of infections.

amphetamine: One of a group of drugs, related to the generic parent drug amphetamine, that stimulates the central nervous system.

analgesic: An agent that relieves pain. Some examples of analgesics include *narcotics, NSAIDs* (which have properties in addition to pain relief), and a varied group of miscellaneous pain relievers, such as acetaminophen.

anaphylaxis: An acute allergic reaction to a drug or venom, such as from a bee sting, that may be marked by swollen airways and severe difficulty breathing.

androgen: A male sex hormone, such as testosterone, that is administered for cancer, certain endocrine disorders, and a few other conditions.

anesthetic: A drug that eliminates the sensation of pain.

angiotensin-converting enzyme inhibitor: See *ACE inhibitor*.

anorectic: A drug that suppresses appetite. Some drugs suppress appetite as a *side effect*.

antacid: A drug that counteracts stomach acids. Antacids are used to relieve indigestion, heartburn, peptic ulcers, and a few other gastrointestinal disorders.

antagonist: A drug or other compound that inhibits chemical activity in specific cells, suppressing particular physiological reactions and bodily processes.

antianginal: A drug, such as a *nitrate,* that relieves the chest pain caused by insufficient flow of heart blood, a characteristic of angina.

antianxiety agent: A psychiatric drug, also called an anxiolytic, that relieves anxiety. These drugs also help relax muscles and to treat insomnia.

antiarrhythmic: A drug used to correct heart rhythm abnormalities.

antiasthmatic: A drug used in the treatment of asthma.

antibacterial: A drug used specifically to combat bacterial infections, as opposed to infections caused by other microorganisms, such as fungi and viruses. Also commonly referred to as an *antibiotic*.

antibiotic: A drug that kills or inhibits the growth of infectious bacteria or other germs. Some antibiotics are naturally produced by bacteria, fungi, and other microorganisms; others are synthetic (man-made).

antibody: A protein produced by the immune system that normally acts to neutralize or eliminate foreign substances in the body. A *drug allergy* is associated with an overactive response of an antibody to a particular drug.

anticancer agent: A drug used to combat cancer.

anticlotting agent: A general term describing a drug that inhibits the clotting of blood. These drugs are sometimes referred to as *anticoagulants*.

anticoagulant: A drug that blocks the activity of certain blood-clotting factors that promote the formation of fibrin, a protein essential in the formation of blood clots. Anticoagulant drugs can either impede the formation of a clot or prevent an already formed clot from breaking away, traveling to a narrow blood vessel, and stopping circulation in a critical organ.

anticonvulsant: A drug used to control seizures or convulsions, typically those brought on by epilepsy.

antidementia drug: A drug that slows the progression of Alzheimer's disease and other related forms of mental deterioration.

antidepressant: A drug that elevates mood and relieves depression. Types of antidepressants include *tricyclic antidepressants, monoamine oxidase (MAO) inhibitors,* and *selective serotonin reuptake inhibitors.*

antidiabetic agent: A drug used to treat diabetes.

antidiarrheal agent: A drug that relieves diarrhea.

antidote: A compound that counteracts *poisoning.*

antiemetic: A drug used to stop or prevent vomiting.

antifungal: A drug that combats fungal infections, such as athlete's foot or nail fungus. *Topical* antifungals are applied externally to the skin, hair, or nails. *Systemic* antifungals are taken orally or by injection; typically, they help fight fungal infections affecting the bloodstream or other internal organs or tissues.

antiglaucoma agent: A drug used to treat glaucoma, the buildup of excessive pressure in the eye. This condition is a common cause of blindness in older people.

antigout agent: A type of drug that serves to relieve gout (a painful arthritic condition of the joints) by limiting the buildup of uric acid, a metabolic waste product.

antihistamine: A drug that blocks the actions of *histamine*. Such drugs relieve allergies, hay fever, hives, rashes, itching, cold symptoms, and motion sickness.

antihypertensive: A drug that lowers blood pressure in people with high blood pressure (hypertension), a condition that increases the risk for stroke, heart disease, and many other ailments. Different types of antihypertensives are prescribed for people with mildly elevated blood pressure and for those with extremely high blood pressure.

antihypotensive: A drug that elevates blood pressure in people who have dangerously low blood pressure (hypotension).

antiinfective: A drug used to treat infections, including those caused by bacteria *(antibacterials)*, fungi *(antifungals)*, viruses *(antivirals)*, parasites *(antiparasitics)*, and other disease-causing microorganisms.

antiinflammatory: A drug used to reduce the swelling, redness, or pain caused by inflammation, an immune reaction to injury that can occur either inside the body (arthritic joints, for example) or on a localized external area (skin rash, for example). Some antiinflammatory drugs are *steroids;* others are nonsteroidal (see *NSAIDs*).

antimalarial: An *antiparasitic* drug used specifically to treat or prevent malaria, a mosquito-borne illness caused by the plasmodia parasite.

antimanic drug: A medication that relieves the mental and physical hyperactivity and incapacitating mania and mood elevation that are characteristic of manic-depressive illness (bipolar disorder).

antimicrobial agent: A general term for a drug used to treat infections caused by microorganisms such as bacteria, fungi, and viruses. This group of drugs includes *antiinfectives, antibiotics, antifungals,* and *antivirals.*

antimigraine drug: A drug that relieves or prevents migraine headaches.

antinauseant: A medication that relieves or prevents the queasy sensations of nausea.

antineoplastic agent: A drug used to counter the growth and spread of tumors and malignant cells.

antiobesity agent: A drug that works to promote weight loss through any of various mechanisms. Some of the antiobesity drugs are *serotonergics.*

antioxidant: A substance that protects cells from the damaging effects of highly reactive oxygen molecules called free radicals. Some antioxidants, such as alpha-lipoic acid, are made by the body; others, such as vitamins C and E, are obtained through diet or supplements.

antiparasitic: A drug used to treat infestations of parasites, including worms and amoebas.

antiparkinsonism agent: A drug used to relieve the trembling and rigidity of Parkinson's disease and other related disorders. These drugs are also called antiparkinsonian agents.

antiplatelet agent: A drug that reduces the tendency of blood cells called platelets to clump together and form clots where the normal flow of blood is disrupted. For example, blood flow may be impaired by fatty deposits in the coronary arteries of someone who has heart disease, predisposing that person to a heart attack. Aspirin, in low doses, is the most widely prescribed antiplatelet drug.

antiproliferative: A drug that suppresses the excess proliferation of skin cells that occurs in certain skin disorders, such as psoriasis.

antipruritic: A drug that is used to relieve itching.

antipsoriatic: A drug used to treat psoriasis, a chronic skin and joint condition marked by scaly red patches. In some cases, this medication is also used for arthritis.

antipsychotic: A drug used to treat severe psychiatric disorders that cause hallucinations or delusions, such as schizophrenia and others.

antipyretic: A drug used to reduce fever (elevated body temperature).

antireflux agent: A drug that alleviates gastroesophageal reflux (commonly known as heartburn).

antirheumatic: A drug used to treat rheumatoid arthritis, a serious, recurring form of arthritis marked by pain and inflammation of the joints.

antiseptic: A drug or other substance that arrests the growth and action of bacteria and other microorganisms. Also called a germicide.

antispasmodic: A drug used to reduce involuntary muscle spasms, such as those that can occur in the gastrointestinal tract or bladder.

antitubercular agent: A type of drug used in the treatment and prevention of tuberculosis.

antitussive: A cough suppressant.

antiurolithic: A drug used in the treatment of kidney stones, a relatively common disorder marked by the formation of small, hard pellets in the urinary tract.

antiviral: A drug used to combat infections caused by viruses, such as influenza or AIDS.

anxiolytic: See *antianxiety agent*.

aplastic anemia: A rare but potentially fatal side effect of certain drugs characterized by suppression of the bone marrow, resulting in the inability to produce adequate amounts of essential blood components.

autonomic nervous system: The part of the nervous system that controls smooth muscle (the type that surrounds blood vessels and other structures), heart muscle, and many of the body's so-called involuntary actions, such as glandular secretions, the motion of the gastrointestinal tract, and the contraction or dilation of blood vessels. Many drugs, such as some used for hypertension, act through the autonomic nervous system. Because this system has such wide-ranging effects, drugs that affect it typically produce a wide variety of side effects in addition to their desired therapeutic actions.

azalide: A type of *antibiotic* used to fight infections.

barbiturate: One of a class of related drugs that are used as *hypnotics*, *sedatives*, and *antispasmodics* to induce sleep, relieve anxiety, and relax the muscles.

behavior modifier: A drug that can facilitate a behavior change, such as stopping excessive drinking or quitting smoking.

benzodiazepine: One of a class of related *antianxiety* drugs used as tranquilizers. Examples include diazepam (brand name Valium) and alprazolam (brand name Xanax); many end with the suffix "-epam" or "-olam."

beta-blocker: A drug that inhibits chemical activity in specialized nervous system structures called beta-receptors, which are found in the heart, the airways, and other areas. Beta-blockers are commonly used as *antihypertensive* drugs; they lower blood pressure by slowing the heart rate and reducing the force of the heartbeat. They are also sometimes used to treat angina, abnormal heart rhythm, anxiety, glaucoma, and other disorders.

bioavailability: A scientific term for the degree and rate at which a substance, such as a drug, is absorbed into the body and becomes available to exert therapeutic effects.

bioequivalent: A scientific term for drugs that have equivalent chemical properties, so that equal amounts of each drug are delivered to the body in a similar time frame. Generic drugs, for example, are bioequivalent to brand name drugs.

bone resorption inhibitor: A drug that suppresses the normal breakdown of bone. These drugs are useful for treating high blood calcium levels (hypercalcemia) or bone disorders such as Paget's disease.

botanical: An herb or plant that has healing properties.

botanical name: The scientific, or Latin, name of an herb or plant.

brand name: The name chosen by a drug manufacturer to market a drug. Prozac, for example, is the brand name for the antidepressant drug with the *generic name* fluoxetine. Advil, for example, is the brand name for the pain reliever with the *generic name* ibuprofen.

brand name drug: A drug that is sold under a registered *brand name.*

broad-spectrum antibiotic: An antibiotic drug that is active against a wide range of infectious bacteria.

bronchodilator: A drug that prompts the bronchial air passages to expand, making it easier to breathe. Bronchodilators are primarily used to treat asthma and related conditions.

calcium channel blocker: A type of *antihypertensive* drug that induces the muscle surrounding blood vessels to relax. It does this by decreasing the movement of calcium ions through muscle cell membranes, thus causing blood vessels to dilate and blood pressure to fall.

caplets: Oblong, capsule-shaped tablets that are generally easier to swallow than round pills.

cardiac glycoside: See *digitalis drug.*

catecholamine: One of a group of chemical messengers that have widespread effects on the body, such as speeding up the heart, raising blood pressure, and increasing respiration. Synthetic catecholamines have been prepared as drugs, primarily for use in emergency situations.

centrally acting: A drug or other agent that works through the *central nervous system* to produce its desired therapeutic effects.

central nervous system (CNS): The part of the nervous system consisting of the brain and spinal cord.

cephalosporin: One of a group of chemically related *antibiotics,* originally derived from a fungus and then enhanced with the production of synthetic versions, that are widely used to treat a variety of infections.

chelating agent: A drug that binds with metals, reducing their concentration in body tissues. Toxic levels of metals can build up in cases of lead poisoning or in conditions such as Wilson's disease, a hereditary disorder marked by the buildup of copper in the body.

chemotherapy: The use of drugs to combat cancer or other conditions.

chronic: Persistent or long term; designates an illness or condition that often requires months or years of treatment for results to be apparent.

clearance: The rate at which a drug is passed through the kidneys and into the urine. The term *renal clearance* is sometimes used instead. ("Renal"

stands for something related to, involving, or affecting the kidneys.)

coenzyme: A substance that acts in concert with enzymes to speed up chemical reactions in the body.

commission E: A special body of scientists, health professionals, and lay experts formed in Germany in 1978. It studies the usefulness and safety of herbal remedies.

complex: A term designating a mixture of vitamins, minerals, herbs, or other nutrients. Examples include vitamin B complex, liver (lipotropic) complex, and amino acid complex.

compress: A soft cotton or flannel cloth or piece of gauze soaked in an herbal tea or other healing substance, then folded and placed on the skin to help reduce inflammation and pain.

contraceptive: A drug or device used to prevent pregnancy.

contraindication: A disease or condition that either completely precludes the use of a certain drug or means that the drug should be used with special caution.

conventional medicine: Also known as allopathic medicine, the approach to healing most commonly practiced in the United States and other Western countries. A doctor diagnoses a problem and typically treats it with drugs or surgery.

corticosteroid: A type of antiinflammatory drug that mimics the actions of powerful naturally occurring substances called *steroids,* which are released by the adrenal glands and have numerous and widespread effects on the body. Corticosteroids are available in many forms, including *inhalant, oph-*

thalmic, otic, topical, and *systemic* preparations. They are used to treat asthma, allergies, skin inflammations, inflammatory bowel disease, some forms of cancer, and other disorders.

cytotoxic drug: A drug that works by killing rapidly dividing cells, typically those associated with cancer.

decongestant: A drug that relieves nasal or sinus congestion resulting from colds or allergies.

dependence: Addiction to a drug because of psychological or physical factors. *Narcotics,* for example, commonly lead to dependence.

desensitization: A medical treatment for a drug allergy that aims to lessen sensitivity and improve *tolerance* to the drug by administering, over time, a series of gradually increased doses.

digitalis drug: A type of drug that slows the heartbeat and increases the force with which the heart beats, thereby improving the pumping action of the heart and relieving the symptoms of congestive heart failure. Also known as a cardiac glycoside.

diuretic: A drug that alters kidney function by drawing water from the body and increasing the total output of urine.

divided doses: Doses of a drug given at intervals that are spaced throughout the day rather than as a single dose.

douche: Herbal teas, acidophilus and water, or other substances that can be used to flush the vagina. This may be recommended for infections.

drug allergy: An allergic reaction to a specific drug, such as *penicillin,* or to a drug component. Responses can

range from mild (a skin rash, for example) to severe (shock, difficulty breathing, and other complications associated with *anaphylaxis*). Those with a drug allergy should avoid use of the drug as well as substances that are chemically related to the drug. Such individuals should also inform their doctors, dentist, and others of the drug allergy (regardless of severity).

drug class: A group of drugs that have similar chemical structures and actions on or in the body. There are many different classes of drugs. Although members of a drug class have similar properties, there are variations among them that may make one particular drug preferable over other drugs in the same class for a specific disorder or patient.

drug fever: An adverse drug reaction marked by elevated body temperature resulting from an allergic reaction or other causes.

drug interaction: Reciprocal activity or influence between two or more drugs that may alter the effects of one or all of the drugs involved. Drug interactions vary widely. They may increase—or decrease—the amount of active drug, the effectiveness of a drug, and the likelihood of adverse side effects. Responses to a drug interaction can range from clinically inapparent or mild to life-threatening.

drug rash: A skin rash resulting from an allergic reaction to a particular medication, usually appearing within a few days after first taking it. Drug rashes can occur with either *topical* or *systemic* preparations.

electrolyte: A chemical, such as calcium, potassium, or sodium, dissolved in blood or cellular fluids, that acts as a vital messenger for many bodily

processes. Electrolytes are essential in maintaining heart rhythm and kidney function, for example. Certain drugs can disrupt electrolyte levels.

elixir: A form of liquid medication that consists of a drug mixed in a flavored alcohol solution.

emollient: A drug preparation or other substance that is applied to the skin to soothe and soften the area. Many emollients can also be applied to the lips and *mucous membranes.*

endorphins: Natural pain-reducing substances released by the pituitary gland, producing an effect similar to that of narcotic pain relievers.

enteric coating: A protective covering that enables a pill to pass intact through the stomach into the small intestine, where the coating dissolves and the contents are best absorbed.

enzyme: A protein that speeds up specific chemical reactions and processes in the body, such as digestion and energy production.

essential fatty acids (EFAs): The building blocks that the body uses to make fats. The body must get various kinds of EFAs through diet or supplements (such as fish oils and flaxseed oil) to ensure proper health.

essential oil: A concentrated oil extracted from herbs or other plants.

estrogen: A female sex hormone, produced by the ovaries, that has multiple effects, including stimulating the reproductive cycle and the development of female secondary sex characteristics. Various forms of estrogen are used as drugs for treating menopause symptoms, breast cancer, and other conditions.

estrogen replacement therapy: The use of supplemental *estrogen,* one of the female sex hormones produced by the ovaries, to relieve the adverse effects of menopause.

expectorant: A type of drug used in cough preparations that promotes the discharge and expulsion of mucus or phlegm from the throat and airways.

extract: A pill, powder, liquid, or other form of an herb that contains a concentrated and usually standard amount of therapeutic ingredients.

Food and Drug Administration (FDA): The U.S. government agency that regulates and monitors food and drug safety. Its functions include ruling on the safety of new drugs before they become available to the public, reclassifying drugs from prescription to *OTC* status, regulating food and drug labeling, and establishing safe limits for additives.

food interactions: An action between a specific food and a drug that may influence the amount of drug available in the body for therapeutic effects. Because of food interactions, some drugs should not be taken with meals in general or with specific foods.

free radicals: Highly reactive and unstable oxygen molecules, generated in the body, that can damage cells, leading to heart disease, cancer, and other ailments. Antioxidants help minimize free radical damage.

g: An abbreviation for *gram.*

generic drug: A copycat version of a *brand name drug.* Generic drugs are chemically equivalent to brand name drugs but cost loss. Generics, which cannot be marketed until the exclusive patent for the brand name drug has

expired (usually after about 20 years), are normally sold under the drug's *generic name.*

generic name: The scientific name for a drug. Generic names, as opposed to *brand names*, are nonproprietary and are recognized worldwide.

gram (g): A metric measure of weight sometimes used in drug dosages. There are about 454 grams in a pound.

growth hormone: A naturally occurring chemical secreted by the pituitary gland that promotes growth by acting through a number of intermediaries on various body tissues. Synthetic versions of the hormone are available as drugs and are usually administered by injection to children. Also called somatotropic hormone or somatotropin.

habituation: A term used to describe psychological dependence on a drug.

herb: A plant or plant part—the leaves, stems, roots, bark, or flowers—that can be used for medicinal or other purposes (such as flavoring foods).

histamine: A compound produced by cells in the stomach, skin, respiratory tract, and elsewhere. Histamine aids digestion by triggering stomach acid secretion. It also plays a central role in allergic reactions, causing inflammation, hives, itching, and constriction of the airways.

histamine (H1) blocker: A type of *antihistamine* used to treat hay fever and other allergies.

histamine (H2) blocker: A drug that binds to a specialized receptor in the stomach wall termed an H2 receptor, thereby preventing the release of *histamine.* In the digestive tract, hist-

amine triggers stomach acid secretion. The drugs in this group are commonly used to treat heartburn, ulcers, and other digestive disorders.

hormone: Chemicals, secreted by various organs, that are typically carried by the bloodstream and exert their effects on cells and tissues throughout the body. Some hormones have been synthesized and are used as drugs to regulate the menstrual cycle, promote growth, combat cancer, and treat other conditions.

hypersensitivity: A drug-related allergic reaction or an exaggerated response to a drug.

hypnotic: A drug that is used primarily to induce sleep (for example, a *benzodiazepine*).

hypoglycemic agent: A drug that lowers blood sugar levels, commonly used in the treatment of diabetes.

immunization: Stimulation of the immune system to produce antibodies against a specific disease, thereby providing protection against it, through the oral or injectable administration of a *vaccine, a toxoid,* or cells or blood serum from infected persons. The term is sometimes used interchangeably with *vaccination.*

immunosuppressant: A drug that suppresses the immune system. Such an effect may be desirable to prevent the immune system from rejecting a new organ following a transplant and in the treatment of certain cancers, the autoimmune disease rheumatoid arthritis, or other serious medical conditions.

implant: A capsule that is implanted under the skin and slowly releases a drug into the body for an extended period.

inactive ingredient: A substance such as a coloring, flavoring, binder, gelatin capsule coating, or preservative that does not have any therapeutic effects but is combined with an active drug compound during the manufacturing process to make a medication. Most manufacturers list the inactive ingredients alphabetically on the label's ingredients list.

indication: The disorder, condition, disease, or symptom for which a drug is prescribed or approved for use by the Food and Drug Administration.

inhalant: A drug preparation that is inhaled through the mouth or nose.

integrative medicine: An approach to healing that utilizes aspects of both conventional and alternative medicine. Also called complementary medicine.

interferon: A naturally occurring substance that activates the body's immune response. Interferons have been synthesized for use as anti-cancer agents and also as drugs for various other purposes.

international unit (IU): A standardized dose measure that provides a set amount of a specific supplement, such as vitamin A, D, or E.

intramuscular: Into the muscle. Some medications and vaccines are formulated as solutions that are injected into a muscle. The body then absorbs the drug from the muscle.

intravenous: Into the vein. Many drugs are formulated as solutions for injection or slow drip into a vein, where they gain immediate access to the bloodstream. The drug is then carried by the blood to other parts of the body.

jaundice: A liver disorder, marked by yellow discoloration of the skin and eyes, that may be the result of liver disease, an allergic reaction to a drug, or even an adverse reaction to a drug that affects the liver. Jaundice is often reversible, but its cause should always be investigated because of the liver's crucial function in the body.

keratolytic: A medication used to treat certain skin conditions, such as acne, that causes the layer of dead skin on its uppermost surface to peel.

kg: An abbreviation for *kilogram*.

kilogram (kg): A metric unit of weight equal to about 2.2 pounds. Some drug doses are prescribed per kilogram of body weight.

laxative: One of a group of drugs that relieves constipation by adding bulk to stools (bulk-forming laxative), softening stools (stool softener), lubricating the gastrointestinal tract (lubricant), or increasing intestinal tract motility (stimulant).

lipid-lowering drug: A medication that lowers harmful blood cholesterol levels and helps reduce the risk of heart disease. Also called a cholesterol-lowering drug.

lipotropic combination: A blend of choline, inositol, methionine, milk thistle, and other nutrients used to promote the health of the liver.

local: An effect that is felt within a restricted portion or area of the body. Drugs that tend to act locally—including most *topical* agents applied to the skin, *inhalants* that act on the airways, and *ophthalmic* preparations applied to the eyes—generally produce less serious *side effects* than *systemic* drugs, which act on sites throughout the body.

loop diuretic: One of a class of *diuretic* drugs commonly prescribed for the treatment of high blood pressure. Loop diuretics act on the part of the kidneys known as the loop of Henle to block the reabsorption of sodium and water into the bloodstream. This action leads to an increased amount of fluid (urine) leaving the body.

macrolide: One of a group of *antibiotics* that are active against various infectious microorganisms and that share a characteristic chemical ring structure.

MAO inhibitor: See *monoamine oxidase inhibitor*.

mast cell stabilizer: A drug that prevents the release of *histamine* from specialized cells (mast cells) in the respiratory passages, thus reducing inflammation of the airways. Mast cell stabilizers are commonly used in the treatment of asthma.

mEq: An abbreviation for *milliequivalent*.

metabolism: The cascading array of chemical reactions through which the body converts food into packets of energy that can be used or stored.

metered-dose inhaler: A device, commonly used by patients with asthma, that converts liquid medicine into an aerosol spray. The spray can then be breathed in through the mouth, delivering a standard dose of medication to the airways.

mg: An abbreviation for *milligram*.

μg: An abbreviation for *microgram*.

microgram (µg): A metric measure of weight, equal to one-millionth of a *gram,* that is sometimes used in drug dosages.

milliequivalent (mEq): A chemical unit of measure that is sometimes used to indicate dosages of vitamins and some drugs.

milligram (mg): A metric measure of weight, equal to one-thousandth of a *gram,* that is commonly used in drug dosages.

milliliter (ml): A metric measure of volume, equal to one-thousandth of a liter, that is sometimes used in dosing recommendations for liquid medications. There are about 5 ml in a teaspoon, 15 ml in a tablespoon, 30 ml in 1 fluid ounce, and 240 ml in 1 cup (8 fluid oz).

mineral: An inorganic substance found in the earth's crust that plays a crucial role for enzyme synthesis, regulation of heart rhythm, bone formation, digestion, and other metabolic processes in the human body. Humans constantly replenish their mineral supply with food and water.

miotic: A drug that causes constriction of the pupils (miosis).

mixed amino acids: A balanced blend (complex) of amino acids, often taken in conjunction with individual amino acid supplements.

ml: An abbreviation for *milliliter.*

monoamine oxidase (MAO) inhibitor: An *antidepressant* drug that elevates mood by blocking the actions of the nervous system enzyme, monoamine oxidase, thereby increasing levels of specialized substances called monoamines in the brain.

mucilage: A gummy, gellike plant substance that, when ingested, forms a protective layer in the throat and digestive tract, suppressing coughs and adding bulk to hard stools.

mucolytic: A type of medication that is used in the treatment of coughs to thin and break up excessive mucous secretions.

mucous membrane: The pink and shiny skinlike layers that line the lips, mouth, vagina, eyelids, stomach, gastrointestinal and urinary tracts, and other cavities and passages in the body. The mucous membranes secrete the thick and slippery fluid called mucus, which lubricates and protects these tissues. Some drugs are formulated as *topical* preparations for application specifically to the mucous membranes.

narcotic: A drug that acts on the *central nervous system* and is used primarily to diminish pain but that has numerous effects on the body, including drowsiness and mental clouding (without loss of consciousness), slowed breathing, and decreased motility of the gastrointestinal tract. Also sometimes called an opiate or opioid.

nebulizer: A device that uses compressed air to convert liquid medications into extremely fine aerosol mists that can deeply penetrate the lungs when inhaled through the mouth or nose. A nebulizer is particularly effective for dilating constricted bronchial tubes, making it easier to breathe. Nebulizers are frequently used in the form of *metered-dose inhalers,* hand-held devices designed to deliver a standardized dose of the medication.

nephrotoxic: Poisonous, or toxic, to the kidneys. A number of medications are considered potentially nephrotoxic, so the function and health of the kidneys should be closely monitored while taking such drugs.

neuropathy: An adverse side effect of certain drugs that is caused by damage to nerves and is marked by burning, tingling, pain, or numbness in the fingers, toes, limbs, or other areas.

neurotoxicity: A scientific term for the nerve damage that can occur as a side effect of certain drugs or *toxins.*

neurotransmitter: Any of various chemicals found in the brain and throughout the body that transmit signals among nerve cells.

nitrates: A group of *antianginal* drugs that dilate the heart's blood vessels, making it easier for blood to flow through them.

nonsteroidal antiinflammatory drug: See *NSAID.*

NSAID: An abbreviation for a nonsteroidal antiinflammatory drug. NSAIDs reduce pain and inflammation in damaged tissues in conditions such as arthritis and headache by blocking the production of specialized *hormone*like fatty acids known as *prostaglandins.*

nutritional supplement: A nutrient synthesized in the laboratory or extracted from plants or animals and taken for medicinal purposes.

off-label use: A common—and legitimate—practice in which a doctor prescribes one or more drugs for a disease, symptom, or condition that has not been specifically approved by the *FDA.* Once a drug has been approved for one *indication,* doctors are then free to prescribe the drug for other purposes.

ointment: A semisolid drug preparation, usually having a greasy or fatty base, typically applied to the skin.

ophthalmic: A drug formulated for administration onto or around the eye.

opiate or opioid: A morphinelike pain-relieving drug chemically related to opium. See *narcotic*.

oral agent: A drug in solid (such as a pill or capsule) or liquid form that is meant to be ingested by swallowing.

orthostatic hypotension: A dramatic drop in blood pressure on sitting or standing up, especially if coming to an upright position quickly. Symptoms include faintness, dizziness, and loss of balance. Various *antihypertensive* agents and other drugs can cause this type of very low blood pressure.

OTC: A common abbreviation for *over-the-counter* drugs.

otic: A drug formulated for administration into or onto the surface of the ear.

ototoxicity: A scientific term for the damage to structures in the ear and loss of hearing that can occur as an adverse reaction to certain drugs (for example, *aminoglycoside antibiotics*) and *toxins*.

over-the-counter (OTC): A drug that is allowed to be sold without a prescription—for example, at a pharmacy, supermarket, or convenience store. An increasing number of drugs that were formerly available only by *prescription* can now be purchased OTC, although the dose is typically lower than that of the prescription version.

overdose: Excessive accumulation of a drug in the body, resulting in toxic levels that can be extremely dangerous. An accidental overdose is of particular concern in children, older adults, and those who have kidney, liver, or other diseases that may impair their ability to process and excrete a drug. An intentional overdose is a concern in depressed patients attempting suicide.

parenteral: A medication that is designed to be administered other than orally (through the gastrointestinal tract), such as by injection into the muscles *(intramuscular)* or veins *(intravenous)* or through the skin *(subcutaneous)*.

parkinsonism: A nervous disorder that can result as a side effect of certain drugs. Symptoms resemble those of Parkinson's disease and include generalized weakness; a rigid, masklike facial expression; trembling or tremors in the hands, arms, or legs; and a rigid posture and shuffling gait.

PCOs (procyanidolic oligomers): A group of antioxidant compounds, also called proanthocyanidins—found in pine bark, grape seed extract, green tea, red wine, and other substances—that may help protect against heart and vascular disease.

penicillin: One of a group of *antibiotics* (first mass-produced for clinical use in the 1940s) that are widely used against a range of infections. Many derivatives of penicillin, such as amoxicillin, have since been synthesized; their names end with the suffix "-illin."

peripherally acting: A drug or other agent that works on or near the surface or periphery of the body, often via the *peripheral nervous system*.

peripheral nervous system: The part of the nervous system outside of the brain and spinal cord, such as the nerves leading to the muscles, skin, and internal organs.

pharmacist: A professional who is licensed to dispense *prescription* medicines.

photosensitivity: An adverse *side effect* of certain medications marked by a decreased tolerance to the sun's ultraviolet rays, resulting in a tendency for exposed skin to sunburn easily.

phytoestrogens: Estrogen-like compounds present in soy and other plants that may help treat symptoms of menopause, certain cancers, and other complaints.

phytomedicines: Therapeutic ingredients found in fruits, vegetables, grains, herbs, and other plants that may help protect against cancer, heart disease, and other ailments.

pioneer drug: The first version of a new *brand name* drug.

placebo: Also called a dummy pill, a substance that contains no medicinal ingredients. It is often used in scientific studies as a control so its effects can be compared with those of the drug or supplement under scrutiny.

poisoning: Illness, injury, or death caused by exposure to a drug or toxin. Depending on the toxic qualities and potency of the substance, small or large amounts can cause poisoning.

potassium-sparing diuretic: A mild *diuretic* drug commonly prescribed for the treatment of high blood pressure. Such drugs act on the kidneys to block the reabsorption of sodium and water by the bloodstream, leading to an increase in the volume of urine. Potassium-sparing diuretics help prevent excessive loss of the electrolyte potassium, a common problem with other types of diuretics.

poultice: A soft, moist substance, spread between layers of cloth or gauze, that is applied (usually heated) to the skin in order to help reduce pain and inflammation.

prescription: An instruction by a physician that directs a pharmacist to dispense a particular drug in a specific formulation and dose. Prescription medications, unlike *over-the-counter* drugs, require the physician's approval, usually in written form.

priapism: A medical term for a condition characterized by prolonged and painful erection of the penis resulting from an obstructed outflow of blood in this organ. In some cases, priapism occurs as a side effect or reaction to a medication and is only relieved once the medication is stopped.

probiotics: "Friendly" bacteria, similar to those found in acidophilus supplements, that are normally present in the intestine and help promote healthy digestion.

progestin: A general term for progesterone, a female sex *hormone* produced by the ovaries that helps regulate menstruation. Synthetic versions of progestin have been prepared as drugs for use as *contraceptives* and in the treatment of menopause, certain cancers, abnormal uterine bleeding, and other conditions.

prolactin: A hormone, secreted by the pituitary gland in the brain, that promotes lactation.

prostaglandin: One of a group of chemicals occurring naturally in the body that produce a wide range of effects, such as inducing pain and inflammation, stimulating contractions of the uterus during labor, and protecting the stomach's lining. Some drugs, such as misoprostol, are synthethic prostaglandins. Other drugs, such as

NSAIDs, counteract the effects of certain prostaglandins.

protease inhibitor drug: A drug that blocks production of a key enzyme, protease, which the virus that causes AIDS (the HIV virus) needs in order to replicate. These drugs have helped keep AIDS from developing in countless HIV-infected individuals.

recommended dietary allowance (RDA): The daily amount of a vitamin or mineral needed by healthy individuals to meet the body's needs and prevent a deficiency. These guidelines are set by the Food and Nutrition Board of the National Academy of Sciences. Also called "recommended daily allowance."

renal clearance: The rate at which a drug is passed through the kidneys and into the urine. "Renal" describes something related to, involving, or affecting the kidneys. Some sources refer to renal clearance as *clearance.*

retinoid: A synthetic derivative of vitamin A used to treat acne, skin wrinkling, and other skin conditions. Tretinoin is a classic example of a retinoid drug.

Reye or Reye's syndrome: A rare but swift and potentially fatal condition affecting children and teenagers that is marked by liver degeneration and swelling of the brain. The illness is thought to be related to the administration of aspirin to children under age 16 who have signs and symptoms of the chicken pox, the flu, or a flulike viral illness.

sedative: A drug that has a calming or tranquilizing effect and is used primarily to reduce anxiety or nervousness.

selective serotonin reuptake inhibitor (SSRI): One of a class of

antidepressant drugs that elevates mood by indirectly increasing the levels of a specialized chemical in the brain (a neurotransmitter) called serotonin. Various SSRI medications are currently being sold (by prescription only) and are used by a large number of individuals. Among the commonly recognized SSRI medications are fluoxetine (Prozac) and sertraline (Zoloft).

serotonergic: A drug that increases the supply of a nervous system chemical in the brain called serotonin. Some serotonergics are used as *antiobesity agents* because they help make the patient feel satiated (full).

serotonin blocker: A drug that blocks activity of the nervous system chemical serotonin in the brain. This effect may help stimulate appetite or relieve certain types of headache.

side effect: A secondary and often adverse effect of a drug. Side effects are known and predictable responses to a specific drug, but usually only a small number of individuals taking the drug will experience them.

soft tissue: A general term for internal body parts other than bones and joints, such as muscles and the tissue under the skin. Soft tissue can become infected by microorganisms such as bacteria; *antiinfectives* are used to treat such infections.

solution: A mixture of one or more drugs that are dissolved in a liquid.

spacer: A device commonly used in conjunction with a *metered-dose inhaler* that attaches to the inhaler's mouthpiece and acts as a reservoir to hold the airborne medicine. The use of a spacer helps ensure that a standard dose of the medication is delivered to the airways.

SPF: An abbreviation for sun protection factor, which indicates the relative ability of a sunscreen to block out the sun's damaging ultraviolet rays. Experts recommend using an SPF of at least 15, which will allow a person to remain in the sun without sustaining ultraviolet burn damage for 15 times longer, on average, than if no sunscreen were applied.

SSRI: See *selective serotonin reuptake inhibitor.*

stability: The chemical properties of a drug that ensure that it will not decompose readily during storage, so it will remain potent and effective through the expiration date.

standardized extract: A concentrated form of an herb that contains a set (standardized) level of active ingredients. Standardization helps guarantee a consistent dosage strength, or potency, from one batch of herb to the next. Standardized extracts are available only for certain herbs, either as pills or liquids or in other forms.

statin: One of a group of drugs that lowers harmful serum cholesterol levels by inhibiting a critical enzyme needed for the manufacture of cholesterol in the liver. Statins are also known as HMG-CoA reductase inhibitors.

steroid: A naturally occurring compound or drug that has far-ranging effects on numerous body processes. Some steroids are *hormones*—either sex hormones (testosterone, for example) or adrenal gland hormones (prednisone, for example). The terms steroid and *corticosteroid* are often used interchangeably.

stool softener: A type of *laxative* that bulks up and softens the consistency of fecal matter, thus easing the passage of stool and relieving constipation, hemorrhoid pain, and related discomforts.

subcutaneous: Under the skin. A number of medications are designed to be injected or surgically inserted just under the skin. Examples include various fertility drugs, anti-HIV medicines, and drugs used to treat chronic headache. When a choice in *parenteral* administration is available, subcutaneous injection is often chosen over *intramuscular injection*, which can be quite painful and not as well absorbed.

sublingual: Beneath the tongue. Some supplements, such as vitamin B_{12}, are formulated to dissolve in the mouth, providing quick absorption into the bloodstream without interference from stomach acids.

sulfa drug: One of a class of bacteria-inhibiting drugs (specifically, *antibiotics*) that is created synthetically in the laboratory and is chemically very closely related to the compound known as sulfanilamide.

sulfonylurea: One of a class of chemically related and commonly used oral medications designed to treat diabetes by means of reducing and controlling the level of sugar in the blood. (Poor blood sugar control is a serious aspect of diabetes that can cause numerous complications.)

superinfection: A dangerous *side effect* of certain *antibiotics* that is marked by the emergence of a secondary infection during the course of antibiotic therapy. It can occur when antibiotics alter the normal balance of microbes in the respiratory, gastrointestinal, or urinary tracts, allowing certain potentially hazardous microorganisms to predominate and flourish.

suspension: A form of liquid medication, often cloudy in appearance, that consists of a solid (typically a powder) that is dispersed into water (or another liquid medium) but in which the solid remains undissolved.

sympatholytic: An *antihypertensive* drug that acts on the *peripheral nervous system* to block nerve signals that trigger the constriction of blood vessels, thus causing the blood vessels to dilate and blood pressure to decline. Drugs that are sympatholytic include the *beta-blockers* and other medications used for treating high blood pressure.

sympathomimetic: A drug that acts on the nervous system and stimulates the involuntary activities of the organs, glands, muscles, and other structures in the body. A sympathomimetic drug such as albuterol dilates the respiratory passages and helps relieve asthma.

syrup: A form of liquid medication consisting of a drug dissolved in a concentrated sugar solution.

systemic: Affecting the body in general, as opposed to a limited *local* area. Drugs taken orally or injected *intravenously,* for example, are sometimes referred to as systemic medications, because they are distributed throughout the body by the bloodstream. In contrast, most medications applied *topically* to the skin or dropped into the ears or eyes would generally be considered nonsystemic, or local, preparations.

tardive dyskinesia: A medical term for an irreversible nervous condition, marked by unusual involuntary movements of the mouth, tongue, neck, lips, and sometimes fingers, that can occur after prolonged treatment with potent *antipsychotic* drugs.

tetracycline: A type of *antibiotic* medication synthesized or derived from a certain *Streptomyces* microorganism. Because tetracycline is effective against a wide range of infections, it is considered a "broad-spectrum" antibiotic.

therapeutic dose: The amount of a vitamin, mineral, herb, nutritional supplement, or drug needed to produce a desired healing effect (as opposed to the minimum amount needed to prevent a deficiency, such as the RDA).

thiazide: A type of *diuretic* drug commonly prescribed for the treatment of high blood pressure. These drugs act on the kidneys to block the bloodstream's reabsorption of sodium and water, leading to an increase in the volume and output of urine.

thrombolytic agent: A drug that dissolves blood clots, also known as thrombi. These medications are typically administered in a hospital by *intravenous* injection—to dissolve a blood clot that is blocking a coronary artery and causing a heart attack, for example.

tolerance: The body's adaptation to a drug, causing the drug's effects to lessen with continued use. Tolerance may work beneficially; for example, a *side effect* may become much less pronounced with continued use of a drug. On the other hand, drugs such as painkillers may become less effective as a person's tolerance develops, and higher and higher doses may be required.

tonic: An herb (such as ginseng) or herbal blend that is used to "tone" the body or a specific organ, imparting added strength or vitality.

topical: Designed to be applied to and act locally on a restricted area of the body, such as the application of a cream medication to the skin, an *ointment* to the eyelid, or an *anesthetic* injection to the gums. Topical drug preparations generally have fewer *side effects* than *systemic* drugs, which are distributed throughout the body.

toxin: A poisonous substance that has adverse effects on the body. Some toxins are produced by disease-causing bacteria or by certain plants (mushrooms, for example) or animals (such as snakes). Affected persons are sometimes inoculated with antitoxins, which neutralize the effects of toxins.

toxoid: A substance derived from bacteria and used for *vaccination* against certain diseases that is capable of combating or neutralizing the toxic effects of certain infectious microorganisms.

tranquilizer: An *antianxiety* drug used to induce sedation and relieve mental disturbance (such as anxiety and tension) in people as well as animals.

transdermal patch: An adhesive bandage containing drugs that is worn on the skin and slowly releases medication over an extended period of time. Examples of drugs widely used in this form include nicotine, which is used for smoking cessation, and nitroglycerin, which controls angina (chest pain).

tricyclic antidepressant: A common type of *antidepressant* medication characterized by a three-ring chemical structure that increases the activity of specialized substances called catecholamines in the brain. Amitriptyline hydrochloride (brand name Elavil) is one of several well-known tricyclic antidepressants.

tyramines: Substances found in certain foods and drinks, including aged cheeses, salami, dark chocolate, over-ripe fruits (especially bananas), and some red wines, that can cause a dangerous elevation of blood pressure in people who take take medications known as *MAO inhibitors*.

uricosuric drug: A drug that prevents recurrent gout attacks by promoting the excretion of uric acid in the urine.

vaccination: The oral or injectable administration of killed or inactivated microorganisms *(vaccines)* for the purpose of conferring immunity against a particular disease. The term is sometimes used interchangeably with *immunization*.

vaccine: A preparation of dead or inactivated bacteria, viruses, or *toxins* that stimulate the immune system to produce long-term *antibodies* against a particular infectious microorganism. By triggering the formation of these antibodies, the vaccine serves to prevent the disease from causing illness in the future. Commonly administered vaccines include the polio vaccine and the measles-mumps-rubella (MMR) vaccine.

vasodilator: A drug that causes the blood vessels to widen (dilate), increasing the amount of blood that can flow through them.

vitamin: An organic substance that plays an essential role in regulating cell functions. Most vitamins must be ingested because the body cannot manufacture them.

xanthine: A type of drug that opens bronchial air passages and makes breathing easier in patients with asthma and related conditions. A commonly used xanthine is theophylline, which is sold under numerous brand names.

ACKNOWLEDGMENTS

▼

PRESCRIPTION AND OVER-THE-COUNTER DRUGS: CONSULTING EDITORS

Eric Wittbrodt, Pharm.D., BCPS, FCCM; Simeon Margolis, M.D., Ph.D.

PRESCRIPTION AND OVER-THE-COUNTER DRUGS: MEDICAL CONSULTANTS

*Chief of Medical
Advisory Board*
Simeon Margolis, M.D., Ph.D.
*Professor of Medicine and
Biological Chemistry
Johns Hopkins
School of Medicine*

Franklin Adkinson, M.D.
Asthma and Allergy Medicine

Frank Anania, M.D.
*Gastroenterology and
Hepatology*

Lawrence Appel, M.D.
Internal Medicine

Paul Auwaerter, M.D.
*Internal Medicine and
Infectious Disease*

William Bell, M.D.
Hematology

Ivan Borrello, M.D.
Oncology

Steven Brant, M.D.
Gastroenterology

Richard Chaisson, M.D.
Infectious Disease

Lawrence Cheskin, M.D.
Gastroenterology and Nutrition

Bernard Cohen, M.D.
Dermatology

David Cromwell, M.D.
Gastroenterology

E. Claire Dees, M.D.
Oncology

Phillip Dennis, M.D.
Oncology

Adrian Dobs, M.D.
Endocrinology

Christopher Earley, M.D.
Neurology

David Essayan, M.D.
Allergy and Immunology

John Flynn, M.D.
*Internal Medicine and
Rheumatology*

Joel Gallant, M.D.
Infectious Disease (HIV/AIDS)

Mary Lawrence Harris, M.D.
Gastroenterology

Bradley Hinz, M.D.
Ophthalmology

Thomas Inglesby, M.D.
*Internal Medicine and
Infectious Disease*

Suzanne Jan de Beur, M.D.
Endocrinology

Christopher Karp, M.D.
Parasitology

Beth Kirkpatrick, M.D.
Infectious Disease

Susan Koch, M.D.
Dermatology

Alan Krasner, M.D.
Endocrinology

Julie Krop, M.D.
Endocrinology and Metabolism

Ralph Kuncl, M.D.
Neurology

John Lawrence, M.D.
Cardiovascular Medicine

Linda Lee, M.D.
Gastroenterology

Ronald Lesser, M.D.
Neurology

John Lipsey, M.D.
Psychiatry

Dan Martin, M.D.
*Internal Medicine and
Rheumatology*

William Moss, M.D.
Immunology

Patrick Murphy, M.D.
Infectious Disease

Philip Norman, M.D.
Allergy and Immunology

Steve O'Connell, M.D.
Ophthalmology

Paul O'Donnell, M.D.
Oncology

Peter Pak, M.D.
Cardiology

Marco Pappagallo, M.D.
*Neurology (Chronic Pain
Management)*

Wendy Post, M.D.
Cardiovascular Medicine

Charles Pound, M.D.
Urology

Thomas Preziosi, M.D.
Neurology

Peter Rabins, M.D.
Neuropsychiatry

Stuart Ray, M.D.
*Internal Medicine and
Infectious Disease*

Jon Resar, M.D.
Cardiovascular Medicine

Beryl Rosenstein, M.D.
Pulmonary Medicine

Walter Royal, M.D.
Neurology and Virology

Christopher Saudek, M.D.
Endocrinology and Metabolism

Eduardo Sotomayor, M.D.
Oncology

Jerry Spivak, M.D.
Hematology

Timothy Sterling, M.D.
Infectious Disease

Francisco Tausk, M.D.
Dermatology

Peter Terry, M.D.
Asthma and Allergy Medicine

Chloe Thio, M.D.
Infectious Disease

Jason Thompson, M.D.
Nephrology

Thomas Traill, M.D.
Cardiovascular Medicine

Glenn Treisman, M.D.
Psychiatry

John Ulatowski, M.D.
Neurology

Edward Wallach, M.D.
Obstetrics and Gynecology

Gary Wand, M.D.
Endocrinology

James Weiss, M.D.
Cardiovascular Medicine

James Weisz, M.D.
Ophthalmology

Elizabeth Whitmore, M.D.
Dermatology

SUPPLEMENTS: MEDICAL CONSULTANTS

 Natural Standard   www.naturalstandard.com

Catherine Ulbricht, Pharm.D.
Massachusetts General Hospital

Ethan Basch, M.D.
Memorial Sloan Kettering Cancer Center

Rita Guldbrandsen, Pharm.D.(c)
Northeastern University

SUPPLEMENTS: MEDICAL BOARD OF ADVISORS

Chief Consultant: David Edelberg, M.D.

Kieth Berndtson, M.D.   Roy R. Hall, M.D.   Tony V. Lu, M.D.   Mark Michaud, M.D.

INDEX

▼

U

V